DATE DUE

OC 15 '96		
AP 14 '97		
MY 07 '97		
MR 2 '98		
SE 11 '0		
OCT 1 0 2005		
APR 1 4 2008		
APR 15 2010		
NOV. 2 9 2010		
JUL 2 4 2013		
NOV 1 2 2013		
DEC 1 0 2013		

Demco, Inc. 38-293

MUSCLES

TESTING AND FUNCTION

Fourth Edition
with POSTURE and PAIN

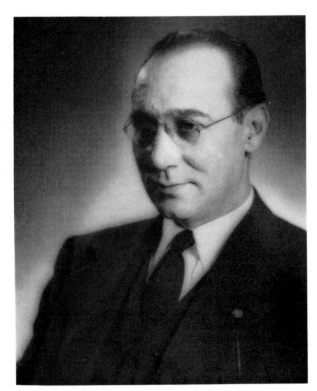

HENRY OTIS KENDALL, P.T. (1898–1979)

Co-author of first and second editions, and *POSTURE AND PAIN*

Former Director of Physical Therapy Department, Children's Hospital, Baltimore, Maryland;
Supervisor of Physical Therapy, Baltimore Board of Education; Instructor in Body
Mechanics, Johns Hopkins School of Nursing; private practice.

MUSCLES
TESTING AND FUNCTION

Fourth Edition
with POSTURE and PAIN

FLORENCE PETERSON KENDALL, P.T., F.A.P.T.A.

Lecturer; Consultant to the Surgeon General, U.S. Army; Consultant to, and Former
Member of, the Maryland State Board of Physical Therapy Examiners. Formerly, Physical
Therapist, Children's Hospital, Baltimore, Maryland; Faculty Member, School of Medicine,
Department of Physical Therapy, University of Maryland; Instructor in Body Mechanics,
Johns Hopkins Hospital, School of Nursing

ELIZABETH KENDALL McCREARY, B.A.

PATRICIA GEISE PROVANCE, P.T.

Clinical Rehabilitation Specialist, Outpatient Physical Therapy Department,
Coordinator, Multiple Sclerosis Rehabilitation Program,
The Union Memorial Hospital, Baltimore, Maryland;
Member, Maryland State Board of Physical Therapy Examiners

· · · ·

Illustrations by
DIANE K. ABELOFF / RANICE W. CROSBY
MARJORIE B. GREGERMAN / WILLIAM E. LOECHEL

Photographs by
PETER J. ANDREWS / CHARLES C. KRAUSE, Jr.

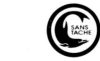

Editor: John P. Butler
Managing Editor: Linda Napora
Copy Editor: S. Gillian Casey
Designer: Dan Pfisterer
Illustration Planner: Ray Lowman
Production Coordinator: Charles E. Zeller

ISBN 0-683-04576-8

90000

9 780683 045765

Printed in the United States of America

First Edition, 1949
Second Edition, 1971
Third Edition, 1983

Library of Congress Cataloging-in-Publication Data

Kendall, Florence Peterson, 1910–
    Muscles, testing and function / Florence Peterson Kendall, Elizabeth
Kendall McCreary, Patricia Geise Provance. —4th ed.
        p. cm.
    Rev. ed. of: Muscles, testing and function, 3rd ed. 1983.
    Includes bibliographical references and index.
    ISBN 0-683-04576-8
    1. Muscles—Examination. 2. Physical therapy. 3. Pain.
4. Posture disorders. 5. Exercise I. McCreary, Elizabeth Kendall.
II. Provance, Patricia Geise . III. Kendall, Florence Peterson, 1910–
Muscles, testing and function. IV. Title.
    [DNLM: 1. Muscles—physiology. 2. Musculoskeletal Diseases—
diagnosis. 3. Musculoskeletal Diseases—therapy. 4. Pain. 5. Posture.
WE500 K326m]
RM701.K46 1993
616.7′40754—dc20
DNLM/DLC
for Library of Congress   92-49150
                                                       CIP

                                        95 96 97
                            4 5 6 7 8 9 10

Dedicated to
Our Families

Foreword

Florence and Henry Kendall have been pioneers in the identification and refinement of techniques for muscle testing, as well as in the critical analysis of posture. For Florence, this is just one of the roles she has played in the ongoing development of Physical Therapy as a profession. I am honored by the request to write the foreword for this text.

The early collaborative observations and writings of the Kendalls provided a foundation for a more scientific approach to the evaluation of muscles and movement. The refinement of this concept and its techniques has been carried forward by Florence with the highest level of commitment to achieving the utmost level of reliability and validity. Furthermore, she has never lost sight of the importance of this information to the patient. This text is a demonstration of the comprehensive body of knowledge she has acquired, her continuing inquisitiveness, and her deep desire to share the knowledge. Through these writings and her extensive teaching, she continues to create a level of excitement for and commitment to thorough evaluation of muscle performance and the interpretation of this evaluation for function.

With the help of two dedicated co-authors, this fourth edition reflects expansion of information, much of it developed by Florence through workshops and teaching, that has not been reflected in her previous writings. It will be a most valuable text for physical therapists, clinicians, and students. The information will challenge the reader to be more thorough and will be a valuable contribution in helping to establish more systematic evaluation of muscle and movement. This book represents a body of knowledge in a major sector of physical therapy and provides a resource that will contribute to the profession's road of progress.

I hope the readers will study this text with an awareness of the intellectual curiosity and excitement demonstrated by the authors in its preparation, and with awareness of the life-long commitment Florence holds for the continued professionalization of physical therapy.

ROBERT C. BARTLETT, P.T.
Professor and Chairman

Department of Physical & Occupational Therapy
Duke University

Preface

This fourth edition of *Muscles, Testing, and Function* is both a text book for students and a reference book for clinicians. Our goal in preparing this work is to provide, in one book, a comprehensive coverage of manual muscle testing, and evaluation and treatment of faulty and painful postural conditions. Parts of *Posture and Pain* were incorporated into the second and third editions, and with this fourth edition the union of the two books is complete. This edition, with its emphasis on fundamentals, purposely includes some historical notes. We hope this text will serve our readers well in the management of musculoskeletal disorders.

The underlying philosophy of this book is that there is a continuing need to "get back to basics." The *science* of manual muscle testing derives from a study of joint motions and muscle origins, insertions, and actions; the *art* of testing evolves through practice and experience under a variety of circumstances. Standards of excellence are maintained by adhering to the principles and rules of procedure required to ensure precision in testing, and by recording the valuable information obtained from experience in this field.

Muscle function, body mechanics, and simple treatment procedures do not change. With respect to muscuolskeletal problems, the underlying purposes of treatment have been—and continue to be—to restore and maintain appropriate range of motion, good alignment, and good muscle balance.

The role of prevention of musculoskeletal problems is destined to become an increasingly important issue in the future. Health practitioners can play an effective role in promoting wellness if they are aware of the adverse effects of muscle imbalance, faulty alignment, and improper exercise. The costs to society for treatment of common problems, such as low back pain, have reached a critical point. Many cases of low back pain are related to faulty posture and are corrected or alleviated by restoring good alignment. A study course (1) relating to the low back mentions the need to improve posture as part of the treatment in ten of the twelve syndromes described.

Musculoskeletal problems are widespread and affect persons of all ages and various occupations. For those who care for patients with these problems, this book will be a valuable resource. The audience encompasses a broad spectrum of practitioners, ranging from medical specialists and therapists, who provide treatment, to those in related fields who administer programs of exercise.

The comprehensive coverage of muscle evaluation procedures contained in previous editions has been retained and enhanced in this edition, and new text, drawings, and photographs have been added. The sequence of the chapters has been planned for the benefit of the student.

Chapter 1 sets the tone for the book by starting with a reference to a *standard*. It has been shortened as a result of moving all the specific information about muscle testing to the appropriate testing chapters. Besides introductory material, it includes a brief discussion about muscle testing devices, and a critique of three physical fitness tests.

Chapter 2 has added a short introductory section, some revised text, and many new drawings that enhance the understanding of planes, axes, and joint motions. A new chart, *Classification of Joints*, at the end of the chapter, shows the relationship of the type of joint tissue to the types and sub-types of articulations.

Chapter 3 is a new chapter devoted specifically to length tests and stretching exercises. Over half of the illustrations (photographs and drawings) are new. Testing procedures are described in detail, with emphasis on precision in performing the tests. The test for length of the fascia lata, precisely as described by Ober in a 1937 issue of the Journal of the American Medical Association, is included.

Chapter 4 on Posture probably contains the most complete analysis of good and faulty posture that is available anywhere. In addition, it includes a section on Developmental Factors and Environmental Influences on Posture. Two pages of exercises appear at the end of the chapter with the notation that permission is granted to reproduce these pages.

Chapter 5 is new to this book. It consists of a limited discussion about scoliosis, including some of the problems associated with past exercise programs. Essentially, it is an appeal for more thorough musculoskeletal evaluation and appropriate follow-up care in the early stages of scoliosis.

Chapter 6 on Trunk Muscles has been rearranged with respect to sequence of tests. Based on the complexity of testing procedures, the less complex extensor tests appear before the more complicated flexor tests. The test for strength of lower abdominals precedes the test for upper abdominals for reasons of emphasis. Testing lower abdominals is often neglected and these muscles are more important than the upper in maintaining good postural alignment. Because widespread misconceptions still exist about the actions of the abdominal and hip flexor muscles during trunk-raising, the detailed analysis of the actions of these muscles remains intact in this edition, but the charts that analyze these movements and muscle actions have been moved to the end of the chapter as a source of reference for those interested in more detailed study.

Chapters 7 and 8 deal with extremity strength tests. All the introductory text material relating to strength testing appears in Chapter 7. New photographs have been added to both chapters, some replacing previous photographs, and numerous legends provide greater detail. The section on grading has been revised for greater clarity and includes a *Key to Grading Symbols*, and a *Key to Muscle Grading*. The latter is based on the fundamental principles and methods of grading that have been in use by physical therapists for many years. We hope that this section will promote better understanding and help to standardize grading procedures. With respect to grading symbols, the use of percentages has been eliminated and the scale of grading changed to 0 to 10, rather than the 0 to 100 as in previous editions. The use of 0 to 10 is highly recommended instead of 0 to 5 in order to avoid the use of fractions or decimals for any statistical study dealing with changes in muscle strength.

Chapter 9 contains all the tests for facial, eye, and neck muscles, and charts of muscles of deglutition and respiration that appeared in previous editions. New text material relating to respiration and respiratory muscles has been added.

Chapters 10 and 11 are new to this edition. They include treatment principles, and approaches to treatment of painful and faulty postural conditions. Much of the material has been taken from *Posture and Pain*, and from lectures and articles by the Kendalls, with updating as needed.

Chapter 12 emphasizes neuromuscular more than musculoskeletal evaluation. New material relating to compression, tension, and impingement syndromes has been added. Color illustrations of cutaneous nerve distribution (from Grant's Atlas of Anatomy) are included in this chapter. A new chart and discussion about muscles that are supplied by nerves that are motor only and those that are supplied by mixed sensory and motor nerves should prove to be an interesting and valuable addition to this book.

The unique Spinal Nerve and Muscle Charts have been made more useful by some additions. An extra horizontal space on the upper extremity chart provided separate lines for the Extensor carpi radialis longus and Extensor carpi radialis brevis, and allowed for grouping the muscles supplied by the posterior interosseus nerve. On the lower extremity chart, an extra column allowed for separating the sciatic nerve into its anterior and posterior divisions.

The charts have been improved, also, by the addition of gray shading that sets off certain areas. The copyright author grants permission to reproduce the charts for personal use but not for sale.

An extensive glossary has been added with numerous cross-references, and the index has been greatly expanded.

Pioneers like Robert W. Lovett and Wilhelmina Wright (2) laid the foundations and paved the way for others who followed in the field of manual muscle testing. In the field of body mechanics, Joel E. Goldthwait (3) was one of the pioneers and a leader who stressed the importance of good posture in relation to health. As we seek to find an appropriate and effective balance between traditional values and technology, it is important that we not forget the teachings of these and the many other dedicated people who have been instrumental in the development of the knowledge so often taken for granted—or worse—overlooked.

Acknowledgements

This book is filled with photographs—not of two or three people posing for several hundred pictures, but of several hundred people, each being a subject for one or more photographs. We acknowledge the contribution so many people have made.

With each edition, volunteer subjects have included hospital staff personnel, physical therapy students, and, not to be overlooked, family members who have been "drafted into service" as subjects, starting with the two who made all "the funny faces" for facial muscle tests. For this fourth edition, we gratefully acknowledge the enthusiastic support by members of the staffs from the in-patient and out-patient Physical Therapy and Sports Medicine Departments at The Union Memorial Hospital in Baltimore. We also wish to thank Stephen Baitch for reviewing the material on foot problems, shoe alterations, and orthoses.

When *Posture and Pain* was being written, the authors had the privilege of selecting posture pictures from one thousand photographs sent to them from the United States Military Academy at West Point. The pictures had been taken on the day of admission to the Academy and showed a wide variety of postural problems. During that same period, many photographs of student nurses were obtained from the Johns Hopkins Hospital School of Nursing. As *Posture and Pain* has been incorporated into the subsequent editions of *Muscles, Testing and Function*, the contributions made by these institutions continue to be significant.

It has been our good fortune to have one of the three artists who worked on the second edition join us for this fourth edition. Diane Abeloff, an outstanding medical illustrator, is as demanding of herself as we are of her. For the photography, the tradition of excellence has been continued in this edition by Peter J. Andrews who, by chance, also became one of our best subjects for a series of pictures. The names of the artists and the photographers for this and earlier editions appear on the Title page.

To Williams & Wilkins, our publisher, we extend our sincere appreciation for the dedication to excellence by all those who have helped in the production and publication of this book.

Contents

chapter 1

Fundamental Principles

Why a plumb line? Because it represents a standard. Based on nature's law of gravity, it is a tool in the science of mechanics. The simple device of a plumb line enables one to see the effects of the force of gravity. Invisible, imaginary lines and planes in space are the absolutes against which variable and relative positions and movements are measured.

In the study of body mechanics, plumb lines represent the vertical planes. With the anatomical position of the body as the basis, positions and movements are defined in relation to these planes. Body mechanics is a science concerned with the static and dynamic forces acting on the body. It is not an exact science but, to the extent that it is possible and meaningful, standards and precision must be incorporated in the study of this science. The ideal alignment of the body may not be attainable in every respect, but it is the standard toward which efforts to attain it are directed.

POSTURE AND PAIN

Good posture is a good habit that contributes to the well-being of the individual. The structure and function of the body provide all the potentialities for attaining and maintaining good posture.

Conversely, bad posture is a bad habit and, unfortunately, is of rather high incidence. Postural faults have their origin in the misuse of the capacities provided, not in the structure and function of the normal body.

If faulty posture were merely an aesthetic problem, the concerns about it might be limited to concerns about appearance. But postural faults that persist can give rise to discomfort, pain, or disability. The range of effect from discomfort to incapacitating disability is related to the severity and persistence of the faults.

The motive for this book springs from a recognition of the prevalence of postural problems, associated painful conditions, and the waste of human resources. This text aims to contribute to a decrease in the incidence of such faults and the resulting pain by defining the concepts of good posture, analyzing postural faults, presenting treatment procedures, and discussing some of the developmental factors and environmental influences that affect posture.

Cultural patterns of modern civilization add to the stresses on the basic structures of the human body by imposing increasingly specialized and limited activity. It is necessary to provide compensatory influences in order to achieve optimum function under the conditions imposed by our mode of life.

The high incidence of postural faults in adults is related to this tendency toward a highly specialized or repetitive pattern of activity. Correction of the existing conditions depends upon understanding the underlying influences and implementing a program of positive and preventive educational measures. Both of the foregoing require an understanding of the mechanics of the body and its response to the stresses and strains imposed upon it.

Inherent in the concept of good body mechanics are the inseparable qualities of alignment and muscle balance. Examination and treatment procedures are directed toward restoration and preservation of good body mechanics in posture and movement. Therapeutic exercises to strengthen weak muscles and stretch tight muscles are the chief means by which muscle balance is restored.

Good body mechanics requires that range of joint motion be adequate but not excessive. Normal flexibility is an attribute, excessive flexibility is not. There is a basic principle regarding joint movements: the more flexibility, the less stability; the more stability, the less flexibility. A problem arises because skilled performance in a variety of sport, dance, and acrobatic activities requires excessive flexibility and muscle length. *Although "the more the better" may apply to improving the skill of performance, it may adversely affect the well-being of the performer.*

The following definition of posture was included in a report of the Posture Committee of the American Academy of Orthopaedic Surgeons in 1947 (4). It is so well stated that it bears repeating.

3

Posture is usually defined as the relative arrangement of the parts of the body. Good posture is that state of muscular and skeletal balance which protects the supporting structures of the body against injury or progressive deformity irrespective of the attitude (erect, lying, squatting, stooping) in which these structures are working or resting. Under such conditions the muscles will function most efficiently and the optimum positions are afforded for the thoracic and abdominal organs. Poor posture is a faulty relationship of the various parts of the body which produces increased strain on the supporting structures and in which there is less efficient balance of the body over its base of support.

Painful conditions associated with faulty body mechanics are so commonplace that most adults have some first-hand knowledge of these problems. Painful low backs have been the most frequent complaint, although cases of neck, shoulder, and arm pain have become increasingly prevalent. With the emphasis on running, foot and knee problems are common.

In discussing pain in relation to postural faults, questions are often asked about why many cases of faulty posture exist without symptoms of pain, and why seemingly mild postural defects give rise to symptoms of mechanical and muscular strain. The answer to both of these questions depends on the constancy of the fault.

A posture may appear to be very faulty, yet the individual may be flexible and the position of the body may change readily. A posture may appear to be good, but the stiffness or muscle tightness that is present may so limit mobility that position cannot change readily. The lack of mobility, which is not apparent as an alignment fault but is detected in tests for flexibility and muscle length, may be the more significant factor.

Basic to an understanding of pain in relation to faulty posture is the concept that the cumulative effects of constant or repeated small stresses over a long period of time can give rise to the same kind of difficulties as a sudden severe stress.

Cases of postural pain are extremely variable in the manner of onset and in the severity of symptoms. There are cases in which only acute symptoms appear, usually as a result of an unusual stress or injury. Some cases have an acute onset and develop chronically painful symptoms, while others exhibit chronic symptoms that later become acute.

Symptoms associated with an acute onset are often widespread. Measures to relieve pain are indicated. Only after acute symptoms have subsided can tests for underlying faults in alignment and muscle balance be done and specific therapeutic measures be instituted.

There are important differences between treatment of an acutely painful condition and that of a chronic one. A given procedure may be recognized and accepted as therapeutic if applied at the proper time. Applied at the wrong time it may be ineffective or even harmful.

Just as an injured neck, shoulder, or ankle may need support, an injured back may need support, also. Nature's way of providing protection is by "protective muscle spasm" or "muscle guarding" in which the back muscles hold the back rigid to prevent painful movements. But muscles can become secondarily involved when they are overburdened by the work of protecting the back. Use of an appropriate support, to immobilize the back temporarily, relieves the muscles of this function and permits healing of the underlying injury. Protective muscle spasm tends to subside rapidly and pain diminishes when a support is applied.

While immobilization is often a necessary expedient for the relief of pain, stiffness of the part is not a desirable end result. The patient should understand that a transition from the acute stage to the stage of recovery requires moving from immobilization to restoration of normal motion. Continuing the use of a support that should have been discarded will act to perpetuate a problem that might otherwise have been resolved.

MANUAL MUSCLE TESTING

This book focuses on the art and science of manual muscle testing—for which there is no substitute. It emphasizes muscle imbalance and the effects of weakness and contracture on alignment and function. It presents the underlying principles involved in preserving muscle testing as an art, and the precision in testing necessary to preserve it as a science.

The care with which an injured part is handled, the positioning to avoid discomfort or pain, the gentleness required in testing very weak muscles, and, when testing for strength, the ability to apply pressure or resistance in a manner that permits the subject to exert the optimal response—all these are part of the art of muscle testing.

Science demands rigorous attention to every detail that might affect the accuracy of muscle testing. Failure to take into account apparently insignificant factors may alter test results. Findings are useful only if they are accurate. Inaccurate test results mislead and confuse and may lead to a misdiagnosis with serious consequences. Muscle testing is a procedure that depends on the knowledge, skill, and experience of the examiner who should not betray, through carelessness or lack of skill, the confidence that others rightfully place in this procedure.

Muscle testing is an integral part of physical examination. It provides information, not obtained by other procedures, that is useful in differential diagnosis, prognosis and treatment of neuromuscular and musculoskeletal disorders.

Many *neuromuscular* conditions are characterized by muscle weakness. Some show definite patterns of muscle involvement; others show spotty weakness without any apparent pattern. In some cases weakness is symmetrical, in others, asymmetrical. The site or level of a peripheral lesion may be determined because the muscles distal to the site of the lesion will show weakness or paralysis. Careful testing and accurate recording of test results will reveal the characteristic findings and aid in diagnosis.

Musculoskeletal conditions frequently show patterns of muscle imbalance. Some patterns are associated with handedness, some with habitually poor posture. Muscle imbalance may also result from occupational or recreational activities in which there is persistent use of certain muscles without adequate exercise of opposing muscles. Imbalance that affects body alignment is an important factor in many painful postural conditions.

The technique of manual muscle testing is basically the same for cases of faulty posture as for neuromuscular conditions, but the range of weakness encountered in faulty posture is less because grades below fair are uncommon. The number of tests used in cases of faulty posture is also less.

Muscle imbalance distorts alignment and sets the stage for undue stress and strain on joints, ligaments, and muscles. Manual muscle testing is the tool of choice to determine the extent of imbalance.

Examination to determine muscle length and strength is essential before prescribing therapeutic exercises because most of these exercises are designed either to stretch short muscles or to strengthen weak muscles.

Muscle *length testing* is done to determine whether the muscle length is limited or excessive, i.e., whether the muscle is too short to permit normal range of motion, or stretched and allowing too much range of motion. When stretching is indicated, tight muscles should be stretched in a manner that is not injurious to the part or the body as a whole. Range of motion should be increased to permit normal joint function unless restriction of motion is a desired end result for the sake of stability.

Muscle *strength testing* is done to determine the capability of muscles or muscle groups to function in movement and their ability to provide stability and support.

Many factors are involved in the problems of weakness and return of strength. Weakness may be due to nerve involvement, disuse atrophy, stretch weakness, pain, or fatigue. Return of muscle strength may be due to recovery following the disease process, return of nerve impulse after trauma and repair, hypertrophy of unaffected muscle fibers, muscular development resulting from exercises to overcome disuse atrophy, or return of strength after stretch and strain have been relieved.

Muscle weakness should be treated in accordance with the basic cause of weakness. If due to lack of use, then exercises; if due to overwork and fatigue, then rest; if due to stretch and strain, then relief of stretch and strain before the stress of additional exercise is thrust upon the weak muscle.

Every muscle is a prime mover in some specific action. No two muscles in the body have exactly the same function. When any one muscle is paralyzed, stability of the part is impaired or some exact movement is lost. Some of the most dramatic evidence of muscle function comes from observing the effects of loss of the ability to contract as seen in paralyzed muscles, or the effect of excessive shortening as seen in a muscle contracture and the resultant deformity.

The muscle testing described in this book is directed toward examination of individual muscles insofar as is practical. The overlap of muscle actions, as well as the interdependence of muscles in movement, is well recognized by those involved in muscle testing. Because of this close relationship in functions, accurate testing of individual muscles requires strict adherence to the fundamental principles of muscle testing and rules of procedure.

Two fundamental components of manual muscle testing are test performance and evaluation of muscle strength or length. To become proficient in these procedures one must possess a comprehensive and detailed knowledge of muscle function. This knowledge must include an understanding of joint motion because length and strength tests are described in terms of joint movements and positions. It must also include knowledge of the agonistic and antagonistic actions of muscles and their role in fixation and in substitution. In addition, it requires the ability to palpate the muscle or its tendon, to distinguish between normal and atrophied contour, and to recognize abnormalities of position or movement.

One who has a comprehensive knowledge of the actions of muscles and joints can learn the techniques necessary to perform the tests. Experience is necessary, however, to detect the substitution

5

movements that occur whenever weakness exists, and practice is necessary to acquire skill in performing the length and strength tests and in accurately grading muscle strength.

The underlying philosophy of this book is that there is a constant need to get "back to basics" in the study of body structure and function. For musculoskeletal problems, accomplishing this entails a review of the anatomy and function of joints, and of the origins, insertions, and actions of muscles. It includes an understanding of the fundamental principles upon which evaluation and treatment procedures are based.

This text stresses the importance of muscle tests, postural examinations, assessment of objective findings, musculoskeletal evaluations, and treatment. In a condition that is primarily musculoskeletal, the evaluation may constitute and determine a diagnosis. In a condition not primarily musculoskeletal, the evaluation may contribute to a diagnosis.

DEMAND FOR OBJECTIVITY

There is increasing demand for objectivity in regard to muscle testing measurements. With the high cost of medical care, the economics of reimbursement requires documentation to prove that there has been improvement as a result of treatment. For proof, there is a demand for numbers. The smaller the improvement, the more important become the numbers so that minimal changes can be documented.

Length tests, performed with precision, can provide objective data through the use of such simple devices as goniometers to measure angles, and rulers or tape measures to measure distance.

Strength tests cannot rely on such simple devices. The problems are very different for measuring strength. Objectivity is based on the examiner's ability to palpate and observe the tendon or muscle response in very weak muscles; to observe the capability of a muscle to move a part through partial or full range of motion in the horizontal plane, or to hold the part in an antigravity position.

Visual evidence of objectivity extends to an observer as well as to the examiner. An observer can see a tendon that becomes prominent (a trace grade), can see movement of the part in the horizontal plane (a poor grade), and can see a part being held in an antigravity position (a fair grade). Even the fair+ grade, based on holding the antigravity position against *slight* pressure by the examiner, is easy to identify. These are the grades of strength for which mechanical devices are not applicable as aids to obtain objectivity.

The ones that remain are the good and normal grades as identified in manual muscle testing. In addition, there is a wide range of strength above the grade of normal. To the extent that determining the higher potentials of muscle strength is necessary, useful, and cost-effective, machines may play a role.

Hand-held devices measure the amount of force exerted manually by the examiner. They are not suitable for measuring the higher levels of maximum effort by the subject.

The value of the objective measurements obtained through the use of present-day machines must be weighed against their limited usefulness and cost.

Under controlled research conditions, isokinetic machines provide technology that can help in obtaining valuable information. At present, however, usefulness in the clinic is limited. There are problems both in testing muscle strength and in exercising. Difficulty is encountered in providing stabilization that is essential for controlling variables and for standardization of testing techniques. Tests lack specificity, and substitution occurs. In addition to the high cost of the machines, setting up patients in the machines is time-consuming. Both are important factors when considering cost-effectiveness of the testing procedures.

The search continues for a suitable hand-held device* that can provide objective data about the amount of force used during manual muscle strength testing. The problem with a hand-held device is that the device comes between the examiner and the part being tested and interferes with the use of the hand. The examiner's hand must not be encumbered for positioning the part, for controlling the specific direction of pressure, and for applying pressure with the fingers, palm, or whole hand, as needed. (Someday there may be a glove that is sensitive enough to register pressure without interfering with the use of the hand.)

With many different types of dynamometers on the market, standardization and establishing reliability of tests is almost impossible. The introduction of new and "better" devices further complicates and compromises all previous testing procedures. The statement by Alvin Toffler may well

---

* Historical Note: In 1941, when the senior author was engaged in a research study for the Foundation for Infantile Paralysis, she described a hand-held device that could measure the force applied during manual muscle testing. The instrument had a pad in the palm of the hand that could transmit force to a gauge. One year later, the device, as proposed, was presented at a symposium on polio. It is possible that this was one of the first, if not the first hand-held dynamometer. (See p. 190.)

apply to this as well as other fields: "Under today's competitive conditions, the rate of product innovation is so swift that almost before one product is launched the next generation of better ones appears"(5).

A review of the literature on dynamometers reveals some of the problems associated with use of these devices. Dynamometer (X) "creates a new set of standards by which a muscle strength examination can be judged"(6). "Other dynamometers measure only perpendicular force in one plane, meaning a slight tip of the dynamometer during testing can alter results"(7). A study of intertester reliability concludes ". . . the hand-held dynamometer shows limited reliability when used by two or more testers"(8). "Hand-held dynamometers (HHD) may underestimate a patient's true maximal isometric strength, due to difficulties in stabilization of the device"(9). "Differences in strength changes between the two systems were large enough, within each patient, as to warrant questioning the use of the HHD to track changes in strength over time"(9). It is evident that the variety of devices used and the many variables preclude the establishment of norms for muscle grading. According to Jules Rothstein, ". . . there may be a danger that fascination with new technology will lead to the clouding of sound clinical judgement" (10).

As tools, our hands are the most sensitive, fine-tuned instruments available. One hand of the examiner positions and stabilizes the part adjacent to the tested part. The other hand determines the pain-free range of motion and guides the tested part into precise test position, giving the appropriate amount of pressure to determine the strength. All the while this instrument we call the hand is hooked up to the most marvelous computer ever created. It is the examiner's very own personal computer and it can store valuable and useful information on the basis of which *judgments* about evaluation and treatment can be made. Such information contains *objective data* that is obtained without sacrificing the art and science of manual muscle testing to the demand for objectivity.

PHYSICAL FITNESS TESTS

Many tests have been designed to evaluate the physical fitness of school children, armed services personnel, athletic teams, and countless others engaged in health and fitness programs. The same movements have been used, also, as exercises to build strength, endurance, and flexibility. Awards, promotions, and accolades are given or withheld on the basis of test results.

In spite of long-standing and widespread use, three tests, in particular, need to be reevaluated: knee-bent sit-ups, push-ups, and sit-and-reach.

The usefulness of these tests depends on their accuracy and on their ability to detect deficiencies. *Unfortunately, these tests have become an evaluation of the performance rather than a measure of physical fitness of the performer.* Emphasis is on excesses—speed of performance, number of repetitions, and extent of stretching—rather than on quality and specificity of movement.

The authors decided to include a discussion of these tests in the introductory chapter of this book because of the need to correct misleading information, and because of the adverse effects of these tests and the test results on both children and adults.

Knee-bent Sit-ups with Feet Held Down. The knee-bent sit-up requires that a person perform as many sit-ups as possible in a period of 60 seconds. The stated purpose of the test is to measure the endurance and strength of the abdominal muscles. The test does not fulfill that purpose. Instead, it measures strength and endurance of hip flexor muscles, aided in their performance by stabilization of the feet.

The sit-up movement requires flexion of the hip joints and this movement can be performed only by hip flexors. Abdominal muscles do not cross the hip joint so they cannot assist in the hip flexion movement.

Abdominal muscles flex the spine, i.e., curl the trunk, and to test for strength of these muscles, the trunk must be curled. If these muscles can *hold the trunk curled* as the movement of hip flexion is performed, there will be indication of good upper abdominal muscle strength.

The problem with using the sit-up movement as a test or exercise lies in the failure to differentiate between a "curled-trunk sit-up" and an "arched-back sit-up." The former involves strong contraction of the abdominal muscles to hold the trunk curled; the latter puts a stretch on the abdominal muscles and a strain on the low back. This strain may be felt by both children and adults when required to perform as many sit-ups as possible in the time period allotted.

Many will start the sit-up with the trunk curled, but the endurance of the abdominal muscles will not be sufficient to maintain the curl and, as the test progresses, the back will arch increasingly. Some will not have the strength to curl the trunk initially and the test will be done with the back arched for the entire 60 seconds. The problem is that *those with weak abdominal muscles can pass this so-called "abdominal muscle test" with a high score.*

The test as advocated requires speed of performance. For accurate testing of abdominal muscle strength, the test must be done slowly, making sure 1) that the trunk curls *before* hip flexion starts, and 2) that the *curl is maintained* when hip flexion starts and while moving to the sitting position.

To have validity, the test should require that credit be given only for the number of sit-ups that can be performed with the trunk curled. Currently, there is no such requirement. Furthermore, the test cannot be done rapidly if there is to be close observation of the position of the trunk. (See *Chapter 6* for extensive coverage of the sit-up movement and testing upper and lower abdominal muscle strength.)

Push-ups. When a push-up is performed properly, the scapulae abduct as the trunk is pushed upward. The scapulae move forward to a position that is comparable to that of reaching the arms directly forward, When the Serratus anterior muscle is weak, the push-up movement still can be performed, but the scapulae do not move into the abducted position as in a properly performed push-up.

If the primary purpose of the push-ups is to test the strength and endurance of arm muscles, it accomplishes that purpose, but, in the presence of Serratus weakness, it does so at the expense of the Serratus muscle. Evidence is seen in the winging of the scapulae and in the inability to complete the range of scapular motion in the direction of abduction. (See p. 292.)

When push-ups are done at the expense of the Serratus muscle, the activity can no longer be considered an index of the physical fitness of the person who engages in the activity.

Sit-and-Reach. Sitting with knees extended, this test is done reaching forward to touch fingertips to toes. For *young* children and *most* adults, it may be considered normal accomplishment to be able to touch the toes in this position. Reaching beyond the toes usually denotes excessive flexibility of the back or excessive length of the Hamstrings or both. The stated purpose of the sit-and-reach test is to evaluate the flexibility of the low back and Hamstrings. Scoring is based on how many inches *beyond* the toes the individual can reach. The distance beyond (ostensibly) equates with good, better, or best flexibility of the back and Hamstrings, with emphasis on "the more the better."

This test fails to address important variables that affect test results. There are variations in "normal" according to age groups, as well as limitations due to imbalances between length of back and Hamstring muscles.

This *inability* to touch toes—much less reach beyond them—at certain ages is normal for many youths between the ages of 10 and 14. They are at a stage of growth when legs are long in relation to the trunk and they should *not* be forced to touch their toes. (See pp. 48, 111, and 112.)

Limited back flexibility can go undetected if Hamstrings are stretched. Individuals with this imbalance may "pass" the test while many children with normal flexibility for their age will "fail." *It would be more accurate to say that the test has failed these children than that the children have failed the test.*

In addition to being told that they have "failed," many young people are then given exercises to increase spine flexibility and/or stretch Hamstrings when such exercises are unnecessary or contraindicated.

Adults will demonstrate numerous variations in the length of Hamstrings and back muscles (see pp. 46 and 47). Like the adolescent, those adults whose legs are long in relation to the trunk may have normal flexibility of the back and Hamstrings, yet be unable to touch their toes.

The extensive use of physical fitness tests and the importance placed on the results makes it imperative that the tests be carefully scrutinized.

chapter 2

Joint Motions

TYPES OF JOINTS

Joints are the mechanisms by which bones are held together. In some cases, the bones are held so close together that there is no appreciable movement; in others, the bones are held loosely together to permit freedom of movement.

Some joints provide great stability; some provide stability in one direction but allow freedom in the opposite direction; and some provide freedom of motion in all directions. Joints are of three types: fibrous or immovable, cartilaginous or slightly movable, and synovial or freely movable.

Joints that offer little or no movement are those that hold the two halves of the body together. The sagittal suture of the skull is considered an *immovable* joint, held together with a strong *fibrous* membrane. The sacroiliac joint and symphysis pubis are considered *slightly movable* joints and are held together by strong *fibrocartilaginous membranes*. Most joints of the body fall into the category of *freely movable* joints, held together by *synovial membranes*.

The elbow and knee joints are essentially hinge joints. The structure of the joint surfaces and the strong lateral and medial ligaments limit sideways movements, and posterior ligaments and muscles limit extension. Hence, there is stability and strength in the extended position, but freedom of motion in flexion. In contrast, the shoulder and wrist joints are movable in all directions and have less stability.

This chapter discusses in detail the freely movable or synovial joints of the body.

ANATOMICAL POSITION, AXES, AND PLANES

Anatomical Position. The anatomical position of the body is an erect posture, face forward, arms at sides, palms of hands forward with fingers and thumbs in extension. This is the position of reference for definitions and descriptions of body planes and axes. It is designated as the *zero position* for measuring joint motions for most of the joints of the body. In the accompanying figure, posterior view, the forearms and hands are in normal, not anatomical, position.

Axes. Axes are lines, real or imaginary, about which movement takes place. Related to the planes of reference seen on the next page, there are three basic types of axes at right angles to each other.

A *sagittal axis* lies in the sagittal plane and extends horizontally from front to back. The movements of abduction and adduction take place about this axis in a coronal plane.

A *coronal axis* lies in the coronal plane and extends horizontally from side to side. The move-

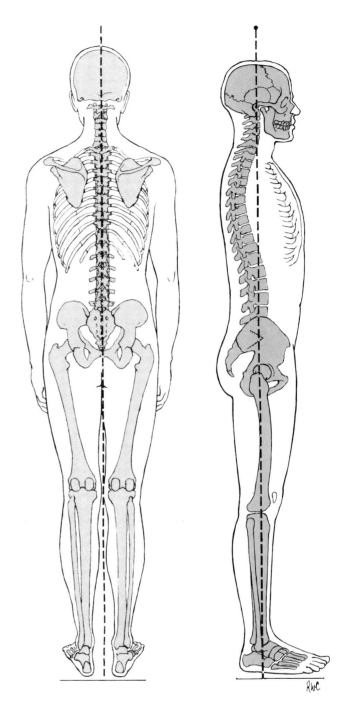

ments of flexion and extension take place about this axis in a sagittal plane.

A *longitudinal axis* is vertical extending in a cranial-caudal direction. The movements of medial and lateral rotation, and horizontal abduction and adduction of the shoulder take place about this axis in a transverse plane.

The exceptions to these general definitions occur with respect to movements of the scapula, clavicle, and thumb (see pp. 16, and 19).

Planes

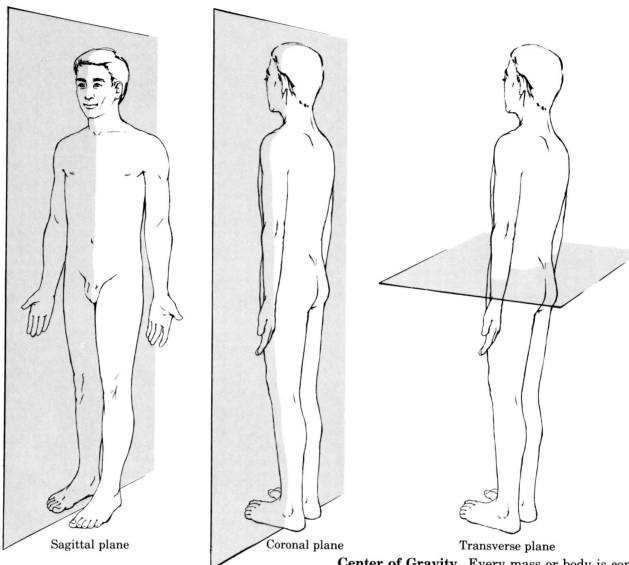

Sagittal plane   Coronal plane   Transverse plane

Planes. The three basic planes of reference are derived from the dimensions in space and are at right angles to each other.

A *sagittal plane* is vertical and extends from front to back, deriving its name from the direction of the sagittal suture of the skull. It may also be called an anterior-posterior plane. The median sagittal plane, *midsagittal*, divides the body into right and left halves.

A *coronal plane* is vertical and extends from side to side, deriving its name from the direction of the coronal suture of the skull. It is also called the frontal or lateral plane, and divides the body into an anterior and a posterior portion.

A *transverse plane* is horizontal and divides the body into upper (cranial) and lower (caudal) portions.

The point at which the three midplanes of the body intersect is the center of gravity.

Center of Gravity. Every mass or body is composed of a multitude of small particles that are pulled toward the earth in accordance with the law of gravitation. This attraction of gravity upon the particles of the body produces a system of practically parallel forces and the resultant of these forces acting vertically downward is the weight of the body. It is possible to locate a point at which a single force, equal in magnitude to the weight of the body and acting vertically upward, may be applied so that the body will remain in equilibrium in any position. This point is called the center of gravity of the body and may be described as the point at which the entire weight of the body may be considered to be concentrated. In an ideally aligned posture in a so-called average adult human being, the center of gravity is considered to be slightly anterior to the first or second sacral segment.

Line of Gravity. The line of gravity is a vertical line through the center of gravity.

FLEXION AND EXTENSION

A *coronal axis* extends horizontally from side to side and lies in the coronal plane. If the coronal *plane* could bend at one of its axes, it could only bend forward and backward. It could not bend sideways nor twist on itself.

The plane cannot bend, but the body can, and in moving forward and backward from this plane (i.e., in a sagittal direction) the movements of *flexion and extension* occur.

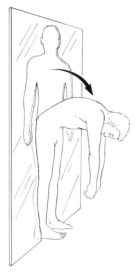

Flexion is movement in the anterior direction for the head, neck, trunk, upper extremity, and hip. *Extension* is movement in the direction opposite flexion. However, flexion of the knee, ankle, and toes is movement in the posterior direction because the developmental pattern of the lower extremities differs from that of the upper extremities.

At an early stage the limbs of the embryo are directed ventrally, the flexor surfaces medially, and the great toes and thumbs cranially. With further development, the limbs rotate 90° at their girdle articulation so that the thumbs turn laterally and the flexor surfaces of the upper extremities ventrally, while the great toes turn medially and the flexor surfaces of the lower extremities dorsally. As a result of this 90° rotation of the limbs in opposite directions, movement which approximates the hand and the anterior surface of the forearm is termed flexion since it is performed by flexor muscles, and movement which approximates the foot and anterior surface of the leg is termed extension since it is performed by extensor muscles. (For alternate terms regarding ankle motion, see p. 22).

Hyperextension. Hyperextension is the term used to describe excessive or unnatural *movement* or *position* in the direction of extension, as in hyperextension of the knees. It is used also in reference to the increased lumbar curvature as in a lordosis with anterior pelvic tilt, or an increased cervical curvature as in a forward head position. In such instances, the range of motion through which the lumbar or cervical spine moves is not excessive, but the position of extension is greater than desirable from a postural standpoint. (See p. 80 and Figure D, p. 91.)

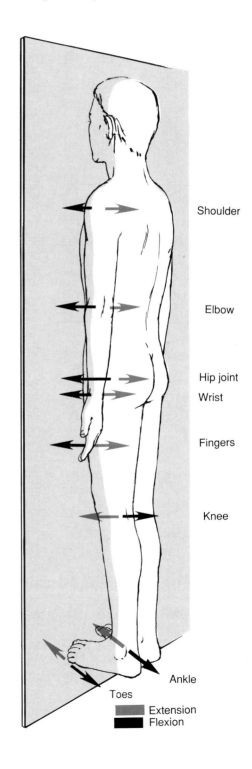

Shoulder

Elbow

Hip joint

Wrist

Fingers

Knee

Ankle

Toes

■ Extension
■ Flexion

ABDUCTION AND ADDUCTION

A *sagittal axis* extends horizontally from front to back and lies in the sagittal plane. If the sagittal *plane* could bend at one of its axes, it could only bend sideways. It could not bend forward or backward or twist on itself.

The plane cannot bend, but the body can, and in moving sideways from this plane (i.e., in a coronal direction) the movements of *adduction and abduction and lateral flexion* take place.

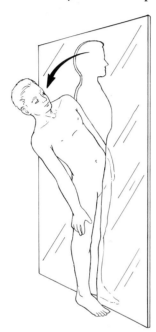

Abduction is movement away from, and adduction is movement toward, the midsagittal plane of the body for all parts of the extremities except the thumb, fingers, and toes. For the fingers, abduction and adduction are movements away from and toward the axial line that extends through the third digit. For the toes, the axial line extends through the second digit. For the thumb, see specific definitions, p. 19.

LATERAL FLEXION

Lateral flexion is the term used to denote lateral movements of the head, neck, and trunk. It occurs about a sagittal axis in a sideways (i.e., coronal) direction.

GLIDING

Gliding movements occur when joint surfaces are flat or only slightly curved and one articulating surface slides on the other.

CIRCUMDUCTION

Circumduction is movement that successively combines flexion, abduction, extension, and adduction in which the part being moved describes a cone. The proximal end of the extremity forms the apex of the cone, serving as a pivot, while the distal end circumscribes a circle. Such movements are possible only in ball-and-socket, condyloid, and saddle types of joints.

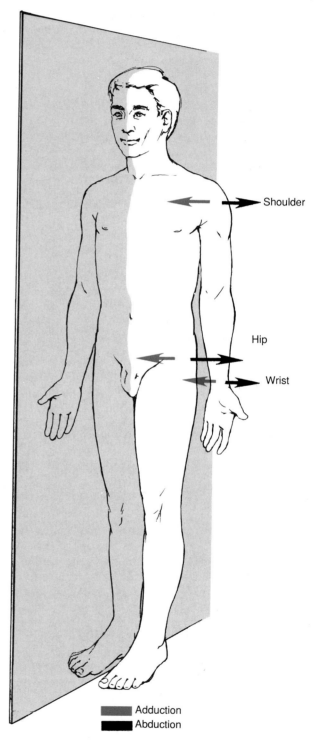

Shoulder

Hip

Wrist

Adduction
Abduction

ROTATION

A *longitudinal* axis is vertical, extending in a cranial-caudal direction. Rotation refers to movement around a longitudinal axis, in a transverse plane, for all areas of the body except the scapula and clavicle.

In the extremities, rotation occurs about the anatomical axis, except in the case of the femur which rotates about a mechanical axis. (See p. 230.) In the extremities, the anterior surface of the extremity is used as a reference area. Rotation of the anterior surface toward the midsagittal plane of the body is *medial* rotation, away from the midsagittal plane is *lateral* rotation.

Since the head, neck, thorax, and pelvis rotate about longitudinal axes in the midsagittal area, rotation cannot be named in reference to the midsagittal plane. Rotation of the head is described as rotation of the face toward the right or left. Rotation of the thorax and pelvis are described, generally, as being clockwise or counterclockwise. With the transverse plane as a reference and 12 o'clock at midpoint anteriorly, clockwise rotation occurs when the left side of the thorax or pelvis is more forward than the right; counterclockwise rotation occurs when the right side is more forward.

TILT

Tilt is a term used to describe certain movements of the head, scapula, and pelvis. The head and pelvis may tilt in an anterior or posterior direction about a coronal axis. Anterior tilt of the head results in flexion (flattening) of the cervical spine, and posterior tilt results in extension. With the pelvis, the opposite occurs. Posterior tilt results in flexion (flattening) of the lumbar spine, and anterior tilt results in extension.

The head and pelvis may tilt laterally, moving about a sagittal axis. Lateral tilt of the head may be referred to as lateral flexion of the neck. Lateral tilt of the pelvis is termed high on one side or low on the other.

Because the pelvis moves as a unit, tilts may be viewed as an anterior, posterior, or lateral tilting of the transverse plane as seen in the accompanying illustration. There may be rotation of the pelvis along with the tilt, more often with anterior and lateral tilt than with posterior tilt. (See also p. 23 for movements of the neck and p. 20 for movements of the pelvis.)

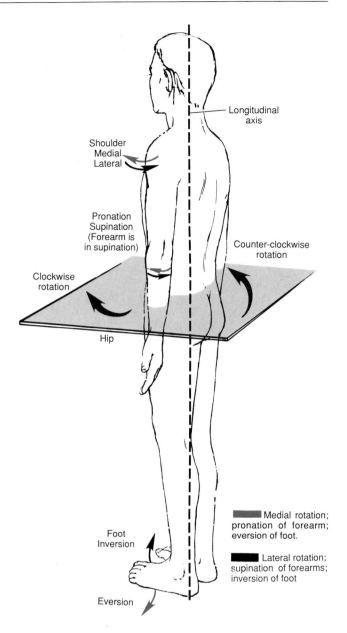

With the scapula in neutral position, there may be anterior tilt but not posterior, except that return from anterior tilt may be referred to as such. (See movements of the scapula, p. 16.)

Movements of Shoulder Girdle and Scapula

SHOULDER GIRDLE

The shoulder girdle is composed of the clavicles and the scapulae. The clavicle articulates laterally with the acromial process of the scapula and medially with the sternum, the latter joint providing the only bony connection with the axial skeleton.

The sternoclavicular joint permits motion in anterior and posterior directions about a longitudinal axis, in cranial and caudal directions about a sagittal axis, and in rotation about a coronal axis. These movements are slightly enhanced and transmitted, by the acromioclavicular joint, to the scapula. Additional motions of the shoulder girdle that will be described are those of the scapula.

The scapula articulates with the humerus at the glenohumeral joint and with the clavicle at the acromioclavicular joint.

In anatomical position, with the upper back in good alignment, the scapulae lie against the thorax approximately between the levels of the second and seventh ribs; the medial borders are essentially parallel and about 4 inches apart.

Muscles that attach the scapula to the thorax and to the vertebral column provide support and motion for it. They are obliquely oriented so that their directions of pull can produce rotatory as well as linear motions of the bone. As a result, the movements ascribed to the scapula do not occur individually as pure movements. Since the contour of the thorax is rounded, some degree of rotation or tilt accompanies abduction and adduction and, to a lesser extent, elevation and depression.

While there are no pure linear movements, seven basic movements of the scapula are described:

> *Adduction* is a gliding movement in which the scapula moves toward the vertebral column.
>
> *Abduction* is a gliding movement in which the scapula moves away from the vertebral column, and following the contour of the thorax assumes a posterolateral position in full abduction.
>
> *Lateral or upward rotation* is movement about a sagittal axis in which the inferior angle moves laterally and the glenoid cavity moves cranially.
>
> *Medial or downward rotation* is movement about a sagittal axis in which the inferior angle moves medially and the glenoid cavity moves caudally.
>
> *Anterior tilt* is movement about a coronal axis in which the coracoid process moves in an anterior and caudal direction while the inferior angle moves in a posterior and cranial direction. The coracoid process may be said to be depressed anteriorly. This movement is associated with elevation.
>
> *Elevation* is a gliding movement in which the scapula moves cranially as in "shrugging" the shoulder.
>
> *Depression* is a gliding movement in which the scapula moves caudally, and is the reverse of elevation and of anterior tilt.

Note: Avoid use of the word "retraction" for adduction, and "protraction" for abduction. (The arm may be protracted by abduction of the scapula, but the scapula is not protracted.)

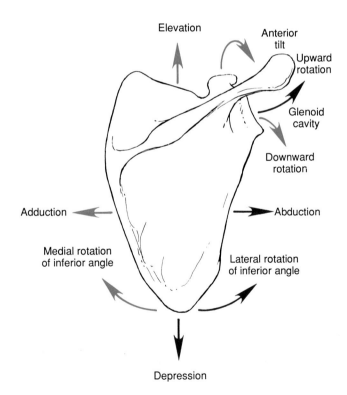

MOVEMENTS OF THE SCAPULA

Elevation

Anterior tilt

Upward rotation

Glenoid cavity

Downward rotation

Adduction

Abduction

Medial rotation of inferior angle

Lateral rotation of inferior angle

Depression

SHOULDER JOINT

The shoulder joint, also called the glenohumeral joint, is a spheroid or ball-and-socket joint formed by the articulation of the head of the humerus and the glenoid cavity of the scapula. In addition to six basic joint movements, it is necessary to define circumduction and two movements in the horizontal plane.

Flexion and extension are movements about a coronal axis. *Flexion* is movement in the anterior direction and may begin from a position of 45° extension (arm extended backward). It describes an arc forward through the zero anatomical position and on to the 180° overhead position. However, the 180° overhead position is attained only by the combined movement of the shoulder joint and the shoulder girdle. The glenohumeral joint can be flexed only to approximately 120°. The remaining 60° is attained as a result of the abduction and lateral rotation of the scapula which allows the glenoid cavity to face more anteriorly and the humerus to flex to a fully vertical position. The scapular motion is at first variable but after 60° of flexion there is a relatively constant relationship between the movement of the humerus and the scapula. Inman et al. found that between the 30° and 170° range of flexion the glenohumeral joint provided 10° and scapular rotation 5° for every 15° of motion (11).

Extension is movement in the posterior direction and technically refers to the arc of motion from 180° flexion to 45° extension. If the elbow joint is flexed, the range of shoulder joint extension will be increased because the tension of the Biceps will be released.

Abduction and adduction are movements about a sagittal axis. *Abduction* is movement in a lateral direction through a range of 180° to a vertical overhead position. This end position is the same as that attained in flexion, and coordinates shoulder girdle and glenohumeral joint movements. *Adduction* is movement toward the midsagittal plane in a medial direction and technically refers to the arc of motion from full elevation overhead through the zero anatomical position to a position obliquely upward and across the front of the body.

Horizontal abduction and adduction are movements in a transverse plane about a longitudinal axis. *Horizontal abduction* is movement in a lateral and posterior direction; *horizontal adduction* is movement in an anterior and medial direction.

The end position of complete horizontal adduction is the same as that for adduction obliquely upward across the body. In one instance, the arm moves horizontally to that position; in the other instance, it moves obliquely upward to that position.

The range of horizontal abduction, being determined to a great extent by the length of the Pectoralis major, is extremely variable. With the humerus in 90° flexion as the zero position for measurement, the normal range should be about 90° in horizontal abduction and about 40° in horizontal adduction, most readily judged by the ability to place the palm of the hand on top of the opposite shoulder.

Medial and lateral rotation are movements about a longitudinal axis through the humerus. *Medial rotation* is movement in which the anterior surface of the humerus turns toward the midsagittal plane. *Lateral rotation* is movement in which the anterior surface of the humerus turns away from the midsagittal plane.

The extent of medial or lateral rotation varies with the degree of elevation in abduction or flexion. For purposes of joint measurement the zero position is one in which the shoulder is at 90° abduction, the elbow is bent at right angles and the forearm is at right angles to the coronal plane. From this position, lateral rotation of the shoulder describes an arc of 90° to a position in which the forearm is parallel with the head. Medial rotation describes an arc of approximately 70° if shoulder girdle movement is not permitted. If the scapula is allowed to tilt anteriorly, the forearm may describe an arc of 90° to a position in which it is parallel with the side of the body.

As the arm is abducted or flexed from the anatomical position, lateral rotation continues to be free but medial rotation is limited. As the arm is adducted or extended the range of medial rotation remains free and that of lateral rotation decreases. In treatment to restore motion in a restricted shoulder joint, one must be concerned with obtaining lateral rotation as a prerequisite to full flexion or full abduction.

Circumduction combines consecutively the movements of flexion, abduction, extension, and adduction as the upper limb circumscribes a cone with its apex at the glenohumeral joint. This succession of movements can be performed in either direction and is used to increase the overall range of motion of the shoulder joint, as in Codman's or in shoulder-wheel exercises.

Movements of Elbow, Wrist, and Fingers

ELBOW JOINT

The elbow is a ginglymus or hinge joint formed by the articulation of the humerus with the ulna and the radius.

Flexion and extension occur about a coronal axis and are the two movements permitted by this joint. *Flexion* is movement in the anterior direction, from the position of a straight elbow, 0°, to a fully bent position, approximately 145°. *Extension* is movement in a posterior direction from the fully bent position to the position of a straight elbow.

RADIOULNAR JOINT

The radioulnar joints are trochoid or pivot joints, formed by the articulations of the radius and ulna, proximally and distally. The axis of motion extends from the head of the radius proximally, to the head of the ulna distally, and allows rotation of the radius about the axis.

Supination and pronation are rotation movements of the forearm. In *pronation*, the distal end of the radius moves from a lateral position, as in the anatomical position, to a medial position; in *supination*, it moves from a medial to a lateral position. The palm of the hand faces anteriorly in supination and posteriorly in pronation.

Shoulder rotation movements can produce movement of the forearm that resemble supination and pronation. To ensure forearm movements only, place the arms directly at the sides of the body with elbows bent at right angles, forearms extended forward. Turn palms directly upward for full supination and directly downward for full pronation.

The neutral or zero position is midway between supination and pronation, that is, from anatomical position with elbow extended the thumb is directed forward; with the elbow bent at right angle, the thumb is directed upward. The normal range of motion is 90° in either direction from zero.

WRIST JOINT

The wrist is a condyloid joint formed by the radius and the distal surface of the articular disc articulating with the scaphoid, lunate, and triquetrum.

Flexion and extension are movements about a coronal axis. From the anatomical position, *flexion* is movement in an anterior direction approximating the palmar surface of the hand toward the anterior surface of the forearm. *Extension* is movement in a posterior direction approximating the dorsum of the hand toward the posterior surface of the forearm. Starting with the wrist straight (as in anatomical position) as zero position, the range of flexion is approximately 80° and that of extension approximately 70°. The fingers will tend to extend when measuring wrist flexion, and to flex when measuring wrist extension.

Abduction (radial deviation) and adduction (ulnar deviation) are movements about a sagittal axis. With the hand in anatomical position, moving it toward the ulnar side is also moving it medially toward the midline of the body and hence, is *adduction*. Moving the hand toward the radial side is *abduction*. With the anatomical position as zero, the range of adduction is approximately 35° and that of abduction approximately 20°.

Circumduction combines the successive movements of flexion, abduction, extension, and adduction of the radiocarpal joint and the midcarpal joint. The movements of these joints are closely related and permit the hand to describe a cone. The movement is not as free as that of the glenohumeral joint; abduction is more limited than adduction because the radial styloid process extends farther caudally than the ulnar styloid process.

CARPOMETACARPAL JOINTS OF FINGERS

The carpometacarpal joints of the fingers are formed by the articulation of the distal row of carpal bones with the second, third, fourth, and fifth metacarpal bones and permit gliding movements. The joint between the hamate bone and the fifth metacarpal is somewhat saddle-shaped and allows, in addition, flexion, extension, and slight rotation.

METACARPOPHALANGEAL JOINTS OF FINGERS

The metacarpophalangeal joints of the fingers are condyloid joints formed by the articulations of the distal ends of the metacarpals with the adjacent ends of the proximal phalanges.

Flexion and extension occur about a coronal axis with *flexion* in an anterior direction and *extension* in a posterior direction. With the extended position as zero, the metacarpophalangeal joints flex to approximately 90°. In most people some extension beyond zero is possible, but for practical purposes the straight extension of this joint, when interphalangeal joints are also extended, is considered normal extension.

Abduction and adduction occur about a sagittal axis. The line of reference for abduction and adduction of the fingers is the axial line through the third digit. *Abduction* is movement in the plane of the palm away from the axial line, spreading fingers wide apart. The third digit may move in abduction both ulnarly and radially from the axial line. *Adduction* is movement in the plane of the palm toward the axial line, that is, closing the extended fingers together sideways.

Circumduction is the combination of flexion, abduction, extension, and adduction movements performed consecutively, in either direction, at the metacarpophalangeal joints of the fingers. Extension in these condyloid joints is somewhat limited so that the base of the cone described by the fingertip is relatively small.

INTERPHALANGEAL JOINTS OF FINGERS

The interphalangeal joints of the fingers are ginglymus or hinge joints formed by articulations of the adjacent surfaces of the phalanges.

Flexion and extension occur about a coronal axis and describe an arc from 0° extension to approximately 100° flexion for the proximal interphalangeal joints and 80° for the distal interphalangeal joints.

CARPOMETACARPAL JOINT OF THUMB

The carpometacarpal joint of the thumb is a reciprocal reception or saddle joint, formed by the articulation of the trapezium with the first metacarpal. The zero position of *extension* is one in which the thumb has moved in a radial direction and is in the plane of the palm. *Flexion* is movement in an ulnar direction with a range of approximately 40° to 50° from zero extension. The thumb can be fully flexed only if accompanied by some degree of abduction and medial rotation.

Adduction and abduction are movements perpendicular to the plane of the palm, *adduction* being toward and *abduction* away from the palm. With the position of adduction as zero, the range of abduction is approximately 80°.

The range of rotation at the carpometacarpal joint is slight and does not occur independently. The *slight rotation*, however, that results from a combination of basic movements is of significance.

In the thumb and little finger, *opposition* is a combination of abduction and flexion with medial rotation of the carpometacarpal joints, and flexion of the metacarpophalangeal joint. To ensure opposition of the thumb and little finger the palmar surfaces (rather than the tips) of the distal phalanges must be brought in contact with each other. Touching the tips of the thumb and little finger to each other can be done without any true opposition.

The movements of opposition are accomplished by the combined actions of the respective opponens and metacarpophalangeal flexors: in the thumb, the Opponens pollicis, Abductor pollicis brevis, and Flexor pollicis brevis; in the little finger, the Opponens digiti minimi, the Flexor digiti minimi, the fourth Lumbricalis, and the fourth Palmar interosseus, assisted by the Abductor digiti minimi.

Circumduction is a movement which includes flexion, abduction, extension, and adduction, performed in sequence, by this saddle joint. With the apex at the carpometacarpal joint, the first metacarpal bone describes a cone and the tip of the thumb describes a circle.

METACARPOPHALANGEAL AND INTERPHALANGEAL JOINT OF THUMB

The metacarpophalangeal joint of the thumb is a condyloid joint formed by the articulation of the distal end of the first metacarpal with the adjacent end of the proximal phalanx. The interphalangeal joint of the thumb is a ginglymus or hinge joint formed by the articulation of the proximal and distal phalanges.

Flexion and extension are movements in an ulnar and radial direction, respectively. The zero position of extension is reached when the thumb moves in the plane of the palm to maximum radial deviation. From the position of zero extension, the metacarpophalangeal joint permits approximately 60° flexion, and the interphalangeal joint, approximately 80° flexion. The metacarpophalangeal joint permits, also, slight abduction, adduction, and rotation.

Movements of Pelvis and Hip Joint

PELVIS

The *neutral position of the pelvis* is one in which the anterior-superior spines are in the same transverse plane, and in which they and the symphysis pubis are in the same vertical plane. An *anterior pelvic tilt* is a position of the pelvis in which the vertical plane through the anterior-superior spines is anterior to a vertical plane through the symphysis pubis. A *posterior pelvic tilt* is a position of the pelvis in which the vertical plane through the anterior-superior spines is posterior to a vertical plane through the symphysis pubis. In a standing position an anterior pelvic tilt is associated with hyperextension of the lumbar spine and flexion of the hip joints, while posterior pelvic tilt is associated with flexion of the lumbar spine and extension of the hip joints. (See pp. 76 and 83–87.)

In a *lateral pelvic tilt* the pelvis is not level from side to side, but one anterior-superior spine is higher than the other. In standing, a lateral tilt is associated with lateral flexion of the lumbar spine and adduction and abduction of the hip joints. For example, in a lateral tilt of the pelvis in which the right side is higher than the left, the lumbar spine is laterally flexed toward the *right* resulting in a curve convex to the *left*. The right hip joint is in adduction, and the left is in abduction.

HIP JOINT

The hip joint is a spheroid or ball-and-socket joint formed by the articulation of the acetabulum of the pelvis with the head of the femur.

Ordinarily, descriptions of joint movement refer to movement of the distal part upon a fixed proximal part. In the upright weight-bearing position, movement of the proximal part upon the more fixed distal part becomes of equal, if not primary, importance. For this reason, movements of the pelvis on the femur are mentioned as well as movements of the femur on the pelvis.

Flexion and extension are movements about a coronal axis. *Flexion* is movement in an anterior direction. The movement may be one of moving the thigh toward the fixed pelvis as in supine alternate-leg raising; or the movement may be one of bringing the pelvis toward the fixed thighs as in coming up from a supine to a sitting position, bending forward from a standing position, or tilting the pelvis anteriorly in standing. *Extension* is movement in a posterior direction. The movement may be one of bringing the thigh posteriorly as in leg-raising backward, or one of bringing the trunk posteriorly as in returning from a standing forward-bent position, or as in tilting the pelvis posteriorly in standing or lying prone.

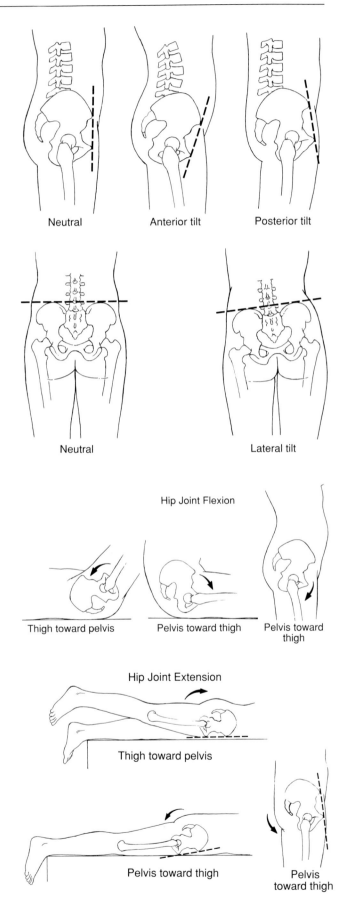

Neutral   Anterior tilt   Posterior tilt

Neutral   Lateral tilt

Hip Joint Flexion

Thigh toward pelvis   Pelvis toward thigh   Pelvis toward thigh

Hip Joint Extension

Thigh toward pelvis

Pelvis toward thigh   Pelvis toward thigh

The range of hip joint flexion from zero is about 125°, the range of extension is about 10°, making a total range of about 135°. The knee joint should be flexed when measuring hip joint flexion to avoid restriction of motion by the Hamstring muscles, and extended when measuring hip joint extension to avoid restriction of motion by the Rectus femoris.

Abduction and adduction are movements about a sagittal axis. *Abduction* is movement away from a midsagittal plane in a lateral direction. In a supine position the movement may be one of moving the thigh laterally on a fixed trunk or moving the trunk so that the pelvis tilts laterally (downward) toward a fixed thigh. *Adduction* is movement of the thigh toward the midsagittal plane in a medial direction. In a supine position, the movement may be one of moving the thigh medially on a fixed trunk or moving the trunk so that the pelvis tilts laterally (upward) away from a fixed thigh. (For abduction and adduction of the hip joints accompanying lateral pelvic tilt, see below.)

From zero, the range of abduction is approximately 45° and of adduction, 10°, making the total range about 55°.

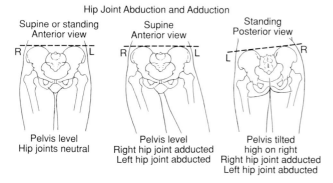

Hip Joint Abduction and Adduction

Supine or standing
Anterior view

Pelvis level
Hip joints neutral

Supine
Anterior view

Pelvis level
Right hip joint adducted
Left hip joint abducted

Standing
Posterior view

Pelvis tilted
high on right
Right hip joint adducted
Left hip joint abducted

Lateral and medial rotation are movements about a longitudinal axis. *Medial rotation* is movement in which the anterior surface of the thigh turns toward the midsagittal plane. *Lateral rotation* is movement in which the anterior surface of the thigh moves away from the midsagittal plane. Rotation may result, also, from movement of the trunk on the femur. For example, when standing with legs fixed, counterclockwise rotation of the pelvis will result in lateral rotation of the right hip joint, and medial rotation of the left.

KNEE JOINT

The knee joint is a modified ginglymus or hinge joint formed by the articulation of the condyles of the femur with the condyles of the tibia and by the patella articulating with the patellar surface of the femur.

Flexion and extension are movements about a coronal axis. *Flexion* is movement in a posterior direction, approximating the posterior surfaces of the leg and thigh. *Extension* is movement in an anterior direction to a position of straight alignment of the thigh and leg (0°). From the position of zero extension, the range of flexion is approximately 140°. The hip joint should be flexed when measuring full knee joint flexion to avoid restriction of motion by the Rectus femoris, but should not be fully flexed when measuring knee joint extension in order to avoid restriction by the Hamstring muscles.

Hyperextension is an abnormal or unnatural movement beyond the zero position of extension. For the sake of stability in standing, the knee normally is expected to be in a position of a very few degrees of extension beyond zero. If extended beyond these few degrees, the knee is said to be hyperextended. (See pp. 95 and 96.)

Lateral and medial rotation are movements about a longitudinal axis. Rotation of the anterior surface of the leg toward the midsagittal plane is *medial rotation*, away from the midsagittal plane is *lateral rotation*.

The extended knee (in zero position) is essentially locked, preventing any rotation. Rotation occurs with flexion, combining movement between the tibia and the menisci as well as movement between the tibia and the femur.

With the thigh fixed, the movement that accompanies *flexion* is medial rotation of the tibia on the femur; with the leg fixed, the movement is lateral rotation of the femur on the tibia.

With the thigh fixed, the movement that accompanies *extension* is lateral rotation of the tibia on the femur; with the leg fixed, the movement is medial rotation of the femur on the tibia.

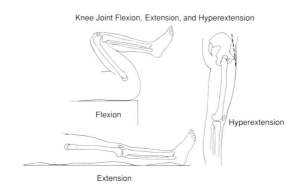

Knee Joint Flexion, Extension, and Hyperextension

Flexion

Hyperextension

Extension

Movements of Ankle, Foot, and Toes

ANKLE JOINT

The ankle joint is a ginglymus or hinge joint formed by the articulation of the tibia and fibula with the talus. The axis about which motion takes place extends obliquely from the posterolateral aspect of the fibular malleolus to the anteromedial aspect of the tibial malleolus.

Flexion and extension are the two movements that occur about the oblique axis. *Flexion* is movement of the foot in which the plantar surface moves in a caudal and posterior direction. *Extension* is movement of the foot in which the dorsal surface moves in an anterior and cranial direction.

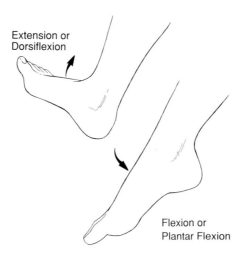

Extension or
Dorsiflexion

Flexion or
Plantar Flexion

Confusion has arisen about the terminology of these two ankle joint movements. An apparent discrepancy occurs because decreasing an angle frequently is associated with flexion while increasing it is associated with extension. Bringing the foot upward to "bend the ankle" seems to connote flexion, while pointing the foot downward to "straighten the ankle" connotes extension. (In a review of 48 authors, 12 of them had the wrong definitions for ankle flexion and extension.) To avoid confusion, there has been rather wide acceptance of the terms *dorsiflexion* for extension, and *plantar flexion* for flexion. This text will adhere to these generally accepted terms.

The knee should be flexed when measuring dorsiflexion. With the knee flexed, the ankle joint can be dorsiflexed about 20°. If the knee is extended, the Gastrocnemius will limit the range of motion to about 10° of dorsiflexion. The range of motion in plantar flexion is approximately 45°.

SUBTALAR JOINT AND TRANSVERSE TARSAL JOINTS

The subtalar joint is a modified plane or gliding joint formed by the articulation of the talus and calcaneus. The talus also articulates with the navicular, and the talonavicular joint is involved in the movements ascribed to the subtalar joint.

Supination and pronation are movements permitted by the subtalar and talocalcaneonavicular joints. *Supination* is rotation of the foot in which the sole of the foot moves in a medial direction; *pronation* is rotation in which the sole of the foot moves in a lateral direction.

The transverse tarsal joints are formed by the articulations of the talus with the navicular, and the calcaneus with the cuboid.

Adduction and abduction of the forefoot are movements permitted by the transverse tarsal joints, *adduction* is movement of the forefoot in a medial direction and *abduction* is movement in a lateral direction.

Inversion is a combination of supination and forefoot adduction. It is more free in plantar flexion than in dorsiflexion.

Eversion is a combination of pronation and forefoot abduction. It is more free in dorsiflexion than in plantar flexion.

METATARSOPHALANGEAL JOINTS

The metatarsophalangeal joints are condyloid, formed by the articulation of the distal ends of the metatarsals with the adjacent ends of the proximal phalanges.

Flexion and extension are movements about a coronal axis. *Flexion* is movement in a caudal direction, *extension* is movement in a cranial direction. The range of motion in adults is variable, but 30° flexion and 40° extension may be considered an average range for good function of the toes.

Adduction and abduction are movements about a sagittal axis. The line of reference for adduction and abduction of the toes is the axial line projected distally in line with the second metatarsal and extending through the second digit. *Adduction* is movement toward the axial line, and *abduction* is movement away from it, as in spreading the toes apart. Because abduction of the toes is restricted by the wearing of shoes, this movement is markedly limited in most adults and little attention is paid to the ability to abduct.

INTERPHALANGEAL JOINTS OF TOES

The interphalangeal joints are ginglymus or hinge joints formed by the articulations of adjacent surfaces of phalanges.

Flexion and extension are movements about a coronal axis with *flexion* being movement in a caudal direction and *extension* movement in a cranial direction.

MOVEMENTS OF VERTEBRAL COLUMN

Vertebral articulations include the bilateral synovial joints of the vertebral arches where the inferior facets of one vertebra articulate with the superior facets of the adjacent vertebra, and the fibrous joints between successive vertebral bodies united by intervertebral fibrocartilaginous discs. Movement between two adjacent vertebrae is slight and is determined by the slope of the articular facets and the flexibility of the intervertebral discs. The range of motion of the column as a whole, however, is considerable and the movements permitted are flexion, extension, lateral flexion, and rotation.

The articulations of the first two vertebrae of the column are exceptions to the general classification. The atlanto-occipital articulation, between the condyles of the occipital bone and the superior facets of the atlas, is classified as a condyloid joint. The movements permitted are flexion and extension with very slight lateral motion. The atlantoaxial articulation is composed of three joints, the two lateral fitting the general description of the joints of the vertebral column. The third, a median joint, formed by the articulation of the dens of the axis with the fovea dentis of the atlas is classified as a trochoid joint and permits rotation.

The normal curves of the spine, anterior in the cervical region, posterior in the thoracic region, and anterior in the lumbar region, are named according to the *convexity* of the curve. Likewise, a lateral curvature is named according to the direction of the convexity, e.g., a left lumbar curve is one which is convex toward the left. To the extent that the spine curves convexly forward or backward during movement, the same rule applies about naming the direction of movement according to the direction of the convexity of the curve.

According to *Stedman's Medical Dictionary*, to flex means to bend, to extend means to straighten (12). With respect to the *thoracic* spine, these meanings apply. The normal *posterior curve is a position of slight flexion*. As the spine moves from flexion to the *straight position, it is in extension*. However, there appears to be an ambiguity when describing the positions and movements of the *cervical* and *lumbar* spines. In each, the normal anterior *curve is a position of slight extension*. As the spine moves from extension to the *straight position, it is in flexion*. Because it is confusing to describe a straight spine as being in flexion, it is better to use the term flat, rather than flexed, when referring to the cervical and lumbar regions.

Flexion of the spine, which occurs in a sagittal plane, is movement in which the head and trunk bend forward as the spine moves in the direction of curving convexly backward. (See below.) From a supine position, normal flexion will allow curling the trunk enough to lift the scapulae from the supporting surface. The seventh cervical vertebra will be lifted upward about 8 to 10 inches.

Flexion varies according to the region of the spine. In the *cervical* region, flexion of the spine is movement in the direction of *decreasing the normal forward curve*. Movement continues to the point of straightening or flattening this region of the spine, but normally does not progress to the point that the spine curves convexly backward. In the *thoracic* region, flexion of the spine is movement in the direction of *increasing the normal backward curve*. In normal flexion, the spine curves convexly backward producing a continuous, gently rounded contour throughout the thoracic area. In the *lumbar* region, flexion of the spine is movement in the direction of *decreasing the normal forward curve*. It progresses to the point of straightening or flattening the low back, but normally the lumbar spine does not curve convexly backward.

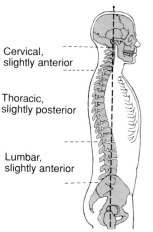

Cervical, slightly anterior

Thoracic, slightly posterior

Lumbar, slightly anterior

Normal curves of spine

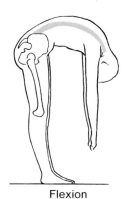

Flexion

Extension of the spine, which occurs in a sagittal plane, is movement in which the head and trunk bend backward while the spine moves in the direction of curving convexly forward. From a prone position, normal extension will allow the head and chest to be raised enough to lift the xiphoid process of the sternum about 2 to 4 inches from the table. (See p. 140.)

Extension varies according to the regions of the spine. In the *cervical* region, extension is movement in the direction of *increasing the normal forward curve*. It occurs by tilting the head back, bringing the occiput toward the seventh cervical vertebra. It may occur, also, in sitting or standing, by slumping into a round upper back, forward-head position—a position that also results in approximating the occiput toward the seventh cervical vertebra. In the *thoracic* region, extension is movement of the spine in the direction of *decreasing the normal backward curve*. Movement may progress to, but normally not beyond, the point of straightening or flattening the thoracic spine. In the *lumbar* region, extension is movement in the direction of *increasing the normal forward curve*. It occurs by bending the body backward or by tilting the pelvis forward.

Hyperextension of the spine is movement beyond the normal range of motion in extension, or may refer to a position greater than the normal anterior curve. Hyperextension may vary from slight to extreme. (See pp. 49 and 80.)

Lateral flexion and rotation are described separately although they occur in combination and are not considered pure movements.

Lateral flexion of the spine, which occurs in a coronal plane, is movement in which the head and trunk bend toward one side while the spine curves convexly toward the opposite side. A curve convex toward the right is the equivalent of lateral flexion toward the left. From a standing position with feet about 4 inches apart, body erect, and arms at sides, normal lateral flexion (bending directly sideways) will allow for the fingertips to reach approximately to the level of the knee.

Lateral flexion varies according to the regions of the spine. It is most free in the cervical and lumbar regions, being restricted in the thoracic region by the rib cage.

Rotation is movement in a transverse plane. It is most free in the thoracic region and slight in the lumbar region. Rotation in the cervical region permits about 90° range of motion of the head and is referred to as rotation of the face toward the right or left. Rotation of the thorax on the pelvis is described as *clockwise* (forward on left side) or *counterclockwise* (forward on right side).

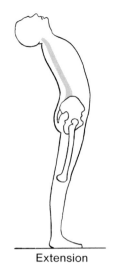

Extension

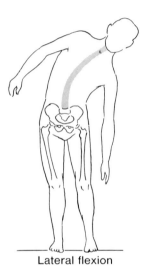

Lateral flexion

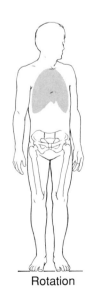

Rotation

JOINT MEASUREMENT CHART

Name...Identification #................................

Diagnosis..Age...

Onset..Doctor..

UPPER EXTREMITY

					Date	Motion*	Average Range	Date						
					Examiner			Examiner						
						Extension	45							
						Flexion	180							
						Range	225							
					Left Shoulder	Abduction	180	Right Shoulder						
						Adduction	0							
						Range	180							
						Lateral Rotation	90							
						Medial Rotation	70							
						Range	160							
					Left Elbow	Extension	0	Right Elbow						
						Flexion	145							
						Range	145							
					Left Forearm	Supination	90	Right Forearm						
						Pronation	90							
						Range	180							
						Extension	70							
						Flexion	80							
					Left Wrist	Range	150	Right Wrist						
						Ulnar Deviation	45							
						Radial Deviation	20							
						Range	65							

LOWER EXTREMITY

					Date	Motion*	Average Range	Date						
					Examiner			Examiner						
						Extension	10							
						Flexion	125							
						Range	135							
					Left Hip	Abduction	45	Right Hip						
						Adduction	10							
						Range	55							
						Lateral Rotation	45							
						Medial Rotation	45							
						Range	90							
					Left Knee	Extension	0	Right Knee						
						Flexion	140							
						Range	140							
					Left Ankle	Plantar Flexion	45	Right Ankle						
						Dorsiflexion	20							
						Range	65							
					Left Foot	Inversion	40	Right Foot						
						Eversion	20							
						Range	60							

*The zero position is the plane of reference. When a part moves in the direction of zero but fails to reach the zero position, the degrees designating the joint motion obtained are recorded with a minus sign and subtracted in computing the range of motion.

Classification of Joints

TISSUE	ACCORDING TO TYPE OF			EXAMPLE
	ARTICULATION		MOVEMENT	
Fibrous	Synarthrosis	Syndesmosis	Immovable	Tibiofibular (distal)
		Sutura	Immovable	Suture of skull
Cartilaginous	Amphiarthrosis	Gomphosis	Immovable	Tooth in bony socket
		Synchondrosis	Slightly movable	First sternocostal
		Symphysis	Slightly movable	Symphysis pubis
Synovial	Diarthrosis	Spheroid or Ball-and-Socket	All joint movements	Shoulder and hip
		Ginglymus or Hinge	Flexion and extension	Elbow
		Modified Ginglymus	Flexion, extension, and slight rotation	Knee and ankle
		Ellipsoid or Condyloid	All except rotation and opposition	Metacarpophalangeal Metatarsophalangeal
		Trochoid or Pivot	Supination, pronation, and rotation	Atlantoaxial and Radioulnar
		Reciprocal-reception or Saddle	All except rotation	Calcaneocuboid and Carpometarcarpal
		Plane or Gliding	Gliding	Head of fibula with lateral condyle of tibia
		Combined Ginglymus and Gliding	Flexion, extension, and gliding	Temporomandibular

Muscle Length Tests and Stretching Exercises

GROSS STRUCTURE OF MUSCLE

The gross structure of muscle helps determine muscle action and affects the way that a muscle responds to stretching. Muscle fibers are arranged in bundles called fasciculi. The arrangement of fasciculi and their attachments to tendons vary anatomically. There are two main divisions of gross structure—fusiform (or spindle), and pennate.

In *fusiform*, fibers are arranged essentially parallel to the line from origin to insertion, and the fasciculi terminate at both ends of the muscle in flat tendons. In *pennate*, fibers are inserted obliquely into the tendon or tendons that extend the length of the muscle on one side or through the belly of the muscle. A third arrangement, the fan-shaped, is probably a modification of the other two, but has a distinct significance clinically

According to Gray's Anatomy, the "arrangement of fasciculi is correlated with the power of the muscles. Those with comparatively few fasciculi, extending the length of the muscle, have a greater range of motion but not as much power. Penniform muscles, with a large number of fasciculi distributed along their tendons, have greater power but smaller range of motion" (13). In all probability the long fusiform muscle is the most vulnerable to stretch. The joint motion is in the same direction as the length of the fiber, and each longitudinal component is dependent on every other one.

The pennate muscles are probably the least vulnerable to stretch because the muscle fiber is oblique to the direction of joint motion and because the fibers and fasciculi are short and parallel, thereby not dependent on other segments for continuity in action.

The fan-shaped muscle has advantages and disadvantages of both of the above. It might be thought of as a group of muscles arranged side by side to form a fan-shaped unit. Each segment is independent in the sense that it has its own origin and insertion. For example, in the fan-shaped Pectoralis major, the clavicular part may be unaffected and the sternal part paralyzed in a cord lesion.

MUSCLE LENGTH TESTS

Muscle length tests are done for the purpose of determining whether the range of muscle length is normal, limited, or excessive. Muscles that are excessive in length are usually weak and allow adaptive shortening of opposing muscles; muscles that are too short are usually strong, and maintain opposing muscles in a lengthened position.

Muscle length testing consists of movements that increase the distance between origin and insertion, elongating muscles in directions opposite to that of the muscle actions.

Accurate testing usually requires that the bone of origin of the muscle be in a fixed position while the bone of insertion moves in the direction of lengthening the muscle. Length tests employ test movements, using passive or active-assisted movements to determine how much the muscle can be elongated.

RANGE OF JOINT MOTION AND RANGE OF MUSCLE LENGTH

The terms "range of joint motion" and "range of muscle length" have specific meanings. *Range of joint motion* refers to the number of degrees of motion present in a joint. In *Chapter 2*, descriptions of joints and the joint measurement charts include references to normal ranges of joint motion. *Range of muscle length*, also expressed in terms of degrees of joint motion, refers to the length of the muscle.

For muscles that pass over *one joint* only, the range of joint motion and range of muscle length will measure the same. Both may be normal, limited, or excessive. Some musculoskeletal conditions exist in which the joint or the muscle is initially involved without restriction by the other.

For muscles that pass over *two or more* joints, the normal range of muscle length will be less than the total range of motion of the joints over which the muscle passes. It is important to understand this difference when dealing with multijoint muscles.

When measuring range of joint motion of the two joints over which a two-joint muscle passes, it is necessary to allow the muscle to be slack over one joint in order to determine the full range of joint motion in the other. For example, when measuring the range of *knee joint flexion*, the hip is flexed to allow the Rectus femoris and Tensor fasciae latae to be slack over the hip joint and permit full range of joint motion at the knee. When measuring range of *hip joint flexion*, the knee is flexed to allow the Hamstrings to be slack over the knee joint and permit full range of joint motion at the hip.

PRINCIPLES

The above explanation can be stated in terms of general principles:

Range of joint motion and range of muscle length may be expressed in degrees.
A normal one-joint muscle possesses sufficient extensibility to lengthen through the full range of motion afforded by the joint over which it crosses.
A normal two-joint muscle does not possess sufficient extensibility to lengthen through the full

range of motion afforded by both joints simultaneously, but it can be elongated fully over one joint if it is not elongated over the other.

By applying the general principles and specific rules of procedure, and by performing tests with precision, muscle length testing can be standardized. A valid test can be obtained if variables are controlled during length testing. (For example: Fix the low back and sacrum flat on a surface that has no soft padding, and keep the knee in extension during the straight-leg-raising test for Hamstring length.)

CORRELATION BETWEEN JOINT RANGE AND MUSCLE LENGTH

An interesting correlation exists between the total range of joint motion and the range of muscle length chosen as a standard for Hamstring and hip flexor length tests. In each case the muscle length adopted as a standard is approximately 80% of the total range of joint motion of the two joints over which the muscles pass.

The following are the joint ranges used as normal: hip—10° extension, 125° flexion, for a total of 135°; knee—0° extension, 140° flexion, for a total of 140°, making the total of both joints 275°.

Hip flexor length test used as a standard (see p. 33): Supine with low back and sacrum flat on table, hip joint extended, the hip flexors are elongated 135° over the hip joint. With the knee flexed over the end of the table at an angle of 80°, the two-joint hip flexors are elongated 80° over the knee joint for a total of 215°. 215° divided by 275° = 78.18%. Range of muscle length is 78% of total joint range.

Hamstring length test used as a standard (see p. 38): Supine with low back and sacrum flat on table, straight-leg raising to 80° angle with table. Hamstrings are elongated 140° over the knee by full extension and 80° over the hip joint by the straight-leg raising for a total of 220°. 220° divided by 275° = 80%. Range of muscle length is 80% of total joint range.

ROLE OF MUSCLES

In addition to their role in movement, muscles have an important role in supporting skeletal structures. A muscle must be long enough to permit normal mobility of the joints and be short enough to contribute effectively to joint stability.

When range of motion is *limited* due to tight muscles, treatment consists of the use of various modalities and procedures that promote muscle relaxation and assist in stretching the muscles. Stretching exercises are one of the most important procedures. Stretching should be gradual and may cause mild discomfort but should not cause pain.

When range of motion is *excessive*, the most important part of treatment is avoiding overstretching. If there is instability with or without pain, it is prudent, in many instances, to apply a support that can allow affected structures to "tighten." It may or may not be necessary to add specific exercises since many muscles weakened by stretching recover with normal activity when overstretching is avoided.

Tests for length of lower extremity and back muscles are presented in this order: hip flexors, Hamstrings, back, Tensor fasciae latae, and Iliotibial band. Because hip flexor shortness can interfere with an accurate test of Hamstring length, it is advisable to test hip flexors prior to testing Hamstrings. Two Hamstring length tests are presented: the straight-leg-raising test, and the sitting, forward-bending test. These tests are followed by the forward-bending test for contour of the back and length of the back muscles. Since this test also involves Hamstring length, it is logical that this test follow the Hamstring length tests. The Tensor fasciae latae is a hip flexor as well as an abductor, and it is observed along with the hip flexor length test, but the length test of the Tensor fasciae latae is done in a side-lying position, using the Ober or modified Ober test. (See p. 57.)

MEASURING JOINT MOTION

For the following muscle length tests, the *low back* must be flat on the table: Latissimus dorsi and Teres major (p. 63), and shoulder medial and lateral rotators (p. 64). For muscle length tests of hip flexors and Hamstrings, the *low back and sacrum* must be flat on the table.

In all of these tests, it is easier and more accurate to use a measuring device that permits the stationary arm of the caliper to rest on the table, and permits the examiner to align the movable arm with the axis of the humerus or femur, as the case may be. The fulcrum will be shifted to permit this change, but the angle will remain the same as if the stationary arm were held parallel to the table along the trunk in line with the shoulder joint or hip joint.

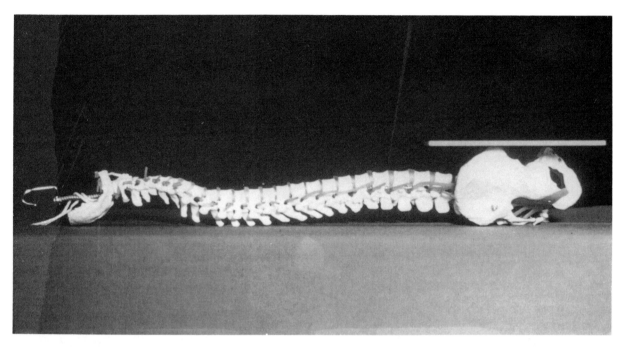

The pelvis is in neutral position and the lumbar spine is in normal anterior curve.

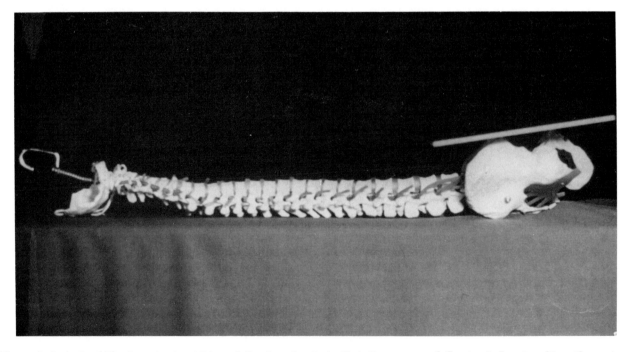

The pelvis is in 10° of posterior tilt and the low back is flat (i.e., normal flexion). In standing there is a corresponding 10° of hip joint extension along with posterior pelvic tilt and flattening of the low back.

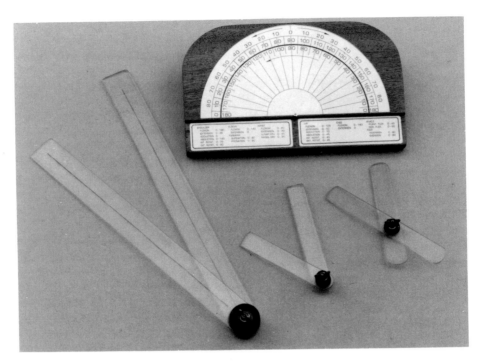

GONIOMETER

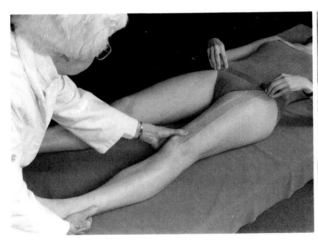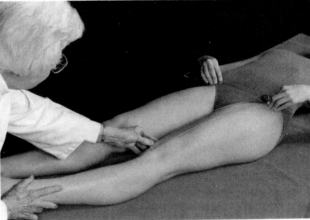

Equipment: Protractor and caliper. The caliper consists of two long arms held together with a set-screw (14).

Starting Position: Subject supine. Pelvis in neutral position. Left leg in neutral position. Right leg placed in enough abduction to allow adduction of left leg. Stationary arm pressed firmly against inferior surface of anterior superior iliac spines.

Movable arm set at 90° angle (as zero) and placed in line with midline of extremity. (Or, movable arm may be set at an angle that coincides with axis of femur (i.e., some adduction), in which case a reading is taken before moving the leg into adduction and the number of degrees is subtracted from the number at completion of adduction.)

Test: The movable arm of the caliper is held in line with the thigh as the left leg is passively moved, *slowly*, into adduction. The moment the pelvis starts to move downward on the side of the adducted leg, the movement of the leg in adduction is stopped and the set-screw is tightened. The caliper is transferred to the protractor for a reading.

Normal Range of Motion: Random testing has disclosed that adduction is often less than 10° and seldom goes beyond 10° in the supine position unless the hip joint is in flexion by virtue of anterior pelvic tilt. (With the hip joint flexed as in sitting, the range of adduction is approximately 20°.) With the thigh maintained in the coronal plane, as in the modified Ober test (see p. 57), the 10° of adduction should be considered normal.

The Psoas major, Iliacus, Pectineus, Adductors longus and brevis, Rectus femoris, Tensor fasciae latae, and Sartorius compose the hip flexor group of muscles. The Iliacus, Pectineus, and Adductors longus and brevis are one-joint muscles. The Psoas major and the Iliacus, as the Iliopsoas, acts essentially as a one-joint muscle. The Rectus femoris, Tensor fasciae latae, and Sartorius are two-joint muscles, crossing the knee joint as well as the hip joint. While all three muscles flex the hip, the Rectus femoris and, to some extent, the Tensor extend the knee, while the Sartorius flexes the knee.

The text for hip flexor length is often referred to as the Thomas Test. (See *Glossary* for definition of the original Thomas Test.)

Tests to distinguish between one-joint and two-joint hip flexor tightness were first described in Posture and Pain in 1952 (15).

Iliopsoas
Action: Hip flexion.
Length test: Hip extension with knee in extension.

Rectus femoris
Action: Hip flexion and knee extension.
Length test: Hip extension and knee flexion.

Tensor fasciae latae
Action: Hip abduction, flexion, and internal rotation, and knee extension.
Length test: See p. 57.

Sartorius
Action: Hip flexion, abduction and external rotation, and knee flexion.
Length test: Hip extension, adduction, and internal rotation, and knee extension. See also p. 36.

Equipment: Table, with no soft padding, and stable so it will not tilt with subject seated at one end.
Goniometer and ruler.
Chart for recording findings.

Starting Position: Subject seated at end of table, thighs half off table.* Examiner places one hand behind subject's back and other hand under one knee, flexing thigh toward chest, and giving assistance as subject lies down. The subject then holds thigh, pulling knee toward chest *only enough* to flatten low back and sacrum on table. (*Do not* bring both knees toward chest because that allows excessive posterior tilt which results in apparent (not actual) hip flexor shortness.)

Reasons: Thighs are half off table in sitting because the body position shifts as subject lies down and brings one knee toward chest. The end position for the start of testing is with the other knee just at edge of table so knee is free to flex, and so thigh can be full length on table.

*Note: If testing for excessive hip flexor length, the hip joint should be at edge of table with thigh off table. (See p. 35.)

Test Movement: If the right knee is flexed toward chest, left thigh is allowed to drop toward table with left knee flexed over end of table. With four muscles involved in the length test, variations occur that require interpretations as described on the following pages.

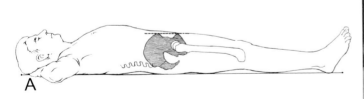

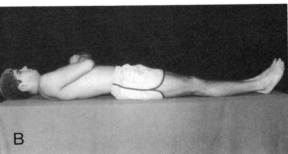

In A, the pelvis is shown in neutral position, the low back in normal anterior curve, and the hip joint in zero position. Normal hip joint extension is considered to be approximately 10°. Normal length of hip flexors permits this range of motion in extension. The length may be demonstrated by moving the thigh in a posterior direction with the pelvis in a neutral position, or moving the

pelvis in the direction of posterior tilt with the thigh in zero position. (See p. 20.)

In a subject with normal length of hip flexors, the low back will tend to flatten in the supine position. If the low back remains in a lordotic position, as in B, there is usually some hip flexor shortness.

Tests for Length of Hip Flexor Muscles

NORMAL LENGTH OF HIP FLEXORS

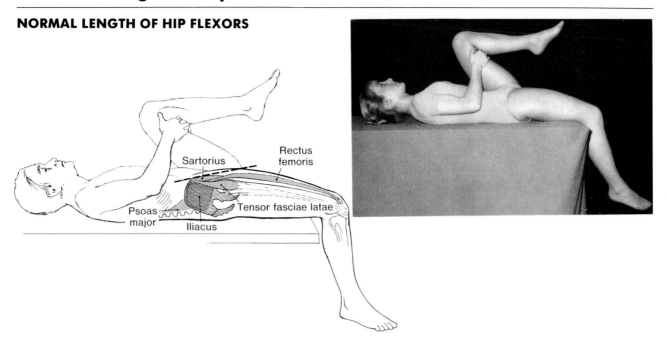

Sartorius

Rectus femoris

Psoas major

Iliacus

Tensor fasciae latae

With low back and sacrum flat on the table, posterior thigh touches the table, and knee flexes approximately 80°. In the figure above, the pelvis is shown in 10° posterior tilt. This is equivalent to 10° hip joint extension, and, with the thigh touching the table, represents normal length of the one-joint hip flexors. In addition, the knee flexion (about 80°) indicates that the Rectus femoris is normal in length and that the Tensor fasciae latae probably is normal. To maintain the pelvis in posterior tilt with the low back and sacrum flat on the table, one thigh is held toward the chest while testing the length of the opposite hip flexors.

SHORTNESS IN BOTH ONE-JOINT AND TWO-JOINT HIP FLEXORS

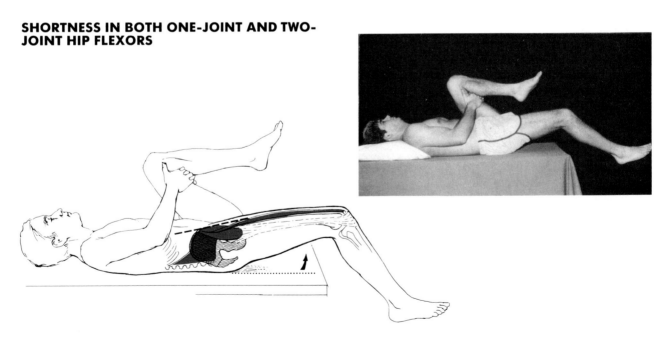

With low back and sacrum flat on the table, posterior thigh does not touch the table, and knee extends. The figures above show shortness of both one-joint and two-joint muscles. If the hip remains in 15° flexion with knee extended, the *one-joint* hip flexors lack 15° of length. If the knee will flex to only 70°, the *two joint* muscles lack 25° of length (15° at the hip plus 10° at the knee).

NORMAL LENGTH OF ONE-JOINT, SHORTNESS IN TWO-JOINT HIP FLEXORS

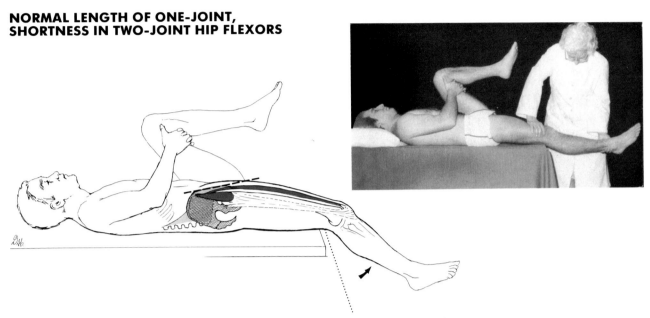

With low back and sacrum flat on the table, and knee in extension, the posterior thigh touches the table. Shortness in the two-joint muscles is determined by holding the thigh in contact with the table and allowing the knee to flex. The angle of knee flexion (i.e., number of degrees less than 80°) determines the degree of shortness. The photograph above shows a subject in whom the hip joint can be extended if the knee joint is allowed to extend. This means that the one-joint hip flexors are normal in length but the Rectus femoris and (probably) the Tensor fasciae latae are short.

EXCESSIVE HIP FLEXOR LENGTH

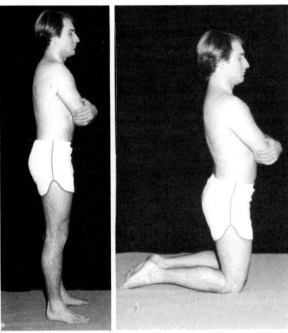

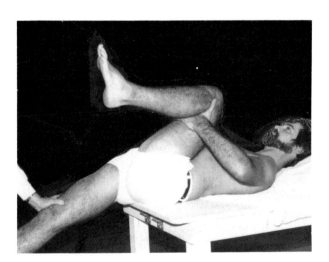

In standing, the subject does not have a lordosis. This fact would indicate that the shortness is *not* in the one-joint hip flexors.

A kneeling position puts a stretch on the short Rectus femoris and Tensor fasciae latae over both the hip joints and knee joints, causing these muscles to pull the pelvis into anterior tilt and the back into a lordotic position.

Subject is tested with low back flat, hip joint at end of table and knee straight. The fact that the thigh drops below table level is evidence of excessive length in the one-joint hip flexors.

Tests for Length of Hip Flexor Muscles

SHORTNESS IN ONE-JOINT, NO SHORTNESS IN TWO-JOINT

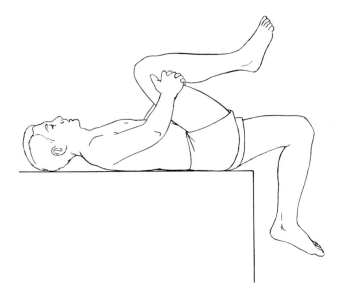

SHORTNESS IN SARTORIUS

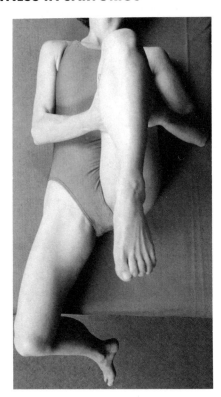

Posterior thigh does not touch the table, and knee can be flexed as many degrees beyond 80° as the hip is flexed. In above figure, thigh is flexed 15° and knee 95°.

SHORTNESS IN TENSOR FASCIAE LATAE

The following variations noted during hip flexor length testing indicate shortness in the Tensor fasciae latae, but do not constitute a length test for this muscle. The length test is done in a side-lying position. (See p. 57.)

> Abduction of thigh as hip joint extends. (Occasionally, the hip joint can be fully extended along with abduction. This finding indicates that there is shortness in the Tensor fasciae latae but not in the Iliopsoas.)
> Lateral deviation of patella. If the hip is not allowed to abduct during extension, there may be a strong lateral pull on the patella due to Tensor fasciae latae shortness. It may also occur even if the hip abducts.
> Extension of knee if thigh is prevented from abducting, or if thigh is passively adducted as hip is extended.
> Internal rotation of thigh.
> External rotation of leg on femur.

A combination of three or more of the following, during hip flexor length test, indicate tightness of the Sartorius: abduction, flexion, and external rotation of the hip; and flexion of the knee.

Shortness in Tensor Fasciae Latae and Sartorius: Similarities and Differences

Tensor fasciae latae	Joint	Sartorius
Abducts	Hip	Abducts
Flexes	Hip	Flexes
Internally rotates	Hip	Externally rotates
Extends	Knee	Flexes

Habitual Positions that Predispose to Bilateral Adaptive Shortening: Sitting in "W" or reverse tailor position favors Tensor fasciae latae shortness; tailor or yoga position favors Sartorius. The habit of sitting with one leg—and always the same one—in one of these positions is conducive to unilateral shortness. Changing postural habits is an important part of treatment.

CORRECT TEST

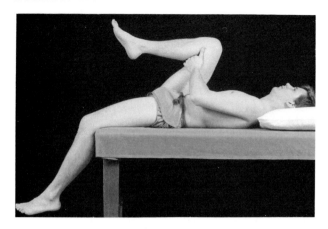

The low back and sacrum are flat on the table. There is normal length of the one-joint hip flexors because the thigh touches the table. The angle of knee flexion indicates that there is some tightness in the two-joint hip flexors. The photograph at the right shows an error in testing the same subject.

ERROR IN TESTING

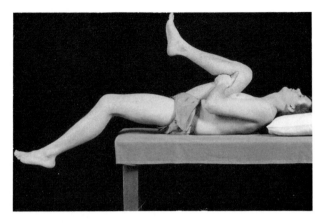

He has excessive back flexibility (see below right). When he pulls the knee too far toward the chest, the buttocks come up from the table and the sacrum is no longer flat on the table. The result is that the one-joint hip flexors, which are normal in length, appear to be tight.

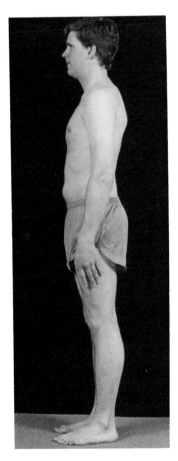

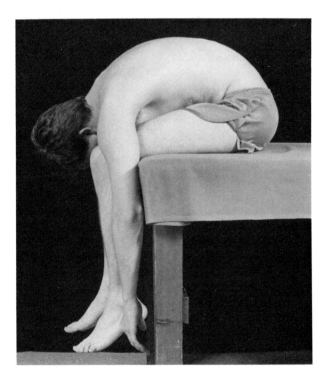

This subject has good postural alignment in standing. Examination of posture in standing does not give a clue to the extent of back flexibility present in this subject.

The excessive flexion in the low back permits the pelvis to go into too much posterior tilt and the low back into too much flexion during the hip flexor length test, as in figure top right above.

Tests For Length of Hamstring Muscles

Muscle length tests consist of movements that elongate the muscles in the direction(s) opposite the muscle actions. The Hamstrings consist of three two-joint muscles and one one-joint muscle.

TEST FOR LENGTH OF ONE-JOINT HAMSTRING

Biceps, short head (and Popliteus)
Action: Knee flexion.
Length test: Knee extension with hip in extension.

Place subject prone with hip in extension to make the two-joint Hamstrings (Semimembranosis, Semitendinosus, and long head of the Biceps) slack over the hip joint to permit them to lengthen over the knee joint. Allow the foot to be relaxed in plantar flexion. If the knee can be fully extended in this position, there is no tightness in the one-joint knee flexors.

TEST FOR LENGTH OF TWO-JOINT HAMSTRINGS

Two tests are recommended for use in Hamstring length testing: the straight-leg-raising test supine, and the forward-bending test in long-sitting.

Semimembranosis, Semitendinosus, and Biceps, long head
Action: Knee flexion and hip extension.
Length test: Hip flexion and knee extension.

STRAIGHT-LEG-RAISING TEST

There are *three variables in the straight-leg-raising test:* the low back, hip joint, and knee joint. The knee joint is controlled by maintaining it in extension. The positions of the low back and pelvis are controlled by keeping the low back and sacrum flat on the table.

Equipment: Table or floor. Folded blanket may be used, but no soft padding.
Reason: Unable to confirm that low back and sacrum are flat on a flat surface if on a soft pad.
Goniometer to measure angle between straight leg and table.
Pillow or towel roll in case of hip flexor shortness.
Chart to record findings.

Starting Position: Supine, legs extended and low back and sacrum flat on table.

Reason: Standardization of the test requires that the knee be in extension, and that there be a fixed position of the low back and pelvis in order to control the variables created by excessive anterior or posterior pelvic tilt.

If low back does not go flat on table due to hip flexor shortness, use pillow or roll under knees to flex hips *just enough* to allow the low back to flatten.

When low back and sacrum are flat, *hold* one thigh firmly down, making use of passive restraint by the hip flexors to prevent excessive posterior pelvic tilt before starting to raise the other leg in the straight-leg-raising test.

Test Movement: With low back and sacrum flat on table and one leg held firmly down, raise the other leg with knee straight, foot relaxed.

Reasons: The knee is kept straight to control this variable. The foot is kept relaxed to avoid Gastrocnemius involvement at the knee. (If the Gastrocnemius is tight, dorsiflexion of the foot will cause the knee to flex, thereby interfering with the test of the Hamstrings.) If the knee starts to bend, lower the leg slightly, and have the subject fully extend the knee and again raise the leg until some restraint is felt and the subject feels slight discomfort. The subject may assist in raising the leg.

NORMAL HAMSTRING LENGTH

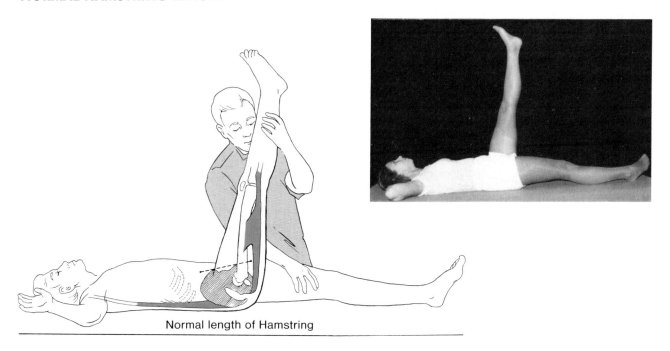

Normal length of Hamstring

No Hip Flexor Shortness Requiring Modification of the Test: Straight-leg raising with subject supine, low back and sacrum flat on table, and the other leg extended and held down.

An angle of approximately 80° between the table and the raised leg is considered normal range of Hamstring length.

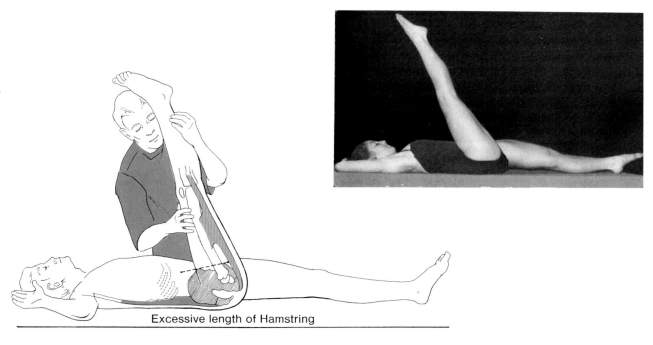

Excessive length of Hamstring

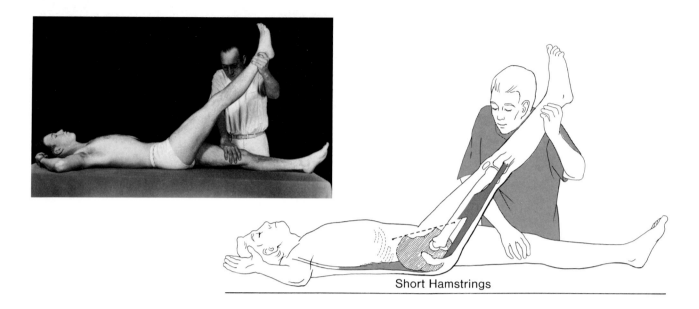

Short Hamstrings

When hip joint flexion has reached the limit of Hamstring length in the straight-leg raise, the Hamstrings exert a downward pull on the ischium in the direction of posteriorly tilting the pelvis. To prevent excessive posterior pelvic tilt and excessive flexion of the back, it is necessary to stabilize the pelvis with the low back in the flat position by holding the opposite leg firmly down. (If there is shortness of hip flexors and a roll or pillow must be put under the knees in order to get the back flat, then the one leg must be held firmly down on the pillow to prevent excessive posterior tilt.)

Excessive posterior tilt of the pelvis allows the leg to be raised slightly higher here than in figures above although the Hamstring length is the same in both instances. With the opposite leg held firmly down, excessive posterior tilt will not occur except in subjects who have excessive length in the hip flexors.

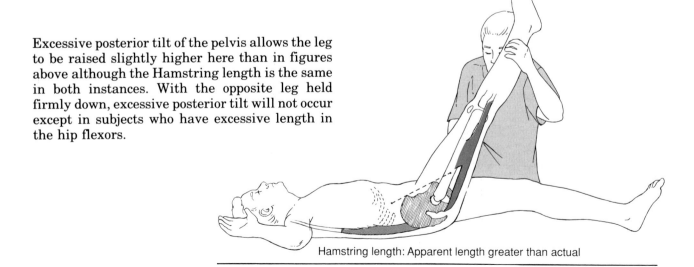

Hamstring length: Apparent length greater than actual

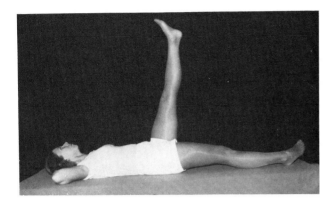

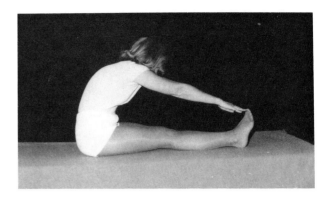

The straight-leg-raising test, with low back flat on the table, shows normal length of Hamstring muscles, which permits flexion of the *thigh toward the pelvis* (hip joint flexion) to an angle of about 80° up from the table.

In forward bending, normal Hamstring length permits flexion of the *pelvis toward the thigh* (hip joint flexion) as illustrated.

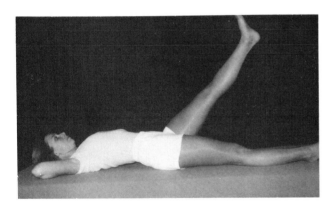

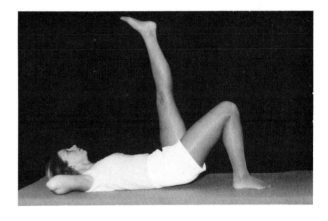

When the low back is hyperextended (arched up from the table), the normal Hamstrings appear to be short.

When the hip and knee are flexed on one side as the opposite straight leg is raised, the back flexes too much, the sacrum is not flat on the table, and the Hamstrings appear to be longer than normal. (This position should not be used for testing or stretching Hamstrings.)

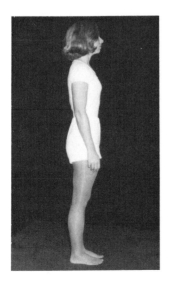

The subject shows good postural alignment in standing, and strength and length tests showed good muscle balance.

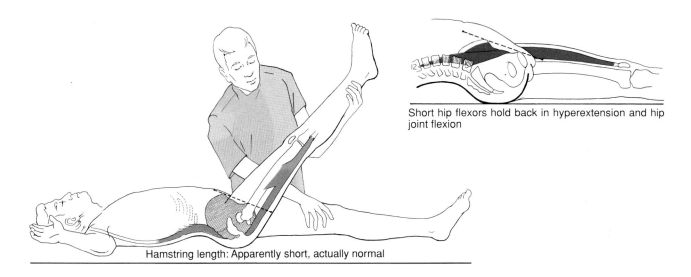

Short hip flexors hold back in hyperextension and hip joint flexion

Hamstring length: Apparently short, actually normal

Hamstring Length Test Modified When There Is Hip Flexor Shortness: In supine position with legs extended, low back hyperextended, and pelvis in anterior tilt, the *hip joint is already in flexion*. If the straight-leg raising test is performed with the low back and pelvis in this position, normal Hamstrings will appear to be short.

Note: With few exceptions, the position of anterior tilt is the result of shortness in the one-joint hip flexors, and the amount of flexion varies with the amount of hip flexor shortness.

If it were possible to determine how many degrees of hip flexion exist by virtue of the pelvic tilt, this number could be added to the number of degrees of straight-leg raise in determining Hamstring length. But it is not possible to measure that amount of flexion. Hence, the position of the low back and pelvis must be standardized. To get the low back and sacrum flat, hips must be flexed, but *only the amount necessary to obtain the desired position*. (See facing page.)

The Hamstring length is the same as in bottom figure on p. 39.

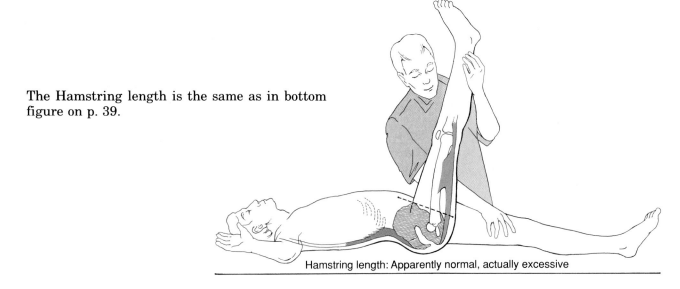

Hamstring length: Apparently normal, actually excessive

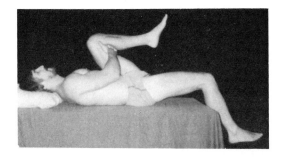

A test for length of hip flexors confirms that there is shortness of these muscles.

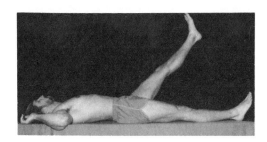

The Hamstrings appear to be short, but the test is not accurate because the low back is not flat on the table. Shortness of the hip flexors on the side of the extended leg holds the back in hyperextension.

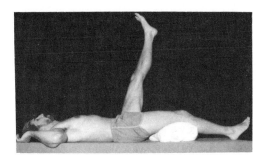

To accommodate for the hip flexor shortness and allow the low back to flatten, the thigh is *passively* flexed by a pillow under the knee, *not actively* held in flexion by the subject. With the back flat, the test accurately shows Hamstrings to be almost normal in length.

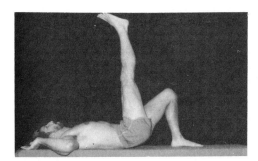

In testing for Hamstring length and in exercising to stretch short Hamstrings, *avoid* placing one hip and knee in flexed position (as illustrated) while raising the other. Flexibility of the low back is added to the range of hip flexion making Hamstrings appear longer than they are. Not infrequently, there is excessive back flexibility along with Hamstring shortness.

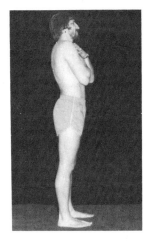

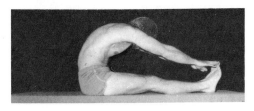

Flexion of the *pelvis toward the thigh* (hip flexion) appears to be almost normal in forward bending. Since both hips are in flexion in forward bending, hip flexor shortness does not interfere with the movement of the pelvis toward the thigh as occurs when one leg is extended in the supine position.

The lordosis in standing is evidence of the hip flexor shortness in this subject.

43

Errors in Testing Hamstring Length

ERROR IN TESTING

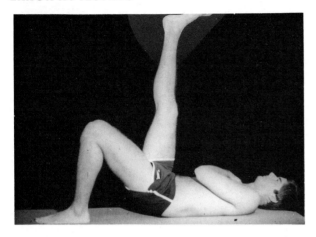

When the straight-leg-raising test is done starting with one knee and hip flexed and the foot resting on the table as the other leg is raised, the pelvis is free to move in the direction of excessive posterior tilt with the sacrum no longer flat on the table. Depending upon the

CORRECT TEST

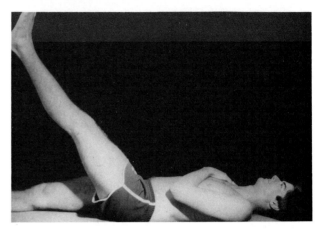

amount of flexibility of the back, the Hamstring length will appear longer than actual because back flexion is added to hip flexion. An individual with as little as 45° of actual Hamstring length can appear to have as much as 90° of length as seen in the photographs above.

NO STANDARDIZATION OF THE LOW BACK AND PELVIS

If the hip and knee are flexed to allow approximately 40° of hip flexion, the position will ensure enough slack in the hip flexors so that they will not cause anterior pelvic tilt. It will not, however, insure against excessive posterior tilting. *Standardization* of the amount of hip and knee flexion will not standardize the position of the low back and pelvis, which must be standardized. Hip flexor shortness is the chief cause of anterior pelvic tilt in the supine position and the degree of shortness varies from one individual to another. In order to stabilize the pelvis with the low back and sacrum flat on the table, one must "give in" to the tight hip flexors by using a pillow or towel roll under the knees, but *only as much as is necessary* to obtain the required position of the pelvis.

THREE VARIABLES, NONE CONTROLLED

Sometimes an effort is made to determine Hamstring length by ascertaining the number of degrees lacking in knee joint extension. The starting position is as follows: One leg is placed in approximately 40° of hip flexion with the knee flexed and the foot resting on the table (giving rise to problems cited above). The thigh of the opposite leg is raised to a position perpendicular to the table (which may or may not be 90° of true hip joint flexion). The knee is then moved in the direction of extension. The length of Hamstrings is stated in the number of degrees the knee joint *lacks* in extension.

MISLEADING TEST

Perhaps the most misleading "test" for Hamstring length is the following: With a subject supine on the table with both legs extended, the examiner slowly raises one leg with the knee straight. The start of posterior pelvic tilt is supposed to indicate the degree of tightness of the Hamstrings. It is relatively easy for both the examiner and the subject to recognize the moment that the pelvis starts tilting posteriorly, and it usually occurs when the leg is raised to about 35° of hip flexion.

It is not uncommon to find that individuals tested in this manner show normal or even excessive range of muscle length. It is extremely rare in the general population to find 35° or 40° of straight-leg raise and the error in this test can best be ascertained by doing an accurate, straight-leg-raising test or a forward-bending test.

Hamstring length is measured by the range of hip joint flexion with the knee in extension. In the straight-leg-raising test, the hip is flexed by moving the thigh toward the pelvis; in the forward-bending test, the hip is flexed by moving the pelvis toward the thigh. In straight-leg raising, the angle between the thigh and the table is measured; in forward bending, the angle between the sacrum and the table is measured. In both cases, it is a measure of the amount of hip joint flexion permitted by Hamstring length.

There are only two variables in the forward-bending test, the knee joint and the hip joint. Movement at the knee is controlled by keeping the knee in extension during the movement of hip flexion.

When no significant difference exists between the length of the right and left Hamstrings, forward bending is an accurate and practical test. When there is a difference, it is necessary to use the straight-leg-raising test.

Equipment: Table (not padded) or floor.
Board 3 inches wide, 12 inches long, and about 1/4 inch thick to place flat against sacrum.
Goniometer to measure angle between sacrum and table.
Chart for recording findings.

Starting Position: Sitting with hips flexed, knees fully extended (long-sitting). Allow feet to be relaxed; avoid dorsiflexion.

Reasons: Keeping knee straight maintains a fixed elongation of the Hamstrings over the knee joint, eliminating movement at the knee as a variable. Avoiding dorsiflexion of the foot prevents the knee flexion that may occur if the Gastrocnemius is tight.

Test Movement: Have subject reach forward as far as possible in the direction of trying to touch fingertips to toes or beyond.

Reasons: Subject will tilt the pelvis forward toward the thighs, flexing the hip joints to the limit allowed by the Hamstring length.

Measuring Arc of Motion: Place board with the 3 inch side on table and the 12 inch side pressed against sacrum when Hamstring length appears normal or excessive. Place the 12 inch side on table and the 3 inch side pressed against sacrum when Hamstrings are tight. Measure the angle between the upright board and the table.

Normal Range of Motion: The pelvis flexes toward the thigh to the point that the angle between the sacrum and the table is approximately 80° (i.e., the same angle as between the leg and the table in the straight-leg-raising test).

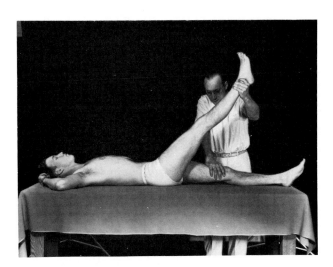

Short Hamstrings limit flexion of the *thigh toward the pelvis* (hip joint flexion).

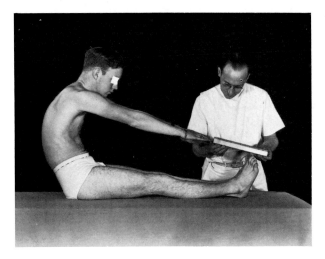

In forward bending, short Hamstrings limit flexion of the *pelvis toward the thigh* (hip joint flexion). Note that the angle of the sacrum with the table is the same as the angle of the posterior thigh with the table in figure at left.

Forward-Bending Test for Length of Posterior Muscles

BACK FLEXIBILITY AND HAMSTRING LENGTH LONG-SITTING, FORWARD BENDING

Equipment: Same as for Hamstring length test plus a ruler. The ruler is used to measure the distance of the fingertips from or beyond the base of the big toe. This measurement is used only as a record to show overall change in forward bending, but in no way indicates where limitation or excessive motion has taken place.

Starting Position: Sitting with legs extended (long-sitting), feet at right angle.

Reason: To standardize the position of the feet and knees.

Test Movement: Have subject reach forward, with knees straight, trying to touch fingertips to base of big toe, or beyond, reaching as far as range of muscle length permits.

Reason: Both back and Hamstrings will elongate to their maximum.

Normal Range of Motion in Forward Bending: Normal *length of Hamstrings* permits pelvis to flex toward thigh to the extent that the angle between the sacrum and the table is approximately 80°. Normal *flexion of lumbar spine* permits the spine to flatten. Normal *flexion of thoracic spine* permits an increase in the posterior convexity, seen as a smooth, continuous curve in this area. The average adult will be able to touch finger tips to toes in forward bending with knees straight if the flexibility of the back and the length of the Hamstrings are both normal. (See figure in left column.)

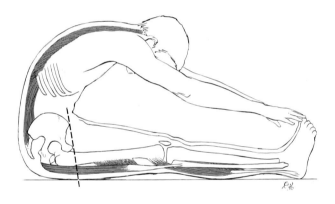

Normal length of back, Hamstring, and Gastroc-soleus muscles.

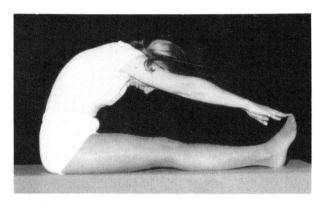

The ability to touch fingertips to toes is a desirable accomplishment for most adults. This subject shows Hamstring length and back flexibility within normal limits.

VARIATIONS IN FORWARD BENDING:

Hamstrings and back, both normal.
Hamstrings and back, both excessively flexible.
Hamstrings and back, both tight.
Hamstrings excessive in length, back tight.
Hamstrings tight, low back excessively flexible.
Hamstrings tight, upper back excessively flexible.
Hamstrings and back normal flexibility, but legs long in relation to trunk. (Seen among adolescents and some adults.)

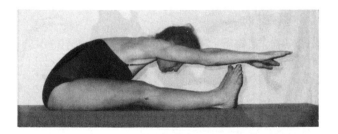

In forward bending, excessive Hamstring length permits excessive flexion of the *pelvis toward the thigh* (hip joint flexion.) This subject has also excessive flexion in the mid-back (thoracolumbar) area.

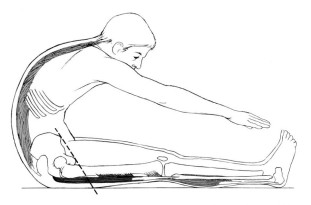

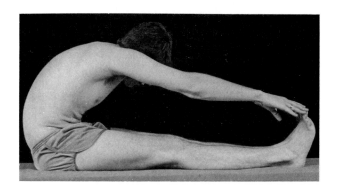

Excessive length of back muscles, short Hamstrings, normal length of Gastroc-soleus.

The excessive flexibility of the back overcompensates for the shortness of the Hamstring muscles.

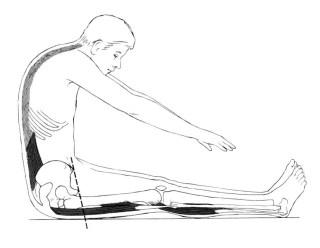

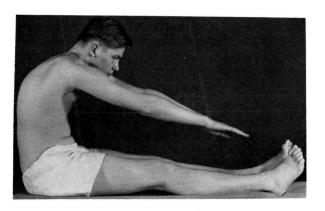

Excessive length of upper back muscles, slight shortness of muscles in mid and lower back, and in Gastroc-soleus. Hamstrings normal in length.

The subject is unable to touch his toes because of slight shortness in the Hamstrings and Gastrocsoleus, and slight limitation of flexibility in the mid-back area. The upper back shows some excessive flexion.

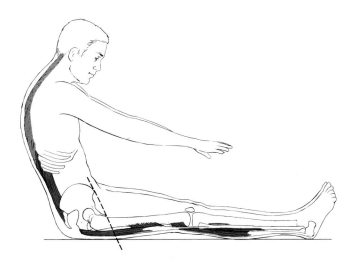

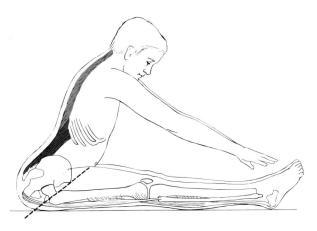

Normal length of upper back muscles, short low back, Hamstring, and Gastroc-soleus muscles.

Normal length of upper back muscles, contracture of low back muscles with paralysis of extremity muscles.

Normal Flexibility According to Age Level

The ability to touch the toes with the finger tips may be considered normal for young children and adults. However, between the ages of 11 and 14 years many individuals who show no signs of muscle or joint tightness are unable to complete this movement. The reason seems to be that the proportionate length of the trunk and lower extremities is different in individuals of this age group from that of younger and older age groups.

The five drawings are representative of the majority of individuals in each of the following age groups: A, 1 to 3 years; B, 4 to 7 years; C, 8 to 10 years; D, 11 to 14 years, and E, 15 years and over.

The change from the apparently extreme flexibility of the youngest child to the apparently limited flexibility of the child in D occurs gradually over a period of years as the legs become proportionately longer in relation to the trunk. Standards of performance for children that involve forward bending should take into consideration the normal variations in the ability to complete the range of this movement.

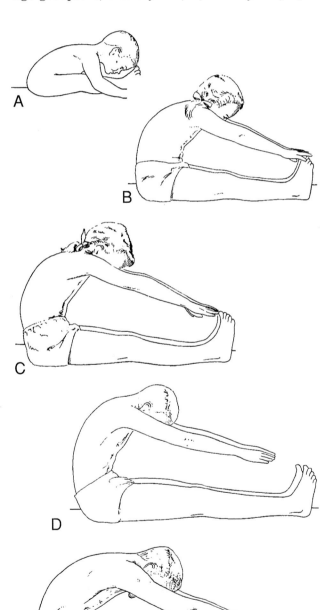

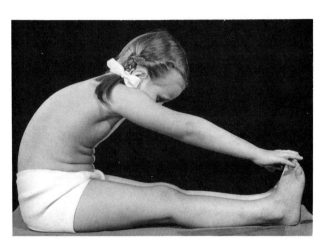

This 6-year-old girl touches her toes easily. There is good contour of the back and normal Hamstring length.

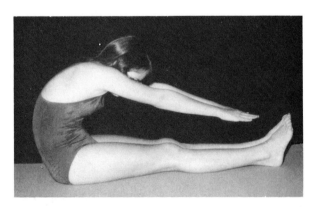

This subject is a 12-year-old girl. The inability to touch the toes is typical of this age. (See also pp. 8, 111, and 112.) Sometimes the leg length is the determining factor; sometimes, as in this case, there is slight shortness of the Hamstrings at this age.

The normal spine exhibits four natural curves, named according to the direction of their convexity. The first three are movable, the sacral is a fixed curve.

Slightly anterior in cervical region.
Slightly posterior in thoracic region.
Slightly anterior in lumbar region.
Slightly posterior in sacral region.

FLEXION OF THORACIC SPINE

In the thoracic region, *flexion* is movement in the direction of increasing the normal posterior curve, resulting in a roundness of the upper back. A position of *excessive flexion* is a kyphosis.

FLEXION OF CERVICAL AND LUMBAR SPINES

In the cervical and lumbar regions, *flexion* is movement in the direction of decreasing the normal anterior curve, resulting in a straight position of the neck and low back. The ability to flatten the neck or low back may be considered *normal flexion.*

In the neck, flexion is obtained by tilting the head forward, and by bending the head forward. (The latter movement also involves some upper back flexion see p. 66.) In the low back, flexion is obtained by trunk forward bending or by posterior pelvic tilt.

Excessive flexion in the neck is seen as a slight posterior convexity. (See Figure B, p. 91.) *Excessive flexion in the low back* may be referred as hyperflexion, or hypermobility in the direction of flexion, or as a position of lumbar kyphosis in sitting. A lumbar kyphosis in standing is not a common finding. An individual with excessive back flexion compensates in standing with the low back in slight anterior curve (see p. 37), or, in some instances, in a sway-back posture (see p. 85).

EXTENSION OF THORACIC SPINE

Normal extension of the thoracic spine means the ability to straighten the upper back. (If a kyphosis becomes fixed, the thoracic spine cannot be extended.) *Excessive extension* is seen as a slight anterior curve in the upper back and is usually a fixed position. It is not a common finding.

EXTENSION OF CERVICAL SPINE

Extension of the cervical spine is an increase in the normal anterior curve and results from tilting the head back, approximating the occiput and the seventh cervical vertebra. It may result, also, from sitting or standing in a typical round-shoulder, forward-head position. (See pp. 66 and 91.)

EXTENSION OF LUMBAR SPINE

Extension of the lumbar spine is an increase in the normal anterior curve. The range of extension is highly variable, as seen in the accompanying photographs, making it difficult to establish a standard for the purpose of measurements. Furthermore, these variations may exist without complaints of pain or disability, making it difficult to determine to what extent limited or excessive motion constitutes a disability. Too often, assessment of back extension is inaccurate or arbitrary.

Excessive extension in the standing position is obtained by anterior pelvic tilt and is a position of lordosis. The range of back extension as seen in testing does not translate, automatically, into the same degree of lordosis in standing. Other factors such as hip flexor length and abdominal muscle strength affect the position.

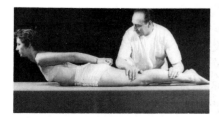

Back extension range of motion, less than average but muscle strength normal.

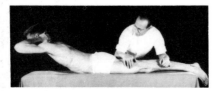

Back extension range of motion, about average. Anterior-superior-iliac spines are in contact with the table.

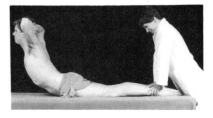

Excessive range of motion in back extension. Subject is a diver and also has excessive flexion. (See p. 37.)

Range of Motion in Trunk Flexion and Extension

Forward bending and backward bending are the movements used to assess the range of motion in flexion and extension of the spine. Several variations of these tests exist.

RANGE OF MOTION IN TRUNK FLEXION

The forward-bending, *long-sitting* position involves hip joint flexion along with back flexion. One must try to disregard the hip joint movement when observing the contour of the back. (See *Normal range of motion*, p. 46.)

Range of motion and contour of the back may be observed, also, by having a subject bend forward from the *standing* position. There are certain disadvantages, however, in using this as a test position. If the pelvis is not level, or if it is rotated, the plane of forward bending will be altered and the test will not be as satisfactory as the test in long-sitting position in which the pelvis is level and in which rotation is better controlled.

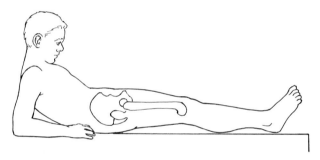

To assess the flexion of the back without associated hip-joint flexion, place a subject *supine*, resting on forearms with elbows at right angle and arms close to the body. If the subject can flex the spine in this position *with the pelvis flat on the table* (i.e., no hip flexion), the range of motion may be considered good.

Sometimes it is necessary to ascertain the range of back flexion passively. With the subject *supine*, the examiner lifts the upper trunk in flexion to completion of the subject's range of motion. The subject must relax in order for the examiner to obtain complete flexion.

Scapular instability and, specifically, Serratus anterior weakness can interfere with the back extension test, as seen in the accompanying photograph.

Note: Push-ups *should not* be done by individuals who exhibit this type of weakness.

RANGE OF MOTION IN TRUNK EXTENSION

Because low back muscles are seldom weak, the range of back extension may be determined by the active strength test in the *prone* position. (See p. 140.) Whether the range of motion is normal, limited, or excessive, the subject is capable of moving through the existing range. The anterior-superior-iliac spines should not be lifted from the table during back extension because doing so adds hip extension to back extension range of motion.

Back extension often is checked in the *standing position*. The test is useful as a gross evaluation, but it is not very specific. Swaying forward at the hips is almost a necessity for balance when bending backward, but it adds the element of hip extension to the test; or the knees must bend somewhat if the hip does not extend.

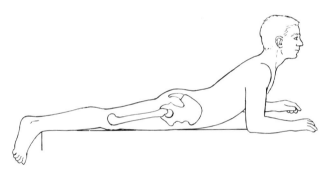

Similar to the test to determine range of motion in spine flexion, a test can be done to determine the range in spine extension. The subject lies *prone* on a table, resting on forearms, elbows bent at right angles, arms close to the body. If the subject can extend the spine enough to prop up on the forearms with pelvis flat on table (i.e., anterior-superior-iliac spines on table), the range of motion in extension may be considered good.

Sometimes it is necessary to determine the amount of passive back extension with the subject *prone* on the table and lifting the subject up in extension through the available range of motion.

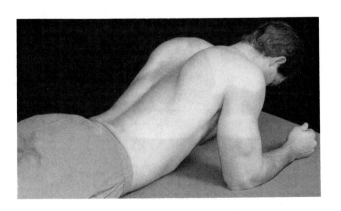

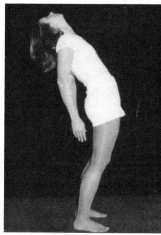

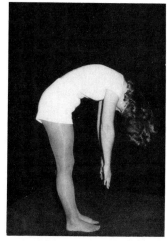

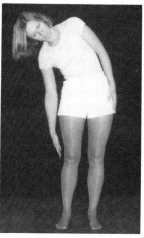

Backward bending in the standing position requires that the pelvis and thighs be displaced forward for balance. Spine extension must be distinguished from backward bending. How far the spine will bend backward depends upon the available range of motion in the spine and upon the length of the abdominal muscles. How far the body will bend backwards depends upon the length of hip flexors in addition to the above.

This subject is not trying to touch finger-tips to the floor (which would require more hip joint flexion), but has fully flexed the spine. There is normal flexion as denoted by the fact that the lumbar spine is straight, and there is a smooth, continuous curve in the thoracic region. (See pp. 47 and 54 for excessive flexion, and p. 47 and 55 bottom right for limited lumbar flexion.)

Lateral flexion of the spine depends upon the available range of motion in the spine and upon the length of the opposite lateral trunk flexors. The amount the body can bend sideways depends upon the length of the opposite hip abductors in addition to the above. To use side bending for measuring lateral flexion requires that the pelvis be level and that the feet be a standardized distance apart.

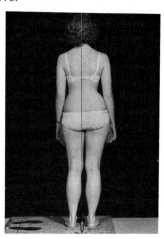

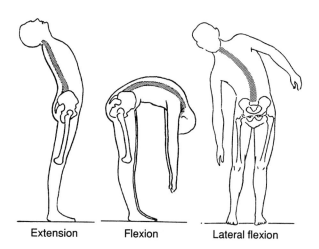

Extension   Flexion   Lateral flexion

The above figure shows a high hip on the right. If this subject were to do side bending and a measurement taken of the distance of finger-tips to floor, the measurement would be less on the right than on the left. If these measurements were then read as lateral flexion of the spine, it would be recorded, incorrectly, as lateral flexion more limited toward right than toward left. By virtue of the high hip on the right, the spine is already in lateral flexion so the shoulder and arm will not move downward as far as would occur if the pelvis were level.

Accurate measurements of spine extension, flexion, and lateral flexion should not include movements in the hip joints which do occur in the bending movements illustrated above. In an effort to localize the measurements to the spine itself, Schober, in 1937, used one marking at the lumbosacral junction and another 10 cm above that point. Measurements between the points were taken in the erect standing position and in full forward bending. The increase in distance between the points indicated the amount of lumbar flexion (16). Macrae and Wright modified the test by placing a third mark 5 cm below the lumbosacral junction and measuring from there to the upper mark (17). (The modified Schober test lacks reliability (18).)

Various devices have been developed with the hope that *meaningful* objective measurements can be obtained. Goniometers, inclinometers, flexible rulers, tape measures, and radiographs are some of the devices used in an effort to establish a suitable method of measuring. Without first defining normal flexion of the lumbar spine, however, measurements may not be meaningful.

Tests for Length of Ankle Plantar Flexors

ONE-JOINT PLANTAR FLEXOR

Soleus

Action: Ankle plantar flexion
Length test: Ankle dorsiflexion with knee in flexion.

Starting Position: Prone, supine with hip and knee flexed, or sitting.

Test Movement: With knee flexed about 90°, to make the two-joint Gastrocnemius and Plantaris slack over the knee joint, dorsiflex the foot.

Normal Range: The foot can be dorsiflexed approximately 20°.

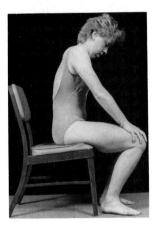

Soleus Stretch: Sitting forward in chair with knees bent and feet pulled back toward chair enough to raise heels slightly from floor. Press down on thigh to help force heel to floor.

TWO-JOINT PLANTAR FLEXORS

Gastrocnemius and Plantaris

Action: Ankle plantar flexion and knee flexion.
Length test: Ankle dorsiflexion and knee extension.

Starting Position: Subject may be supine, or may sit with knees extended unless Hamstring tightness causes the knee to flex.

Test Movement: With knee in extension to elongate the gastrocnemius and plantaris over the knee joint, dorsiflex the foot.

Normal Range: With knee fully extended, the foot can be dorsiflexed approximately 10°.

Notes: The 20° of dorsiflexion listed as normal (under Soleus above and in the chart on p. 25) is with the knee *flexed*, and should not apply to this test, nor to the standing Gastrocnemius stretch.

When stretching to restore joint range of motion, two-joint muscles must be slack over one joint in order to obtain the best possible range of motion over the other joint.

Tightness in the Soleus muscles may be found among women who habitually wear high-heeled shoes. Some patients who have had surgery on a lower extremity develop tightness in muscles that

TREATMENT OF MUSCLE LENGTH PROBLEMS

If muscle length is excessive, *avoid* exercises that stretch, and avoid postural positions that maintain elongation of the already stretched muscles. Work to correct faulty posture. Because the stretched muscles are usually weak, strengthening exercises are indicated. However, for most active individuals, strength will improve simply by avoiding over-stretching.

Supports are indicated to prevent excessive range if the problem cannot be controlled through positioning and corrective exercise. For example, marked knee hyperextension, which is unavoidable in weight bearing, should be prevented by an appropriate support to allow the posterior knee joint ligaments and muscles to shorten.

A low back that is excessively flexible will be stretched further if sitting in a "slumped" position, but usually will not be stretched in the standing position (see figures p. 37). Proper positioning and support by chairs *may* be adequate to prevent further stretching. However, the lack of proper support from many chairs and car seats calls for the wearing of a back support when excessive flexion cannot be avoided and, particularly, if a painful condition has developed.

When muscle shortness exists and stretching exercises are indicated, they must be done with precision to insure that the tight muscles are the ones actually being stretched and to avoid adverse effects on other parts of the body.

flex the knee and plantar flex the ankle. When a patient is required to keep the hip, knee, and ankle flexed to ensure that no weight will be borne by the extremity, adaptive shortening can develop in both the one-joint and the two-joint muscles. To restore range of motion, both groups must be treated.

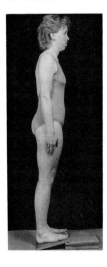

Gastrocnemius Stretch: Stand erect on board inclined at 10° angle with feet at approximately 8° to 10° out-toeing.

Begin with supine position, low back held flat by keeping one knee toward chest with other leg extended. Subject should contract gluteals to actively extend the hip joint, bringing thigh down toward table or floor *without* arching the back. **Note:** In a setting where no table is available, this is the only hip flexor stretching exercise that can be done in supine position. The stretching will affect the one-joint hip flexors only.

To stretch both one-joint and two-joint hip flexors, the test position may be used. If there is much tightness, care should be taken to progress *gradually* with stretching. A little bit of stretching can cause soreness that may be felt more the next day. Also, it is *important* to remember that the Psoas muscle is attached to the bodies, transverse processes, and intervertebral discs of the lumbar spine, and too vigorous stretching can create or aggravate a problem with the low back.

The prone position on a table or floor is an unsatisfactory position for stretching hip flexors because the low back, already in anterior curve, cannot be held flat or controlled in any fixed position. If a table is available, the subject may lie with trunk prone at the end of the table with legs hanging down, knees bent as necessary, and feet on the floor. Have subject raise one leg in hip extension, high enough to put a stretch on the hip flexors, with knee straight for a one-joint stretch; knee bent about 80° for one- and two-joint stretch.

When two-joint hip flexors are short, avoid the kneeling lunge. (The kneeling lunge may be used to stretch the one-joint muscles, provided the two-joint hip flexors are not tight.) Be cautious in the use of the kneeling lunge because of potential strain on the sacroiliac joint as well as on the low back.

AVOID

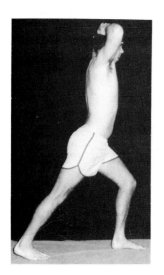

When one-joint hip flexors are short, *avoid* the lunge. Since the low back is not stabilized, tight hip flexors pull it into a lordosis. In supine position the low back is held flat and tightness appears at the hip joint.

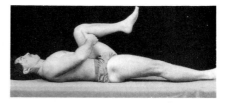

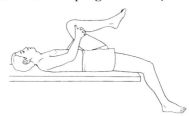

Exercise to stretch the one-joint hip flexors. Contract the Gluteus maximus to pull the thigh toward the table (or floor), maintaining the knee in extension and *keeping the back flat.*

To stretch one-joint and two-joint hip flexors on right, lie on back with right lower leg hanging over end of table. Pull left knee toward chest just enough to flatten low back and sacrum on table. With hip flexor tightness, thigh will be up from table. *Keeping back flat and knee bent*, press right thigh down toward table by pulling with buttock muscle. If stretching one-joint hip flexors only, passive extension of knee is permitted. To stretch left hip flexors, reverse the procedure. (To stretch two-joint hip flexors, see pp. 118 and 352.)

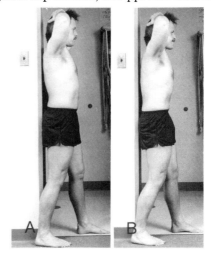

An effective stretch of one-joint hip flexors can be done standing by a door frame. Place one leg forward to help brace the body against the door frame, and place the other back to extend the hip joint. In starting position (A), the low back will be arched due to hip flexor tightness. Keep the hip extended and pull up and in with lower abdominal muscles to tilt the pelvis posteriorly and stretch hip flexors (B). This exercise requires a *strong* pull by the abdominals and is useful in building the strength of these muscles which are direct opponents of hip flexors in standing.

Hamstring Stretching

Straight-Leg Raising: As illustrated by figure at right, Hamstring stretching may be performed as a passive exercise or as an active-assisted exercise.

Or: It may be performed as an active exercise if not contraindicated because of tightness of hip flexors.

Or: The exercise may be performed by placing the leg in a position that places a stretch on Hamstrings: Supine on floor with one leg extended, other leg raised and heel resting on back of a chair, or lying in an open doorway area with one leg extended and the other raised, heel resting against wall. To increase the stretch, move body closer to chair or wall. *Avoid* placing both legs in the raised position at the same time because low back will be stretched instead of Hamstrings. Keeping one leg extended prevents excessive posterior tilt of the pelvis and excessive lower back flexion.

Knee Extension in Sitting Position: Sit with back against a wall as illustrated by figure at right: With back kept straight and buttocks touching the wall, raise one leg, extending the knee as much as possible.

Hip Flexion Sitting at Desk: With heel resting on the floor (if Hamstrings are very tight, or on low stool if moderately tight), straighten one knee. While keeping the *knee straight*, bend forward at the hips with the *back straight*. This exercise may be done with both knees straight providing the back is kept straight and the bending is all at the hip joints.

Forward Bending in Long-Sitting Position: Forward bending to stretch Hamstrings may be used for mild tightness provided the back is not excessively flexible, but should be *avoided* when there is excessive flexion of the back as seen in the figure below.

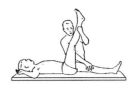

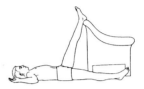

To stretch the right Hamstrings, lie on the table with legs extended and have an assistant hold the left leg down and gradually raise the right with the knee straight. (To stretch the left Hamstrings, apply the same procedure to the left leg.)

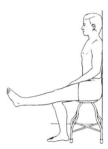

Lie on floor behind a sturdy chair.

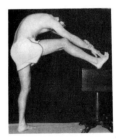

Sit on a stool with the back against a wall.

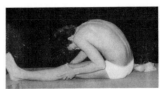

Avoid the standing position, with one heel on a stool or table and forward bending. For patients with pain or disability, it is a risky position. It is also impossible to control the pelvic position to insure proper Hamstring stretching. Furthermore, the exercise has an adverse effect on anyone who has a kyphosis of the upper back. Exercise should be localized to stretching the Hamstrings.

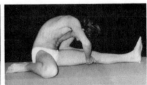

Avoid the "hurdler's position" for stretching Hamstrings. Excess strain is placed on the bent knee, and the low back is excessively stretched.

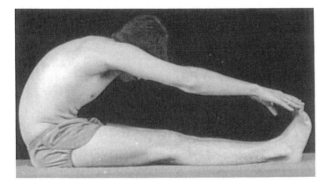

Normal flexion of the lumbar spine is movement in the direction of straightening the low back and is achieved if the low back flattens. A low back that straightens out to a flat back position does not need stretching. A curve which is convex posteriorly denotes excessive flexion. A low back that has excessive flexion should not be stretched.

The upper back seldom needs stretching in flexion since problems of the upper back usually involve excessive flexion (kyphosis). Most often the need is for exercises to stretch the shortened anterior chest and upper abdominal musculature to allow the upper back to extend.

Back stretching, if indicated, should be localized to the lower back. When possible, the stretching should be preceded by gentle heat to relax the tight musculature. Whether positional (such as prone over pillow), assisted, or active (pelvic tilt), exercises should be done slowly, and the stretched position held several seconds.

The standing or long-sitting forward-bending position should be *avoided* in two common combinations of muscle length imbalance: 1) persons with stretched Hamstrings and tight low back muscles and 2) persons with marked Hamstring shortness and excessive low back flexion. True to the law of least resistance, the muscles that are already stretched will just stretch further.

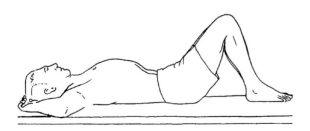

Lying in a prone position, place a firm pillow under the abdomen and a rolled blanket under the ankles.

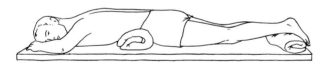

Lying in a supine position, bend the knees and place the feet flat on the table. With the hands up beside the head, tilt the pelvis to flatten the low back on the table. If the low back flattens to touch the table, the low back muscles are not tight.

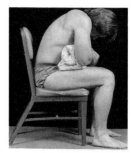

Sitting on a chair (not on side of table) with feet resting on the floor, place a rolled-up pillow on lap and bend forward over the pillow.

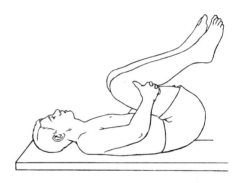

Lying in a supine position, grasp one leg at a time under the knee, then pull both knees slowly toward the chest. Try to keep the stretch localized to the low back, and avoid straining the neck or shoulders.

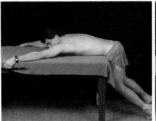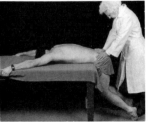

Lie face down at the end of a sturdy table or counter top with legs hanging down as in the photograph above. The low back will feel a stretch if the position is right. The position provides a strong stretch and should be used cautiously. An assistant may give some added pressure downward on the pelvis but should *avoid* a vigorous stretch. There may be a sensation of "a weak feeling in the back" following even a mild stretch.

Tensor Fasciae Latae and Iliotibial Band

HISTORICAL NOTE ABOUT THE OBER TEST

In the Journal of the American Medical Association, May 4, 1935, there appeared an article by Frank Ober of Boston, entitled "Back Strain and Sciatica" (19). In it he discussed the relationship of a contracted Tensor fasciae latae and Iliotibial band to low back and sciatic pain. The test for tightness was described, but did not mention anything about avoiding hip flexion or internal rotation as the thigh is allowed to drop in adduction.

After the article appeared in the Journal, Henry O. Kendall* physical therapist at Children's Hospital School in Baltimore, expressed concern about the test to his medical director, George E. Bennett. The concern was that allowing the thigh to drop in flexion and internal rotation would "give in" to the tight Tensor and not accurately test it for length. At some point in late 1935 or early 1936, Dr. Ober visited Children's Hospital School and Mr. Kendall expressed concerns about the test to him.

In the Journal of the American Medical Association of August 21, 1937, another article appeared in which Dr. Ober again described his test, this time cautioning the examiner to avoid hip flexion and internal rotation as the thigh is allowed to adduct (20).

It may be that, subsequently, some people who have described the test had access to the first article but not the second. A well-known text describes positioning the leg in abduction, hip neutral, and knee flexed 90°, and then *releasing* the abducted leg. The text also states that the normal iliotibial band will allow the thigh to drop to the adducted position (as illustrated by the knee touching the other leg or the table) (21).

A Tensor fasciae lata of normal length will not permit the thigh to drop to table level unless the hip goes into some internal rotation and flexion.

---

*Senior author of 1st and 2nd editions of *Muscles, Testing and Function.*

In the first article, Ober states, "The thigh is abducted and extended in the coronal plane of the body." With respect to what should be considered "normal" range of motion in the direction of adduction, this article states, "If there is no contraction present, the thigh will adduct beyond the median line." It must be noted that this statement referred to the test in which there was no reference to preventing flexion and internal rotation.

In the second article, he does not specifically refer to the coronal plane, but does say, "The thigh is allowed to drop toward the table in this plane" and by the description it is the coronal plane. Maintaining the thigh in the coronal plane prevents hip-joint flexion.

The second article makes no mention of how far the thigh should drop toward the table. (See below for further discussion about normal range of motion in adduction).

Before deciding what may be considered normal range of adduction in the Ober Test, it is necessary to review normal range of motion of the hip joint. Contrary to the information in several books (22–26), the normal range of hip joint adduction from the anatomical position (i.e., in the coronal plane) is, and should be, limited to about 10°.

Limitation of range of motion provides stability by preventing excessive motion. Limitation of knee-joint extension prevents hyperextension; limitation of hip joint extension prevents the pelvis from swaying forward abnormally in standing; limitation of hip-joint adduction provides stability for standing on one leg at a time.

If adduction is limited to 10°, then in side-lying position, with the pelvis in neutral position, the extended extremity should not drop more than 10° below the horizontal if kept in the coronal plane. In flexion and internal rotation, the range in adduction is greater, but *such a position is no longer a test for length of the Tensor fasciae latae.* The action of the muscle is abduction, flexion, and internal rotation of the hip, and assisting in extension of the knee. By "giving in" to flexion and internal rotation, the muscle is *not being lengthened.*

OBER TEST

Below is the test (which Ober called "The Abduction Test") quoted directly from the 1937 article in order to provide the reader with the author's exact description.

The Abduction Test

1. The patient lies on his side on a table, the shoulder and pelvis being perpendicular to the table.
2. The leg on which he is lying is flexed at the knee, and the hip is flexed and kept flexed to flatten the lumbar curve.
3. If the patient is on his left side, the examiner places his left hand over the patient's hip in the region of the trochanter to steady him.
4. The right leg is flexed to a right angle at the knee and is grasped just below the knee with the examiner's right hand, the leg and ankle being allowed to extend backward under his forearm and elbow.
5. The right thigh is abducted widely then hyperextended in the abducted position, the lower part of the leg being kept level and care being taken to keep the hip joint in a neutral position as far as rotation is concerned.
6. The examiner slides his right hand backward along the leg until it grasps the ankle lightly but with enough tension to keep the hip from flexing.
7. The thigh is allowed to drop toward the table in this plane. (Caution: Do not bear down on the leg.) If the fascia lata and the iliotibial band are tight the leg will remain more or less permanently abducted. If the hip is allowed to flex or internally rotate, the iliotibial band becomes relaxed and the leg falls from its own weight.
8. The same procedure for the opposite side is followed in every case.

MODIFIED OBER TEST

A modification of the Ober Test was first recommended by the Kendalls in *Posture and Pain*. The reasons for modifying the test are valid: less strain medially in the area of the knee joint; less tension on the patella; less interference by a tight Rectus femoris; and, for a muscle that has multiple actions like the Tensor fascia latae, it is not necessary to stretch in reverse of all actions when testing for length.

Place the subject in a side-lying position with the underneath leg flexed at hip and knee to flatten the low back, thereby stabilizing the pelvis against anterior pelvic tilt. Anterior pelvic tilt is the equivalent of hip flexion and is to be avoided because it "gives in" to the tightness.

The pelvis must also be stabilized to prevent lateral pelvic tilt downward on the tested side. Downward lateral tilt is the equivalent of hip joint abduction, and such a movement of the pelvis would "give in" to a tight Tensor. For most people, the lateral trunk will be in contact with the table in the side-lying position. People with wide hips and narrow waists will be the exceptions.

On the tested side, the examiner places one hand laterally on the subject's pelvis just below the iliac crest and pushes upward enough to stabilize the pelvis and keep the lateral trunk in contact with the table. The examiner does not externally rotate the thigh, but keeps it from internally rotating, and brings it back in extension. If the Tensor is tight, it will be necessary to abduct the leg in order to bring it into extension. Keep the leg extended in line with the trunk (i.e., in the coronal plane) and allow the leg to drop in adduction toward the table.

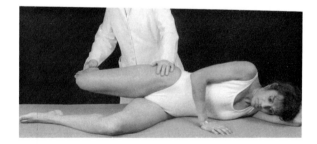

Ober Test—Normal Length: With the knee maintained at a right angle, the thigh drops *slightly* below horizontal.

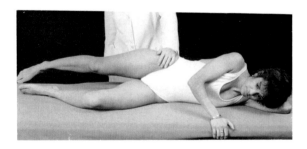

Modified Ober Test—Normal Length: With the knee straight and the pelvis in neutral position, the thigh drops about 10° below the horizontal. If the pelvis is laterally tilted upward on the tested side, there will be slightly less than 10° adduction.

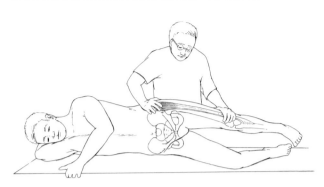

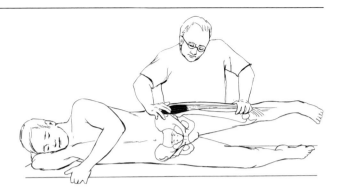

In the above figure, the pelvis is in neutral position, the hip is neutral between medial and lateral rotation, the leg is in the coronal plane, and allowed to drop in adduction. It drops 10° below the horizontal, which may be considered normal length for the Tensor fasciae latae. If the pelvis tilts upward on the side of the upper leg, there will be some hip joint adduction due to the pelvic tilt and the leg will drop less than 10° for normal length.

As seen in the figure above, the leg fails to drop when the pelvis is fixed, indicating a tightness of the Tensor fasciae latae and iliotibial tract. At times it is advisable to apply some pressure to be sure the subject is not holding the leg in abduction in an effort to avoid an uncomfortable stretch on the Tensor fasciae latae and Iliotibial band.

In the 1937 article, Ober also stated: ". . . when the maximum amount of fascial contracture is on the side and in front of the femur, the spine is held in lordosis, and that if the contracture is posterolateral, the lumbar curve is flattened. The former condition is common; the latter is rare. Either condition may be associated with pain low in the back and sciatica. Unilateral contracture may produce lateral curvature of the spine" (20).

To test for tightness of the posterolateral Iliotibial band the hip is slightly flexed and medially rotated along with the adduction. Tightness of this band can be a factor in a straight-leg-raising test for Hamstring length.

Three fourths of the Gluteus maximus inserts into the Iliotibial band, but the fibers are oblique to the band and do not have the direct line of pull as does the Tensor fasciae latae. Furthermore, the Gluteus maximus is seldom tight.

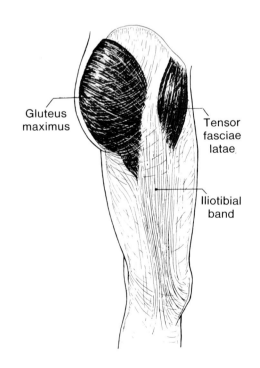

Gluteus maximus

Tensor fasciae latae

Iliotibial band

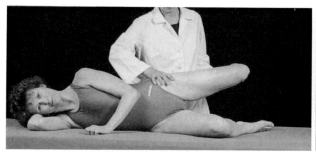 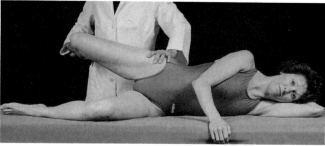

BILATERAL TIGHTNESS OF TENSOR FASCIAE LATAE: POSITIVE OBER TEST

The range of motion in adduction may be considered normal if the thigh drops slightly below horizontal with the thigh in neutral rotation in the coronal plane, and with the knee flexed 90°. This subject's thighs remain in marked abduction due to bilateral tightness of the Tensor fasciae latae and Iliotibial band.

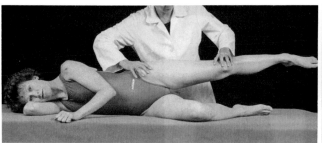 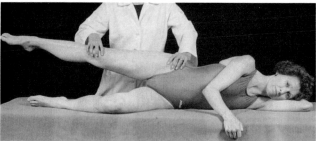

BILATERAL TIGHTNESS OF TENSOR FASCIAE LATAE: MODIFIED OBER TEST

The range of motion in adduction may be considered normal if the leg drops 10° below the horizontal with the thigh in neutral rotation in the coronal plane, and the knee extended. In this test, this subject's legs do not drop to the horizontal because of the tightness in the Tensor fasciae latae and Iliotibial band.

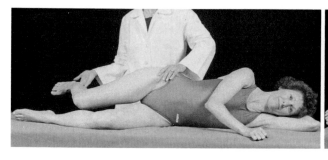 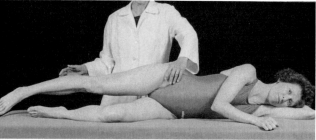

ERRORS IN TESTING FOR TIGHTNESS OF TENSOR FASCIAE LATAE AND ILIOTIBIAL BAND

According to one reference, the leg, with the knee bent, is maneuvered into correct Ober test position *and then released* (21). As seen in the photographs above, the hip internally rotates and flexes when not controlled by the examiner. The thigh must be kept in the coronal plane and prevented from internally rotating in order to test accurately for tightness of the Tensor fasciae latae and Iliotibial band.

Tensor Fasciae Latae Stretching

Tightness, or even contracture, of the iliotibial band is frequently seen. The relationship to painful conditions is discussed in Chapter 11 (see p. 361.). The following deals with *exercises* to stretch the Tensor fasciae latae and the anterolateral iliotibial band.

The Tensor fasciae latae abducts, flexes, and internally rotates the hip joint, and assists in knee extension. When a muscle has multiple actions, it is not necessary to elongate the muscle in all directions opposite its actions in order to stretch it. An exercise may include two or three movements in the direction of stretching. Most of all, it is important that the stretching be specifically directed to the area in need of stretch. Some commonly prescribed exercises are not meeting this requirement.

Standing with legs crossed puts the hip joints in adduction. However, in this position, the hips are usually in internal rotation and in some degree of flexion by virtue of the pelvis being tilted anteriorly. If, besides standing in a position of adduction, the person sways sideways toward a wall or table, the stretch will often affect the posterior Gluteus medius more than the Tensor.

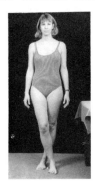 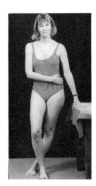

Crossing legs places hip joint in flexion (by anterior pelvic tilt) and in internal rotation.

Swaying sideways, with hip internally rotated and flexed, stretches Gluteus medius more than Tensor fasciae latae.

Better control and more precision in the stretching can be obtained by moving the pelvis in relation to the femur. To understand the mechanism, it is necessary to describe the effect of pelvic tilt on the hip joints.

When legs are of equal length and the pelvis is level in standing, both hip joints are neutral as far as adduction and abduction are concerned. If the person sways sideways, the position of the hip joints changes. Swaying toward the left results in adduction of the left hip joint. Likewise, if a lift is placed under the left foot, the left side of the pelvis will be elevated and the left hip joint will be in adduction without swaying sideways.

To stretch a tight left Tensor and anterior Iliotibial band, stand with a board, book, or magazine, under the left foot, the thickness of such a raise to be determined by the amount tolerated. Keep weight on both feet, and keep feet and knees (i.e., femurs) in good alignment, i.e., the feet out-toeing approximately 8° to 10° on each side, and patellae facing straight ahead. Then attempt to posteriorly tilt the pelvis. Posterior pelvic tilt results in extension of the hip joint. The range of motion will be slight but the stretch should be felt very specifically in the area of the left Tensor fasciae latae. The Tensor will be stretched by adduction and extension of the hip joint without allowing internal rotation. The stretching can be done, also, by removing the right shoe (if the heel is not too high), instead of putting a lift under the left foot.

For bilateral tightness, place the lift alternately under left and right, or alternately remove one shoe, and hold the stretch position for a comfortable length of time (1 to 2 minutes).

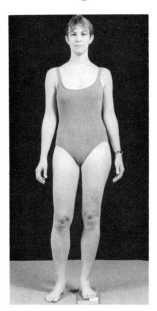

Standing with a raise under the left foot places the left hip joint in adduction. Posterior pelvic tilt adds hip joint extension, providing a stretch on the left Tensor fasciae latae and Iliotibial band. The subject makes an effort to control rotation, keeping the patellae facing straight ahead. Standing with slight out-toeing of the feet also helps control rotation.

When tightness is unilateral, a lift (1/4 inch heel pad) in the shoe on the side of tightness will serve to passively stretch the Tensor. Make sure that it is worn in all shoes and bedroom slippers, and that the person avoids any bad habit of standing on the opposite leg. *A lift will not do any good unless the person stands with weight evenly distributed over both feet.* (For assisted stretching of a tight Tensor fasciae latae, see p. 117, and for treatment of a stretched Tensor fasciae latae, see p. 362.)

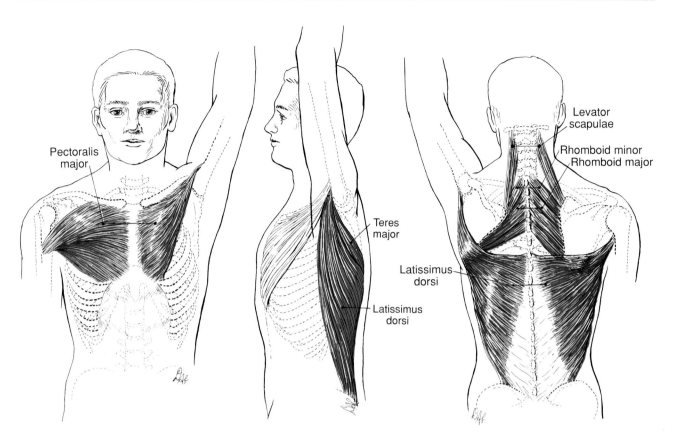

Full range of scapulohumeral and scapular motion for normal overhead elevation of the arm in flexion or in abduction requires adequate length in the following muscles: Pectoralis major, Pectoralis minor, Latissimus dorsi, Teres major, Subscapularis, and Rhomboids.

Full range of motion in lateral rotation requires normal length of medial rotators, namely, Pectoralis major, Latissimus dorsi, Teres major, and Subscapularis. Full range of motion in medial rotation requires normal length of lateral rotators, namely, Teres minor, Infraspinatus, and Posterior deltoid.

To test accurately for the various movements, there must be no substitution by movements of the trunk. The trunk position must be standardized with the subject supine, knees bent, and low back flat on a flat surface. The table should not have a soft pad but may have a folded blanket for the comfort of the subject.

If the *low back arches* up from the table, the amount of shoulder flexion or lateral rotation will appear to be *greater*, and medial rotation will appear to be *less*, than the actual range of shoulder and scapular motion. If the *chest is depressed*, the amount of shoulder flexion and external rotation will appear to be *less*, and medial rotation will appear to be *greater*, than the actual range motion.

If the trunk *bends laterally* with convexity toward the tested side, abduction will appear *greater* than the actual range of shoulder and scapular motion.

Tests for Length of Glenohumeral and Scapular Muscles

TESTS FOR LENGTH OF PECTORALIS MAJOR

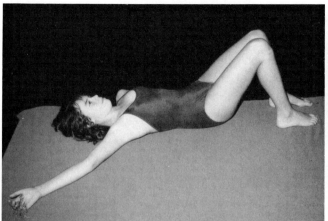

Normal length of lower fibers.

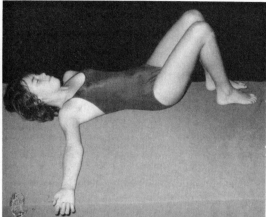

Normal length of upper fibers.

PECTORALIS MAJOR

Equipment: Firm table, no soft padding.

Starting Position: Supine, knees bent, low back flat on table

Test Movement for Lower (Sternal) Part: Examiner places arm in a position of approximately 135° abduction (in line with the lower fibers), with elbow extended. The shoulder will be in lateral rotation.

Normal Length: Arm drops to table level with low back remaining flat on table.

Shortness: The extended arm does not drop down to table level. Limitation may be recorded as slight, moderate, or marked; or measured in degrees using a goniometer; or measured in inches using a ruler to record the number of inches from the lateral epicondyle to the table.

Test Movement for Upper (Clavicular) Part: Examiner places arm in horizontal abduction with elbow extended and shoulder in lateral rotation (palm upward).

Normal Length: Full horizontal abduction with lateral rotation, arm flat on table, without trunk rotation.

Shortness: Arm does not drop down to table level. Limitation may be recorded as slight, moderate or marked; or measured in degrees using a goniometer; or measured in inches using a ruler to record the number of inches between the table and the lateral epicondyle. Marked limitation is seldom found in this length test.

Note: Tightness of acromioclavicular fascia can interfere with length testing of the clavicular portion.

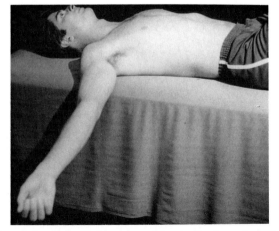

Excessive length in upper (clavicular) part of Pectoralis major.

Excessive Length: To test for excessive length, position the subject with the shoulder joint at the edge of table so the arm can drop below table level. Record excessive range as slight, moderate, or marked; or measure in degrees using a goniometer. Excessive range of motion is not uncommon.

TEST FOR SHORTNESS OF PECTORALIS MINOR

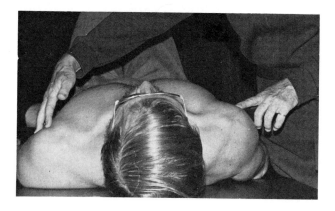

Left, normal length; right, short, holding shoulder forward.

Equipment: Firm table, unpadded.

Starting Position: Supine, arms at sides, elbows extended, palms upward, knees bent, and low back flat on table.

Test: Examiner stands at head of table and observes the position of the shoulder girdle. This figure shows normal length of the left Pectoralis minor and shortness of the right. The amount of tightness is measured by the extent to which the shoulder is raised from the table, and by the amount of resistance to downward pressure on the shoulder. Tightness may be recorded as slight, moderate, or marked.

TERES MAJOR, LATISSIMUS DORSI, RHOMBOID MAJOR AND MINOR

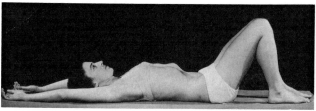 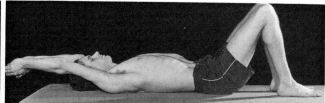

Equipment: Firm table, unpadded

Starting Position: Supine, arms at sides, elbows extended, knees bent, and low back flat on table.

Test Movement: Subject raises both arms in flexion overhead, keeping arms close to the head and bringing arms down toward the table, (maintaining low back flat).

Normal Length: The ability to bring arms down to table level, keeping them close to the head.

Shortness: Indicated by the inability to get the arms to table level. Record measurements as slight, moderate, or marked; or measure angle between table and humerus to determine the number of degrees of limitation; or measure the number of inches between the table and the lateral epicondyle.

Note: Tightness of upper abdominals will depress the chest and tend to pull the shoulder forward, interfering with the test. Likewise, a kyphosis of the upper back will make it impossible to get the shoulder down on the table.

A contracted Pectoralis minor tilts the scapula anteriorly pulling the shoulder girdle down and forward. With the change of alignment of the shoulder girdle, flexion of the glenohumeral joint will appear to be limited, even if range is normal, because the arm cannot be brought down to touch the table.

Tightness of the Pectoralis minor is an important factor in many cases of arm pain. With attachment of the Pectoralis minor on the coracoid process, tightness of this muscle depresses the coracoid anteriorly causing pressure and impingement on the cords of the brachial plexus and the axillary blood vessels that lie between the coracoid and the rib cage (see p. 343).

Tests for Length of Shoulder Rotators

TEST FOR LENGTH OF MEDIAL ROTATORS

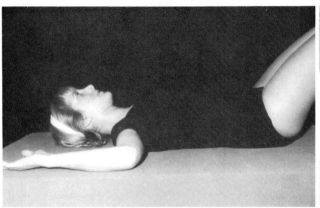

Equipment: Firm table, no soft padding.

Starting Position: Supine, low back flat on table, arm at shoulder level (90° abduction), elbow at edge of table and flexed to 90°, forearm perpendicular to table.

Test for Length of Medial Rotators: Lateral rotation of shoulder, bringing forearms down toward table level, parallel with head. (Do not allow back to arch up from table.)

Normal Range of Motion: 90° (forearm flat on table, while maintaining low back flat on table).

Note: If the test for tightness of Teres major and Latissimus dorsi (p. 63) shows limitation, but external rotation (as above) shows normal range, then tightness is in the Latissimus dorsi but not in the Teres major.

TEST FOR LENGTH OF LATERAL ROTATORS

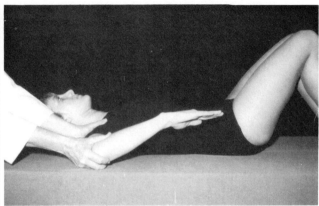

Equipment: Firm table, no soft padding.

Starting Position: Supine, low back flat on table, arm at shoulder level (90° abduction), elbow at edge of table and flexed to 90°, forearm perpendicular to table.

Test for Length of Lateral Rotators: Medial rotation of shoulder, bringing forearms downward toward table, while examiner holds shoulder down to prevent substitution by the shoulder girdle. (Do not allow forward thrust of shoulder girdle.)

Normal Range of Motion: 70° (forearm at 20° angle with table).

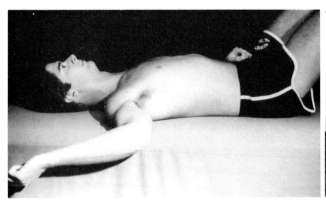

To test for excessive range of motion in lateral rotation, it is necessary to have elbow slightly beyond edge of table to allow forearm to drop below table level. Excessive lateral rotation is found frequently.

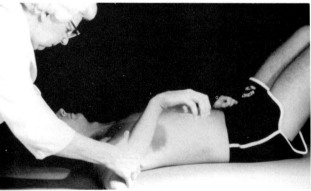

This subject demonstrated marked limitation of medial rotation and excessive lateral rotation—an imbalance often seen in baseball players.

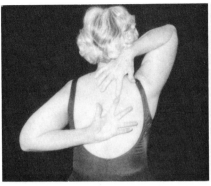
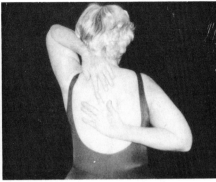

Placing hands behind back, as illustrated, requires normal range of shoulder joint rotation without abnormal shoulder girdle movement.

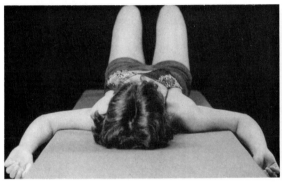
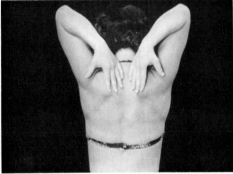

Slightly excessive shoulder joint lateral rotation. Hands can be placed easily on upper back.

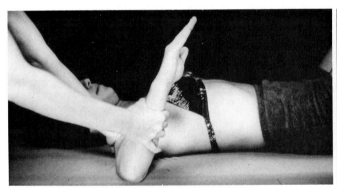
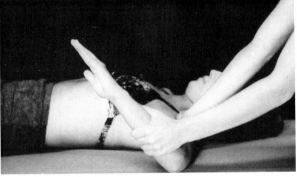

Shoulder joint medial rotation limited, right more than left. Shoulder girdle is held down to prevent substitution of shoulder girdle motion for shoulder joint motion.

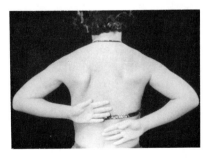

Substitution by shoulder girdle motion permits subject to place hands behind back. However, encouraging or permitting such substitution has adverse effects by contributing to over-development of the Pectoralis minor. (See Pectoralis minor, p. 278.)

65

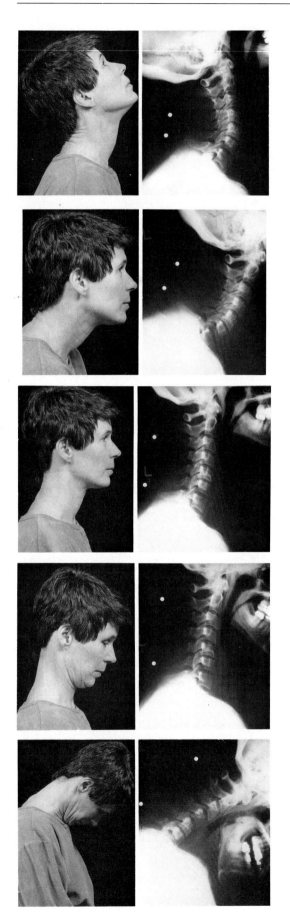

In the following example, a subject with normal flexibility was photographed and x-rayed in five positions of the neck. "Markers" were placed at the hair line and over C-7.

Cervical spine extension by tilting the head in a posterior direction. Note the approximation of the markers on the x-ray.

Cervical spine extension in a typical forward head posture. Note the similarity in curve and position of markers to the example above. (Often this slumped posture is mistakenly referred to as flexion of the lower cervical spine and extension of the upper.) Actually, the extension is more pronounced in the lower cervical region than in the upper.

Good alignment of the cervical spine.

Flexion (flattening) of the cervical spine by tilting the head in an anterior direction.

Flexion of the cervical spine plus flexion of the upper thoracic spine occurs when bringing the chin toward the chest.

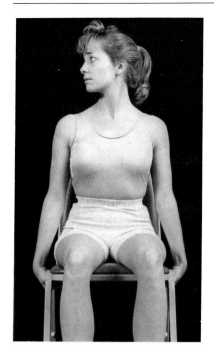

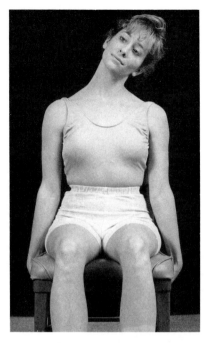

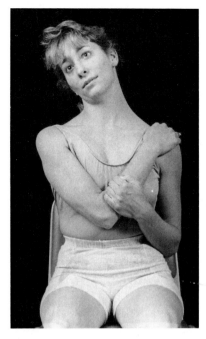

Stretch Neck Rotators
Sit on chair with hands grasping seat of chair to keep shoulders down and level. Without tilting head, turn toward each side (using opposite neck rotators).

Stretch Lateral Neck Flexors
Sit on chair with shoulders back and hands grasping seat of chair to hold shoulders down and level. Tilt head directly sideways to stretch opposite lateral neck flexors. Exercises for lateral neck stretching may be modified to tilt antero-laterally to stretch opposite posterolateral muscles.

Stretch Lateral Neck Flexors
Seated or standing, place right hand on left shoulder to hold it down. Give assistance with left by grasping right forearm near elbow and pulling downward. Tilt head directly sideways toward right to stretch left lateral neck flexors. Reverse the hands and neck position to stretch the right side.

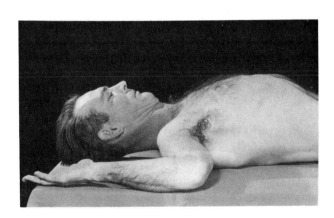

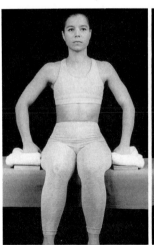

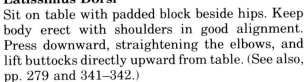

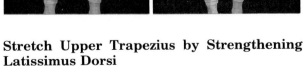

Stretch Neck Extensors
Lie supine (or sit on stool with back to wall). With hands up beside head and low back flat, press head back with chin down and in, using anterior neck flexors to straighten (flatten) the neck.

Stretch Upper Trapezius by Strengthening Latissimus Dorsi
Sit on table with padded block beside hips. Keep body erect with shoulders in good alignment. Press downward, straightening the elbows, and lift buttocks directly upward from table. (See also, pp. 279 and 341–342.)

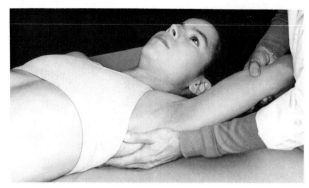

Assisted Stretch of Teres Major and Latissimus Dorsi

Supine, with hips and knees flexed, feet flat on table and low back flat. Hold scapula to prevent excessive abduction to localize stretch to shoulder joint adductors and prevent excessive stretch of Rhomboids. Therapist provides traction on the arm while stretching arm overhead.

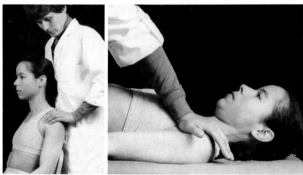

Stretch of Pectoralis Minor

With subject seated, assistant pulls shoulder(s) back and down. With subject supine, assistant presses shoulder back and down. Hand should be "cupped" around shoulder to allow firm, uniform pressure that helps to rotate the shoulder girdle back.

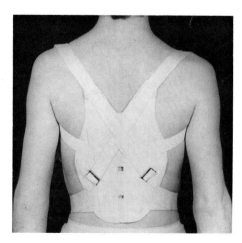

Shoulder support with stays in back to help correct roundness of upper back as well as correcting forward shoulders.

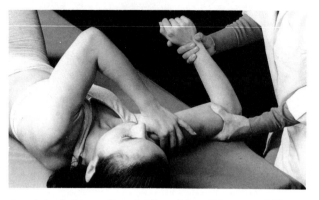

Assisted Stretch of Shoulder External Rotators

Supine, with hips and knees flexed, feet flat on table, low back flat, and arm at shoulder level. Starting with elbow bent at right angle and forearm in vertical position, have subject hold (right) shoulder down with firm pressure by left hand to *prevent shoulder girdle motion*. Therapist provides *traction* on the arm and helps the subject medially rotate the shoulder.

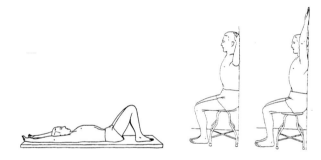

Stretch of Shoulder Adductors

Supine, or sitting, with hands and upper back against wall or table, place arms at shoulder level to stretch upper part of Pectoralis major by pulling back with Middle trapezius. Place arms diagonally overhead to stretch lower part of Pectoralis major by pulling back with Lower trapezius. Place arms directly overhead to stretch Teres major and Latissimus dorsi by pressing arms toward wall or table. Hold each position while pulling up and in with lower abdominals to flatten low back and prevent substitution of trunk by arching the back.

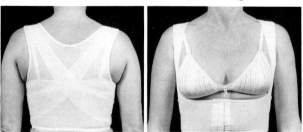

Elastic vest-type support that helps hold shoulders back without the discomfort of straps that loop around under the arms.

chapter 4

Posture: Alignment and Muscle Balance

Muscle Balance: Opposing Muscles

The following is a brief outline of muscles that oppose each other or work in combination with others in anteroposterior, lateral, and rotary movements and positions of the trunk and lower extremities. The muscles are grouped according to action or the main ones in the action are named.

FOOT

Anteroposterior: Dorsiflexors oppose plantar flexors.
Lateral and rotary: Tibials oppose peroneals.

KNEE

Anteroposterior: Hamstrings, Gastrocnemius, and Popliteus oppose Quadriceps.

HIP

Anteroposterior: Iliopsoas, Rectus femoris, Tensor fasciae latae, and Sartorius oppose Gluteus maximus and Hamstrings.
Lateral: Unilaterally, abductors oppose adductors. Bilaterally, right abductors and left adductors oppose left abductors and right adductors.
Rotary: Unilaterally, internal rotators oppose external rotators. Bilaterally, right internal rotators and left external rotators oppose left internal and right external rotators.

TRUNK

Anteroposterior: Low back muscles oppose anterior abdominal muscles.
Lateral: Lateral trunk muscles oppose each other.
Rotary: Muscles that produce clockwise rotation oppose those that produce counterclockwise rotation.

PELVIS

With the pelvis pivoting on the femora, the opposing groups of muscles act not only in straight anteroposterior opposition, but combine their pulls diagonally to tilt the pelvis forward or backward and laterally. There are four main groups of muscles in *anteroposterior opposition*:

1. Erector spinae, Quadratus lumborum, and other posterior back muscles attached to the posterior superior part of the pelvis, exert an *upward pull posteriorly*.
2. The anterior abdominals, especially the Rectus abdominis with its insertion on the symphysis pubis and the External oblique with attachment on the anterior iliac crest, exert an *upward pull anteriorly*.
3. The Gluteus maximus and Hamstrings, with attachments on the posterior ilium, sacrum, and ischium, exert a *downward pull posteriorly*.
4. The hip flexors, including the Rectus femoris, Tensor fasciae latae, and Sartorius with attachments on the anterior superior and inferior spines of the ilium, and the Iliopsoas with attachment on the lumbar spine and inner surface of the ilium, *exert a downward pull anteriorly*.

The low back muscles act with the hip flexors (especially the Psoas with its direct pull from the lumbar spine to the femur) to tilt the pelvis down and forward (anterior tilt). They are opposed in action by the combined pull of the anterior abdominals pulling up anteriorly, and the Hamstrings and Gluteus maximus pulling down posteriorly to level the pelvis from a *position of anterior tilt*.

There are two main groups in *lateral opposition*:

1. Leg abductors (mainly the Gluteus minimus and medius), which arise from the lateral surface of the pelvis, pull down on the pelvis when the leg is fixed as in standing.
2. Lateral trunk muscles, attached to the lateral crest of the ilium, pull up laterally on the pelvis.

Hip abductors on one side and lateral trunk muscles on the other side combine in action to tilt the pelvis laterally: right abductors pull *downward* on the right side of the pelvis as left lateral trunk muscles pull *upward* on the left side, and vice versa. These actions are assisted by hip adductors on the same side as the lateral trunk muscles.

In combination, right hip abductors, left hip adductors and left lateral trunk muscles *oppose* left hip abductors, right hip adductors and right lateral trunk muscles.

PRINCIPLES

Posture is a composite of the positions of all the joints of the body at any given moment, and static postural alignment is best described in terms of the positions of the various joints and body segments. The two preceding chapters have provided basic information on anatomical positions, axes, planes, movements of joints, and tests of muscle length. This information is essential when analyzing postural alignment.

Posture may be described, also, in terms of muscle balance. This chapter describes the muscle balance or imbalance associated with static postural positions.

Evaluating and treating postural problems requires an understanding of basic **principles** relating to alignment, joints, and muscles:

- Faulty alignment results in undue stress and strain on bones, joints, ligaments, and muscles.
- An assessment of joint positions indicates which muscles are in an elongated and which are in a shortened position.
- A correlation exists between alignment and muscle test findings if posture is habitual.
- Muscle weakness allows separation of the parts to which the muscle is attached.
- Muscle shortness holds the parts to which the muscle is attached closer together.
- Stretch weakness can occur in one-joint muscles that remain in an elongated condition.
- Adaptive shortening can develop in muscles that remain in a shortened condition.

THE STANDARD POSTURE

As is true in all testing, there must be a standard when evaluating postural alignment. The ideal skeletal alignment used as a standard is consistent with sound scientific principles, involves a minimal amount of stress and strain, and is conducive to maximal efficiency of the body. It is essential that the standard meet these requirements if the whole system of posture training that is built around it is to be sound. Basmajian states "... among mammals, man has the most economical of antigravity mechanisms once the upright posture is attained. The expenditure of muscular energy for what seems to be a most awkward position is actually extremely economical" (27).

In the **standard posture**, the spine presents the normal curves, and the bones of the lower extremities are in ideal alignment for weight bearing. The "neutral" position of the pelvis is conducive to good alignment of the abdomen and trunk, and that of the extremities below. The chest and upper back are in a position that favors optimal function of the respiratory organs. The head is erect in a well-balanced position that minimizes stress on the neck musculature.

The body contour in the illustrations of the standard posture shows the relationship of skeletal structures to surface outline in ideal alignment. There are variations in body type and size, and shape and proportions of the body are factors in weight distribution. Variations in contour are correlated to some degree with variations in skeletal alignment. This is essentially true regardless of body build. An experienced observer can estimate the position of the skeletal structures by observing the contours of the body.

The intersection of the sagittal and coronal midplanes of the body forms a line that is analogous to the **gravity line.** Around this line, the body is hypothetically in a position of equilibrium. Such a position implies a balanced distribution of weight, and a stable position of each joint.

When viewing a posture in standing, a **plumb line** is used to represent a line of reference. A plumb line is a cord with a plumb bob attached to provide an absolute vertical line—standard for measuring deviations. The point in line with which a plumb line is suspended must be a standard **fixed point.** Since the only fixed point in the standing posture is at the base where the feet are in contact with the floor, the point of reference must be at the base. A movable point is not acceptable as a standard. The position of the head is not stationary and using the lobe of the ear as a point in line with which to suspend a plumb line is not appropriate.

In *lateral view,* the fixed reference point is slightly anterior to the outer malleolus and represents the base point of the midcoronal plane of the body in ideal alignment. In *posterior view,* the point is midway between the heels and represents the base point of the midsagittal plane of the body in ideal alignment.

The standing position may be regarded as the composite alignment of a subject from four views: front, back, right side, and left side. It involves the position and alignment of many joints and parts of the body. It is not expected that any individual should match the standard in every respect, nor have the authors seen anyone who has.

The standard posture is illustrated in front, back, and side views by line drawings and photographs. In *back view,* the line of reference in the drawings and the plumb line in the photographs represent a projection of the gravity line in the midsagittal plane. Beginning midway between the heels, it extends upward midway between the lower extremities, through the midline of the pelvis, spine, sternum, and skull. The right and left halves of the skeletal structures are essentially symmetrical and by hypothesis the two halves of the body exactly counterbalance. (See p. 88.)

In *side view*, the line of reference in the drawings and the plumb line in the photographs represent a projection of the gravity line in the midcoronal plane. This plane hypothetically divides the body into front and back sections of equal weight. These sections are not symmetrical and there is no obvious line of division on the basis of anatomical structures.

The *plumb line test* is used to determine whether the *points of reference* of the individual being tested are in the same alignment as are the corresponding points in the standard posture. The deviations of the various points of reference from the plumb line reveal the extent to which the subject's alignment is faulty.

For the purpose of testing, the subject steps up to a suspended plumb line. In back view, he stands with the feet equidistant from the line. In side view, a point just in front of the lateral malleolus is in line with the plumb line.

Deviations from plumb alignment are described as slight, moderate, or marked, rather than in terms of inches or degrees. In routine examinations, it is not practical to try to determine exactly how much each point of reference deviates from the plumb line.

With the ideal alignment as the standard, the positions of the low back, pelvis, lower extremity, head, neck, thoracic spine, and shoulder girdle are described in the following pages.

Listed below and in the accompanying drawings are the points that coincide with the line of reference in lateral view, ideal alignment.

> Slightly anterior to lateral malleolus.
> Slightly anterior to axis of knee joint.
> Slightly posterior to axis of hip joint.
> Bodies of lumbar vertebrae.
> Shoulder joint.
> Bodies of most of cervical vertebrae.
> External auditory meatus.
> Slightly posterior to apex of coronal suture.

Pelvis and Low Back

The relationship of the pelvis to the line of reference is determined to a great extent by the relationship of the pelvis to the hip joints. Since the side-view line of reference represents the plane passing slightly posterior to the axes of the hip joints, the pelvis will be intersected at the acetabula. But these points of reference are not sufficient to establish the position of the pelvis because the pelvis can tilt anteriorly or posteriorly about the axes through the hip joints.

It is, therefore, necessary to define the *neutral position of the pelvis* in the standard posture. The neutral position used as standard in this text is one in which the anterior superior spines are in the same horizontal plane, and the anterior superior spines and the symphysis pubis are in the same vertical plane. From the standpoint of the action of muscles attached to the anterior spines and the symphysis pubis, opposing groups of muscles have an equal mechanical advantage in a straight line of pull. The Rectus abdominis with its attachment on the pubis extends upward to the sternum, and Rectus femoris, Sartorius, and Tensor fasciae latae with their attachments on the anterior iliac spines extend downward to the thigh.

To describe neutral position of the pelvis on the basis of a specific anterior point and a specific posterior point being in the same horizontal plane is not practical because of structural variations of the pelvis. The anterior superior spines and the posterior superior spines are approximately in the same plane, however.

In *neutral position* of the pelvis, there is a *normal anterior curve* in the low back; in *anterior tilt*, a *lordosis*; and in *posterior tilt*, a *flat back*.

Without minimizing the importance of proper foot positions that establish the base of support, it may be said that the position of the pelvis is the key to good or faulty postural alignment. The muscles that maintain good alignment of the pelvis, both anteroposteriorly and laterally, are of utmost importance in maintaining good overall alignment. Imbalance between muscles that oppose each other in standing changes the alignment of the pelvis and adversely affects the posture of the parts of the body above and below.

Hip and Knee Joints

The side-view line of reference through the lower extremities passes slightly posterior to the center of the hip joint and slightly anterior to the axis of the knee joint representing a stable position of these joints.

If the center of the weight-bearing joint coincides with the line of gravity, there is an equal tendency for the joint to flex or to extend. This on-center position of the joint is not a stable one for weight bearing. The slightest force exerted in either direction will cause it to move off center unless stabilized by constant muscular effort. If the body must call on muscular effort to maintain a stable position, there is an unnecessary expenditure of energy.

If the hip joint and knee joint moved freely in extension as well as in flexion, there would be no stability and constant effort would be required to resist movement in both directions. A stable off-center position for a joint is dependent upon limitation of joint motion in one direction. For the hip and knee, extension is limited. Ligamentous structures, strong muscles, and tendons are the restraining force preventing hyperextension. Stability in the standing position is obtained by this normal limitation of joint motion.

There should be careful scrutiny of exercises or manipulations that tend to hyperextend the knee or hip joint, or that excessively stretch such muscles as Hamstrings. The normal restraining influence of the ligaments and muscles helps to maintain good postural alignment with a minimum of muscular effort. When muscles and ligaments fail to offer adequate support, the joints exceed their normal range and posture becomes faulty with respect to positions of knee and hip hyperextension. (See pp. 85, 95, and 96.)

Ankle

The line of reference passes slightly anterior to the outer malleolus, and approximately through the apex of the arch, designated laterally by the calcaneocuboid joint. Dorsiflexion at the ankle with the knee extended is normally about 10°. This means that standing barefoot with feet in a position of slight out-toeing and with knees straight, the lower leg cannot sway forward on the foot more than about 10°. Forward deviation of the body (dorsiflexion at the ankle) is checked by the restraining tension of strong posterior muscles and ligaments. However, this element of restraint is materially altered with changes in heel height that place the ankle in varying degrees of plantar flexion, and appreciably altered if the knees are flexed.

Feet

In the standard posture, the position of the feet is one in which the heels are separated about three inches, and the forepart of the feet separated so that the angle of out-toeing is about 8° to 10° from the midline on each side, making a total of 20° or less.

This position of the feet refers only to the static and barefoot position. Elevation of the heels and motion affect the foot position.

In establishing a standard position of the feet, and determining where, if at all, out-toeing should occur, it is necessary to consider the foot in relation to the rest of the lower extremity. The out-toeing position cannot occur at the knee because there is no rotation in extension.

In ideal alignment, the axis of the extended knee joint is in a frontal plane. With the knee joint in this plane, out-toeing cannot take place from the hip joint level. There can be a position of out-toeing as a result of outward rotation of the

hip, but the entire extremity would be outwardly rotated and the degree of out-toeing would be exaggerated.

This makes the question of whether there should be rotation of the foot into an out-toeing position dependent on the relationship of the foot to the ankle joint. The ankle joint permits flexion and extension only, no rotation. Unlike the knee joint, the ankle joint is not in a frontal plane. According to anatomists, it is in a slightly oblique plane. The line of obliquity is such that it extends from slightly anterior at the medial malleolus to slightly posterior at the lateral malleolus. The angle at which the axis of the ankle joint deviates from the frontal plane suggests that the foot is normally in a position of slight out-toeing in relation to the lower leg.

The foot is not a rigid structure. The movements of the subtalar and transverse tarsal joints permit pronation and supination of the foot and abduction and adduction of the forefoot. The combination of pronation and forefoot abduction is seen as *eversion* of the foot, and the combination of supination and forefoot adduction as *inversion*. (See p. 22.) Passive or active movements of the foot and ankle reveal that the foot tends to move *outward as it moves upward, and inward as it moves downward.*

In the standing position, the foot usually is not fully dorsiflexed on the leg nor is it in full eversion. However, the person who stands with flexed knees and marked out-toeing of the feet will be in dorsiflexion and eversion—a position that results in stress and strain on the foot.

It is not possible to determine the degree of eversion or inversion of the foot that corresponds with each degree of dorsal or plantar flexion. The two are not so correlated that an exact relationship exists, but it may be assumed that the movement from eversion in the dorsiflexed position to inversion in the plantar flexed position is relatively uniform.

When influenced by shoes with heels, the standing position represents varying degrees of plantar flexion of the foot based on the heel height. As heel height is increased, the tendency toward a parallel position or in-toeing increases.

The relationship of heel height to out-toeing or in-toeing of the foot is analogous to the position of the foot in standing, walking, and running. In barefoot standing, a slight degree of out-toeing is natural. Standing with heels raised or walking fast, the feet tend to become parallel. As speed increases from walking to sprinting, the heels do not contact the ground, and the weight is borne on the anterior part of the foot entirely. There is then a tendency for the print of the forefoot to show in-toeing.

Head and Neck

The position of the head and neck in ideal alignment is one in which the head is in a well-balanced position and maintained with minimal muscular effort. In side view, the line of reference coincides with the lobe of the ear and the neck presents the normal anterior curve. In posterior view, the line of reference coincides with the midline of the head and with the cervical spinous processes. The head is not tilted upward nor downward, it is not tilted sideways nor rotated, and the chin is not retracted.

Good alignment of the upper back is essential to good alignment of the head and neck; faulty alignment of the upper back adversely affects the head and neck position. If the upper back slumps into a rounded position in sitting or standing, there will be a compensatory change in the position of the head and neck.

If the head position were to remain fixed with the neck held in its normal anterior curve as the upper back flexed into a position of round upper back, the head would be inclined forward and downward. But "eyes seek eye level" and the head must be raised from that position by extending the cervical spine. In normal extension of the cervical spine, there is an approximation of the occiput and the seventh cervical vertebra. As the head is raised to seek eye level, the distance between the occiput and the seventh cervical is reduced remarkably. Compared to the separation between the two points in ideal alignment, there may be as much as 2 or 3 inches difference between the two positions.

The forward head position is one in which the neck extensors are in a shortened position and strong, and the potential exists for the development of adaptive shortening in these muscles. The anterior vertebral neck flexors are in an elongated position and give evidence of weakness when tested for strength. (See below and x-rays on pp. 66 and 91.)

Thoracic spine

In ideal alignment, the thoracic spine curves slightly in a posterior direction. Just as the positions of the head and neck are affected by the positions of the thoracic spine, so the thoracic spine is affected by the positions of the low back and pelvis. With the pelvis and lumbar spine in ideal alignment, the thoracic spine can assume ideal position. If a normally flexible individual assumes a position of lordosis of the low back (i.e., increased anterior curve), the upper back tends to straighten, decreasing the normal posterior curve. On the other hand, habitual positions and repetitive activities may give rise to the development of a lordosis-kyphosis posture in which one tends to compensate for the other. In a sway-back posture, the position of increased posterior curvature of the upper back compensates for a forward deviation of the pelvis.

Shoulder Joint and Shoulder Girdle

In ideal alignment of the shoulder joint, the side-view line of reference passes midway through the joint. But the position of the arm and shoulder joint depends upon the position of the scapula. In good alignment, the scapulae lie flat against the upper back, approximately between the second and seventh thoracic vertebrae, and about 4 inches apart (more or less, depending upon the size of the individual). Faulty positions of the scapulae adversely affect the position of the shoulder joint, and malalignment of this joint can predispose to injury and chronic pain.

A drawing of the standard posture appears on the facing page. Legends indicate the skeletal structures that coincide with the line of reference. For comparison, beside the drawing is a photograph showing a subject whose alignment closely approaches that of the standard posture.

In the side-view drawing of the standard posture, the artist has attempted to present a composite of male and female pelves, and to show an average in regard to shape, length of sacrum, coccyx, and other measurements.

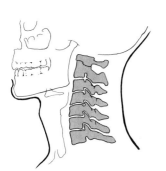

Good alignment of cervical spine.

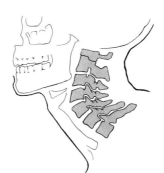

Extension of cervical spine in faulty posture with round upper back and forward head.

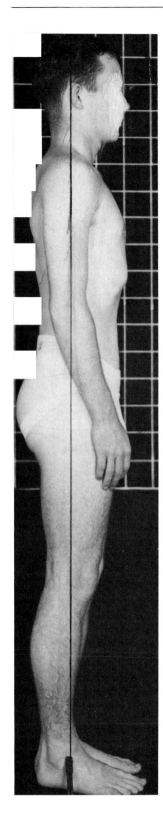

Through lobe of the ear (head is slightly forward)

Slightly posterior to apex of coronal suture

Through external auditory meatus

Through bodies of cervical vertebrae

Through odontoid process of axis

Through shoulder joint (provided arms hang in normal alignment in relation to thorax)

Approximately midway through trunk

Through bodies of lumbar vertebrae

Through sacral promontory

Approximately through greater trochanter of femur

Slightly posterior to center of hip joint

Slightly anterior to a midline through knee

Slightly anterior to axis of knee joint

Slightly anterior to lateral malleolus.

Through calcaneocuboid joint

Surface landmarks that coincide with the plumb line. (This subject shows excellent alignment except that the head is slightly forward.)

Anatomical structures that coincide with the line of reference.

Four Types of Postural Alignment

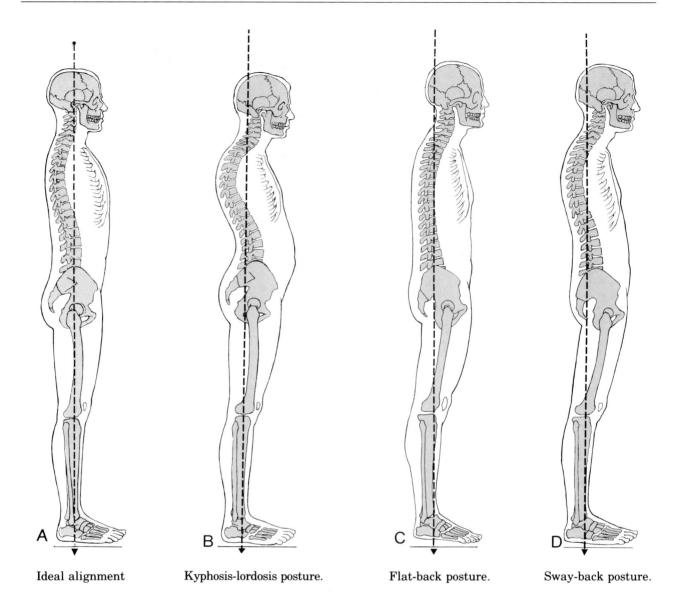

A	B	C	D
Ideal alignment	Kyphosis-lordosis posture.	Flat-back posture.	Sway-back posture.

The *normal curves of the spine* consist of a curve convex forward in the neck (cervical region), convex backward in the upper back (thoracic region), and convex forward in the low back (lumbar region). These may be described as slight extension of the neck, slight flexion of the upper back, and slight extension of the low back. When there is a normal curve in the low back the *pelvis is in a neutral position*. In Figure A, the bony prominences at the front of the pelvis are in the same vertical plane indicating that the pelvis is in neutral position.

In faulty postural position, the pelvis may be in anterior, posterior, or lateral tilt. Any tilting of the pelvis involves simultaneous movements of the low back and hip joints. In *anterior pelvic tilt*, Figure B, the pelvis tilts forward decreasing the angle between the pelvis and the thigh anteriorly, resulting in flexion of the hip joint; the low back arches forward creating an increased forward curve (lordosis) in the low back. In *posterior pelvic tilt*, Figures C and D, the pelvis tilts backward, the hip joints extend and the low back flattens. In *lateral pelvic tilt*, one hip is higher than the other and the spine curves with convexity toward the low side. (For lateral pelvic tilt, see pp. 89, 90, 126, and 222–224.)

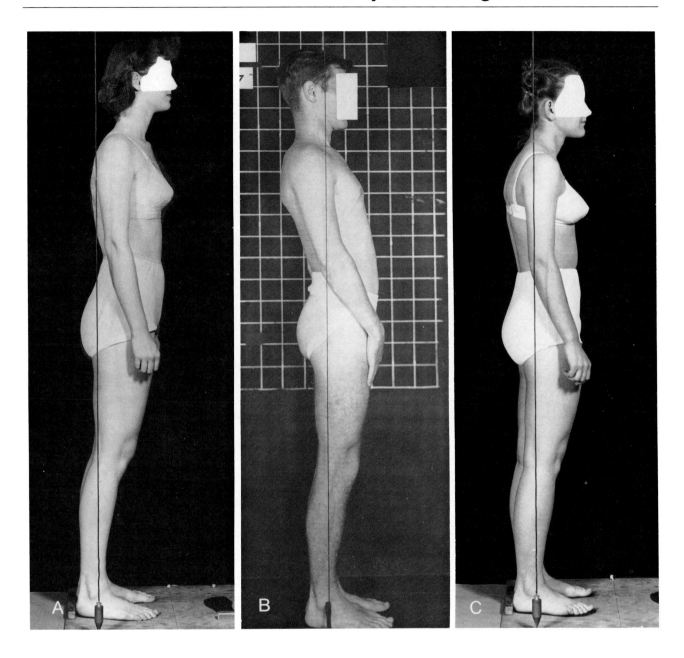

Figure A shows a marked anterior deviation of the body in relation to the plumb line, seen most frequently among tall slender individuals, with body weight carried forward over the balls of the feet. Subjects who habitually stand this way may exhibit strain on the anterior part of the foot with calluses under the ball of the foot and even under the great toe. Metatarsal arch supports may be indicated along with correction of the overall alignment. The ankle joint is in slight dorsiflexion because of the forward inclination of the leg, and the slight flexion of the knee. Posterior muscles of the trunk and lower extremities tend to remain in a state of constant contraction and the alignment must be corrected to achieve relaxation of these muscles effectively.

Figure B shows a marked posterior deviation of the upper trunk and head. The knees and pelvis are displaced anteriorly to counterbalance the posterior thrust of the upper part of the body.

Figure C shows a counterclockwise rotation of the body from the ankles to the cervical region. The deviation of the body from the plumb line appears different from the right and left sides in subjects who have such rotation. The body is anterior from the plumb line as seen from the right, but would show fairly good alignment from the left. From both sides, the head would appear forward.

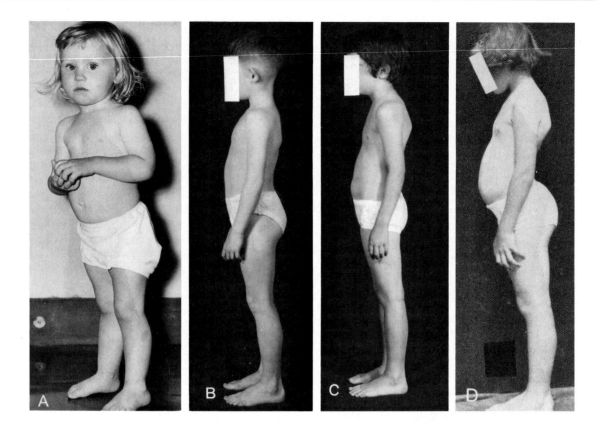

Figure A shows the posture of a small child. The flexed hips and wide stance of this 18-month-old child suggest the uncertain balance associated with this age. Although it is not very evident in the picture, the subject had at this time a mild degree of knock-knees. (This deviation gradually decreased without any corrective measures so that at the age of 6 years, this child's legs were in good alignment.) The development of the longitudinal arch is very good for a child this age.

Figure B shows a 7-year-old child who has very good posture for his age.

Figure C shows poor posture in a 6-year-old child. There is forward head, kyphosis, depressed chest, and there is a tendency toward sway-back posture. Prominence of the scapulae is evident in side view.

Figure D shows a marked lordosis in an 8-year-old child. A corset to hold the back in good alignment and to support the abdomen is needed along with therapeutic exercises when alignment is this faulty.

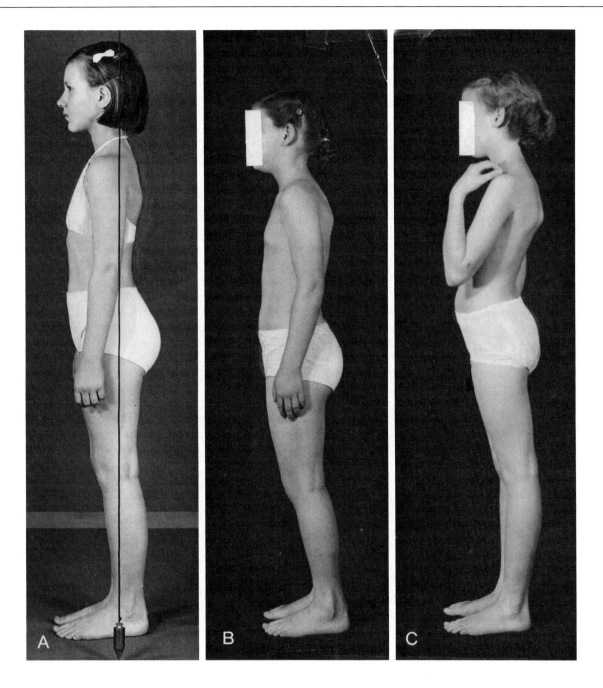

Figure A shows a 10-year-old child who has very good posture for this age. The posture resembles the normal adult posture more than that of the younger child. The curves of the spine are nearly normal and the scapulae are less prominent. It is characteristic of small children to have a protruding abdomen, but there is a noticeable change about the age of 10 to 12 years when the waistline becomes relatively smaller and the abdomen no longer protrudes.

Figure B shows a 9-year-old child whose posture is about average for this age.

Figure C is an 11-year-old child whose posture is very faulty with forward head, kyphosis, lordosis, anterior pelvic tilt, and hyperextended knees.

Lordosis

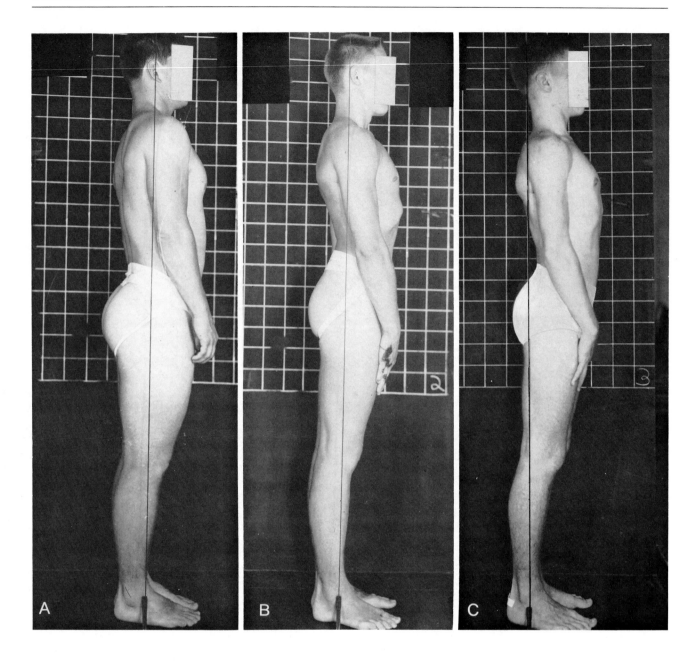

Figure A shows a marked anterior pelvic tilt and a curve that is sharply convex forward in the lumbosacral area. This degree of tilt and lordosis is often associated with marked shortness of the Iliopsoas (hip flexor) muscles. There is slight counterclockwise rotation of the pelvis and trunk.

Figure B shows a high and rather marked lordosis. The lumbar spine is inclined forward to the level of about the second lumbar vertebra. Above this level, there is a sharp deviation backward. This type of posture suggests weakness of the anterior abdominal muscles and shortness of the hip flexors.

Figure C shows an anterior deviation from the plumb line in addition to a marked anterior pelvic tilt and lordosis. This forward deviation from the plumb line compounds the problem of muscle imbalance associated with the segmental alignment faults, and puts strain on the forefoot (see also Figure B (side view), p. 82). (Note the difference in appearance of the feet in Figure C compared to A and B).

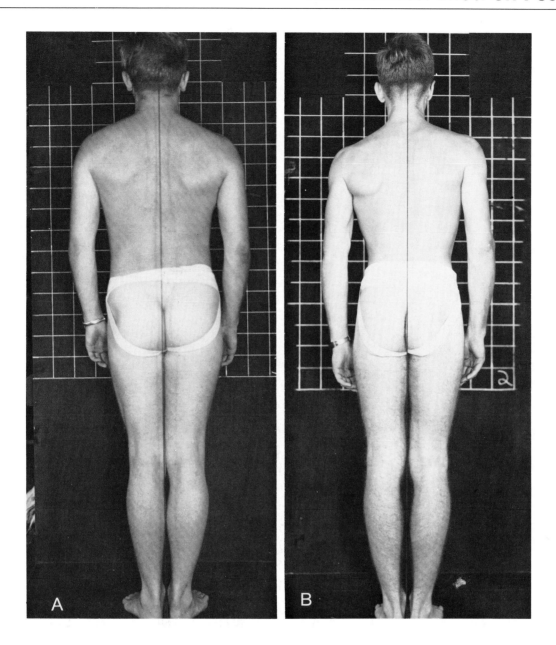

HANDEDNESS PATTERNS

Each of the above figures illustrates a typical pattern of posture as related to handedness. In Figure A, the right shoulder is lower than the left, the pelvis is deviated slightly toward the right, and the right hip appears slightly higher than the left. This pattern is typical of right-handed people. Usually there is a slight deviation of the spine toward the left, and the left foot is more pronated than the right. The right Gluteus medius is usually weaker than the left.

Handedness patterns related to posture may begin at an early age. The slight deviation of the spine toward the side opposite the higher hip may appear as early as age 8 or 10 years. There tends to be a compensatory low shoulder on the side of the higher hip. In most cases, the low shoulder is less significant than the high hip. Usually shoulder correction tends to following correction of lateral pelvic tilt, but the reverse does not necessarily occur.

Figure B shows the opposite pattern, which is typical of left-handed individuals. Usually, however, the low shoulder is not quite as marked as in this subject.

Faulty Posture: Side and Back Views

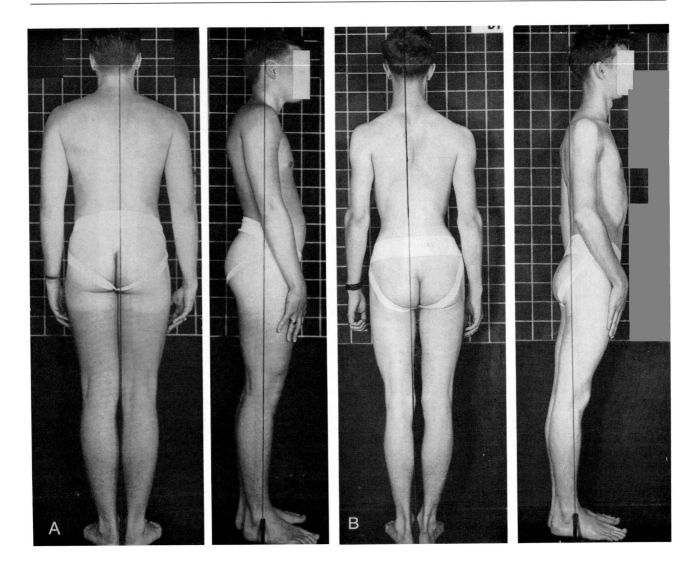

Figure A is an example of posture that appears good in back view but is very faulty in side view.

The side view posture shows marked segmental faults but the anterior and posterior deviations compensate for each other so that the plumb alignment is quite good. The contour of the abdominal wall almost duplicates the curve of the low back.

Figure B shows a posture that is faulty in both side and back views. The back view shows a marked deviation of the body to the right of the plumb line, a high right hip, and a low right shoulder.

In side view, the plumb alignment is worse than the segmental alignment. The knees are posterior, the pelvis, trunk, and head are markedly anterior. Segmentally, the anteroposterior curves of the spine are only slightly exaggerated. The knees, however, are quite hyperextended.

This type of posture may result from the effort to follow such misguided but common admonitions as "Throw your shoulders back" and "Stand with your weight over the balls of your feet."

The result in this subject is so much forward deviation of the trunk and head that the posture is most unstable and requires a good deal of muscular effort to maintain balance.

An individual with this type of fault might appear as one with good posture when fully clothed.

In this, as in the right-hand figure on p. 80, the anterior part of the foot shows evidence of strain.

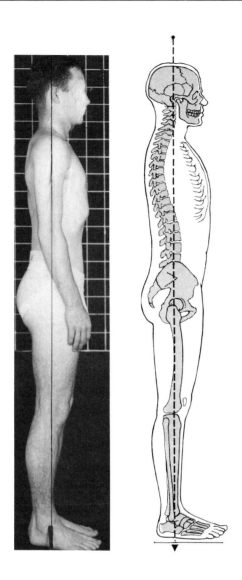

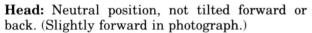

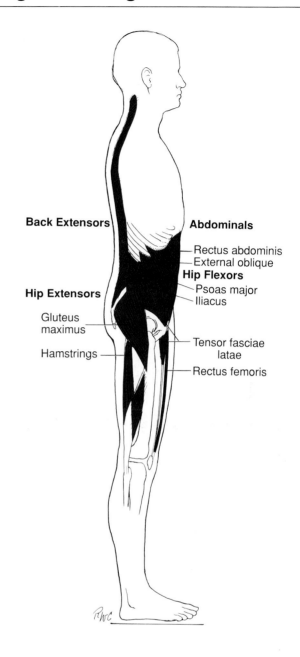

Back Extensors

Abdominals
Rectus abdominis
External oblique
Hip Flexors
Psoas major
Iliacus

Hip Extensors
Gluteus maximus
Tensor fasciae latae
Hamstrings
Rectus femoris

Head: Neutral position, not tilted forward or back. (Slightly forward in photograph.)

Cervical Spine: Normal curve, slightly convex anteriorly.

Scapulae: As seen in the photograph, appear to be in good alignment, flat against upper back.

Thoracic Spine: Normal curve, slightly convex posteriorly.

Lumbar Spine: Normal curve, slightly convex anteriorly.

Pelvis: Neutral position, anterior superior spines in same vertical plane as symphysis pubis.

Hip Joints: Neutral position, neither flexed nor extended.

Knee Joints Neutral position, neither flexed nor hyperextended.

Ankle Joints: Neutral position, leg vertical and at right angle to sole of foot.

In lateral view, the anterior and posterior muscles attached to the pelvis maintain it in ideal alignment. Anteriorly, the abdominal muscles pull upward and the hip flexors pull downward; posteriorly, the back muscles pull upward and the hip extensors pull downward. Thus, the anterior abdominal and hip extensor muscles work together to tilt the pelvis posteriorly; the low back and hip flexor muscles work together to tilt the pelvis anteriorly.

Kyphosis-Lordosis Posture

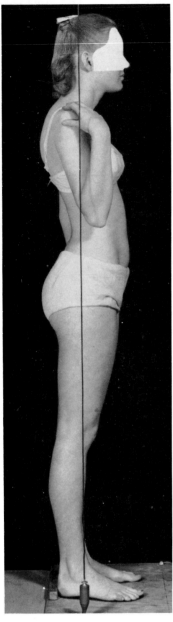
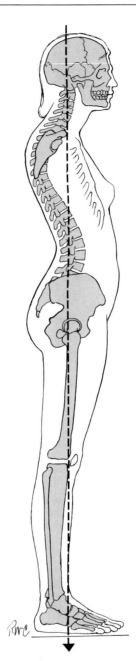
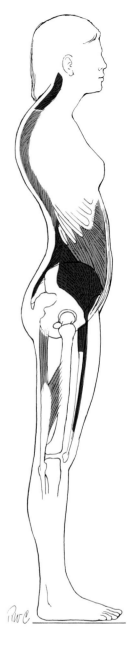

Head: Forward.

Cervical Spine: Hyperextended.

Scapulae: Abducted.

Thoracic Spine: Increased flexion (kyphosis).

Lumbar Spine: Hyperextended (lordosis).

Pelvis: Anterior tilt.

Hip Joints: Flexed.

Knee Joints: Slightly hyperextended.

Ankle Joints: Slight plantar flexion because of the backward inclination of the leg.

Short and Strong: Neck extensors and hip flexors. The low back is strong and may or may not develop shortness.

Elongated and Weak: Neck flexors, upper back Erector spinae, External oblique. Hamstrings are slightly elongated but may or may not be weak.

The Rectus abdominis is not necessarily elongated because the depressed position of the chest offsets the effect of the anterior pelvic tilt.

The lordotic posture in standing and the sitting posture place one-joint hip flexors in a shortened position; sitting allows the low back muscles to elongate as the back flattens. This combination of circumstances has a bearing on the fact that low back muscle shortness is less prevalent than hip flexor shortness in this type of posture.

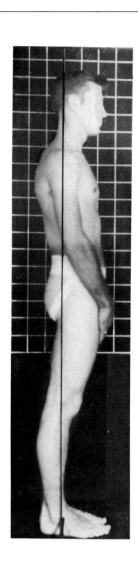
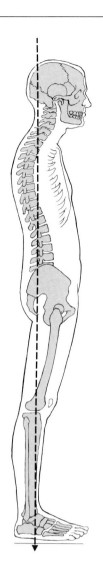

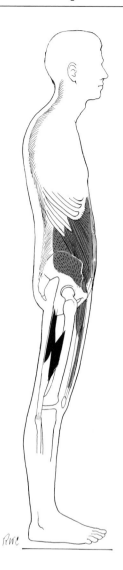

Head: Forward.

Cervical Spine: Slightly extended.

Thoracic Spine: Increased flexion (long kyphosis) with posterior displacement of upper trunk.

Lumbar Spine: Flexion (flattening) of low lumbar area.

Pelvis: Posterior tilt.

Hip Joints: Hyperextended with anterior displacement of pelvis.

Knee Joints: Hyperextended.

Ankle Joints: Neutral. Knee joint hyperextension usually results in plantar flexion of the ankle joint but that does not occur here because of anterior deviation of the pelvis and thighs.

Elongated and Weak: One-joint hip flexors, External oblique, upper back extensors, neck flexors.

Short and Strong: Hamstrings, upper fibers of Internal oblique. Strong but not short: Low back muscles.

The pelvis is in posterior tilt and sways forward in relation to the stationary feet causing the hip joint to extend. The effect is equivalent to extending the leg backward with the pelvis stationary. With posterior pelvic tilt, the lumbar spine flattens and hence there is no lordosis although the long curve in the thoracolumbar region, (which is due to the backward deviation of the upper trunk) is sometimes mistakenly referred to as a lordosis. (The term sway-back posture is an appropriate label and requires that the word "sway-back" not be used synonymously with the word "lordosis.")

85

"Military-Type" Posture

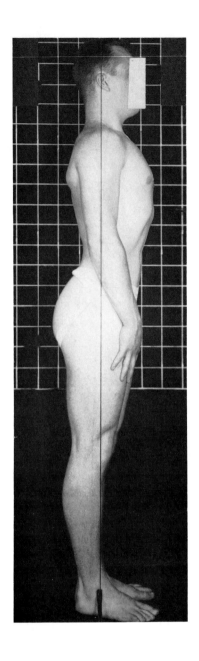
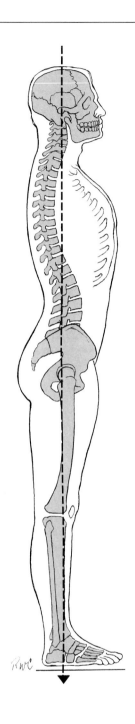
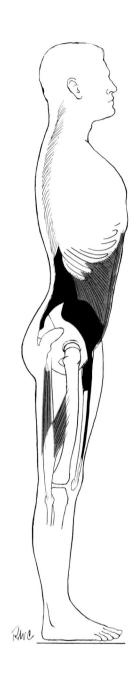

Head: Neutral position.

Cervical Spine: Normal curve, slightly anterior.

Thoracic Spine: Normal curve, slightly posterior.

Lumbar Spine: Hyperextended (lordosis).

Pelvis: Anterior tilt.

Knee Joints: Slightly hyperextended.

Ankle Joints: Slightly plantar flexed.

Elongated and Weak: Anterior abdominals. Hamstring muscles are somewhat elongated but may or may not be weak.

Short and Strong: Low back and hip flexors muscles.

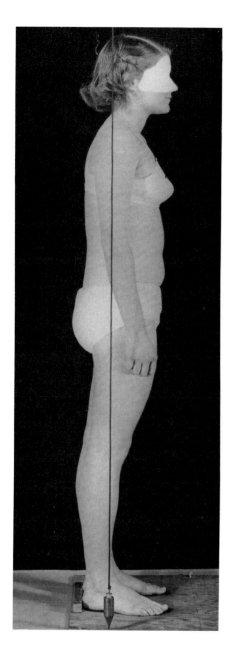

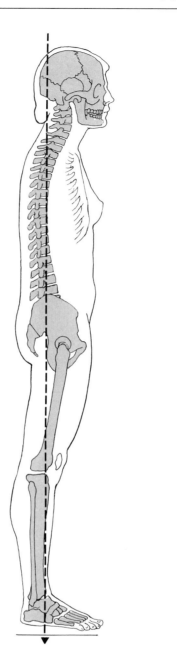

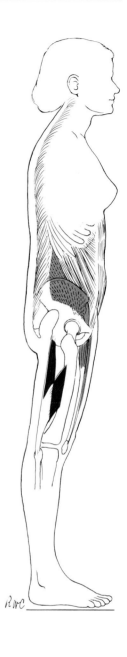

Head: Forward.

Cervical Spine: Slightly extended.

Thoracic Spine: Upper part increased flexion; lower part, straight.

Lumbar Spine: Flexed (straight).

Pelvis: Posterior tilt.

Hip Joints: Extended.

Knee Joints: Extended.

Ankle Joints: Slight plantar flexion.

Elongated and Weak: One-joint hip flexors.

Short and Strong: Hamstrings.

Frequently, abdominal muscles are strong. Although back muscles are slightly elongated when the normal anterior curve is eliminated, they are not weak. Sometimes knees are slightly flexed rather than hyperextended along with the flat-back posture.

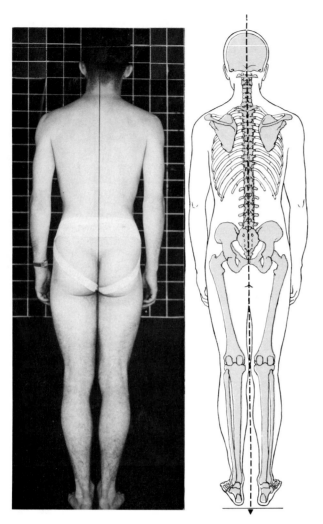

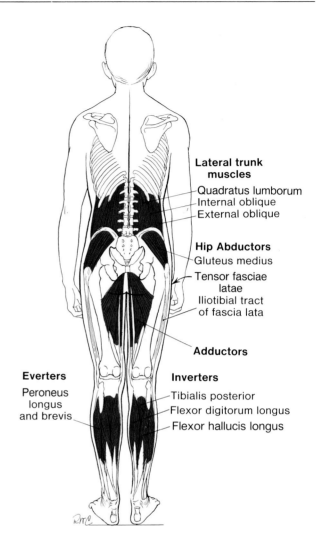

Lateral trunk muscles
Quadratus lumborum
Internal oblique
External oblique

Hip Abductors
Gluteus medius
Tensor fasciae latae
Iliotibial tract of fascia lata

Adductors

Everters
Peroneus longus and brevis

Inverters
Tibialis posterior
Flexor digitorum longus
Flexor hallucis longus

Head: Neutral position, neither tilted nor rotated. (Slightly tilted toward right in photograph.)

Cervical Spine: Straight in drawing. (Slight lateral flexion toward right in photograph.)

Shoulders: Level, not elevated or depressed.

Scapulae: Neutral position, medial borders essentially parallel and about 3 to 4 inches apart.

Thoracic and Lumbar Spines: Straight.

Pelvis: Level, both posterior superior iliac spines in same transverse plane.

Hip Joints: Neutral position, neither adducted nor abducted.

Lower Extremities: Straight, neither bowed nor knock-kneed.

Feet: Parallel or toeing out slightly. Outer malleolus and outer margin of sole of foot in same vertical plane so that foot is not pronated or supinated. (See p. 94.) Tendo calcaneus should be vertical when seen in posterior view; in photograph, alignment suggests slight pronation.

Laterally, the following groups of muscles work together in stabilizing the trunk, pelvis, and lower extremities:

Right lateral trunk flexors
Right hip adductors
Left hip abductors
Right Tibialis posterior
Right Flexor hallucis longus
Right Flexor digitorum longus
Left Peroneus longus and brevis

Left lateral trunk flexors
Left hip adductors
Right hip abductors
Left Tibialis posterior
Left Flexor hallucis longus
Left Flexor digitorum longus
Right Peroneus longus and brevis

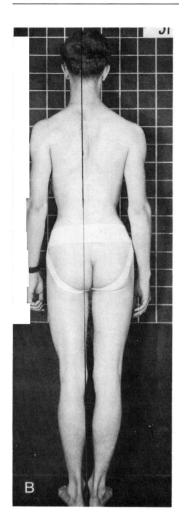

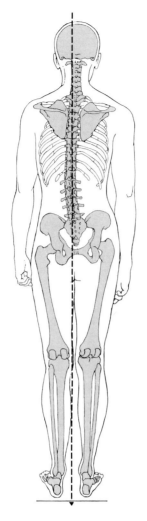

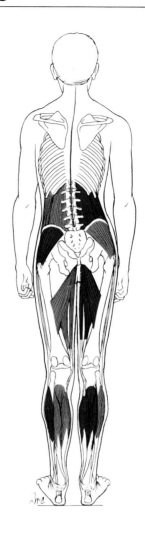

Head: Erect, neither tilted nor rotated. (Slightly tilted and rotated right in photograph.)

Cervical Spine: Straight.

Shoulders: Right low.

Scapulae: Adducted; right slightly depressed.

Thoracic and Lumbar Spines: Thoracolumbar curve convex toward *left*.

Pelvis: Lateral tilt, high on right.

Hip Joints: Right adducted and slightly medially rotated, left abducted.

Lower Extremities: Straight, neither bowed nor knock-kneed.

Feet: In the photograph, the right is slightly pronated as seen in the alignment of the Tendo calcaneus. The left is in a position of slight postural pronation by virtue of the deviation of the body toward the right.

Elongated and Weak: Left lateral trunk muscles, right hip abductors (especially posterior Gluteus medius), left hip adductors, right Peroneus longus and brevis, left Tibialis posterior, left Flexor hallucis longus, left Flexor digitorum longus. The right Tensor fasciae latae may or may not be weak.

Short and Strong: Right lateral trunk muscles, left hip abductors, right hip adductors, left Peroneus longus and brevis, right Tibialis posterior, right Flexor hallucis longus, right Flexor digitorum longus. The left Tensor fasciae latae is usually strong and there may be tightness in the Iliotibial band.

The right leg is in "postural adduction" and the position of the hip gives the appearance of a longer right leg.

This posture is typical of right-handed individuals.

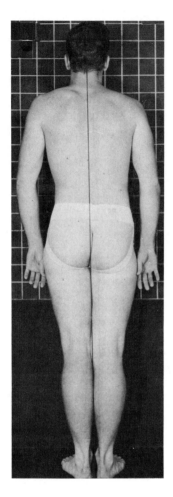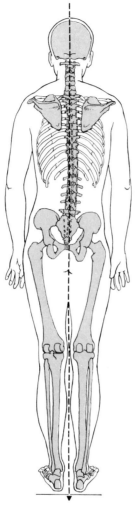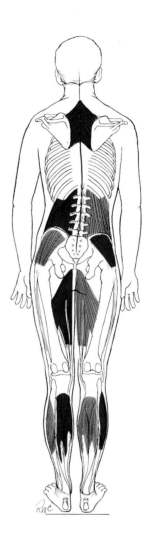

Head: Erect, neither tilted nor rotated.

Cervical spine: Straight.

Shoulders: Elevated and adducted.

Shoulders Joints: Medially rotated as indicated by position of hands facing posteriorly.

Scapulae: Adducted and elevated.

Thoracic and Lumbar Spines: Slight thoracolumbar curve convex toward *right*.

Pelvis: Lateral tilt, higher on left.

Hip Joints: Left adducted and slightly medially rotated, right abducted.

Lower Extremities: Straight, neither bowed nor knock-kneed.

Feet: Slightly pronated.

Elongated and Weak: Right lateral trunk muscles, left hip abductors (especially posterior Gluteus medius), right hip adductors, right Tibialis posterior, right Flexor hallucis longus, right Flexor digitorum longus, left Peroneus longus and brevis.

Short and Strong: Left lateral trunk muscles, right hip abductors, left hip adductors, left Tibialis posterior, left Flexor hallucis longus, left Flexor digitorum longus, right Peroneus longus and brevis. With the elevation and adduction of the scapulae, the Rhomboids are in a shortened position.

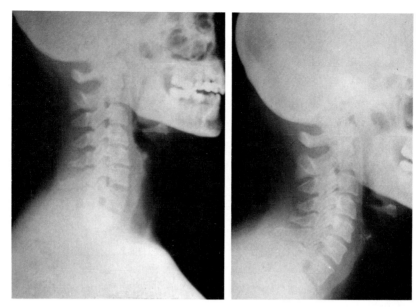

X-rays of a Cervical Spine in Good and Faulty Positions. For the x-ray shown at left, the subject sat erect with the head and upper trunk in good alignment. The x-ray shown on right is the same subject sitting in a typically slumped position with a round upper back and forward head. As illustrated, the cervical spine is in extension.

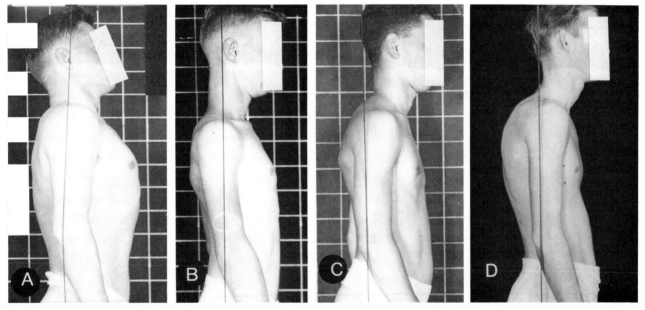

Head, Posterior Tilt. In Figure A, the head tilts backward and there is hyperextension of the cervical spine. The chest and shoulder are held high.

Head, Anterior Tilt. In Figure B, the head is tilted forward and the cervical spine is in flexion.

A posture in which the normal anterior curve of the cervical spine tends to reverse, as it does in this subject is abnormal and unusual.

Forward Head with Attempted Correction. The subject in Figure C is apparently trying to correct what is basically a forward position. The curve of the neck begins in a typical way in the low cervical region, but a sharp angulation occurs at about the sixth cervical vertebra. Above this level, the curve seems very much decreased. The chin is pressed against the front of the throat. This distorted, rather than corrected, position of the neck results from a failure to correct the related faulty position of the upper trunk.

Forward Head, Marked. In Figure D, the subject shows an extremely faulty alignment of the neck and thoracic spine. The degree of deformity in the thoracic spine is suggestive of an epiphysitis. This patient was treated for pain in the posterior neck and occipital region.

Shoulders and Scapulae

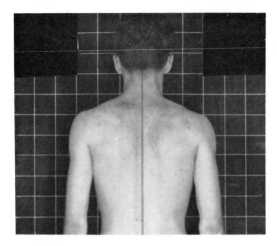

Shoulders and Scapulae, Good Position. This subject illustrates a good position of the shoulders and scapulae.

The scapulae lie flat against the thorax and no angle or border is unduly prominent. Their position is not distorted by unusual muscular development or misdirected efforts at postural correction.

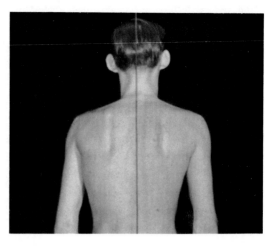

Scapulae, Abducted and Slightly Elevated. In this subject, both scapulae are abducted, the left one more than the right. They are slightly elevated. This kind of elevation goes with round shoulders and round upper back. (For side view of this subject see p. 91, Figure D.)

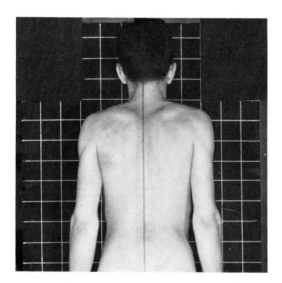

Shoulders Elevated, Scapulae Adducted. In this subject, both shoulders are elevated with the right slightly higher than the left. The scapulae are adducted. The upper Trapezius and other shoulder elevators are tight.

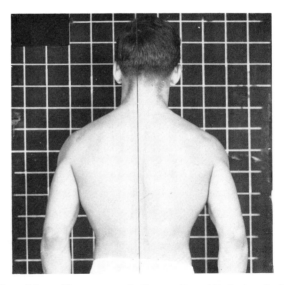

Shoulders Depressed, Scapulae Abducted. In this subject, the shoulders slope downward sharply, accentuating their natural broadness. The marked abduction of the scapulae also contributes to this effect.

Exercises to strengthen the Trapezius muscles, especially the upper part, are needed to correct the faulty posture of the shoulders.

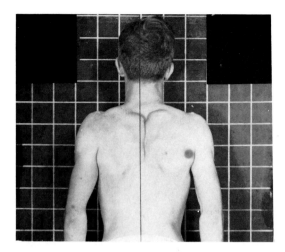

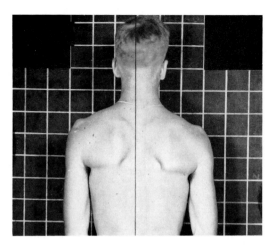

Scapulae, Adducted and Elevated. In this subject, the scapulae are completely adducted and considerably elevated.

The position illustrated appears to be held by voluntary effort but, if this habit persists, the scapulae will not return to normal position when the subject tries to relax.

This position is the inevitable end result of engaging in the military practice of "bracing" the shoulders back.

Scapulae, Abnormal Appearance. This subject shows abnormal development of some of the scapular muscles with a faulty position of the scapulae.

The Teres major and Rhomboids, that are clearly visible, form a V at the inferior angle. The scapula is rotated so that the axillary border is more nearly horizontal than normal. The appearance suggests weakness of either the Serratus anterior or the Trapezius or both.

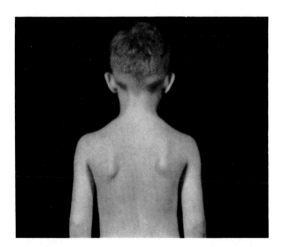

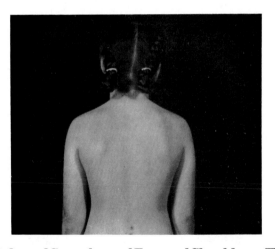

Adducted and Slightly Winged Scapulae. This subject shows a degree of scapular prominence that is seen rather frequently among children of this age (8 years). Slight prominence and slight abduction need not be a matter of concern at this age but this subject is borderline and there is a difference in the level of the scapulae that indicates additional muscle imbalance.

Abducted Scapulae and Forward Shoulders. This subject is a 9-year-old girl who is rather mature for her age. The forward position of the shoulders is typical of that assumed by many young girls at the time of beginning development of the breasts. When such a postural habit persists, it may result in a fixed postural fault. See page 79B for sideview of this subject.

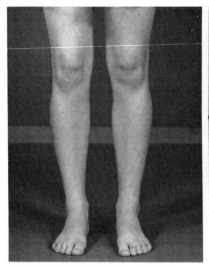

Good Alignment of Feet and Knees. The patellae face directly forward and the feet are neither pronated nor supinated.

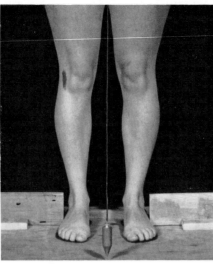

Pronation of Feet and Medial Rotation of Femurs. The distance between the lateral malleolus and the foot board indicates a moderate pronation of the feet, and the position of the patellae indicates a moderate degree of medial rotation of the femurs.

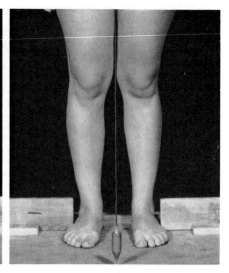

Pronation of Feet and Knock-knees. The feet are moderately pronated; there is slight knock-knee position, but no medial or lateral rotation.

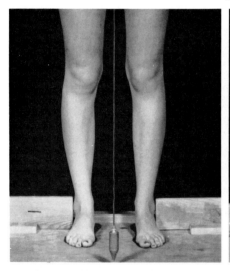

Feet Good, Knees Faulty. The alignment of the feet is very good but there is medial rotation of the femurs as indicated by the position of the patellae. This fault is harder to correct by use of shoe corrections than one in which pronation accompanies the medial rotation.

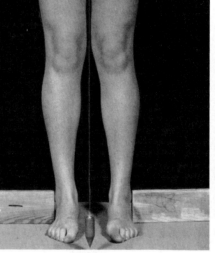

Supinated Feet. The weight is borne on the outer borders of the feet, and the long arches are higher than normal. The perpendicular foot board touches the lateral malleolus, but is not in contact with the outer border of the sole of the foot.

It appears as if an effort were being made to invert the feet because the anterior tibial muscles are so prominent, but the position shown is the natural posture of this subject's feet.

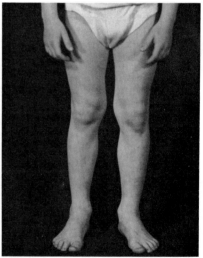

Lateral Rotation of the Legs. The lateral rotation of the legs as seen in this subject is the result of lateral rotation at the hip joint.

This position is more typical of boys than of girls. It may or may not have serious effects, although persistence of such a pattern in walking as well as in standing puts undue strain on the longitudinal arches.

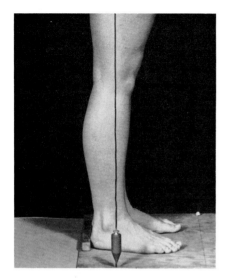

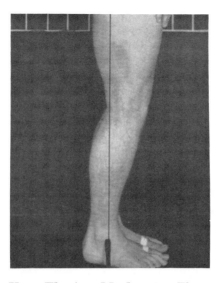

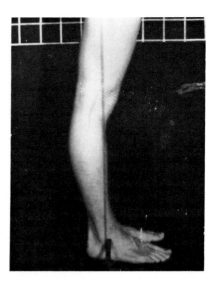

Knees, Good Alignment. In good alignment of the knees in side view, the plumb line passes slightly anterior to the axis of the knee joint.

Knee Flexion, Moderate. Flexion of the knees is seen less frequently than hyperextension in cases of faulty posture. The flexed position requires constant muscular effort by the Quadriceps. Knee flexion in standing may result from hip flexor tightness. When hip flexors are tight there must be compensatory alignment faults of the knees or the low back or both. Attempting to reduce a lordosis by flexing the knees in standing is not an appropriate solution when hip flexor stretching is needed.

Knee Hyperextension. With marked hyperextension of the knee, the ankle joint is in plantar flexion.

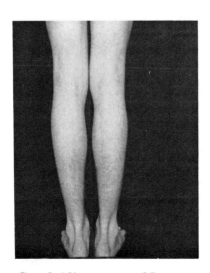

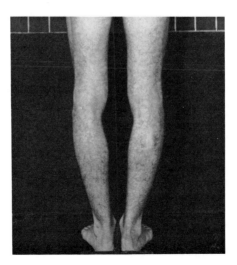

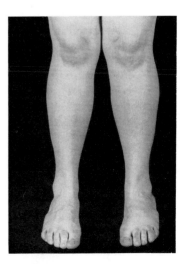

Good Alignment of Legs.

Bowlegs. This figure shows a mild degree of structural bowlegs (genu varum).

Knock-knees. This figure shows a moderate degree of structural knock-knees (genu valgum).

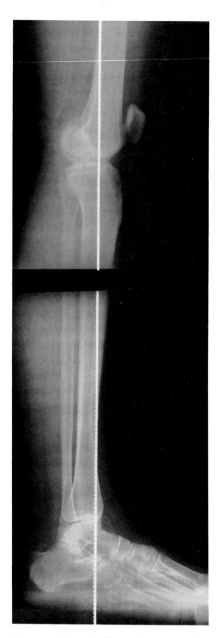 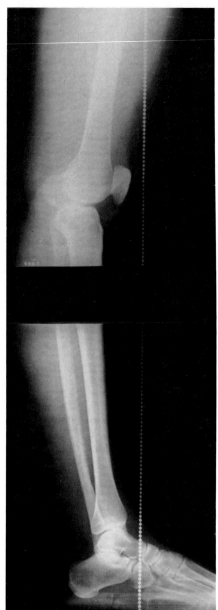 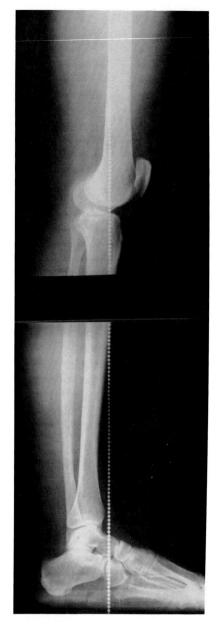

For each of the photographs above, a beaded metal plumb line was suspended beside the subject when the x-ray was taken. Two x-ray films were in position for the single exposure. The above illustration shows the relationship of the plumb line to the bones of the foot and lower leg, with the subject standing in a position of good alignment.

This is an x-ray of a subject who had a habit of standing in hyperextension. The plumb line was suspended in line with the standard base point while the x-ray was taken. Note the change in position of the patella, and the compression anteriorly of the knee joint.

The above x-ray is of the same subject shown in center figure. As an adult, she attempted to correct her hyperextension fault. The alignment through the knee joint and femur are very good, but the tibia and fibula show evidence of posterior bowing. (Compare with the good alignment of these bones as seen in the figure at far left.)

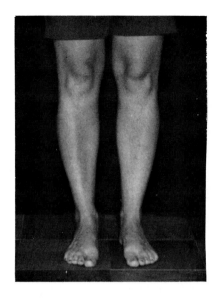
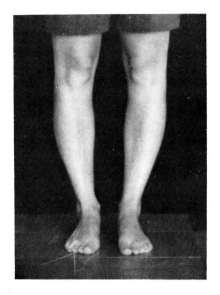
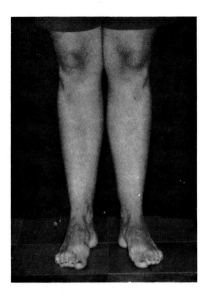

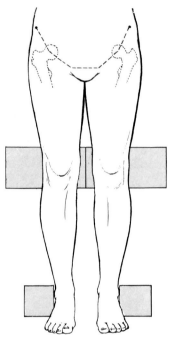
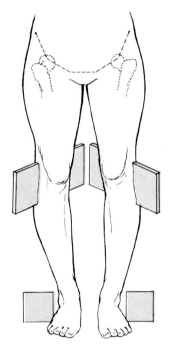
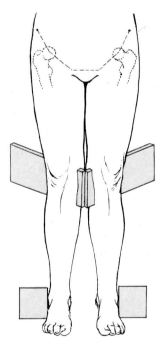

IDEAL ALIGNMENT   **POSTURAL BOWLEGS**   **POSTURAL KNOCK-KNEES**

In ideal alignment, the hips are neutral in rotation as evidenced by the position of the patellae facing directly forward. The axis of the knee joint is in the coronal plane and flexion and extension occur in the sagittal plane. The feet are in good alignment.

Postural bowlegs results from a combination of medial rotation of the femurs, pronation of the feet, and hyperextension of the knees. When femurs medially rotate, the axis of motion for flexion and extension is oblique to the coronal plane. From this axis, hyperextension occurs in a posterolateral direction, resulting in a separation at the knees and apparent bowing of the legs.

Postural knock-knees results from a combination of lateral rotation of the femurs, supination of the feet, and hyperextension of the knees. With lateral rotation, the axis of the knee joint is oblique to the coronal plane and hyperextension results in adduction at the knees.

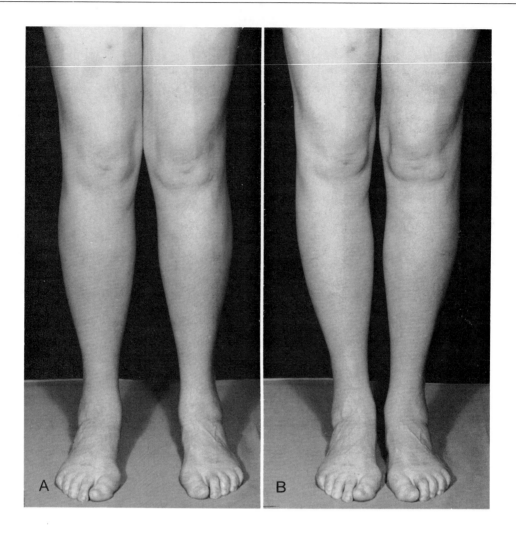

Mechanism of Postural Bowing Compensatory for Knock-Knees.

Figure A shows the position of knock-knees that the subject exhibits when the knees are in good anteroposterior alignment.

Figure B shows that by hyperextending her knees, the subject is able to produce enough postural bowing to accommodate for the 4-inch separation of her feet in Figure A.

See Figure A on the previous page for the extent of postural bowing that can be produced by hyperextension in an individual who has no knock-knee condition.

Children are often embarrassed by the appearance of knock-knees, and it is not uncommon for them to compensate if the knock-knee condition persists. Sometimes they "hide" the knock-knee position by flexing one knee and hyperextending the other so the knees can be close together. Rotation faults may result if the same knee is habitually flexed while the other is hyperextended.

The appearance of postural bowlegs and postural knock-knees also may result from the combination of knee flexion with rotation, but is not illustrated. With lateral rotation and slight flexion, legs will appear slightly bowed, and with medial rotation and slight flexion, there will appear to be a position of knock-knees. These variations associated with flexion are of less concern than those associated with hyperextension because flexion is a normal movement while hyperextension is an abnormal one.

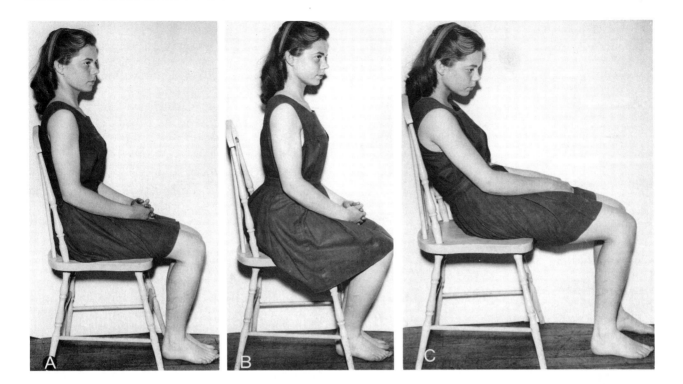

Maintaining good alignment of the body in the sitting position can reduce or prevent pain associated with posture-related problems. In Figure A there is good alignment. This allows for the greatest ease since the least amount of muscle energy is expended. Figure B is sometimes mistakenly considered a correct sitting position. The low back is in a lordosis, the back muscles fatigue, and this position can be maintained only with effort. The familiar slumped position in Figure C results in strain from lack of support for the low back and results in very faulty position of upper back, neck, and head.

Generally people are advised to sit with feet flat on the floor or with feet crossed, and to avoid crossing knees. If knees are crossed, they should be alternated so that they are not always crossed in the same manner. While some people, especially those with problems of poor circulation in the legs, should avoid sitting with knees crossed, there is good reason why so many people sit this way. Unless a person is sitting in a chair that gives adequate support to the low back, there is a tendency, when sitting erect, for the pelvis to tilt forward to the point of arching the low back. If the knees are crossed, the pelvis does not tilt forward, and the hips and low back are in a stable position.

Some people may be comfortable in a chair with a pad in the lumbar area. Others may experience discomfort and even pain from such a lumbar support. Certain people find that a contoured pad in the sacroiliac area, or a chair that is rounded to conform to the body in that area, will enable them to sit without discomfort.

There is no one correct chair. The height and depth of the chair must be appropriate to the individual. The chair should be of a height that allows the feet to rest comfortably on the floor and thereby avoid pressure on the back of the thighs. In a chair that is too deep from front to back, either the back will be unsupported or there will be undue pressure against the lower leg. Hips and knees should be at approximately a 90° angle and the back of the chair should incline about 10°. The sitting position can be comfortable if the chair and additional props maintain the body in good alignment.

Procedure for Postural Examination

Postural examination consists of three essential parts: 1) examination of the alignment in standing; 2) tests for flexibility and muscle length; and 3) tests for muscle strength.

EQUIPMENT

The equipment used (see facing page) consists of the following:

Posture Boards. These are boards on which footprints have been drawn. Footprints may be painted on the floor of the examining room, but the posture boards have the advantage of being portable. (See lower photograph on facing page.)

Plumb Line. The plumb line is suspended from an overhead bar, and the plumb bob is hung in line with the point on the posture board that indicates the standard base point, i.e., anterior to lateral malleolus in side view, midway between the heels in back view.

Folding Ruler with Spirit Level. This is used to measure the difference in level of posterior iliac spines. It may be used also to detect any differences in shoulder level. A background with squares (as shown in many of the photographs) is a more practical aid in detecting differences in shoulder level.

Set of Six Blocks. These measure 4 inches by 10 inches and are of the following thicknesses: 1/8, 1/4, 3/8, 1/2, 3/4, and 1 inch. They are used for the purpose of determining the amount of lift needed to level the pelvis laterally. This method is preferred to the use of leg length measurement for this purpose (see discussion p. 103).

Marking Pencil. The pencil is used for marking the spinous processes in order to observe the position of the spine in cases of lateral deviation.

Tape Measure. This may be used in taking leg length measurements, and for measuring forward bending in reaching fingertips toward, or beyond, toes.

Chart for Recording Examination Findings. (See p. 105.)

Appropriate Clothing. Clothing, such as a two-piece bathing suit for girls or trunks for boys, should be worn by subjects for a postural examination. Postural examination of school children is unsatisfactory when attempts are made to examine children clothed in ordinary gym suits.

In hospital clinics, gowns or other suitable garb should be provided.

ALIGNMENT IN STANDING

The subject stands on the posture boards with feet in the position indicated by the footprints.

Anterior View. Observe the position of the feet, knees, and legs. Toe positions, appearance of the longitudinal arch, alignment in regard to pronation or supination of the foot, rotation of the femur as indicated by the position of the patella, knock-knees or bowlegs should be noted. Any rotation of the head, or abnormal appearance of the ribs should also be noted. Findings are recorded on the chart under "Segmental Alignment."

Lateral View. With the plumb line hung in line with a point just anterior to lateral malleolus, the relationship of the body as a whole to the plumb line is noted and recorded under "Plumb Alignment." It should be observed from both right and left sides for the purpose of detecting rotation faults. Such descriptions as the following may be used in recording findings: "Body anterior from ankles up," "pelvis and head anterior," "good except lordosis," "upper trunk and head posterior."

Segmental alignment faults may be noted with or without the plumb line. Observe whether the knees are in good alignment, hyperextended, or flexed; note the position of the pelvis as seen from side view; whether the anteroposterior curves of the spine are normal or exaggerated; head position, forward or tilted up or down; chest position, whether normal, depressed, or elevated; and the contour of the abdominal wall. Findings are recorded on the chart under "Segmental Alignment."

Posterior View. With the plumb line hung in line with a point midway between the heels, the relationship of the body or parts of the body to the plumb line are expressed as good, or as deviations toward the right or left, and are so recorded on the chart. *In examining scoliosis patients, it is especially important to observe the relationship of the overall posture to the plumb line.* Suspending a plumb line in line with the seventh cervical vertebra, or the buttocks crease (as is frequently done) may be useful in ascertaining the curvature of the spine itself, but does not reveal the extent to which the spine may be compensating for a lateral shift of the pelvis or other postural faults that contribute to lateral pelvic tilt and associated spinal deviations.

From the standpoint of segmental alignment, one should note the alignment of the tendo calcaneous, postural adduction or abduction of the hips, relative height of the posterior iliac spines, lateral pelvic tilt, lateral deviations of the spine, position of the shoulders and of the scapulae. For example, a lateral pelvic tilt may occur as a result of one foot being pronated or one knee being habitually flexed, see p. 367, allowing a dropping of the pelvis on that side in standing. In scoliosis

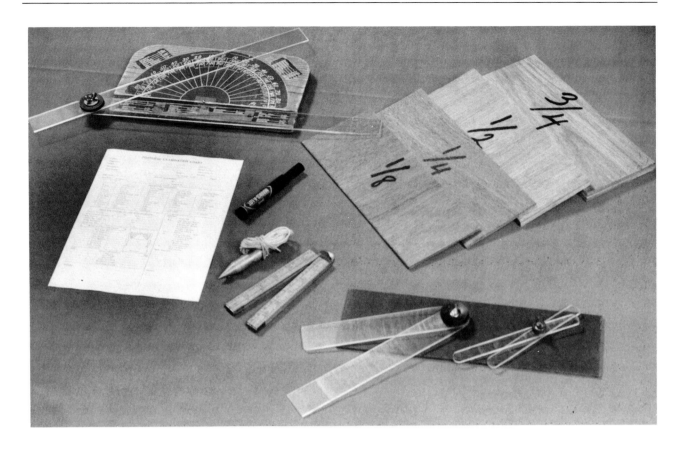

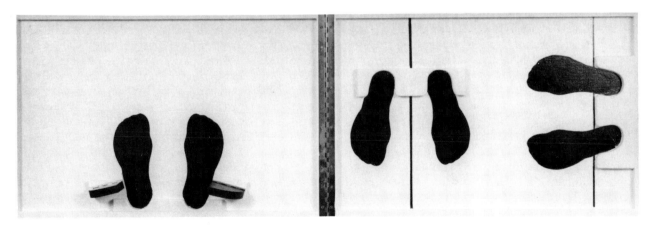

Equipment used for postural examination: Postural examination chart, plumb line, set of blocks, ruler with spirit level, protractor and calipers, board for measuring angle of sacrum with table, marking pencil and posture boards.

patients, it is important to observe any asymmetrical segmental faults that may give rise to lateral pelvic tilts and accompanying deviations of the spine. Rotation of the spine or thorax, as seen in scoliosis cases, is observed with the patient bending forward. When forward bending from a standing position, rotation of the bodies of the vertebrae is seen as a fullness or prominence on the side of convexity in a structural (fixed) curve of the spine. However, in a functional curve, there may be no evidence of rotation in forward bending. This is especially true if the functional curve is associated with hip abductor imbalance resulting in lateral pelvic tilt, or of anterior abdominal muscle imbalance because the effects of these imbalances on the spine are minimized in forward bending. Findings are recorded under "Segmental Alignment."

TESTS FOR FLEXIBILITY AND MUSCLE LENGTH

In this group are the tests for muscle length as described in Chapter 3. Findings are recorded on the chart in the space provided. Forward bending is recorded as "Normal," "Limited," or "Normal +," with the number of inches from, or beyond, the toes recorded. (See p. 48 and charts p. 112 regarding normal for various ages in this test.) On the chart, "Bk" indicates back, "H.S.," Hamstrings, and "G.S.," Gastroc-soleus.

Forward bending may be checked in the standing or sitting position, but the authors consider the test in sitting more indicative of flexibility. If flexibility is normal in sitting and limited in standing, there is usually some rotation or lateral tilt of the pelvis resulting in rotation of the lumbar spine, which in turn restricts the flexion in the standing position.

Findings in regard to the arm overhead elevation tests may be recorded as normal or limited, and, if limited, as slight, moderate, or marked.

Trunk extension is the movement of backward bending, and may be done in the standing position to help differentiate the flexibility of the back from the strength of the back muscles as done in the prone position. (See discussion, p. 50.) Normally the back should arch in the lumbar region. If hyperextension is limited, the subject may try to simulate the backward bending by flexing knees and leaning backward. Knees should be kept straight during the test.

Lateral flexion movements are used to test for lateral flexibility of the trunk. The length of the left lateral trunk muscles permit range of motion for trunk bending toward the right, and vice versa. In other words, if flexibility of the trunk toward the right is limited it should be interpreted as some muscle tightness of the left lateral trunk muscles unless, of course, there is the element of limited spinal motion due to ligamentous or joint tightness.

Among other things, the variation among individuals in length of torso and in space between the ribs and iliac crest make for differences in flexibility. It is impractical to try to measure the degree of lateral flexion. Range of motion is considered to be normal for the individual when the rib cage and iliac crest are closely approximated in side bending. Most people can bring the fingertips to about the level of the knee when bending directly sideways (See discussion, p. 51.)

MUSCLE STRENGTH TESTS

Muscle tests essential in postural examinations are described in Chapters 6, 7, and 8. They include tests of the upper, lower, and oblique abdominals, lateral trunk flexors, back extensors, middle and lower Trapezius, Serratus anterior, Gluteus medius, Gluteus maximus, Hamstrings, hip flexors, Soleus and toe flexors.

In problems of anteroposterior deviations in postural alignment, it is especially important to test the abdominal muscles, back muscles, the hip flexors and extensors, and the Soleus. In problems of lateral deviation of the spine or lateral tilt of the pelvis, it is especially important to test the oblique abdominal muscles, lateral trunk flexors, and the Gluteus medius.

INTERPRETATION OF TEST FINDINGS

In the usual case of faulty posture, the pattern of faulty body mechanics as determined by the alignment test will be confirmed by the muscle tests if both procedures have been accurate. At times, there may be an apparent discrepancy in test findings. The inconsistency may be based on such things as the following: The effects of an old injury or disease may have altered the alignment pattern particularly as related to handedness patterns; effects of a recent illness or injury may have been superimposed on an established pattern of imbalance; or a child with a lateral curvature of the spine may be in a transition stage between a C-curve and an S-curve.

Except in flexible children, the postural faults seen at the time of examination will usually correspond with the habitual faults of the individual. With children it is necessary and advisable to do repeated tests of alignment, and to obtain information regarding the habitual posture from the parent and teacher who see them frequently. It is also advisable to keep photographic records of children's posture for a really worthwhile evaluation of postural changes in growing children.

It is of particular importance that girls between the ages of 10 and 14 years have periodic examination of the spine because more spinal curvatures occur in girls than in boys, and usually appear between these ages.

LEG LENGTH MEASUREMENTS

So-called "actual leg length" is a measurement of length from the anterior-superior spine of the ilium to the medial malleolus. Obviously such a measurement is not an absolutely accurate determination of leg length because the points of measurement are from a landmark on the pelvis to one on the leg. Since it is impossible to palpate a point on the femur under the anterior superior spine, it is necessary to use the landmark of the pelvis. It becomes necessary, therefore, to fix the alignment of the pelvis in relation to the trunk and legs before taking measurements to insure the same relationship of both extremities to the pelvis. Pelvic rotation or lateral tilt will change the relationship of the pelvis to the extremities enough to make a considerable difference in measurement. To obtain as much accuracy as possible, the patient lies supine on a table with trunk, pelvis, and legs in straight alignment and legs close together. The distance from the anterior superior spine to the umbilicus is measured on right and left to check against lateral pelvic tilt or rotation. If there is a difference in measurements, the pelvis is leveled and any rotation corrected so far as possible before leg length measurements are taken.

"Apparent leg length" is a measurement from the umbilicus to the medial malleolus. This type of measurement is more often a source of confusion than an aid in determining differences in length for the purpose of applying a lift to correct pelvic tilt. The confusion arises because the picture in standing is the reverse of that in lying, and occurs when the pelvic tilt is due to muscle imbalance rather than actual leg length difference.

In *standing*, a fault in alignment will result when a weak muscle fails to provide adequate support for weight bearing. For example, a weakness of the right Gluteus medius allows the pelvis to deviate toward the right and elevate on that side, giving the appearance of a *longer* right leg. If the postural fault has been of long standing, there is usually an associated imbalance in the lateral trunk muscles in which the right laterals are shorter and stronger than the left. (See p. 89.)

In *lying,* a fault in alignment will more often result from the pull of a strong muscle. In the supine position, an individual with the type of imbalance described above (i.e., a weak right Gluteus medius and strong right laterals) will tend to lie with the pelvis higher on the right, pulled up by the stronger lateral abdominal muscles. This position in turn draws the right leg up so that it appears *shorter* than the left.

It is recommended that the need for an elevation on a shoe be determined by measurements in the standing rather than lying position. The boards of various thicknesses (see p. 100) are used for this purpose. (See, also, apparent leg length discrepancy due to muscle imbalance, p. 224.)

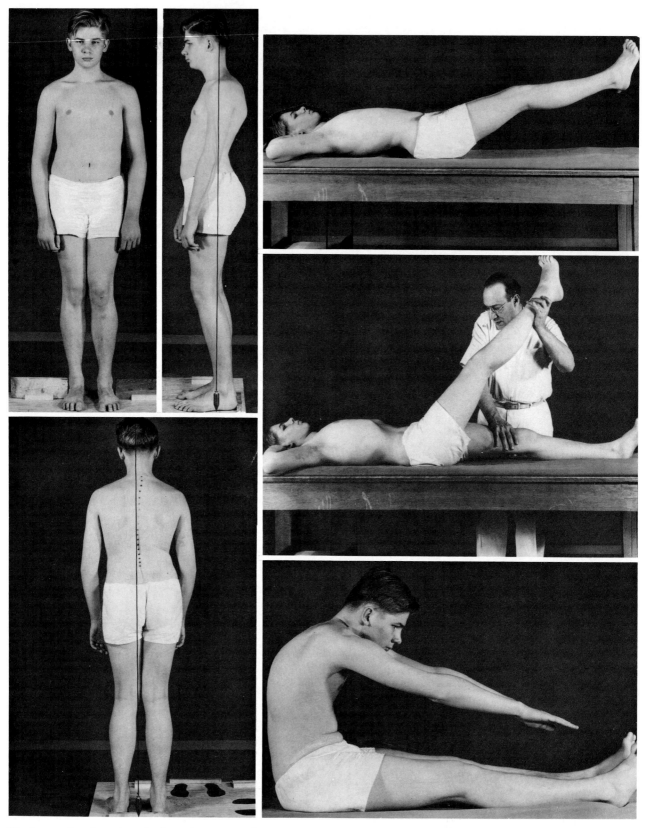

Photographs showing faulty alignment, limitation of motion in flexibility tests, and abdominal muscle weakness. Examination findings in this case are recorded on the *Postural Examination Chart* on the facing page.

POSTURAL EXAMINATION CHART

Name *D.L.*   Doctor ⎯

Diagnosis *Faulty posture*   Date of 1st Ex. ⎯

Onset   Date of 2nd Ex. ⎯

Occupation *High school student*   Height ⎯ Weight ⎯

Handedness *Right*   Age *17*   Sex *M*   Leg length: Left ⎯   Right ⎯

PLUMB ALIGNMENT

Side view: Lt. *Knee, pelvis, and head anterior* Rt. *(Same as from left)*

Back view: Deviated lt.   Deviated rt. *Body from feet upward*

SEGMENTAL ALIGNMENT

	Feet	X	Hammer toes		Hallux valgus		Low ant. arch			Ant. foot varus
		L	Pronated >		Supinated		Flat long. arch			Pigeon toes
		B	Med. rotat *R > L*		Lat. rotat.	B	Knock-knees *slight*			Tibial torsion
	Knees		Hyperext. >	B	Flexed *L > R*		Bowlegs			Tibial torsion
	Pelvis	R	Leg in postural add.		Rotation	Ant.	Tilt	Ant.	Deviation
	Low back	X	Lordosis *marked*		Flat		Kyphosis			Operation
	Up. back	X	Kyphosis		Flat	B	Scap. abducted *R>L*			Scap. elevated
	Thorax	X	Depressed chest		Elevated chest		Rotation	Post.	Deviation *slight*
	Spine		Total curve	L	Lumbar *– Thoracic*		Thoracic	R	Cervical *– Thoracic*
	Abdomen	X	Protruding *slight*		Scars					
	Shoulder		Low		High	B	Forward	B	Med. rotated
	Head	X	Forward		Torticollis		Tilt			Rotation

TESTS FOR FLEXIBILITY AND MUSCLE LENGTH

Forward bending: *Limited 7"* Bk. *Tight* H.S. *Tight* G.S. *Sl. tight*

Arm overhead elevation: Lt. *Slightly limited* Rt. *Normal length*

Hip flexors: Lt. *Marked tightness* Rt. *Marked tightness*

Tensor fas. lata: Lt. *Slight tightness* Rt. *Normal length*

Trunk extension: *Normal range*

Trunk lat. flex.: To lt. *Slightly limited* To rt. *Normal range*

MUSCLE STRENGTH TESTS

L		R
7	Mid. trapezius	7
(6)	Low. trapezius	6
10	Back extensors	10
10	Glut. medius	7
10	Glut. maximus	10
10	Hamstrings	10
10	Hip flexors	10
8	Tib. posterior	10
Weak	Toe flexors	Weak

R   9   TRUNK RAISING   *Slight weakness*   5   LEG LOWERING   L

SHOE CORRECTION

Left		Right
1/8"	(Wide Heel) Inner wedge (Narrow heel)	
3/16"	Level heel raise	
Medium, bar	Metatarsal support	Medium, bar
	Longitudinal support	

NOTES:

TREATMENT

Exercises:

Bk. Lying	Pel. tilt and breath.	X
	Pel. tilt and leg sl.	X
	Head and sh. raising	(omit)
	Shoulder add. stretch	X
	Straight leg-raise	X
	Hip flex. stretch	X
Sd. Lying	Stretch *left* tensor	X
Sitting	Forward bending	
	To stretch low bk.	X
	To stretch h. s.	X
	Wall-sitting	
	Middle trapezius	X
	Lower trapezius	X
Standing	Foot and knee ex.	X
	Wall-standing	X

Other Exercises:

Stretching toe extensors

Cross-sectional exercise for left

External oblique and right

Internal oblique

Support:

Key: *Segmental Alignment:* X, postural defect present; L, left; R, right; B, both; Ant., anterior; Post., posterior. *Tests for Flexibility and Muscle Length:* Bk., back; H.S., Hamstring; G.S., Gastroc-soleus.

105

Faulty Posture, Side View: Analysis and Treatment

Postural Fault	Anatomical Position of Joints	Muscles in Shortened Position	Muscles in Lengthened Position	Treatment procedures, if indicated on the basis of tests for alignment and muscle length and strength tests
Lordosis posture	Lumbar spine hyperextension Pelvis, anterior tilt Hip joint flexion	Low back Erector spinae Hip flexors	Abdominals, especially External oblique Hip extensors	Stretch low back muscles, if tight. Strengthen abdominals by posterior pelvic tilt exercises, and if indicated, by trunk curl. Avoid situps because they shorten hip flexors. Stretch hip flexors, when short. Strengthen hip extensors, if weak. Instruct regarding proper body alignment. Depending upon degree of lordosis and extent of muscle weakness and pain, use support (corset) to relieve strain on abdominals, and to help correct the lordosis.
Flat-back posture	Lumbar spine flexion Pelvis, posterior tilt Hip joint extension	Anterior abdominals Hip extensors	Low back Erector spinae Hip flexors (one-joint)	Low back muscles are seldom weak, but if they are weak, do exercises to strengthen them and to restore normal anterior curve. Tilt pelvis forward, bringing low back into anterior curve. *Avoid* prone hyperextension because it increases posterior pelvic tilt and stretches hip flexors. (See p. 355.) Instruct in proper body alignment. If back is painful and in need of support, apply corset that holds the back in a position of normal anterior lumbar curve. Strengthen hip flexors to help produce normal anterior lumbar curve. Stretch Hamstrings, if tight.
Sway-back posture (Pelvis displaced forward, upper trunk backward)	Lumbar spine position depends on level of posterior displacement of upper trunk Pelvis, posterior tilt Hip joint extension	Upper anterior abdominals especially upper Rectus and Internal oblique Hip extensors	Lower anterior abdominals especially External oblique Hip flexors (one-joint)	Strengthen lower abdominals (stress External oblique). Stretch arms overhead and do deep breathing to stretch tight intercostals and upper abdominals. Instruct in proper body alignment. Wall-standing exercise is particularly useful. Stretch Hamstrings, if tight. Strengthen hip flexors, if weak, using alternate hip flexion in sitting, or alternate leg raising from supine position. *Avoid* double leg-raising exercises because of strain on abdominals.

Note: Common painful conditions associated with imbalance of anteroposterior trunk and hip joint muscles: low back pain.

Faulty Head and Shoulder Positions: Analysis and Treatment

Postural Fault	Anatomical Position of Joints	Muscles in Shortened Position	Muscles in Lengthened Position	Treatment procedures, if indicated on the basis of tests for alignment and muscle length and strength tests
Forward head	Cervical spine hyperextension	Cervical spine extensors Upper Trapezius and Levator	Cervical spine flexors	Stretch cervical spine extensors, if short, by trying to flatten the cervical spine. Strengthen cervical spine flexors, if weak. A forward head position is usually the result of faulty upper back posture. If neck muscles are not tight posteriorly, the head position will usually correct as the upper back is corrected. Strengthen the thoracic spine extensors. Do deep breathing exercises to help stretch the intercostals and the upper parts of abdominal muscles. Stretch Pectoralis minor. Stretch shoulder adductors and internal rotators, if short. Strengthen middle and lower Trapezius. Use shoulder support when indicated, to help stretch Pectoralis minor and relieve strain on middle and lower Trapezius. (See exercises and supports, pp. 67 and 68 and 117 and 118. See also Chapter 10.)
Kyphosis and Depressed chest	Thoracic spine flexion Intercostal spaces diminished	Upper and lateral fibers of Internal oblique Shoulder adductors Pectoralis minor Intercostals	Thoracic spine extensors Middle Trapezius Lower Trapezius	
Forward shoulders	Scapulae abducted and (usually) elevated	Serratus anterior Pectoralis minor Upper Trapezius	Middle Trapezius Lower Trapezius	

Faulty Posture, Back View: Analysis and Treatment

Postural Fault	Anatomical Position of Joints	Muscles in Shortened Position	Muscles in Lengthened Position	Treatment procedures, if indicated on basis of tests for alignment and muscle length and strength tests
Slight left C-curve Thoracolumbar scoliosis	Thoracolumbar spine: Lateral flexion, convex toward left	Right lateral trunk muscles	Left lateral trunk muscles	*If present without lateral pelvic tilt,* stretch right lateral trunk muscles, if short, and strengthen left lateral trunk muscles, if weak. *If present with lateral pelvis tilt,* see below for additional treatment procedures. Correct faulty habits that tend to increase the lateral curve: *Avoid* sitting on left foot in manner that thrusts spine toward left; *Avoid* lying on left side, propped up on elbow, to read or write. If weak, exercise right Iliopsoas in sitting position. See p. 127.
	Opposite for right C-curve.			
		Left Psoas major	Right Psoas major	
Prominent or high right hip	Pelvis, lateral tilt, high on right	Right lateral trunk muscles	Left lateral trunk muscles	Stretch right lateral trunk muscles, if short. Strengthen left lateral trunk muscles, if weak. Stretch left lateral thigh muscles and fascia, if short. Specific exercises to strengthen right Gluteus medius *are not required* to correct slight postural weakness; functional activity will suffice if the alignment is corrected and maintained. The subject should: Stand with weight evenly distributed over both feet, with pelvis level. *Avoid* standing with weight on right leg, causing right hip to be in postural adduction. Temporarily use straight raise on heel of left shoe (usually about 3/16 inch), or pad inside heel of shoe and in bedroom slippers.
	Right hip joint, adducted Left hip joint, abducted	Left hip abductors and Fascia lata Right hip adductors	Right hip abductors, especially Gluteus medius Left hip adductors	
	Opposite for posture with right C-curve and high left hip.			

Faulty Leg, Knee, and Foot Positions: Analysis and Treatment

Postural Fault	Anatomical Position of Joints	Muscles in Shortened Position	Muscles in Lengthened Position	Treatment procedures, if indicated on the basis of tests for alignment and muscle length and strength tests
Hyper-extended knee	Knee hyperextension Ankle plantar flexion	Quadriceps Soleus	Popliteus Hamstrings at knee	Instruct regarding overall postural correction with emphasis on avoiding knee hyperextension. In hemiplegics, short-leg brace with right-angle stop.
Flexed knee	Knee flexion Ankle dorsiflexion	Popliteus Hamstrings at knee	Quadriceps Soleus	Stretch knee flexors, if tight. Overall postural correction. Knee flexion may be secondary to hip flexor shortness. Check length of hip flexors; stretch if short.
Medially rotated femur (often associated with pronation of foot, see below.)	Hip joint medial rotation	Hip medial rotators	Hip lateral rotators	Stretch hip medial rotators, if tight. Strengthen hip lateral rotators, if weak. Young children should *avoid* sitting in reverse tailor fashion ("W" position). (See below for correction of any accompanying pronation.)
Knock-knee (Genu valgum)	Hip joint adduction Knee joint abduction	Fascia lata Lateral knee joint structures	Medial knee joint structures	Inner wedge on heels, if feet are pronated. Stretch Fascia lata, if indicated.
Postural bowlegs	Hip joint medial rotation Knee joint hyperextension Foot pronation	Hip medial rotators Quadriceps Foot everters	Hip lateral rotators Popliteus Tibialis posterior and long toe flexors	Exercises for overall correction of foot, knee, and hip positions. *Avoid* knee hyperextension. Strengthen hip lateral rotators. Inner wedges on heels to correct foot pronation.
		Stand with feet straight ahead and about 2 inches apart. Relax the knees into an "easy" position, i.e., neither stiff nor bent. Tighten the muscles which lift the arches of the feet, rolling the weight *slightly* toward the outer borders of the feet. Tighten the buttocks muscles to rotate the legs slightly outward (until kneecaps face directly forward).		
Pronation	Foot eversion	Peroneals and toe extensors	Tibialis posterior and long toe flexors	Inner wedges on heels. (Usually 1/8 inch on wide heels, and 1/16 inch on medium heels.) Overall correction of posture of feet and knees. Exercises to strengthen the inverters. Instructions in proper standing and walking.
Supination	Foot inversion	Tibials	Peroneals	Outer wedge on heels. Exercise for peroneals.
Hammer toes and low metatarsal arch	Metatarsophalan-geal joint hyperextension Proximal interphalangeal joint flexion	Toe extensors	Lumbricales	Stretch metatarsophalangeal joints by flexion; stretch interphalangeal joints by extension. Strengthen lumbricales by metatarsophalangeal joint flexion. Metatarsal pad or bar.

Developmental and Environmental Effects on Posture

The preceding pages have dealt with posture, primarily in relation to the adult. This segment introduces a variety of concepts dealing with the development of postural habits in the growing individual and with a variety of influences that affect such development. No attempt is made to give the various concepts either exhaustive or equal treatment. The authors hope that the material presented will be useful in a preventive sense and that it will create, through a recognition of factors involved in postural development, a more positive approach toward providing, within available limits, the best possible environment for good posture.

While it is important to observe and recognize marked or persistent postural deviations in the growing individual it is equally important to recognize that children are not expected to conform to an adult standard of alignment. This is true for a variety of reasons but primarily because the developing individual exhibits much greater mobility and flexibility than the adult.

Most postural deviations in the growing child fall in the category of developmental deviations; when patterns become habitual they may result in postural faults. Developmental deviations are those that appear in many children at about the same age and that improve or disappear without any corrective treatment, sometimes even despite unfavorable environmental influences. Whether or not a deviation in a child is becoming a fault should be determined by repeated or continued observation, not by a single examination. If the condition remains static, or if the deviation increases, corrective measures are indicated. Any faults which are *severe* need treatment as soon as they are observed regardless of the age of the individual.

A young child is not likely to have habitual faults and can be harmed by corrective measures that are not needed. Overcorrection may lead to atypical faults more harmful and difficult to deal with than the ones that caused the original concerns.

Some of the differences between children and adults are due to the fact that in the years between birth and maturity the structures of the body grow at varying rates, and in general grow rapidly at first and then at a gradually reduced rate. An example of this is the increase in size of the bones. Associated with increased overall length of the skeleton is a change in the proportionate lengths of its various segments. This change in proportions occurs as first one part of the skeleton and then another has the most rapid rate of growth. The gradual tightening of ligaments and fascia and strengthening of muscles is a significant developmental factor. Its effect is to gradually limit the range of joint motion toward that typical of maturity. The increase in stability that results is advantageous because it decreases the danger of strain from handling heavy objects or from other strenuous activities. Normal joint range for adults should provide an effective balance between motion and stability. A joint that is either too limited in range or not sufficiently limited is vulnerable to strain.

The child's greater range of joint motion makes possible momentary and habitual deviations in alignment that would be considered distortions in the adult. At the same time the flexibility serves as a protection against developing *fixed* postural faults.

Since the primary functions of muscles are to move the body and to contribute to its support, the degree of muscular strength needed has a direct relation to the size and weight of the body and its various parts. Thus, though a child's musculature may be normally strong at any given age, strength must continue to develop as height and weight increase. In general, then, muscle strength in children and adults is not equal, but the relative strength of the various muscles is comparable.

Beginning in infancy there is a persistent imbalance between the strength of the anterior and posterior muscles of the trunk and neck. The greater strength of the posterior muscles permits the child to raise the head and trunk backward long before being able to raise either forward without assistance. Although the abdominal and neck flexor muscles never do match the strength of their opponents, they are much stronger relatively in the adult than in the child. Thus in this regard an individual should not be expected to conform to the adult standard until approaching maturity.

Good postural development is dependent upon good structural and functional development of the body which, in turn, is highly dependent upon adequate nutrition. The influence of nutrition upon the proper structural development of skeletal and muscular tissues is of particular significance. Rickets, for example, which is often responsible for severe skeletal deformities in children, is known to be a deficiency disease.

After growth is completed, poor nutrition is less likely to cause structural faults that directly affect posture. At this stage deficiencies are more likely to interfere with physiological function and to be represented posturally in positions of fatigue. The body uses food not only for growth, but also for fuel, transforming it into heat and energy. If the fuel is insufficient there is a loss of energy output and a decrease in general physiological efficiency. Nutritional deficiencies in the adult are most likely to occur when unusual physiological demands are made upon the individual over a period of time.

There are physical defects, diseases and disabilities that have associated postural problems; these conditions can be roughly divided into three groups insofar as attention to posture is of importance in their treatment.

The first group consists largely of physical defects in which the postural aspects are more potential than actual in the initial stages, and become a problem only if the defect cannot be completely corrected by medical or surgical means. These defects may be visual, auditory, skeletal such as clubfoot or dislocation of the hip, neuromuscular such as brachial plexus injury, or muscular such as wry neck.

The second group includes conditions that are in themselves potentially disabling, but in which continuing attention to posture from the early stages can minimize the disabling effects. In an arthritic condition of the spine, (like Marie-Strümpell, for example), if the body can be kept in good functional alignment during the time that fusion of the spine is taking place, the individual may have little obvious deformity and only moderate disability when the fusion is complete. If the postural aspect is disregarded, the trunk is usually in marked flexion when fusion of the spine is complete. This is a position of severe deformity and of associated severe disability.

In the third group are conditions in which a degree of permanent disability exists as a result of injury or disease, but in which added postural strain can greatly increase the disability. An amputation of the lower extremity, for example, throws an unavoidable extra burden on the remaining weight-bearing structures. A postural alignment that minimizes, as much as possible, the mechanical strains of position and motion does much to keep these structures from breaking down.

A consideration of normal and abnormal variations in the posture of children can be discussed both from the standpoint of overall posture, and from the standpoint of the deviations of the various segments. Variations in overall posture of children at approximately the same age are illustrated on pp. 78 and 79.

A small child's foot is normally flat when beginning to stand and walk. The bones are in a formative stage and the arch structure is incomplete. The arch develops gradually along with the development of the bones, and with the strengthening of muscles and ligaments. By the age of 6 or 7 years one may expect good arch formation. Footprints taken at regular intervals help to gauge the amount of change that has occurred in the arch. These can be taken with a podograph, or if this is not available, the sole of the foot can be painted with Vaseline and a footprint made on paper. As the arch increases in height, less of the sole of the foot in the area of the arch will be seen in the footprint.

Flat longitudinal arches may persist as a fixed fault or they may recur because of foot strain at any age. Improper shoes or a habit of standing and walking with the feet in an out-toeing position may cause such strain. If a child's foot is very flat, is pronated, and toes out in a manner that allows the body weight to be borne constantly on the inner side of the foot, it may be necessary to use a slight correction such as inner heel-wedge or small longitudinal pad in the shoe quite soon after the child begins to stand and walk. In most cases, however, it is advisable to institute corrective measures only after a period of observation. There are individuals who fail to develop a longitudinal arch and have what is termed a static flat foot. Usually, however, the alignment of the foot is not faulty in regard to pronation or out-toeing, and there are no symptoms of foot strain. The corrective measures usually indicated for flat arches are not indicated in such cases.

A degree of knock-knee is common in children, and is usually first observed when the child begins to stand. The height and build of the child must be taken into consideration when judging whether the deviation is a fault, but in general it may be said that a fault exists if the ankles are more than 2 inches apart when the knees are touching. (See p. 95.) Knock-knee should be showing definite improvement before and be nonexistent by the age of 6 or 7 years. (See figure A, p. 78.)

In some cases, knock-kneed children may stand with one knee (often the right) slightly flexed and the other slightly hyperextended so that the knees overlap in order to keep the feet together. Knock-knees may persist; in adults this fault is more prevalent among women than among men.

Records of the change in the degree of knock-knee can be kept by drawing an outline of the legs on paper while the child is lying or standing with knees touching each other. Mild to moderate knock-knee conditions are usually treated by shoe corrections, while bracing or even surgery may be required for the more severe.

Bowlegs is an alignment fault in which there is separation of the knees when the feet are together. It may be a postural or a structural fault. Postural bowing is a deviation associated with knee hyperextension and hip medial rotation. (See p. 97.) As the posterior ligaments tighten and hyperextension decreases, this type of fault tends to become less pronounced. If it persists as a postural habit the child should be given instruction in order to correct the alignment faults. This fault is less easy to correct as the individual approaches maturity, although some degree of correction may be obtained in young adults who are very flexible.

Postural bowlegs may be compensatory for knock-knees. If a knock-kneed child stands with legs thrust back into hyperextension, the resultant postural bowing of the legs will let the feet be brought together without having the knees overlap. In this position, the knock-knee fault may be obscured, but it will become obvious if the legs are brought into a neutral position of knee extension. (See p. 98.)

Postural bowing usually disappears when an individual is recumbent, while structural bowing does not. Structural bowing requires early treatment, or in later stages may require surgery.

Drawings to record the change in structural bowlegs can be made while the child is in a back-lying position with feet together. Since postural bowing shows up only in standing, the drawing of this for record must be made in standing. It can be done by placing the paper on a wall behind the standing child.

Inward rotation of the femur, seen as a turning inward of the patella, is the most common alignment fault of the knees and may occur at any age. It frequently occurs in combination with other faults such as pronation of the feet, hyperextension of the knees, postural bowlegs and less often with knock-knees. When inward rotation of the femur is associated with postural bowlegs it usually disappears when the legs are brought forward out of hyperextension. (See figure, p. 97.) Permanent improvement depends upon the correction of the faulty habit of hyperextension.

Children may stand in a position of external rotation of the feet and knees. (See p. 370.) Such a position is more typical of boys than of girls. It may or may not have serious effects, although persistence of such a pattern in walking as well as in standing puts undue strain on the longitudinal arches.

Hyperextension is a fairly common fault, usually associated with lack of firm ligamentous support. It tends to disappear as the ligaments tighten, but if it persists as a postural habit an effort should be made to correct it by postural training.

It is characteristic of small children to have a protruding abdomen. (See p. 78.) For the most part, the contour of the abdominal wall changes gradually but there is a noticeable change about the age of 10 to 12 years when the waistline becomes relatively smaller, and the abdomen no longer protrudes.

Posture of the back varies somewhat with the age of the child. A small child may stand bent slightly forward at the hips (see p. 78), and with feet apart for better balance. Children of early school age appear to have a typical deviation of the upper back in which the shoulder blades are quite prominent. Beginning about the age of 9 years there seems to be a tendency for increased forward curve or lordosis of the low back. The deviations should tend to become less pronounced as the child grows older.

As early as 8 or 10 years of age, handedness patterns related to posture may appear. The slight deviation of the spine to the side opposite the higher hip makes an appearance early. There tends to be a compensatory low shoulder on the side of the higher hip. In most cases the low shoulder is a less significant factor. Usually shoulder correction tends to follow correction of lateral pelvic tilt, but the reverse does not occur. No attempts should be made to raise the shoulder into position by constant muscular effort.

The ability of individuals to touch the toes with the fingertips while sitting with legs extended shows interesting and significant variations according to age. The chart on p. 112 and a series of figures on p. 48 indicate what is apparently normal accomplishment in this movement at different ages, (see also *Chapter 1*, p. 8.)

The activities in which an individual engages may have favorable or adverse influence on posture. The nature of the activities, the time expended in them, and whether the effect of habitual movements is reinforced or counteracted by habitual positions determine to a great extent the effect on posture.

The activities of an individual must be considered as a whole in gauging the effect on posture. Concentration on one type of activity provides a high potential for muscle imbalance. A secretary who engages in sedentary activities such as piano playing during leisure time has no real change in type of activity from the postural standpoint.

Activities which cause lateral deviations in the alignment may or may not cause fixed postural faults. Sometimes the deviations to the left and right tend to counteract each other. However, the tendency to assume positions that consistently cause a deviation to the same side may result in a fixed lateral curve.

Some deviations of alignment have no obvious relation to the activities of the individual, but are constant enough to be habitual faults, e.g., standing with one knee flexed. (See p. 367.).

If changes of activity are to be compensatory they must give variety in position and movement.

FLEXIBILITY TEST # I, TOUCHING FINGER-TIPS TO TOES (28)
Measurements of 5115 Individuals

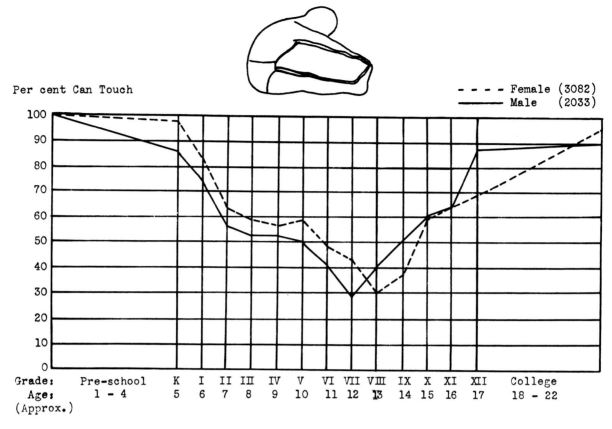

Per cent Can Touch

- - - - Female (3082)
——— Male (2033)

Grade:	Pre-school	K	I	II	III	IV	V	VI	VII	VIII	IX	X	XI	XII	College
Age: (Approx.)	1 - 4	5	6	7	8	9	10	11	12	13	14	15	16	17	18 - 22

FLEXIBILITY TEST # I: TOUCHING FINGER-TIPS TO TOES
Measurements of 5115 Individuals

MALE Range of Limitation	Mean	% Can Touch	Total Ex'd.	Grade Age	Total Ex'd.	% Can Touch	Mean	FEMALE Range of Limitation
$\frac{1}{2}"$ - 9"	$2\frac{3}{4}"$	86%	102	K 5	102	98%	$3\frac{3}{4}"$	$3\frac{1}{2}"$ - 4"
1" - 10"	4"	74%	125	I 6	108	83%	3"	$\frac{1}{2}"$ - 4"
$\frac{1}{2}"$ - $10\frac{1}{2}"$	3"	56%	147	II 7	152	63%	$3\frac{1}{2}"$	$\frac{1}{2}"$ - $10\frac{1}{2}"$
$\frac{1}{2}"$ - $9\frac{1}{2}"$	$3\frac{1}{2}"$	52%	150	III 8	192	59%	4"	1" - $8\frac{1}{2}"$
$\frac{1}{2}"$ - $10\frac{1}{2}"$	$4\frac{1}{2}"$	52%	150	IV 9	158	57%	$4\frac{1}{2}"$	1" - $13\frac{1}{2}"$
1" - 10"	$4\frac{1}{2}"$	50%	158	V 10	174	59%	4"	$\frac{1}{2}"$ - 8"
1" - $11\frac{1}{2}"$	$4\frac{1}{4}"$	41%	140	VI 11	156	49%	$4\frac{1}{2}"$	$\frac{1}{2}"$ - 10"
$\frac{1}{2}"$ - $9\frac{1}{2}"$	4"	28%	100	VII 12	100	43%	6"	$\frac{1}{2}"$ - $11\frac{1}{2}"$
$1\frac{1}{2}"$ - 13"	$4\frac{1}{2}"$	40%	151	VIII 13	115	30%	5"	$\frac{1}{2}"$ - 10"
$\frac{1}{2}"$ - 10"	$4\frac{1}{2}"$	50%	222	IX 14	108	37%	$5\frac{1}{2}"$	2" - 13"
$\frac{1}{2}"$ - $12\frac{1}{2}"$	$3\frac{1}{2}"$	60%	100	X 15	498	59%	5"	$\frac{1}{2}"$ - 12"
$\frac{1}{2}"$ - $12\frac{1}{2}"$	5"	64%	100	XI 16	507	64%	5"	1" - 12"
1" - 12"	3"	87%	113	XII 17	405	69%	5"	1" - 14"
1" - 11"	4"	90%	275	18-22	307	95%	3"	1" - $6\frac{1}{2}"$
Total number tested: 2033					3082 :Total number tested			

112

For anyone who has to sit long hours at a desk, whether in school or at work, shifts of position or simple extension movements are usually possible and desirable. A sitting position keeps the hips, the knees, and usually the back in flexion. Relaxing against the back of the seat is a small but useful change from sitting with the trunk held forward as for writing at a desk. A true change of position would involve extension of the body as in standing up or lying down.

The principle that activities should be varied for the sake of good posture is subject to sensible limitations in its application. It is not logical to assume that an individual's primary consideration in choosing activities will be postural. However, it may be possible to eliminate or minimize unfavorable postural influences intrinsic to activities engaged in if postural implications are known and adjustments made whenever practical.

A fault sometimes seen in adults as a result of several years of gymnastics at an early age is a flattening or reversal of the normal backward curve of the spine in the upper back. It results from repeated hyperextension movements of the spine through an extreme range of motion persisted in during the period of growth when the bones are still in the formative stage. Individuals who begin dancing at a later age when the spinal curves are less susceptible to distortion rarely show this particular fault.

Activities that are rather neutral in the effect on posture are games or sports in which walking or running predominates. Sports that exert an influence toward muscle imbalance are the predominantly one-sided games, such as those involving the use of a racket.

The play activities of young children usually are varied enough so that no problem of muscle imbalance or habitual alignment fault is present. However, when a child becomes old enough to engage in competitive athletics a point may be reached where further development of skill through intensive practice requires a sacrifice of some degree of good muscle balance and good skeletal alignment. Although seemingly unimportant at the time, the faults acquired may progress until a painful condition results.

Specific exercises may be needed to maintain range of joint motion and to strengthen certain muscles if opposing muscles are being overdeveloped by the activity. These exercises must be specific for the part and therapeutic for the body as a whole.

Vocational activity is a more influential factor in the posture of the average adult than is recreational activity. The repeated movements involved in a specialized occupation are the equivalent of repeated exercises, and thus may be responsible for overdevelopment of certain muscle groups. If the effect of poor position reinforces that of repeated activity, the muscle imbalance is greatly increased.

There are a number of environmental factors that influence the development and maintenance of good posture. These environmental influences should be made as favorable to good posture as is practical; when no major adjustment is possible, small adjustments will often contribute considerably. The following discussion takes into account such factors as chairs, desks, and beds because they illustrate environmental influences on posture in the sitting and lying positions. After a child starts school, the amount of time spent in the sitting position increases considerably and the school seat is an important environmental factor.

Both the chair and desk should be adjusted to fit the child. The child should be able to sit with both feet flat on the floor with knees bent to about a right angle. If the chair is too high or too low, either there is lack of support for the feet, or the hips and the knees are bent into too much flexion. The seat of the chair should be deep enough from front to back to support the thighs adequately, but the depth should not interfere with the bending of the knees. The back of the chair should provide support for the child's back. It should also incline backward a few degrees so that the child can relax against the back of the chair. (See illustration of sitting postures p. 99.)

The top of the desk should be about elbow level when the child is sitting in a good position, and may be slightly inclined. The desk should be close enough so that arms can rest upon it without the need to lean too far forward or sit forward on the seat of the chair.

The type and size of a chair is important to anyone who spends many hours in a sitting position. Whenever possible a chair that gives a maximum of comfort and support should be selected. Not all chairs are conducive to good sitting position. So-called posture chairs which support the back only in the lumbar region tend to cause an increase in the lumbar curve and are often undesirable. While it is advisable that the back of a chair be inclined slightly backward, it is not good to have too great an angle of backward tilt. Sitting for long periods of time in a swivel chair which tilts back may contribute to a very faulty position of the upper back and head.

Automobile seats that are too low or that have been tilted backward for the comfort of the passengers may be unsatisfactory for the driver. Pain and fatigue in the neck and shoulder region, which are frequently associated with long periods of driving, can be traced to the need to hold the head in a forward or tilted position. A long wedge-

113

shaped pillow (with wider part at the top) can be used to decrease the inclination of the back of the seat behind the driver.

The qualifications for the height and proximity of the school desk apply to almost any work surface for a sedentary worker. Whenever it is practical, tools and equipment should be placed where they may be reached without undue stretch or torsion. Computer monitors should be at eye level, and easels used to hold paperwork should be next to the computer or typewriter, whenever possible. The light provided for any activity should be of adequate intensity for the purpose and located so that it falls correctly on the work space. It should be free from glare, bright reflections, or unnecessary shadows. Those who must spend extended periods of time using the telephone should consider using a headphone and mouthpiece to avoid undue tension in the neck and shoulder.

The firmness of a mattress is an important factor in the consideration of posture in the lying position. A good sleeping position involves having the various parts of the body in about the same horizontal plane. Either sagging springs or too soft a mattress may permit poor body alignment.

Many people who have experienced postural back pain have found that pain has been decreased or eliminated by changing from a sagging to a firm level bed. Others who have been accustomed to sleeping on a firm mattress have found that acute pain may be brought on by sleeping on a soft or sagging bed. A pillow under the waist when sleeping on the abdomen, or between the knees in a side-lying position can assist in maintaining more normal alignment and relieving stress on the lower back. If marked hip flexor tightness is present, a pillow under the knees, when backlying, can also relieve strain on the back.

For some individuals, particularly those who have fixed structural faults of alignment such as exaggerated curves of the spine, a softer mattress may be necessary for sleeping comfort because the mattress will give more support and comfort if it conforms to the curves than if it "bridges" them.

An infant should have a bed with a firm mattress. It may be somewhat softer than the mattress used by an adult because the weight of the infant does not cause the mattress to sag. The infant should sleep without a pillow.

An adult might be comfortable without a pillow when sleeping on the back or abdomen, but would probably not be comfortable in a side-lying position. Use of too high a pillow or more than one pillow may contribute to faulty head and shoulder positions. However, a person who is used to sleeping with the head high should not change abruptly to using a low pillow or none at all. A person who has a *fixed* postural fault of forward head and round upper back should not sleep without a pillow. It is important to have a pillow high enough to compensate for the round upper back and forward head position. Without a pillow or if the pillow is too low, the head will drop back in hyperextension of the neck.

POSTURE INSTRUCTION

Good posture is not an end in itself but a part of general well-being. Ideally, posture instruction and training should become a part of general experience rather than be a separate discipline. To the extent that parents and teachers are cognizant of good postural habits and able to recognize the influences and habits that tend toward development of good or faulty posture, they will be able to contribute to this aspect of well-being in the daily life of the growing individual. Nevertheless, posture instruction and training should not be neglected in a good program of health education; attention should be paid to observable faults. When instruction is given, it should be simple and accurate; while it must not be neglected, neither should it be overemphasized. It should be given in such a manner as to capture the interest and cooperation of the child.

While correction of postural defects requires the use of special therapeutic measures, the prevention of faults depends largely on teaching the fundamentals of good alignment. The tables on pp. 115 and 116 describes posture in relation to the various segments of the body in terms of both good and faulty alignment. An attempt has been made to present the material in a manner that makes it useful for the layman.

Good and Faulty Posture: Summary Chart

Good Posture	Part	Faulty Posture
In standing, the longitudinal arch has the shape of a half dome. Barefoot or in shoes without heels, the feet toe out slightly. In shoes with heels the feet are parallel. In walking with or without heels, the feet are parallel and the weight is transferred from the heel along the outer border to the ball of the foot. In sprinting the feet are parallel or toe in slightly. The weight is on the balls of the feet and toes because the heels do not come in contact with the ground.	Foot	Low longitudinal arch or flat foot. Low metatarsal arch, usually indicated by calluses under the ball of the foot. Weight borne on the inner side of the foot (pronation). "Ankle rolls in." Weight borne on the outer border of the foot (supination). "Ankle rolls out." Toeing-out while walking, or while standing in shoes with heels ("slue-footed"). Toeing-in while walking or standing ("pigeon-toed").
Toes should be straight, that is, neither curled downward nor bent upward. They should extend forward in line with the foot and not be squeezed together or overlap.	Toes	Toes bend up at the first joint and down at middle joints so that the weight rests on the tips of the toes (hammer toes). This fault is often associated with wearing shoes that are too short. Big toe slants inward toward the midline of the foot (hallux valgus). "Bunion." This fault is often associated with wearing shoes that are too narrow and pointed at the toes.
Legs are straight up and down. Kneecaps face straight ahead when feet are in good position. Looking at the knees from the side, the knees are straight, i.e., neither bent forward nor locked backward.	Knees and Legs	Knees touch when feet are apart (knock-knees). Knees are apart when feet touch (bowlegs.) Knee curves slightly backward (hyperextended knee). "Back-knee." Knee bends slightly forward, that is, it is not as straight as it should be (flexed knee). Kneecaps face slightly toward each other (medially rotated femurs). Kneecaps face slightly outward (laterally rotated femurs).
Ideally, the body weight is borne evenly on both feet, and the hips are level. One side is not more prominent than the other as seen from front or back, nor is one hip more forward or backward than the other as seen from the side. The spine does not curve to the left or the right side. (A *slight* deviation to the left in right-handed individuals and to the right in left-handed individuals is not uncommon. Also, a tendency toward a *slightly* low right shoulder and *slightly* high right hip is frequently found in right-handed people, and vice versa for left-handed.)	Hips, Pelvis, and Spine Back view	One hip is higher than the other (lateral pelvic tilt). Sometimes it is not really much higher but appears so because a sideways sway of the body has made it more prominent. (Tailors and dressmakers often notice a lateral tilt because the hemline of skirts or length of trousers must be adjusted to the difference.) The hips are rotated so that one is farther forward than the other (clockwise or counterclockwise rotation).

Good and Faulty Posture: Summary Chart

Good Posture	Part	Faulty Posture
The front of the pelvis and the thighs are in a straight line. The buttocks are not prominent in back but slope slightly downward. The spine has four natural curves. In the neck and lower back the curve is forward, in the upper back and lowest part of the spine (sacral region) it is backward. The sacral curve is a fixed curve while the other three are flexible.	Spine and Pelvis Side view	The low back arches forward too much (lordosis). The pelvis tilts forward too much. The front of the thigh forms an angle with the pelvis when this tilt is present. The normal forward curve in the low back has straightened. The pelvis tips backward as in sway-back and flat-back postures. Increased backward curve in the upper back (kyphosis or round upper back). Increased forward curve in the neck. Almost always accompanied by round upper back and seen as a forward head. Lateral curve of the spine (scoliosis); toward one side (C-curve), toward both sides (S-curve).
In young children up to about the age of 10 the abdomen normally protrudes somewhat. In older children and adults it should be flat.	Abdomen	Entire abdomen protrudes. Lower part of the abdomen protrudes while the upper part is pulled in.
A good position of the chest is one in which it is slightly up and slightly forward (while the back remains in good alignment). The chest appears to be in a position about halfway between that of a full inspiration and a forced expiration.	Chest	Depressed, or "hollow-chest" position. Lifted and held up too high, brought about by arching the back. Ribs more prominent on one side than on the other. Lower ribs flaring out or protruding.
Arms hang relaxed at the sides with palms of the hands facing toward the body. Elbows are slightly bent, so forearms hang slightly forward. Shoulders are level and neither one is more forward or backward than the other when seen from the side. Shoulder blades lie flat against the rib cage. They are neither too close together nor too wide apart. In adults, a separation of about 4 inches is average.	Arms and Shoulders	Holding the arms stiffly in any position forward, backward, or out from the body. Arms turned so that palms of hands face backward. One shoulder higher than the other. Both shoulders hiked-up. One or both shoulders drooping forward or sloping. Shoulders rotated either clockwise or counterclockwise. Shoulder blades pulled back too hard. Shoulder blades too far apart. Shoulder blades too prominent, standing out from the rib cage (winged scapulae).
Head is held erect in a position of good balance.	Head	Chin up too high. Head protruding forward. Head tilted or rotated to one side.

LOW BACK STRETCHING

☐ In face-lying position, place a firm pillow under abdomen and a rolled towel under ankles. Lying on a firm pillow puts low back muscles in a position of slight stretch.

☐ In back-lying position, slowly pull both knees toward chest lifting buttocks up slightly from table to gently stretch the low back.

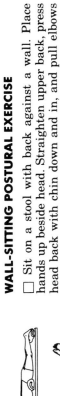

LOWER ABDOMINAL EXERCISE AND LOW BACK STRETCHING

☐ In back-lying position, bend knees and place feet flat on table. With hands up beside head, tilt pelvis to flatten low back on table by *pulling up and in with lower abdominal muscles.* Keep low back flat and slide heels down along table. Straighten legs as much as possible with back held flat. Keep back flat and return knees to bent position, *sliding one leg back at a time.* (Do NOT lift feet from table.)

LOWER ABDOMINAL EXERCISE

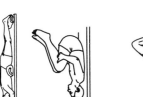

☐ In back-lying position, place a rolled towel or small pillow under knees. With hands up beside head, tilt pelvis to flatten low back on table by *pulling up and in with lower abdominal muscles.* Hold back flat and breathe in and out easily, relaxing upper abdominal muscles. There should be good chest expansion during inspiration, but back should not arch. Do NOT use buttock muscles to tilt the pelvis.

UPPER ABDOMINAL EXERCISE

☐ In back-lying position, tilt pelvis to flatten low back on table by *pulling up and in with lower abdominal muscles.* With arms forward, raise head and shoulders up from table. Do NOT attempt to come to sitting position, but raise upper trunk as high as back will bend. As strength progresses, arms may be folded across chest, and later placed behind head to increase resistance during the exercise.

POSTERIOR NECK STRETCHING

☐ In back-lying position, bend knees and place feet flat on table. With elbows bent and hands up beside head, tilt pelvis to flatten low back on table. Press head back, with chin down and in, trying to flatten neck against table.

SHOULDER ADDUCTOR STRETCHING

☐ With knees bent and feet flat on table, tilt pelvis to flatten low back on table. Hold low back flat, place both arms overhead and try to reach arms to the table with elbows straight. Bring upper arms as close to sides of head as possible. (Do NOT allow the back to arch.)

WALL-SITTING POSTURAL EXERCISE

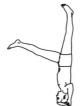

☐ Sit on a stool with back against a wall. Place hands up beside head. Straighten upper back, press head back with chin down and in, and pull elbows back against wall. Flatten low back against wall by *pulling up and in with lower abdominal muscles.* Keep arms in contact with wall and slowly move arms to a diagonally overhead position.

PASSIVE HAMSTRING STRETCHING

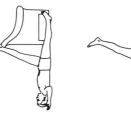

☐ Lie on floor behind a sturdy chair. Place one leg out straight beside chair, the other in a position of straight-leg-raise, resting ankle against back of chair. As muscles relax, move closer to chair, raising leg higher and giving added stretch to Hamstrings. (This stretch also may be done by an indoor doorway.)

ACTIVE HAMSTRING STRETCHING

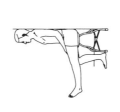

☐ To stretch right Hamstrings, lie on table with legs extended, hold left leg down and gradually raise right leg with knee straight. (Reverse the procedure to stretch left Hamstrings.)

☐ Sit on a stool with back against a wall. Keep one knee bent and straighten other leg. A stretch should be felt under the knee and along Hamstring muscles.

ASSISTED TENSOR FASCIAE LATAE STRETCHING

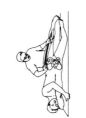

☐ To stretch left Tensor fasciae latae, have subject lie on right side with right hip and knee bent. Relax left leg on pillows placed between thighs and lower legs. Apply heat and massage to left lateral thigh. Remove the pillows. Bend right hip and knee enough to flatten low back. Stabilize the pelvis firmly with one hand, draw the thigh slightly back, and press gently (on thigh, not leg) downward toward table, stretching the muscles and fascia between the hip and knee. (The knee should not be allowed to rotate inward, and care should be taken to avoid strain at the knee joint.)

☐ To stretch right Tensor, have subject lie on left side and reverse the procedure.

☐ For mild to moderate unilateral Tensor fasciae latae tightness, place a heel lift of 1/8 to 3/16 inch thickness in shoe on the side of tightness to level the pelvis and provide a gradual stretch in the standing position.

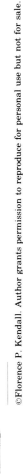

Treatment of Postural Faults: Individual Instructions

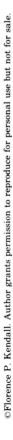

The general and specific instructions on these pages are given to help you carry out the necessary follow-up treatment for correction of your postural faults.

The exercises and other treatment selected for you on the basis of your posture examination are indicated by an X in the box beside the paragraphs describing the exercises you should do at home.

Gentle heat and massage are used to help relax tight muscles and should precede the *stretching* exercises. (Avoid using heat on weak, overstretched muscles.) There should be a conscious effort to relax the muscles being stretched. Stretching should be gradual, and sufficient to cause *mild* discomfort but not pain. Return the part *slowly* from the stretched position.

Exercises in the lying position should be done on a firm table or on the floor. For comfort, a thin pad or folded blanket should be placed on the hard surface.

Strengthening exercises should be done *slowly* and you should try to get a strong pull by the muscles that are being exercised. The completed position should be held for several seconds before relaxing. The exercises should be repeated the number of times indicated by your therapist.

Specific exercises are done to improve muscle balance. To be effective they should be done every day, and continued for a period of weeks until normal length has been restored to the tight muscles, and until the weak muscles have regained strength. The purpose of treatment is to restore good posture. This involves the specific treatment outlined to restore muscle balance plus daily practice in assuming and maintaining good posture until it becomes a habit.

While working to correct muscle imbalance, it is usually advisable to AVOID the following exercises: Lying on the back and raising both legs at the same time; lying on the back and coming up to a sitting position with the feet held firmly down; lying on the back, with most of the weight resting on the upper back, and doing the "bicycling" exercise; standing or sitting with knees straight, reaching forward to touch toes. Those who have an increased forward curve in the low back, should AVOID the exercise of raising the trunk to arch the back from a face-lying position.

HIP FLEXOR STRETCHING AND HIP EXTENSOR STRENGTHENING

☐ To stretch right hip flexors, lie on back with right lower leg hanging over end of a *sturdy table*. Pull left knee firmly toward chest to flatten (low back on table. (When there is hip flexor tightness, this position will bring right thigh up from table.) *Keeping back flat and knee bent,* stretch right hip flexors by pulling thigh downward with the right buttock muscle, trying to touch thigh to table.

☐ To stretch left hip flexors, pull right knee toward chest and apply the stretch to left thigh as described above.

Note: This exercise can be done at the top of a flight of stairs if no sturdy table is available.

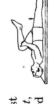

ONE-JOINT HIP FLEXOR STRETCHING

☐ In back-lying position, pull one knee toward chest until low back is flat on table. *Keeping back flat,* press other leg, with knee straight, down toward table by tightening the buttock muscle.

TWO-JOINT HIP FLEXOR STRETCHING

☐ Stand with back against a doorframe, weight on one leg, other knee bent and resting on a stool. This position puts a stretch on the two-joint hip flexors. Add stretching by pulling up and in with lower abdominal muscles to posteriorly tilt the pelvis and flatten the low back against the doorframe.

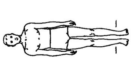

CORRECTION OF PRONATION AND INTERNAL ROTATION

☐ Stand with feet about 4 inches apart and toeing-out slightly. Relax knees into an "easy" position, i.e., neither stiff nor bent. Tighten muscles that lift the arches of the feet, rolling the weight *slightly* toward outer borders of feet. Tighten buttock muscles to rotate legs slightly outward (until kneecaps face directly forward).

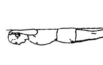

WALL-STANDING POSTURAL EXERCISE

☐ Stand with back against a wall, heels about 3 inches from wall. Place hands up beside head with elbows touching wall. If needed, correct feet and knees as in above exercise, then tilt pelvis to flatten low back against wall by *pulling up and in with the lower abdominal muscles.* Keeping arms in contact with wall, move arms slowly to a diagonally overhead position.

chapter 5

Scoliosis

SCOLIOSIS

Scoliosis is a lateral curvature of the spine. The spine has normal curves in an anterior-posterior direction, but a curve in a lateral direction is considered abnormal. Since the vertebral column cannot bend laterally without also rotating, scoliosis involves both lateral flexion and rotation.

There are many *known causes* of scoliosis. It may be congenital or acquired; it may result from disease or injury. Some of the causes of scoliosis involve changes in bony structure such as a wedging of a vertebral body, some relate to neuromuscular problems directly affecting the musculature of the trunk, and some relate to impairment of an extremity such as shortness of one leg, or impairment of vision or hearing.

There are also many cases of scoliosis for which there is *no known cause*. They are referred to as *idiopathic*. In spite of the battery of tests that are available to help establish a cause, a high percentage of cases fall into this category.

This section on scoliosis deals chiefly with idiopathic scoliosis. Muscle imbalance that exists as a result of disease, such as poliomyelitis, is readily recognized as a cause of scoliosis when it affects the musculature of the trunk. However, muscle imbalance is present in so-called "normal" individuals, but often goes unrecognized except by those who employ muscle testing when examining cases of faulty posture. A basic problem in the management of idiopathic scoliosis is failure to accept the fact that muscle imbalance, which can exist without known cause, plays an important role in the etiology.

The purpose of the following discussion is to focus on one segment of this subject that deserves more attention than it has received, namely, the care of early scoliosis patients for whom *proper* exercises and supports can make a difference in the outcome. Scoliosis literature is devoid of specific procedures for testing overall postural alignment and muscle imbalance. Analysis of postural alignment appears in *Chapter 4*, length tests in *Chapter 3*, and strength tests in *Chapters 6, 7, and 8*.

EXERCISE PROGRAMS

Throughout the years, elaborate programs of exercise have been instituted in response to the treatment needs of scoliosis patients. The creeping exercises advocated by Klapp were discarded when problems with children's knees forced the discontinuance of such a program (29). Exercises that overemphasized flexibility created problems by making the spine more vulnerable to collapse. When treating patients with S-curves, one must avoid exercises that adversely affect one of the curves, while attempting to correct the other.

It is not surprising, therefore, that the usefulness of exercises in cases of scoliosis has been questioned. For many years, the attitude has been that exercises are of little or no value. The idea is not new. The following is a statement made years ago by Risser: "It was customary at the scoliosis clinic at . . . Orthopedic Hospital, as late as 1920–1930, to send new patients with scoliosis to the gymnasium for exercises. Invariably the patients who were 12 to 13 years of age showed an increase of the scoliosis . . . it was therefore assumed that exercises and spinal motion made the curve increase" (30).

Except in some isolated instances, programs of exercises for scoliosis patients continued to be looked upon with scepticism. In the American Academy of Orthopedic Surgeons 1985 Lecture series, this statement appears: "Physical therapy cannot prevent a progressive deformity, and there are those who believe specific spinal exercise programs work in a counterproductive fashion by making the spine more flexible than it ordinarily would be and by so doing making it more susceptible to progression" (31).

Overemphasis on flexibility was wrong. Adequate musculoskeletal evaluation has been lacking, and as a result there has been little scientific basis upon which to justify the selection of therapeutic exercises. Scoliosis is a problem of asymmetry. To restore symmetry requires the use of asymmetrical exercises along with appropriate support. Stretching of tight muscles is desirable, but overall flexibility of the spine is not. It is better to have stiffness in the best attainable position than to have too much flexibility of the back.

Examination

Instead of abandoning the use of exercises in the treatment of scoliosis, attention should be focused on a more scientific approach to evaluation and selection of appropriate exercises. Musculoskeletal evaluation should include alignment and muscle tests.

Postural *alignment* tests, both plumbline and segmental, in back, side, and front views should be included (see pp. 75–90.).

Muscle *length* tests should include, but not be limited to, the following: Hip flexor (see pp. 33–37); Hamstring (see pp. 38–45); forward bending for contour of back and length of posterior muscles (see pp. 46–48); Tensor fasciae latae and Iliotibial band (see pp. 56–60); and Teres and Latissimus dorsi (see pp. 63 and 64).

Muscle *strength* tests should include: Back extensors (see p. 140); upper and lower abdominals (see pp. 162 and 154); lateral trunk (see p. 144); oblique abdominal muscles (see p. 146); hip flexors (see pp. 214 and 215); hip extensors; (see p. 226); hip abductors and Gluteus medius (see pp. 220–223); hip adductors (see p. 229); and middle and lower Trapezius (see pp. 284 and 286).

An essential part of examination is observation of the back *during movement*. The examiner stands behind the subject and has the subject bend forward, and then return *slowly* to the upright position. If there is a structural curve, there will be some fullness (prominence) on the side of the convexity of the curve. The fullness will be on one side only if there is a single curve, or C-curve. In a double curve, or S-curve, as in a right thoracic, left lumbar, there will be fullness on the right in the upper back and fullness on the left in the low back area.

The fullness caused by rotation may also be observed in side view as seen in the photograph below.

For most people, the curves in the spine are "functional," they do not become fixed or "structural." When curves do become fixed, they also tend to change and become "compensatory," that is, change from a single C-curve to an S-curve. Usually, a single curve toward the left stays as a left curve in the low back and changes to a right curve in the upper back.

In an ordinary C-curve, the shoulder is low on the side of the high hip. *If the shoulder is high on the same side as the high hip, there probably is an S-curve.*

In some cases, faulty alignment appears to be limited to the spine. The accompanying figure shows a simple C-curve in which overall plumb alignment of the body is good. Segmentally, the right shoulder is low along with the C-curve.

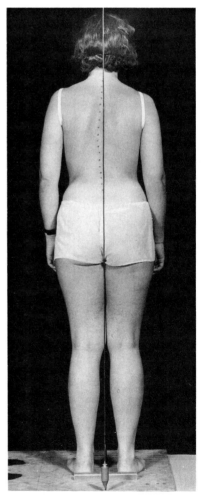

For this patient, a shoe lift is not indicated because the pelvis is level. Exercise is indicated for right External oblique and left Internal oblique by shifting upper trunk toward right without any lateral movement of the pelvis (p. 127).

The lessons learned from treating polio patients were easily understood because of the obvious effects of the disease on the functions of muscles. People who treated these patients appreciated the fact that deformities could develop where muscle imbalance existed. They saw the devastating effects of muscle weakness and the subsequent tightness or contractures in opposing muscles, not the least of which were the devastating effects on the spine. Some potentially severe problems were helped by appropriate intervention.

The accompanying photographs show the marked weakness of the right abdominal musculature and the associated lateral curve. This patient had polio at the age of 1 year and 4 months, but was not admitted to a hospital for treatment until the age of 8 years and 8 months. She was placed on a flexed frame to relax the abdominal muscles with a pullover strap pulling in the direction of the right External oblique. Specific exercises were given to the weak muscles of the trunk in addition to the support from the pullover strap. Seven months after treatment was started, the strength of the abdominal muscles had improved with the right External oblique showing an increase from a poor − to a good grade.

In treating polio patients, it became obvious, in many instances, that weakness due to stretching had been superimposed on the initial weakness caused by the disease. As in the case illustrated, the muscles were not reinnervated by relieving stretch and strain on them. Innervation existed as a latent factor, but the stretched muscles were incapable of response until the stretch and strain were relieved by adequate support, and stimulated by proper exercise.

BEFORE
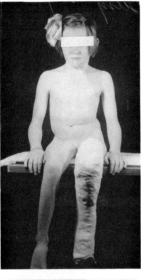

BEFORE
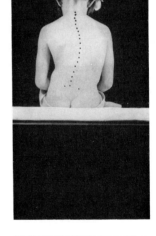

AFTER
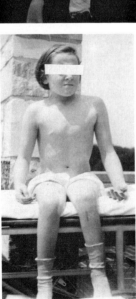

AFTER
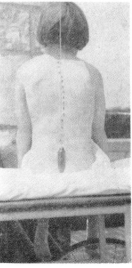

Scoliosis Cases and Test Findings

The accompanying photographs show four subjects with varying types and degrees of scoliosis, none of which are severe. Information about the type of curve, flexibility, muscle length, and muscle strength for each of the subjects is recorded below.

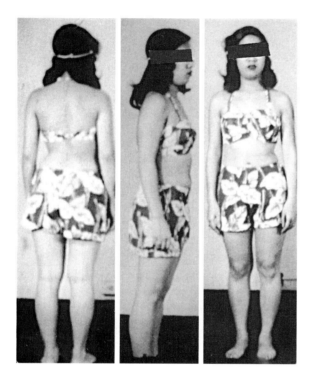
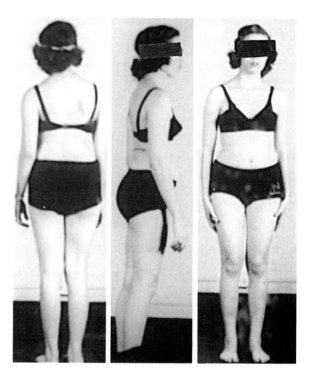

Scoliosis: Right Thoracolumbar	
Test	Result
Forward bending (sitting)	(−) 3 inches
Back contour	Slightly excessive flexion, mid-back
Hamstrings	Slightly limited
Gastroc-soleus	Normal
Lower abdominals	6
Upper abdominals	10
Obliques, left	10
Obliques, right	10
Back extensors	10
Psoas, left	—
Psoas, right	—
Gluteus medius, left	7
Gluteus medius, right	10
Anterior pelvic tilt	No
Lateral pelvic tilt	Slightly low on right

Note: Subject had actual shortness of right leg. Straight raise of 1/4 inch placed on right heel. Fullness in right lumbar area in forward bending.

Scoliosis: Right Thoracic, Left Thoracolumbar	
Test	Result
Forward bending (sitting)	Normal
Back contour	Tight low back
Hamstrings	Normal
Gastro-soleus	Normal
Lower abdominals	6
Upper abdominals	4
Obliques, left	3
Obliques, right	5
Back extensors	10
Psoas, left	10
Psoas, right	8
Gluteus medius, left	10
Gluteus medius, right	8
Anterior pelvic tilt	Moderate
Lateral pelvic tilt	No

Note: Marked counterclockwise rotation. Low back tight. Right Psoas exercise in sitting indicated. Straight raise of 3/16 inch placed on left heel. (See exercises, p. 127.)

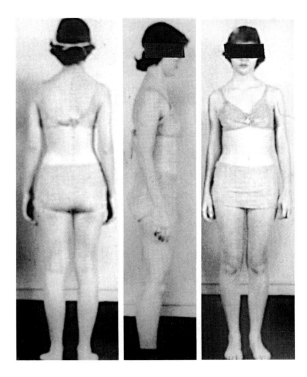

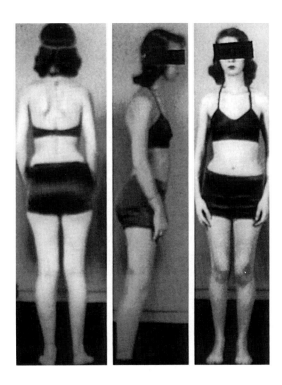

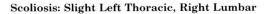

| Scoliosis: Slight Left Thoracic, Right Lumbar ||
Test	Result
Forward bending (sitting)	+ 4 inches
Back contour	Slightly excessive flexion, low back
Hamstrings	Normal +
Gastroc-soleus	Normal
Lower abdominals	10
Upper abdominals	10
Obliques, left	—
Obliques, right	—
Back extensors	10
Psoas, left	8
Psoas, right	10
Gluteus medius, left	10
Gluteus medius, right	10
Anterior pelvic tilt	No
Lateral pelvic tilt	Slightly low on right

Note: Left Psoas exercise in sitting. Cross-sectional exercise contracting left External and right Internal oblique (See exercises, p. 127.)

| Scoliosis: Left Lumbar ||
Test	Result
Forward bending (sitting)	(−) 6 inches
Back contour	Good
Hamstrings	Tight (60°)
Gastroc-soleus	Slight tightness
Lower abdominals	7
Upper abdominals	10
Obliques, left	10
Obliques, right	10
Back extensors	—
Psoas, left	8
Psoas, right	10
Gluteus medius, left	7
Gluteus medius, right	7
Anterior pelvic tilt	Moderate
Lateral pelvic tilt	No

Note: Subject a dancer and acrobat. Always did split with right leg forward. Posture shows counterclockwise rotation. Also did cartwheels in manner that encouraged same rotation. Slight anterior curve in high thoracic area.

SCOLIOSIS AND LATERAL PELVIC TILT

If the pelvis tilts laterally, the lumbar spine moves with the pelvis into a position of lateral curve, convex toward the low side. An *actual leg length difference* causes a lateral tilt in standing, low on the side of the shorter leg. A temporary position of lateral tilt can be demonstrated by standing with a lift under one foot.

An example of a muscle problem that was recognized as a contributing cause of scoliosis among polio patients is *unilateral tightness* of the Tensor fasciae latae and Iliotibial band. The effect of such tightness is to produce a lateral tilt of the pelvis, low on the side of tightness. The existence of unilateral tightness of these structures is not limited to persons with some known etiology; it is common among so-called normal individuals.

Less understood, but equally important, is the fact that *unilateral weakness* can result in a lateral pelvic tilt. Weakness of the right hip abductors as a group or, more specifically, of the right posterior Gluteus medius, will allow the pelvis to ride upward on the right side, tilting downward on the left side. Likewise, weakness of the left lateral trunk muscles will allow the left side of the pelvis to tilt downward. These weaknesses may be present separately or in combination—more often in combination (see pp. 89 and 224).

In the sitting position, lateral pelvic tilt accompanied by a lateral curve in the spine will result from unilateral weakness and atrophy of the Gluteus maximus muscle.

HANDEDNESS IN RELATION TO SCOLIOSIS

The combination of pronation of the left foot, *tightness* of the left iliotibial band, and *weakness* of the right Gluteus medius, left hip adductors, and left lateral abdominals is seen frequently among right-handed individuals who also exhibit a functional left curve. Most people do not develop a scoliosis, but of those who do, there is predominance of right thoracic, left lumbar curves. There is also a predominance of right-handed people in our society and many activities and postural positions predispose these people to problems of muscle imbalance that are only discovered by precise and adequate manual muscle testing. Among left-handed individuals, the patterns tend to be the opposite but with somewhat less frequency, probably because these people must conform to so many activities or positions that are designed for right-handed use. Muscle imbalance as related to handedness is illustrated on pp. 81 and 89.

FAULTY POSTURAL HABITS

It is important to be cognizant of the postural habits of a child in the various positions of the body in standing, sitting, and lying. For a right-handed individual seated at a desk to write, the position is one in which the body (or upper body) is turned slightly counterclockwise, the paper is turned diagonally on the desk and the right shoulder is slightly forward.

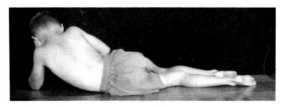

Sometimes children assume a side-lying position on the floor or bed to do their homework. A right-handed person will lie on the left side so the right hand is free to write or turn pages in a book. Such a position places the spine in a left curve.

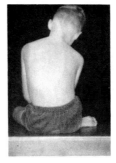

Sitting on one foot (e.g., left foot) will cause the pelvis to tilt downward on the left and upward on the right because the right buttock is raised by resting on the left foot. The spine curves left.

If a book bag is carried by a strap over the left shoulder, and the child keeps that shoulder raised to keep the strap from slipping off, there will be a tendency for the spine to curve toward the left.

Children who are engaged in repetitive asymmetrical activities, vocational or recreational, are prone to develop muscle imbalance problems that can lead to lateral deviations of the spine.

When the spine habitually curves toward the same side in the various postural positions, it becomes a matter of concern with respect to correction or prevention of early scoliosis.

Not to be overlooked are problems associated with pronation of one foot and not the other, or the habit of standing with one knee slightly bent—a problem, if it is always the same knee that is bent (see p. 367). Logically, the imbalance in hip musculature and faulty foot or leg positions, which result in lateral pelvic tilts, are more closely related to primary lumbar or thoracolumbar curves than to primary thoracic curves.

Exercises should be carefully selected on the basis of examination findings. There must be adequate instruction to ensure that exercises will be performed with precision. If possible, a parent or other individual in the home should monitor the performance until the child becomes capable of doing the exercise without supervision. The object is to use asymmetrical exercises to bring about optimal symmetry. Following is an example:

Along with other findings, it has been determined that the right Iliopsoas is weak. The subject is a dancer. One of the stretching exercises she performs is a split in which one leg is forward and the other back. Routinely, the right leg has been forward and left back. There is a left lateral curve in the lumbar region and right curve in the thoracic area.

Because the Psoas muscle attaches to the lumbar vertebrae, transverse processes, and the intervertebral discs, this muscle can pull directly on the spine. If the spine is still flexible, it can be influenced by an exercise, carefully performed, that helps to correct the lateral deviation. The exercise is done in sitting at the side of a table with the knees bent and legs hanging down. *(It is not done in a supine position.)* A strong effort is made as if to lift the right thigh in flexion, but enough resistance is applied (by an assistant or by the subject) to prevent movement of the thigh. By so doing, the force is not dissipated by movement of the thigh but is exerted on the spine, pulling it toward the right.

The accompanying photographs show (A) the S-curve of the subject in sitting, (B) the somewhat adverse effect of exercising the left Iliopsoas, (C) the correction that takes place with the exercise of the right Iliopsoas, and (D) the overall correction when the appropriate exercise to correct the thoracic curve is added.

Regarding the thoracic curve correction, the subject reaches in a diagonally upward direction, slightly forward from the coronal plane, sitting tall with spine in as good anteroposterior alignment as possible. The aim is to practice holding the corrected position in order to develop a new kinesthetic sense of what is straight. The faulty position has become so customary that the straight position feels abnormal.

The person who monitors this exercise should stand behind the subject as the exercise is being performed to be sure that both curves are being corrected at the same time. Because curves vary greatly, close monitoring is necessary to avoid emphasis on the correction of one curve at the expense of the other.

In a right thoracic, left lumbar scoliosis, there is often weakness of the posterolateral part of the right External oblique muscle, and shortness of the upper anterior part of the left External oblique. In the supine position, the subject places the right hand on the right lateral chest wall, and the left hand on the left side of the pelvis. Keeping the hands in position, the object of the exercise is to bring the two hands closer by contracting the

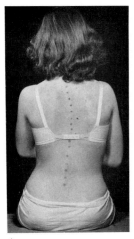

A

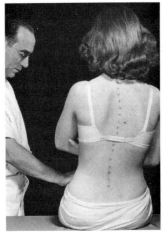

B

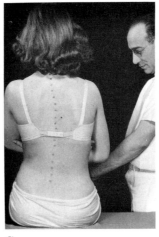

C

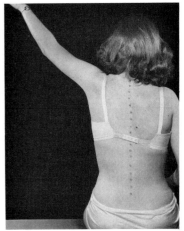

D

abdominal muscles, without flexing the trunk. It is as if the upper part of the body shifts toward the left, and the pelvis shifts toward the right. By not allowing trunk flexion, and contracting the posterior lateral fibers of the External oblique, there will be a tendency toward some counter-clockwise rotation of the thorax in the direction of correcting the thoracic rotation that accompanies a right thoracic curve.

All too often, early cases of lateral curvature are "treated" merely by observation and x-rays at specified intervals. Early tendencies toward a lateral curvature are potentially more serious than the anteroposterior deviations seen in the usual faulty postures. Instruction in good body mechanics and appropriate postural exercises, plus the necessary shoe alteration to mechanically assist in correction of alignment constitutes more rational treatment than mere observation.

Correction of lateral pelvic tilt associated with a lateral curvature can be helped by proper heel lifts. Cooperation by the subject is of utmost importance. The lifts need to be used in all shoes and bedroom slippers. But no amount of lift can help if the subject continues to stand with weight predominantly on the leg with the higher hip and with knee flexed on the side of the lift.

For use of a lift in connection with a tight Tensor fasciae latae and Iliotibial band, see p. 60. See p. 224 regarding use of lift in heel of opposite shoe to relieve strain on a weak Gluteus medius.

Along with the use of appropriate exercises, it is important to avoid those exercises that would have an adverse effect. There is an inherent danger in increasing overall flexibility of the spine. *Gains in flexibility in the direction of correcting the curves are indicated, provided that strength is also increased in order to maintain the corrections.* If the subject has the potential for gaining in strength, and is dedicated to a strict program of strengthening exercises and the wearing of a support, exercises that increase flexibility can have a desirable end result.

A subject who is developing a kyphoscoliosis along with a lordosis should not do back extension exercises from a prone position. In an effort to obtain better extension in the upper back, the low back problem increases. Extension of the upper back may be done sitting on a stool with the back against a wall, but the low back must not arch in an effort to make it appear that the upper back is straight. In this same instance, "upper" abdominal exercises by the trunk curl or sit-up should be avoided even if upper abdominals are weak. The exercise would be counter-productive because curling the trunk is rounding the upper back. If there is a developing kyphoscoliosis, such an exercise would increase the kyphotic curve. Exercise of the lower abdominals, in the form of pelvic tilt, or pelvic tilt and leg-sliding, emphasizing the action by the External oblique, would, however, be strongly indicated. (See p. 158.)

The significance of muscle imbalance and overall faulty posture as etiological factors in idiopathic scoliosis should not be overlooked. Scoliosis is a complex postural problem. As such, it calls for thorough evaluation procedures to determine the existence of weakness or tightness of muscles that results in distortion of alignment. Verification can come only from repeated testing, but the testing must be done with precision. There must be adherence to the principles upon which manual muscle testing is founded. (See p. 179.) Using a long lever whenever appropriate is vitally important in order to distinguish differences in strength of some of the large muscles (e.g., hip abductors) when comparing one side with the other.

SUPPORTS

In addition to exercises and proper shoe corrections, many early scoliosis patients need some support. It may be that only a corset type of support is needed or, as in more advanced cases, a more rigid support. The Kendalls made many of these rigid supports.

In the illustration opposite, the subject is shown wearing a removable cellulose jacket of the type often used for scoliosis cases. The procedure for making this jacket follows.

The subject was placed in a standing position with head traction from a Sayre head sling. A heel raise was used to level the pelvis and strips of adhesive tape or moleskin were placed diagonally from rib cage to opposite iliac crest to obtain the best possible correction of the trunk position before the original plaster cast was made. For girls, a brassiere with small extra padding was put on under the stockinet in order to allow room for development of the breasts.

After the positive plaster mold was poured and dry, further adjustments were made by shaving down slightly on the side of convexity and adding an equal amount of plaster at places of concavity at the same level to maintain the necessary circumference measurements. The jacket was then made over the plaster mold.

Today, there are newer materials that provide greater versatility and ease of handling, but the basic principles for use of supports remain with little change: Obtain the best possible alignment; allow for expansion in the area of concavity; apply pressure in the area of convexity to the extent tolerated without adverse effects or discomfort.

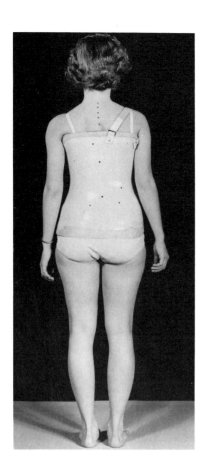

IMPORTANCE OF EARLY INTERVENTION

Instead of waiting to see if a curve gets worse before deciding to do something about it, why not treat the problem to help prevent the curve from getting worse?

Doing something in the very early stages of treating a lateral curve does not mean getting involved in a vigorous, active program of exercises, but, rather, prescribing a few carefully selected exercises that help to establish a kinesthetic sense of good alignment. It means providing good instruction to the patient and the parents in how to avoid habitual positions or activities that clearly are conducive to increasing the curvature.

It may mean taking a picture of the child's back in the usual sitting or standing position and taking another in a corrected position so the child can see the effect that the exercise has on the posture. It also means providing incentives that help keep the person interested and cooperative because achieving correction is an ongoing project.

For those in whom the curve has become more advanced, it is necessary and advisable, in many instances, to provide some kind of a support in order to help maintain the improvement in alignment that has been gained through an exercise program.

Historical Note

Henry O. Kendall was the first physical therapist at the Children's Hospital School in Baltimore, beginning work there in June, 1920. The following is a quote from some handwritten notes made by him in the early 1930s regarding scoliosis.

Symmetrical exercises should not be attempted. A careful muscle examination should be made and muscles graded according to their strength. If one group or one muscle is too strong for its antagonist, that muscle or group should be stretched and the weaker antagonist built up to sufficient strength to compete with it.

In examination of more than one hundred cases of lateral curvature, I have yet to find a case with weak erector spinae muscles, each and every case was able to hyperextend the spine against gravity and in most cases against resistance as well.

The muscle weakness was almost always found in the lateral abdominals, anterior abdominals, pelvic, hip and leg muscles. This weakness caused the body to deviate from either the lateral median plane or the anterior-posterior median plane, causing the patient to compensate for the deviation by substituting other muscles in order to maintain equilibrium. In doing the substituting, the patient invariably develops muscles which cause lateral rotatory movements and it is easy to see why we have lateral curvature with rotation.

By correcting muscle imbalance we get at the primary cause of many cases of lateral curvature.

chapter 6

Trunk Muscles, Strength Tests and Exercises

TRUNK MUSCLES

Trunk muscles consist of back extensors that bend the trunk backward, lateral flexors that bend it sideways, and anterior abdominals that bend it forward. All of these muscles play a role in stabilizing the trunk, but the back extensor muscles are the most important. The loss of stability that accompanies paralysis or marked weakness of back muscles offers dramatic evidence of their importance. Fortunately, marked weakness of these muscles occurs very seldom. In persons who have faulty posture with roundness of the upper back, weakness may exist in the extensors of the upper back, but the low back muscles are very seldom weak. The term "weak back" as frequently used in connection with low back pain mistakenly suggests that there is weakness of the low back muscles. The feeling of weakness that occurs along with a painful back is associated with the faulty alignment the body assumes and is often caused by weakness of abdominal muscles.

Despite the fact that the low back muscles are the most important, relatively little space will be devoted to them in this chapter as compared to the detailed discussion of abdominal muscles. Testing back muscles is less complicated than testing abdominal muscles, and in the field of exercise, there are few errors regarding back exercises, while there are many misconceptions and errors regarding proper abdominal exercises. Furthermore, in contrast to back muscles, weakness of abdominal muscles is prevalent. It is important to know how to test for strength and how to prescribe proper exercises for the abdominal muscles because of the effect that weakness of these muscles has on overall posture and the relationship to painful postural problems.

Illustrations, definitions, and descriptions of basic concepts are used to help achieve this purpose. The illustrations of the trunk muscles that follow, and the accompanying text, provide information in detail about the origins, insertions, and actions of these muscles. This information is essential to understanding the functions of these important trunk muscles.

The tests for evaluating strength of trunk muscles are presented in the following order:

Back extensors
Lateral trunk flexors
Oblique trunk flexors
Anterior trunk flexors
    Lower abdominal muscles
    Upper abdominal muscles

Back extensors are tested by back extension in the prone position. This test is neither complicated nor difficult to administer. (See p. 140.)

Lateral trunk flexors are tested by trunk raising sideways from a sidelying position. Oblique trunk flexors are tested by holding a position of trunk flexion and rotation. These two tests are more difficult to administer and more strenuous for the subject than the back extension test. They are not recommended for routine use. (See pp. 144 and 146.)

The tests for anterior abdominal muscles are divided into tests for strength of upper and lower abdominal muscles. These terms are useful in describing the muscle actions that are involved in flexing the upper trunk as in the trunk curl (upper abdominals), and in holding the pelvis in posterior tilt with low back flat during leg lowering (lower abdominals). The terms do not imply cranial and caudal segments of abdominal muscles.

Emphasis is being placed on the test for strength of the lower abdominals by having the description of this test precede the more familiar trunk-raising test. From the standpoint of good posture, the lower abdominals are more important than the upper. The test is less difficult to administer than the trunk-raising test, but achieving a good score is difficult for the subject because of the high incidence of weakness in the lower abdominal muscles.

The trunk-raising test for the upper abdominal muscles is a valuable test when performed correctly. However, when the ability to perform a sit-up—*regardless of how it is done*—is equated with good abdominal strength, the test loses its value. (See discussion, pp. 7 and 162.)

Definitions and Descriptions of Terms

The following definitions relate to the trunk and hip joints and are considered essential to understanding the functions of the trunk muscles.

The *trunk*, or torso, is the body excluding the head, neck, and limbs. The *thorax* (rib cage), the *abdomen* (belly), the *pelvis* (hip bones), and the *low back* are all parts of the trunk. The term *trunk raising* may be used to describe raising the trunk against gravity from various positions: from face-lying (prone), trunk raising backward; from side-lying, trunk raising sideways; from back-lying (supine), trunk raising forward. The term may also apply, in standing, to raising the trunk from positions of forward bending, side bending, or backward bending to the erect position.

The thorax is *elevated* (chest lifted up and forward) by straightening the upper back, bringing the rib cage out of a slumped position. The thorax is *depressed* when sitting or standing in a slumped position or it may be pulled downward by action of certain abdominal muscles.

The trunk is joined to the thighs at the hip joints. The movement of *hip flexion* means bending forward at the hip joint. It may be done by bringing the front of the thigh closer to the pelvis, as in leg raising, or by tilting the pelvis forward toward the thigh as in the sit-up movement. (Positions of the pelvis in good and faulty postural alignment are illustrated on pp. 20 and 76.)

In addition to understanding pelvic tilts in relation to the upright posture, it is necessary to understand how the pelvis tilts during such exercises as sit-ups and double leg raising. *During a curled trunk sit-up* with legs extended, the pelvis first tilts posteriorly, accompanied by flattening of the low back and *extension* of the hip joints. After the trunk curl phase is completed, the pelvis tilts anteriorly (forward) toward the thigh in hip flexion but still remains in posterior tilt in relation to the trunk, maintaining the flat-back position (see figures C and D on p. 173). *During a sit-up with low back arched*, on the other hand, the pelvis tilts anteriorly toward the thigh as the sit-up begins and remains tilted anteriorly.

During double leg raising, if abdominal muscles are weak, the pelvis tilts anteriorly as the legs are lifted, causing the low back to arch. When abdominal muscles are strong, the pelvis can be held in posterior tilt with the low back flat as the legs are lifted. (See pp. 137 and 155.)

Extension of the spine moves the head and trunk in a backward direction. In the neck and low back, extension results in an increase in the normal curves as the spinal column bends backward; in the upper back it results in a decrease of

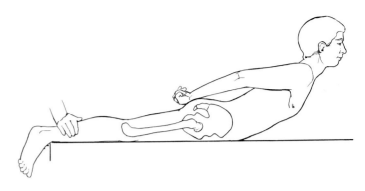

the normal curve and straightening the spine since this part does not bend backward. When done against gravity, as in lifting the head and shoulders from a face-lying position, the movement is performed by back extensor muscles with fixation of the pelvis by hip extensors.

Hyperextension of the spine is movement beyond the "normal" range of motion or may refer to a position that is greater than the normal anterior curve. Hyperextension may vary from slight to extreme.

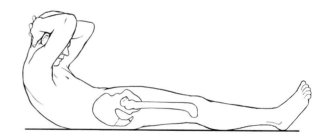

Flexion of the spine moves the head and trunk in a forward direction. In the upper back, the spine normally curves convexly backward. Flexion increases this curve resulting in a rounding of the upper back. In the neck, the spine normally curves convexly forward. Flexion, by *tilting* the head forward, usually results only in straightening the cervical spine. Seldom does flexion continue to the point that the neck curves convexly backward. Similarly, in the low back, the spine normally curves convexly forward. When a person bends the trunk forward in flexion, the forward curve in the low back *straightens* and the low back appears flat. In the neck and low back, straightening the spine may be considered normal flexion. This concept results in some confusion because one tends to think of a straight spine being extended. It is, therefore, easier to understand if one speaks in terms of the motion in low back ranging from a lordotic to a flat-back position.

Trunk curl refers to flexion of the spine only (i.e., upper back curves convexly backward, and low back straightens). When abdominal muscles are strong and hip flexor muscles are very weak, only the trunk curl can be completed when attempting to do a sit-up. The subject illustrated below has strong abdominal muscles but the hip flexors are paralyzed. (Leg braces were left on so legs could be propped in the knee-bent position for two of the photographs.)

Sitting position is one in which the trunk is upright and the hips are flexed. To *sit down* means to move from an upright to a sitting position by

flexing at the hip joints but may not require hip flexor muscle action. To *sit up* means to move from a reclining to a sitting position by flexing at the hip joints and, when done unassisted, can be performed only by hip flexor muscles. *Alone or in combination, the word "sit" should be used only in connection with movement that involves hip joint flexion.*

The *sit-up exercise*, therefore, is the movement of coming from a supine to a sitting position by flexing the hip joints, and is performed by hip flexors. It may be combined with various trunk and leg positions as illustrated on the following page.

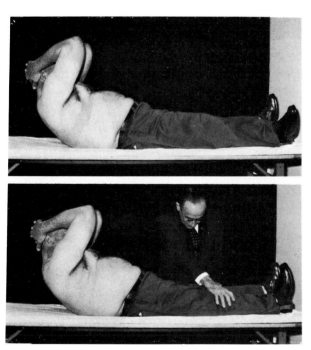

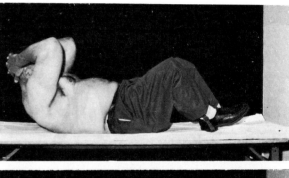

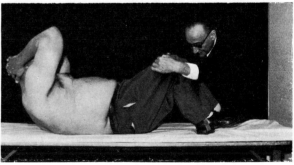

A subject with *strong abdominal muscles* and *paralyzed hip flexor muscles* can perform only the trunk curl. Flexing the trunk toward the thighs (i.e., hip joint flexion) requires action by muscles that cross the hip joint, namely, the hip flexors. Since the abdominal muscles do not cross the hip joint, they cannot assist in the movement.

It does not matter whether legs are extended or flexed, or whether legs are held down, no flexion can

occur at the hip joints in the absence of hip flexors.

It may be noted that the subject does not raise the trunk as high from the table with legs flexed as with legs extended. The pelvis moves more freely in posterior tilt with legs flexed. As the abdominal muscles shorten, both the pelvis and thorax move with the result that the thorax is not raised as high from the table as would occur if the pelvis were stabilized by the legs being in extension.

Definitions and Descriptions of Terms

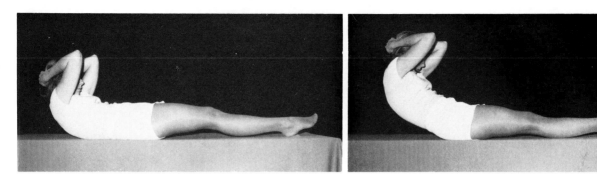

Curled-trunk sit-up with legs extended consists of flexion of the spine (trunk curl), performed by abdominal muscles, followed by flexion of the hip joints (sit-up), performed by hip flexors.

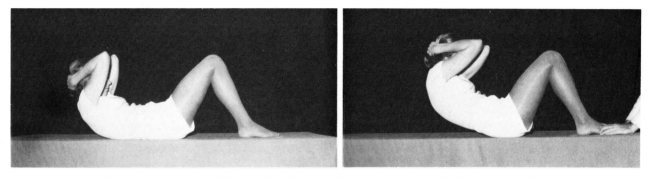

Curled-trunk sit-up with hips and knees flexed (knee bent sit-up), starts from a position of hip flexion (flexion of thigh toward pelvis) and consists of flexion of the spine (trunk curl) performed by abdominal muscles, followed by further flexion of the hip joints (by flexion of pelvis toward thigh) performed by hip flexors.

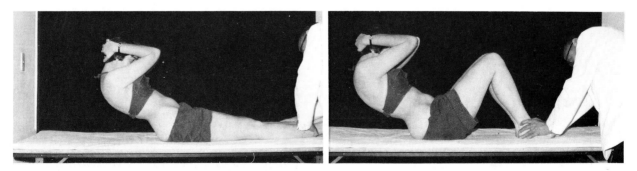

Sit-up with low back arched (with legs extended or flexed) occurs when the abdominal muscles are very weak and consists of flexion of the hip joints by action of the hip flexors, accompanied by hyperextension of the low back (lordosis). With strong hip flexors, the entire trunk-raising movement can be performed. (Compare with photographs on the preceding page in which no hip joint flexion occurs in absence of hip flexors.)

Double leg raising from a supine position is flexion of the hips with knees extended. With the knee extensors holding the knees straight, the hip flexors raise the legs upward. *No abdominal muscles cross the hip joints*, so these muscles cannot assist directly in the leg-raising movement. The role of the hip flexors is made very clear by observing the loss of function when hip flexors are paralyzed, as seen in the drawing below. The role of the abdominal muscles is illustrated in the photographs below.

In order to perform the double-leg raising movement from a supine position, the pelvis must be stabilized in some manner. Although the abdominal muscles cannot enter directly into the leg-raising movement, the strength or weakness of these muscles directly affects the trunk position and the way in which the pelvis is stabilized. Leg raising through hip flexor action, exerts a strong pull downward on the pelvis in the direction of tilting it anteriorly. The abdominal muscles pull upward on the pelvis in the direction of tilting it posteriorly.

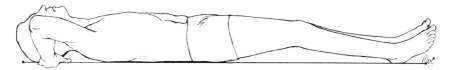

A subject with *strong abdominal muscles and very weak or paralyzed hip flexors* cannot begin to lift the legs upward from a supine position. The only active movement that occurs in attempting to raise the legs is that the pelvis is drawn forcefully into posterior tilt. Passively, the thighs may be raised slightly from the table secondary to the tilting of the pelvis, as illustrated above, or they may remain flat on the table if anterior hip joint structures are relaxed.

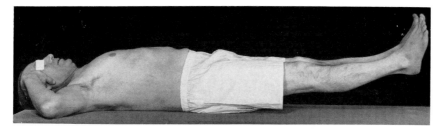

If the subject has strong abdominal muscles, the back can be held flat on the table by the abdominals holding the pelvis in posterior tilt during the leg-raising movement.

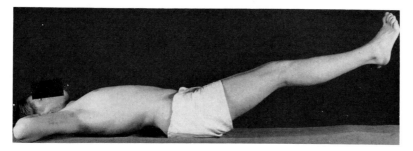

If the abdominal muscles are weak, the pelvis tilts anteriorly as the legs are lifted. As this tilt occurs, the back hyperextends, often causing pain, and the weak abdominal muscles are put on a stretch and vulnerable to strain.

137

Origins and Insertions of Neck and Back Extensors

	Origin	Insertion
Erector spinae (Superficial) Iliocostalis: lumborum	Common origin from anterior surface of broad tendon attached to medial crest of sacrum, spinous processes of lumbar and 11th and 12th thoracic vertebrae, posterior part of medial lip of iliac crest, supraspinous ligament, and lateral crests of sacrum.	By tendons into inferior borders of angles of lower six or seven ribs.
thoracis	By tendons from upper borders of angles of lower six ribs.	Cranial borders of angles of upper six ribs, and dorsum of transverse process of seventh cervical vertebra.
cervicis	Angles of third, fourth, fifth, and sixth ribs.	Posterior tubercles of transverse processes of fourth, fifth, and sixth cervical vertebrae.
Longissimus: thoracis	In lumbar region it is blended with Iliocostalis lumborum, posterior surfaces of transverse and accessory processes of lumbar vertebrae, and anterior layer of thoracolumbar fascia.	By tendons into tips of transverse processes of all thoracic vertebrae, and by fleshy digitations into lower nine or 10 ribs between tubercles and angles.
cervicis	By tendons from transverse processes of upper four or five thoracic vertebrae.	By tendons into posterior tubercles of transverse processes of second through sixth cervical vertebrae.
capitis	By tendons from transverse processes of upper four to five thoracic vertebrae, and articular processes of lower three or four cervical vertebrae.	Posterior margin of mastoid process.
Spinalis: thoracis	By tendons from spinous processes of first two lumbar and last two thoracic vertebrae.	Spinous processes of upper four to eight (variable) thoracic vertebrae
cervicis	Ligamentum nuchae, lower part; spinous process of seventh cervical.	Spinous process of axis and, occasionally, into spinous processes of C3 and C4.
capitis	Inseparably connected with Semispinalis capitis.	See below.
Transversospinalis (Deep) Semispinalis: (First layer) thoracis	Transverse processes of lower thoracic vertebrae.	Spinous processes of upper four thoracic and lower two cervical vertebrae.
cervicis	Transverse processes of upper five or six thoracic vertebrae.	Cervical spinous processes, second through fifth.
capitis	Tips of transverse processes of upper six or seven thoracic and seventh cervical vertebrae, and articular processes of cervical fourth, fifth, and sixth.	Between superior and inferior nuchal lines of occipital bone.
Multifidi (Second layer)	*Sacral region:* Posterior surface of sacrum, medial surface of posterior superior iliac spine, and posterior sacroiliac ligaments. *Lumbar region:* ⎫ *Thoracic region:* ⎬ Transverse processes of L5 *Cervical region:* ⎭ through C4.	Spanning two to four vertebrae, inserted into spinous process of a vertebra above.
Rotatores (Third layer)	Transverse processes of vertebrae.	Lamina of the vertebra above.
Interspinales	Placed in pairs between spinous processes of contiguous vertebrae. *Cervical:* six pairs. *Thoracic:* two or three pairs; between first and second, (second and third), and 11th and 12th. *Lumbar:* four pairs.	
Intertransversarii	Small muscles placed between transverse processes of contiguous vertebrae in cervical, thoracic, and lumbar regions.	
Splenius cervicis	Spinous processes of third through sixth thoracic vertebrae.	Posterior tubercles of transverse processes of first two or three cervical vertebrae.
capitis	Caudal one half of ligamentum nuchae; spinous process of seventh cervical vertebra; spinous processes of first three or four thoracic vertebrae.	Mastoid process of temporal bone, and on occipital bone inferior to lateral one third of superior nuchal line.

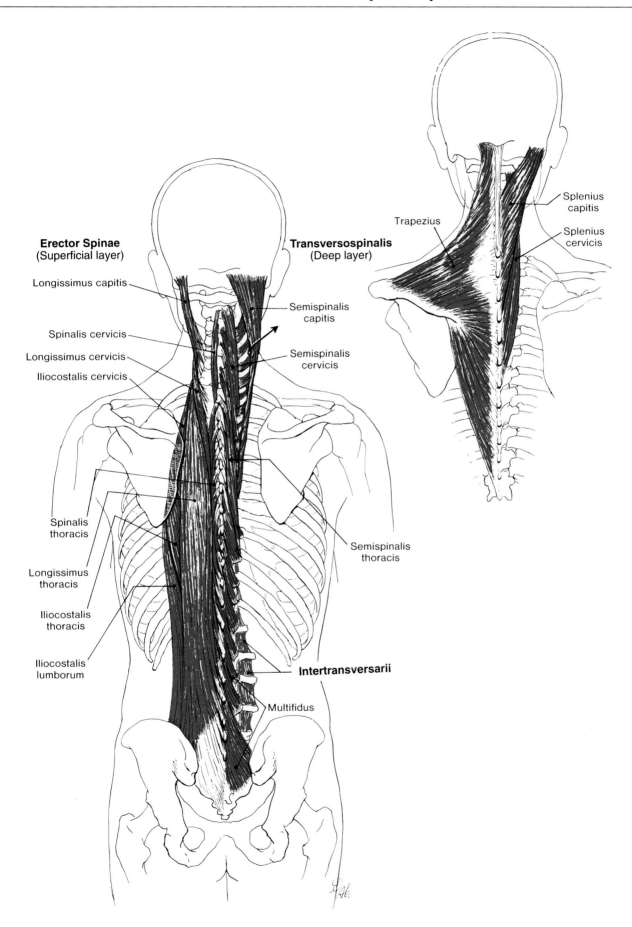

Erector Spinae
(Superficial layer)

Longissimus capitis

Spinalis cervicis

Longissimus cervicis

Iliocostalis cervicis

Spinalis
thoracis

Longissimus
thoracis

Iliocostalis
thoracis

Iliocostalis
lumborum

Transversospinalis
(Deep layer)

Semispinalis
capitis

Semispinalis
cervicis

Semispinalis
thoracis

Intertransversarii

Multifidus

Trapezius

Splenius
capitis

Splenius
cervicis

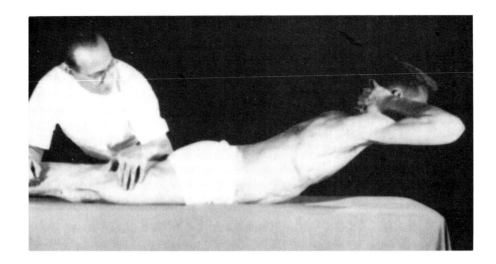

In the trunk extension test, the Erector spinae muscles are assisted by the Latissimus dorsi, Quadratus lumborum, and Trapezius.

In prone position, the low back will assume a normal anterior curve except in the presence of tight hip flexors when it will assume a degree of extension (lordosis) commensurate with the amount of hip flexor tightness. In other words, the low back will be in extension before beginning the trunk extension movement. In such a case, the subject will be *limited in the height* to which the trunk can be raised, and the mistaken interpretation may be that the back muscles are weak.

A similar situation may arise if hip extensor muscles are weak. For strong extension of the back, the hip extensors must stabilize the pelvis toward the thighs. If the hip extensors cannot provide this stabilization, the pelvis will be pulled upward by the back extensors into a position of back extension. Again, as in the case of hip flexor tightness, if the back is already in some extension before the trunk-raising movement is started, the trunk will not be raised as high from the table as it would be if the pelvis were fixed in extension on the thighs. (See pp. 141 and 142.)

To avoid false interpretations of the test, it may be necessary to perform some preliminary tests. It is not necessary to do so routinely because close observation of the subject in prone position and of the movements taking place during trunk extension will indicate if preliminary tests for length of hip flexors (p. 33) and strength of hip extensors (p. 226) should be done.

Patient: Prone with hands clasped behind buttocks (or hands clasped behind the head).

Fixation: Hip extensors must give fixation of the pelvis to the thighs, and the examiner stabilizes the legs firmly on the table.

Test: Trunk extension to the subject's full range of motion. If range appears to be limited, a second person should hold the legs down (or legs should be held down with straps) as the examiner passively raises the subject's trunk in extension to that individual's completion of spine extension.

If hip extensors are weak, it is possible that the examiner can stabilize the pelvis firmly in the direction of posterior tilt toward the thighs, provided the legs are also firmly held down by another person or by straps. (See p. 142.) Or, the subject may be placed at the end of the table, trunk prone, legs hanging down with knees bent as needed. Examiner stabilizes the pelvis and asks subject to raise trunk in extension and hold against pressure.

Pressure: If performed with hands behind the head, no pressure need be added; if performed with hands behind the back, the examiner places one hand against the subject's mid-back and exerts pressure, while stabilizing the legs with the other arm.

Grading: The ability to complete the movement and hold the position with hands behind the head or behind the back may be considered normal strength. The low back muscles are seldom weak, but if there appears to be weakness, the hip flexor tightness and/or hip extensor weakness must first be ruled out. Actual weakness can usually be determined by having the examiner raise the subject's trunk in extension (to the subject's maximum range) and asking the subject to hold the completed test position. The inability to hold will indicate weakness. Weakness is best described as slight, moderate, or marked, for purpose of grading, based on the judgment of the examiner.

Weakness: *Bilateral* weakness of the back extensor muscles results in a lumbar kyphosis and an increased thoracic kyphosis. *Unilateral* weakness results in a lateral curvature with convexity toward the weak side.

Contracture: *Bilateral* contracture of the low back muscles results in a lordosis. *Unilateral* contracture results in a scoliosis with convexity toward the opposite side.

For back extensors to raise the trunk from a prone position, the hip extensors must fix the pelvis in extension on the thigh.

Normally, extension of the hip joints and extension of the lumbar spine are initiated simultaneously and not as two separate movements.

The illustrations on this page show the variations that occur depending upon the strength of the two primary muscle groups.

If slight tightness exists in hip flexors, there is no range of extension in the hip joint, and all the movement in the direction of leg raising backward is accomplished by lumbar spine hyperextension and pelvic tilt.

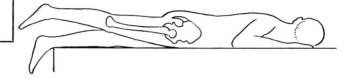

For hip extensors to raise the extremity backward from a prone position through the few degrees of true hip joint extension (approximately 10°) the back extensors must stabilize the pelvis to the trunk.

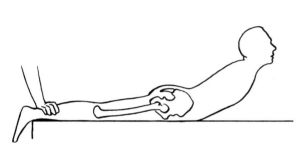

A subject with *strong back extensor muscles* and *strong hip extensor muscles* can raise the trunk in extension.

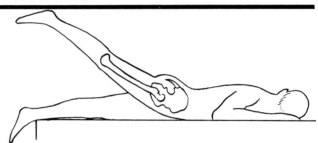

Raising the extremity higher is accomplished by hyperextension of the lumbar spine and anterior tilting of the pelvis. In this latter movement, the back extensors are assisted by hip flexors on the opposite side, helping to tilt the pelvis anteriorly.

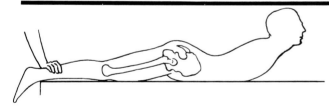

A subject with *strong back extensor muscles* and *markedly weak or paralyzed hip extensor muscles,* can hyperextend the lumbar spine, but the trunk cannot be lifted high from the table.

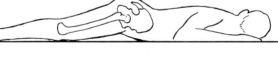

In an effort to lift the extremity, the back muscles contract to fix the pelvis on the trunk, but, with little or no strength in the hip extensors, the thigh cannot be extended on the pelvis. The unopposed pull of the back muscles results in hyperextension of the back, and the hip joint is passively drawn into flexion despite the effort to extend it.

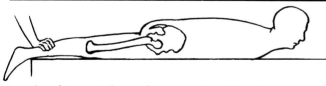

A subject with *weak or paralyzed back extensor muscles* and *strong hip extensor muscles* cannot raise the trunk in extension. The hip extensors, in their action to fix the pelvis, are unopposed, the pelvis tilts posteriorly, and the lumbar spine flexes.

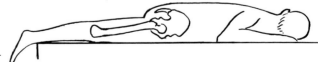

In an effort to lift the extremity, the hip extensors contract, but the extremity cannot be lifted because the back muscles are unable to stabilize the pelvis. The pelvis tilts posteriorly by the pull of the hip extensors and the weight of the extremity, instead of tilting anteriorly as it would if the back extensors were normal.

Treatment for Weakness of Back Muscles

An individual should be able to raise the trunk backward from a face-lying position to the extent that range of motion of the back permits. If a person does not have the strength to perform this movement, and if there is no contraindication, then back-extension exercises would be appropriate. Adequate strength in back muscles is important for maintenance of upright posture.

Marked weakness of Erector spinae muscles is not seen except in connection with neuromuscular problems. Even in cases of extensive involvement in some neuromuscular conditions, the back extensor muscles are often spared.

When there is severe involvement, a support is necessary. The type, rigidity, and length of the support depend upon the severity of the weakness. Entire trunk musculature is usually involved if Erector spinae are weak. The collapse of the trunk takes place anteroposteriorly and laterally.

Exercises to build up strength in extensors must be gauged according to the patient's tolerance and response. Good alignment must be preserved in recumbent positions, and support must be provided in sitting or standing positions to help maintain any benefit from exercises.

Weakness of the low back is seldom seen in ordinary faulty posture problems. The back muscles are an exception to the general rule that muscles that are elongated beyond normal range tend to show weakness. For a striking example, see p. 37 for photographs of a subject who has excessive flexion, but normal back strength (p. 49, right).

Weakness of the upper back Erector spinae develops as shoulders slump forward and the upper back becomes rounded. If the back has not become fixed in the faulty position, exercises are indicated to help strengthen the upper back extensors and stretch opposing anterior trunk muscles if they have begun to shorten. Proper shoulder supports are indicated during the period when muscles are very weak.

The middle and lower portions of the Trapezius muscles reinforce the upper back extensors and help to hold the shoulders back. The manner in which these muscles are exercised is very important. (The wall-sitting and wall-standing exercises are illustrated on pp. 68 and 117–118.)

It is necessary to check whether there is opposing tightness that limits the range of motion before attempting to do the exercises. Tests for length of Latissimus dorsi and Teres major, Pectoralis major, and Pectoralis minor should be done. (See pp. 62 and 63.) Tightness in upper anterior abdominal muscles, and restriction of chest expansion will also interfere with efforts to straighten the upper back.

As a general rule, exercises for the Rhomboid muscles are not indicated. Although these muscles pull the shoulders back, they do so in a manner that elevates the shoulder girdle and tends to tip it forward in a faulty postural position. Besides, the Rhomboids are usually strong.

WEAKNESS OF GLUTEUS MAXIMUS

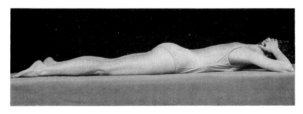

Lying prone on table, subject exhibits normal anterior curve in low back.

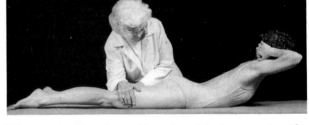

When extension is continued, subject can raise the trunk farther but not to completion of the range of motion.

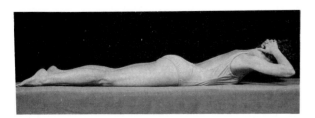

The moment that back extension is *initiated*, the curve in the low back increases because of weakness in the Gluteus maximus.

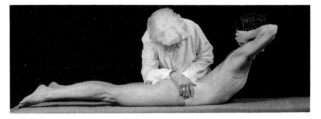

Holding the pelvis in the direction of posterior pelvic tilt, in the manner provided by a strong Gluteus maximus, enables the subject to complete the full range of motion.

142

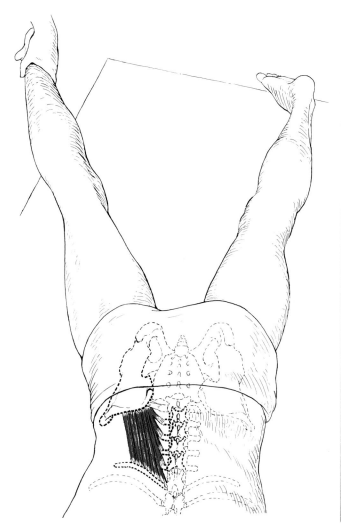

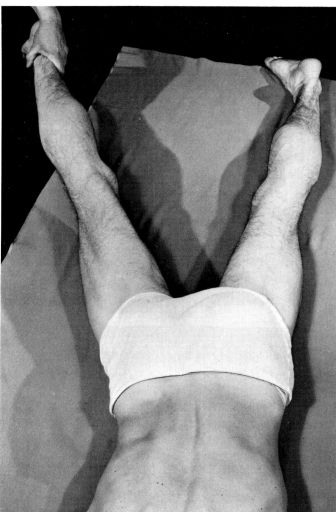

Origin: Iliolumbar ligament, iliac crest. Occasionally from upper borders of transverse processes of lower three or four lumbar vertebrae.

Insertion: Inferior border of last rib and transverse processes of upper four lumbar vertebrae.

Action: Assists in extension, laterally flexes the lumbar vertebral column, and depresses the last rib. Bilaterally, acting together with the diaphragm fixes the last two ribs during respiration.

Nerve: Lumbar plexus, T12, L**1, 2, 3.**

Patient: Prone.

Fixation: By muscles which hold the femur firmly in the acetabulum.

Test Movement: Elevation of the pelvis laterally. The extremity is placed in slight extension and in the degree of abduction that corresponds with the line of fibers of the Quadratus lumborum.

Resistance: Given in the form of traction on the extremity, directly opposing the line of pull of the

Quadratus lumborum. If hip muscles are weak, pressure may be given against the posterolateral iliac crest opposite the line of pull of the muscle.

The Quadratus lumborum acts along with other muscles in lateral trunk flexion. It is difficult to palpate this muscle because it lies deep beneath the Erector spinae. Although the Quadratus lumborum enters into the motion of elevation of the pelvis in the standing position or in walking, the standing position does not offer a satisfactory position for testing. Elevation of the right side of the pelvis in standing, for example, depends as much, if not more, on the downward pull by the abductors of the left hip joint as it does on the upward pull of right lateral abdominals.

The test illustrated should not be considered as limited to Quadratus lumborum action, but as giving the most satisfactory differentiation that can be obtained. This text does not recommend attempting to grade numerically the strength of this muscle but merely to record whether it appears weak or strong.

Lateral Trunk Flexors

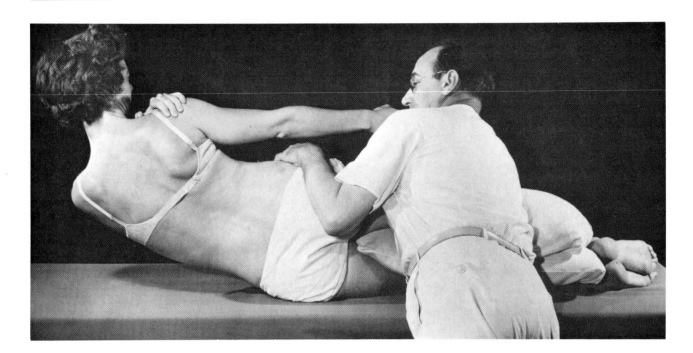

Before doing the test for lateral trunk muscles, one should test the strength of hip abductors, adductors, and lateral neck flexors; and test for the range of motion in lateral flexion.

Trunk raising sideways is a combination of lateral trunk flexion and hip abduction (the latter produced by downward tilting of the pelvis on the thigh). The lateral trunk muscles entering into the movement are the lateral fibers of the External and Internal obliques, the Quadratus lumborum, the Latissimus dorsi, and the Rectus abdominis on the side being tested.

Patient: Side-lying with pillow between thighs and legs, and with head, upper trunk, pelvis, and lower extremities in a straight line. The top arm is extended down along the side, and fingers are closed so patient will not hold onto the thigh and attempt to assist with the hand. The under arm is forward across the chest with the hand holding the upper shoulder to rule out assistance by pushing up with the elbow.

Fixation: Hip abductors must fix the pelvis to the thigh. The opposite adductors also help stabilize the pelvis. The legs must be held down by the examiner to counterbalance the weight of the trunk, but must not be held so firmly as to prevent the upper leg from moving slightly downward to accommodate for the displacement downward of the pelvis on that side. If the pelvis is pushed upward or not allowed to tilt downward, the subject will be unable to raise the trunk sideways even if the lateral abdominal muscles are strong.

Test Movement: Trunk raising directly sideways without rotation.

Resistance: The body weight offers sufficient resistance.

Normal (10) Grade:* The ability to raise the trunk laterally from a side-lying position to a point of maximum lateral flexion.

Good (8) Grade: Same as above except underneath shoulder is about 4 inches up from table.

Fair (5) Grade: Same as above except underneath shoulder is about 2 inches up from table. See p. 176 for tests and grades in cases of marked weakness of lateral trunk muscles.

Note: Test of the lateral trunk muscles may reveal an imbalance in the oblique muscles. In trunk raising sideways, if the legs and the pelvis are held steady, that is, not permitted to twist forward or backward from the direct side-lying position, the thorax may be rotated forward or backward as the trunk is laterally flexed. A forward twist of the thorax denotes a stronger pull by the External oblique, while a backward twist denotes a stronger pull by the Internal oblique. If the back hyperextends as the patient raises the trunk, the Quadratus lumborum and the Latissimus dorsi show a stronger pull, indicating that anterior abdominal muscles cannot counterbalance this pull to keep the trunk in straight line with the pelvis.

The test for strength of the lateral trunk flexors is important in cases of scoliosis.

---

*See numerical equivalents for word symbols used in grading, p. 188; and *Key to Muscle Grading*, p. 189.

STRONG LATERAL TRUNK MUSCLES AND STRONG HIP ABDUCTOR MUSCLES

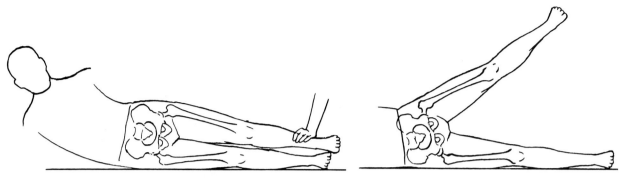

Lateral trunk flexion through subject's full range of motion.

Hip abduction through subject's full range of motion.

STRONG LATERAL TRUNK MUSCLES AND PARALYZED HIP ABDUCTOR MUSCLES

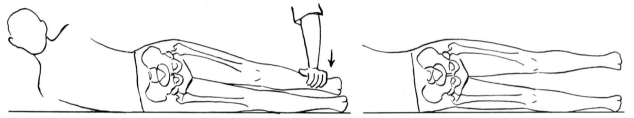

Subject can laterally flex the trunk but the underneath shoulder will scarcely be raised from the table. The pelvis will be drawn upward as the head is raised laterally and the iliac crest and costal margin will be approximated.

In attempting to raise the extremity in abduction, the movement that occurs is elevation of the pelvis by the lateral trunk muscles. The extremity may be drawn upward into the position as illustrated, but the hip joint is not abducted. Actually the thigh has dropped into a position of adduction and is held there by the joint structures rather than by hip muscle action.

WEAK LATERAL TRUNK MUSCLES AND STRONG HIP ABDUCTOR MUSCLES

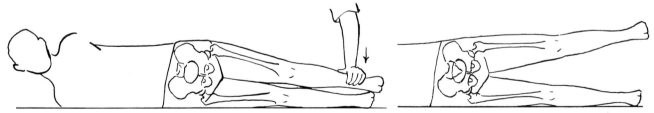

Subject cannot raise the trunk in true lateral flexion. Under certain circumstances the patient may be able to raise the trunk from the table laterally even though lateral trunk muscles are quite weak. If the trunk can be held rigid, the hip abductor muscles may raise the trunk in abduction on the thigh. The rib cage and iliac crest will not be approximately laterally as they are when the lateral trunk muscles are strong. By decreasing the pressure providing fixation for the hip abductors, the examiner can make it necessary for the lateral abdominals to attempt initiation of the movement.

The extremity can be lifted in hip abduction, but without the fixation by the lateral abdominal muscles, it cannot be raised high from the table. Due to the weakness of the lateral trunk muscles, the weight of the extremity tilts the pelvis downward.

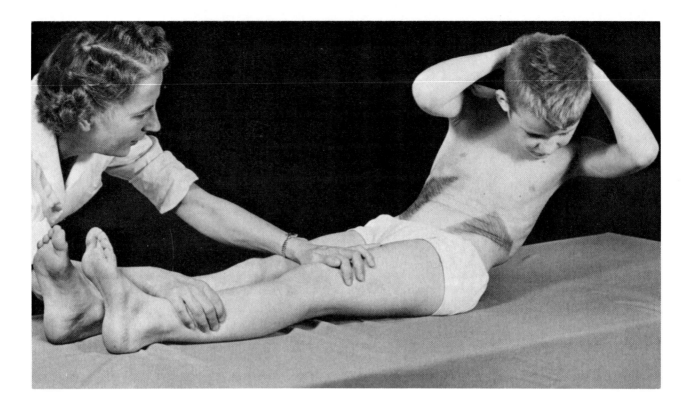

Raising the trunk obliquely forward combines trunk flexion and rotation. It is accomplished by action of the Rectus abdominis, and by the External oblique on one side combined with the Internal oblique on the opposite side.

The oblique trunk flexion test is usually performed after tests for upper and lower abdominals have been done.

Patient: Supine. (For arm position, see below under *Grading*.)

Fixation: Assistant stabilizes the legs as examiner places the patient in test position. (Examiner not shown in photograph.)

Test: Patient clasps hands behind head. Examiner *places* patient in precise test position of trunk flexion and rotation, and asks patient to hold that position. If the muscles are weak, the trunk will derotate and extend. There may be increased flexion of the pelvis on the thighs in an effort to hold the extended trunk up from the table.

Resistance: None in addition to the weight of the trunk. Resistance is varied by position of the arms.

Normal (10) Grade:* The ability to hold the test position with the hands clasped behind the head.

Good (8) Grade: Same as above except with arms folded across the chest.

Fair+ (6) Grade: Same as above except with arms extended forward. (See illustration of arm positions p. 163.)

Fair (5) Grade: Ability to hold trunk in enough flexion and rotation to raise both scapular regions up from the table. See p. 176 for tests and grades in cases of marked weakness of oblique trunk muscles.

Note: The test for strength of the oblique abdominal muscles is important in cases of scoliosis.

---

*See numerical equivalents for word symbols used in grading, p. 188; and *Key to Muscle Grading*, p. 189.

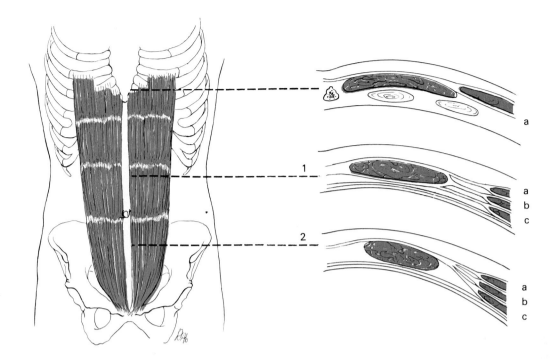

Origin: Pubic crest and symphysis.

Insertion: Costal cartilages of fifth, sixth, and seventh ribs, and xiphoid process of sternum.

Direction of Fibers: Vertical.

Action: Flexes the vertebral column by approximating the thorax and pelvis anteriorly. With the pelvis fixed, the thorax will move toward the pelvis; with the thorax fixed, the pelvis will move toward the thorax.

Nerve: T5–T12, ventral rami.

Weakness: A weakness of this muscle results in a decrease in the ability to flex the vertebral column. In the supine position, the ability to tilt the pelvis posteriorly or to approximate the thorax toward the pelvis is decreased, making it difficult to raise the head and upper trunk. In order for anterior neck flexors to raise the head from a supine position, it is essential that anterior abdominal muscles, particularly the Rectus abdominis, fix the thorax. With marked weakness of abdominal muscles an individual may not be able to raise the head even though neck flexors are strong. In the erect position, weakness of this muscle permits an anterior pelvic tilt and a lordotic posture (increased anterior convexity of the lumbar spine).

Note: Cross Sections of Rectus Abdominis and its Sheath:

(1) Above the arcuate line the aponeurosis of the Internal oblique (b) divides. Its anterior lamina fuses with the aponeurosis of the External oblique (a) to form the ventral layer of the Rectus sheath. Its posterior lamina fuses with the aponeurosis of the Transversus abdominis (c) to form the dorsal layer of the Rectus sheath.

(2) Below the arcuate line the aponeuroses of all three muscles fuse to form the ventral layer of the Rectus sheath, and the transversalis fascia forms the dorsal layer. (See also p. 151.)

External Oblique

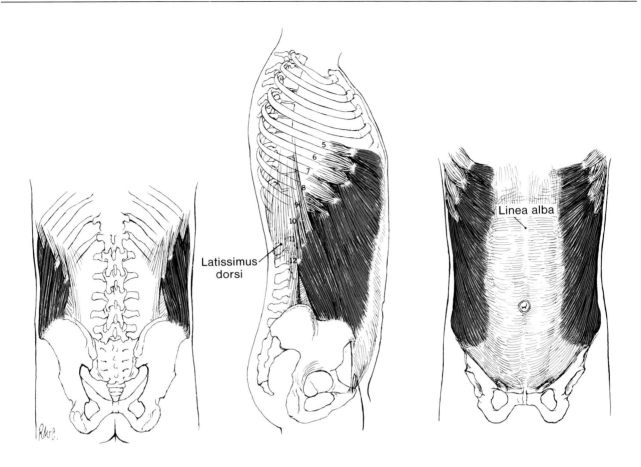

Latissimus dorsi

Linea alba

EXTERNAL OBLIQUE, ANTERIOR FIBERS

Origin: External surfaces of ribs five through eight interdigitating with Serratus anterior.

Insertion: Into a broad, flat aponeurosis, terminating in the linea alba, a tendinous raphe which extends from the xiphoid.

Direction of Fibers: The fibers extend obliquely downward and medialward with the uppermost fibers more medialward.

Action: Acting *bilaterally*, the anterior fibers flex the vertebral column approximating the thorax and pelvis anteriorly, support and compress the abdominal viscera, depress the thorax, and assist in respiration. Acting *unilaterally* with the anterior fibers of the Internal oblique on the opposite side, the anterior fibers of the External oblique rotate the vertebral column, bringing the thorax forward (when the pelvis is fixed), or the pelvis backward (when the thorax is fixed). For example, with the pelvis fixed, the right External oblique rotates the thorax counterclockwise, and the left External oblique rotates the thorax clockwise.

Nerves to anterior and lateral fibers: T5, 6, T7–12.

EXTERNAL OBLIQUE, LATERAL FIBERS

Origin: External surface of ninth rib, interdigitating with Serratus anterior; and external surfaces of 10th, 11th and 12th ribs, interdigitating with Latissimus dorsi.

Insertion: As the inguinal ligament, into anterior superior spine and pubic tubercle, and into the external lip of anterior one half of iliac crest.

Direction of Fibers: Fibers extend obliquely downward and medialward, more downward than the anterior fibers.

Action: Acting *bilaterally*, the lateral fibers of the External oblique flex the vertebral column, with major influence on the lumbar spine, tilting the pelvis posteriorly. (See also action in relation to posture, p. 161.) Acting *unilaterally* with the lateral fibers of the Internal oblique on the same side, these fibers of the External oblique laterally flex the vertebral column, approximating the thorax and iliac crest. These External oblique fibers also act with the Internal oblique on the opposite side to rotate the vertebral column. The External oblique, in its action on the thorax, is comparable to the Sternocleidomastoid in its action on the head.

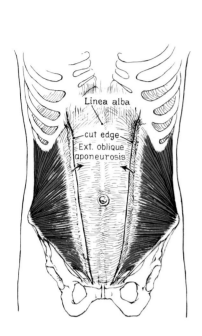
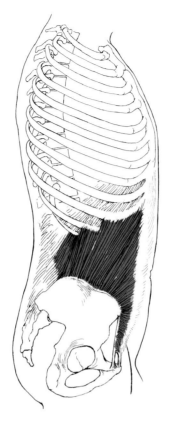
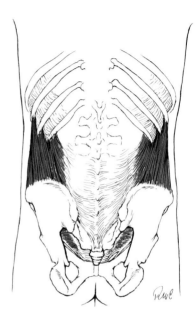

INTERNAL OBLIQUE, LOWER ANTERIOR FIBERS

Origin: Lateral two thirds of inguinal ligament, and short attachment on iliac crest near anterior superior spine.

Insertion: With Transversus abdominis into crest of pubis, medial part of pectineal line, and into linea alba by means of an aponeurosis.

Direction of Fibers: Fibers extend transversely across lower abdomen.

Action: The lower anterior fibers compress and support the lower abdominal viscera in conjunction with the Transversus abdominis.

INTERNAL OBLIQUE, UPPER ANTERIOR FIBERS

Origin: Anterior one third of intermediate line of iliac crest.

Insertion: Linea alba by means of aponeurosis.

Direction of Fibers: Fibers extend obliquely medialward and upward.

Action: Acting *bilaterally,* the upper anterior fibers flex the vertebral column, approximating the thorax and pelvis anteriorly, support and compress the abdominal viscera, depress the thorax, and assist in respiration. Acting *unilaterally,* in conjunction with the anterior fibers of the External oblique on the opposite side, the upper anterior fibers of the Internal oblique rotate the vertebral column, bringing the thorax backward (when the pelvis is fixed), or the pelvis forward (when the thorax is fixed). For example, the right Internal oblique rotates the thorax clockwise, and the left Internal oblique rotates the thorax counterclockwise on a fixed pelvis.

INTERNAL OBLIQUE, LATERAL FIBERS

Origin: Middle one third of intermediate line of iliac crest, and thoracolumbar fascia.

Insertion: Inferior borders of 10th, 11th, and 12th ribs and linea alba by means of aponeurosis.

Direction of Fibers: Fibers extend obliquely upward and medialward, more upward than the anterior fibers.

Action: Acting *bilaterally,* the lateral fibers flex the vertebral column, approximating the thorax and pelvis anteriorly, and depress the thorax. Acting *unilaterally* with the lateral fibers of the External oblique on the same side, these fibers of the Internal oblique laterally flex the vertebral column, approximating the thorax and pelvis. These fibers also act with the External oblique on the opposite side to rotate the vertebral column.

Nerves to anterior and lateral fibers: T7–11, T12, Iliohypogastric and ilioinguinal, ventral rami.

149

External and Internal Obliques

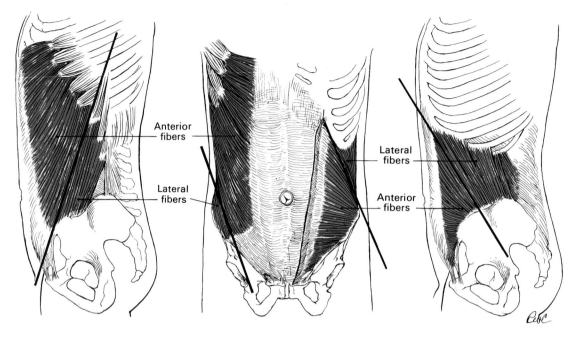

External oblique   Internal oblique

Weakness: Moderate or marked weakness of both External and Internal obliques decreases respiratory efficiency and decreases support of abdominal viscera.

Bilateral weakness of External obliques decreases the ability to flex the vertebral column and tilt the pelvis posteriorly. In standing, it results in either anterior pelvic tilt, or in an anterior deviation of the pelvis in relation to the thorax and lower extremities. (See p. 161.)

Bilateral weakness of Internal obliques decreases the ability to flex the vertebral column.

Cross-sectional weakness of External oblique on one side, and Internal oblique on the other allows separation of costal margin from opposite iliac crest resulting in rotation and lateral deviation of the vertebral column. With weakness of the right External oblique and left Internal oblique (as seen in a right thoracic, left lumbar scoliosis) there is a separation of the right costal margin from the left iliac crest. The thorax deviates toward the right and rotates posteriorly on the right. With weakness of the left External and right Internal obliques the reverse occurs.

Unilateral weakness of lateral fibers of External oblique and Internal oblique on the same side allow separation of the thorax and iliac crest laterally, resulting in a C-curve convex toward the side of weakness. Weakness of the lateral fibers of the left External and Internal obliques gives rise to a left C-curve.

Shortness: *Bilateral shortness of anterior fibers of External and Internal oblique* muscles causes the thorax to be depressed anteriorly contributing to flexion of the vertebral column. In standing, this will be seen as a tendency toward kyphosis and depressed chest. In a kyphosis-lordosis posture, the lateral portions of the Internal oblique are shortened, and the lateral portions of the External oblique are elongated. These same findings occur in a sway-back posture with anterior deviation of the pelvis and posterior deviation of the thorax.

Cross-sectional shortness of External oblique on one side and Internal oblique on the other causes rotation and lateral deviation of the vertebral column. Shortness of left External oblique and right Internal oblique, as seen in advanced cases of right thoracic, left lumbar scoliosis, causes rotation of the thorax forward on the left.

Unilateral shortness of lateral fibers of External oblique and Internal oblique on same side causes approximation of the iliac crest and thorax laterally resulting in a C-curve convex toward the opposite side. Shortness of the lateral fibers of the right Internal and External obliques may be seen in a left C-curve.

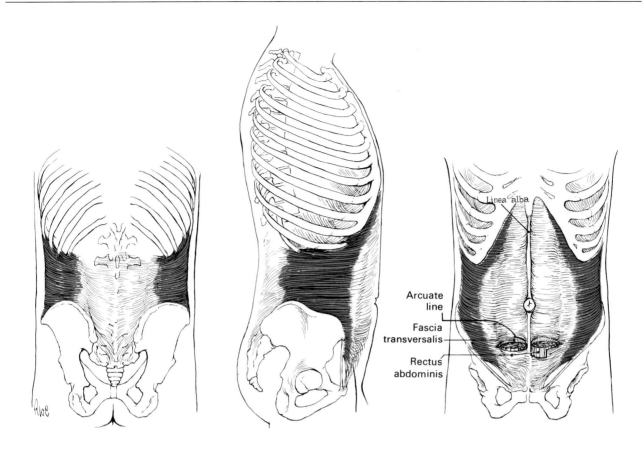

Origin: Inner surfaces of cartilages of lower six ribs, interdigitating with the Diaphragm; thoracolumbar fascia; anterior three fourths of internal lip of iliac crest; and lateral one third of inguinal ligament.

Insertion: Linea alba by means of a broad aponeurosis, pubic crest and pecten pubis.

Direction of Fibers: Transverse (horizontal).

Action: Acts likes a girdle to flatten the abdominal wall and compress the abdominal viscera; upper portion helps to decrease the infrasternal angle of the ribs as in expiration. This muscle has no action in lateral trunk flexion except that it acts to compress the viscera and stabilize the linea alba, thereby permitting better action by anterolateral trunk muscles.

Nerve: T7–T12, Iliohypogastric, ilioinguinal, ventral divisions.

Weakness: Permits a bulging of the anterior abdominal wall, thereby indirectly tending to affect an increase in lordosis. (See accompanying photograph.) During flexion in the supine position, and hyperextension of the trunk in the prone position, there tends to be a bulging laterally if the Transversus abdominis is weak.

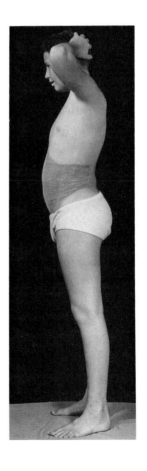

Differentiating Upper and Lower Abdominals

The use of the terms "upper" and "lower" differentiates two important strength tests for abdominal muscles. More often than not, there is a difference between the grades of strength attributed to upper abdominals as compared to lower.

If the same muscles entered into both tests, and the difference in strength were due to a difference in the difficulty of the tests, then there should be a fairly constant ratio between the two tests.

In the order of frequency, the following combinations of strength and weakness are found:

Upper strong and lower weak
Upper and lower both weak
Upper and lower both strong
Lower strong and upper weak

The difference in strength may be remarkable. A subject who can perform as many as fifty or more curled-trunk sit-ups may grade less than fair on the leg-lowering test. The same subject can build up the strength of the lower abdominals to normal by doing exercises specifically localized to the External oblique.

Because the oblique abdominal muscles are essentially fan-shaped, a part of one muscle may function in a somewhat different role than another part of the same muscle. A consideration of the attachments and the line of pull of the fibers, coupled with clinical observations of patients with marked or spotty weakness as well as those with normal musculature, leads to certain conclusions regarding the action of the various muscles or segments of abdominal muscles.

The Rectus abdominis does enter into both tests, but there is a distinct difference between the actions of the Internal oblique and that of the External oblique as exhibited by the two tests.

When analyzing which muscles or parts of muscles enter into the various tests, it is necessary to observe the movements that take place and the line of pull of the muscles that enter into the movement.

As trunk flexion is initiated by *slowly* raising the head and shoulders from a supine position, it will be observed that the chest is depressed and the thorax is pulled toward the pelvis. Simultaneously, the pelvis tilts posteriorly. These movements obviously result from action of the Rectus abdominis muscle. (See figure below.)

Along with depression of the chest, the ribs flare outward and the infrasternal angle is increased. These movements are compatible with the action of the Internal oblique.

No test movement can cause an approximation of parts to which the lower transverse fibers of the Internal oblique are attached since these fibers extend across the lower abdomen from ilium to ilium like the lower fibers of the Transversus abdominis. In posterior pelvic tilt and in trunk-raising movements, however, this part of the Internal oblique will act with the Transversus to compress the lower abdomen.

Electromyographic studies may either confirm or modify the conclusions drawn from clinical observations.

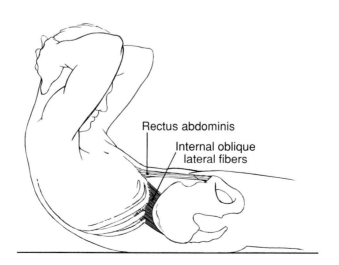

Rectus abdominis

Internal oblique
lateral fibers

As the trunk curl is completed and the movement enters the hip flexion phase, one will observe that the rib cage that had flared outward is now being pulled inward and the infrasternal angle decreases. The anterior fibers of the External oblique come into play.

If the Internal oblique and Rectus are strong (as indicated by the ability to perform numerous curled-trunk sit-ups), and if part of the External oblique is also brought into action during this movement, where is the weakness that accounts for the marked difference in tests of upper and lower abdominals?

The probability is that the posterior lateral fibers of the External oblique are actually elongated as the thoracic spine flexes in completion of the trunk curl. (See figure below.) These fibers of the External oblique help to draw the *posterior rib cage* toward the *anterior iliac crest* and, in so doing, tend to extend, not flex, the thoracic spine. The photographs on p. 161 indicate the line of pull of the posterolateral fibers of the External oblique in good alignment, and the elongation of these fibers in faulty position.

The action of the External oblique may also be observed in cases of scoliosis in which muscle imbalance exists between the right and left External oblique muscles. It is not uncommon to observe that flexion of the spine may begin with a rather symmetrical pull; however, as the effort is made to raise the trunk in flexion toward the thighs, there will be forward rotation of the thorax, with extension of the thoracic spine on the side of the stronger External oblique.

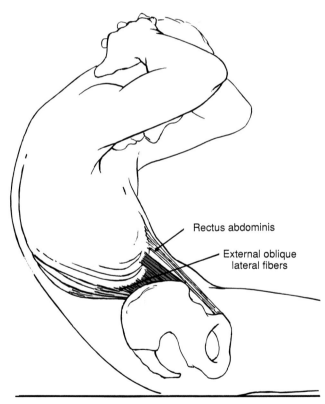

Rectus abdominis

External oblique
lateral fibers

With the trunk held in flexion during the hip flexion phase of trunk raising, the Rectus abdominis, anterior fibers of the External oblique, and the upper anterior and lateral fibers of the Internal oblique shorten. The posterolateral fibers of the External oblique elongate.

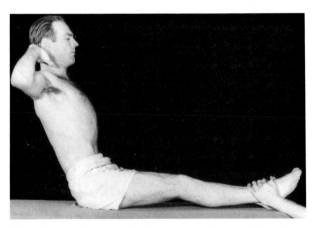

The above photograph shows a subject, with strong External oblique muscles, doing a sit-up with the trunk held straight and the lower abdomen pulled up and in. This is in sharp contrast to a curled-trunk sit-up like figure on left, or to an arched-back sit-up like subject on p. 165.

153

Anterior Trunk Flexors: Lower Abdominal Muscle Test

Anterior trunk flexion by lower abdominal muscles focuses on the ability of these muscles to flex the lumbar spine by flattening the low back on the table, and holding it flat against the gradually increasing resistance provided by the leg-lowering movement.

Patient: Supine on a firm surface. A folded blanket may be used, but no soft pad. Forearms are folded across the chest to ensure that the elbows are not resting on the table for support.

Fixation: None should be applied to the trunk because the test is to determine the ability of the abdominal muscles to fix the pelvis in approximation to the thorax against resistance by the leg lowering. Giving stabilization to the trunk would be giving assistance. Allowing the patient to hold on to the table, or to rest hands or elbows on the table would also provide assistance.

Test: The examiner assists the patient in raising legs to a vertical position, or has the patient raise them *one at a time* to that position, keeping the knees straight. (Hamstring tightness will interfere with obtaining the full starting position.)

Have the subject tilt the pelvis posteriorly to flatten the low back on the table by contracting the abdominal muscles, and *hold it flat* while slowly lowering the legs. Attention is focused on the position of the low back and pelvis as the legs are lowered. The subject should not raise the head and shoulders during the test.

Resistance: The force exerted by the hip flexors and the *lowering of the legs* tends to tilt the pelvis anteriorly and acts as a *strong resistance against the abdominal muscles* which are attempting to hold the pelvis in posterior tilt. As the legs are lowered by the eccentric (lengthening) contraction of the hip flexors, leverage increases and provides increasing resistance against the abdominal muscles for the purpose of grading the strength of these muscles.

Grading: Strength is graded based on the ability to keep the low back flat on the table while slowly lowering both legs from the vertical (90° angle).

The angle between the extended legs and the table is noted *at the moment* that the pelvis starts to tilt anteriorly and the low back arches from the table. To help detect the moment this occurs, the examiner may place one hand at (but not under) the low back and the other hand with the thumb just below the anterior-superior spine of the ilium. However, when testing patients with weakness or pain, place the thumb of one hand just below the anterior-superior spine and leave the other hand free to support the legs the moment the back starts to arch.

The leg-lowering test for abdominal strength is not applicable to very young children. The weight of the legs is small in relation to the trunk, and the back does not arch as legs are raised or lowered. Furthermore, at the age of 6 or 7 years when the test would have some significance, it is not easy for a child to differentiate muscle action and try to hold the back flat while lowering the legs. From about age 8 or 10 years, it is possible to use the test for many children. As adolescence approaches and the legs grow long in relation to the trunk, the picture reverses from that of early childhood and the leverage exerted by the legs as they are lowered is greater in relation to the trunk. At this age, grades of fair+ or good− on the leg-lowering tests should be considered "normal for age" for many children, especially those who have grown tall very quickly. After the ages of 14 to 16, males should have the strength to grade normal, and females should grade good. Because of the distribution of body weight, men have an advantage in the leg-lowering test, and women have an advantage in the trunk-raising test.

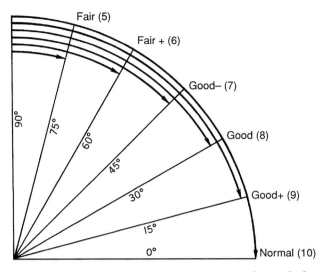

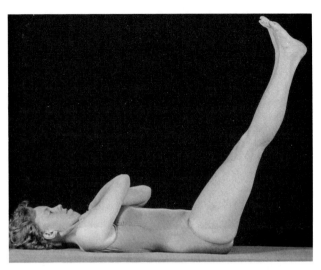

See numerical equivalents for word symbols used in grading, p. 188; and *Key to Muscle Grading*, p. 189.

Fair+ (6) Grade: With arms folded across chest, the subject is able to keep the low back flat on the table while lowering the legs to an angle of 60° with the table.

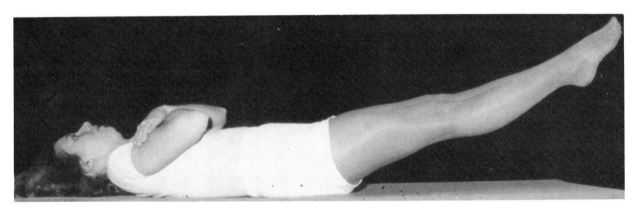

Good (8) Grade: With arms folded across the chest, the subject is able to keep the low back flat while lowering the legs to an angle of 30° with the table. (In this illustration, the legs are at a 20° angle.)

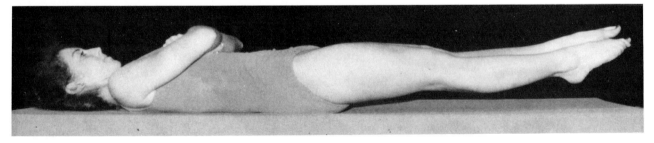

Normal (10) Grade: With arms folded across the chest, the subject is able to keep the low back flat on the table while lowering the legs to table level. (The legs are elevated a few degrees for the photograph.)

155

Abdominal Muscle Action During Leg Lowering

When discussing the actions of the abdominal muscles, it should be recognized that various segments of the abdominal musculature are closely allied and interdependent. However, the External oblique is essentially fan-shaped and different segments may have different actions. The pelvis can be tilted posteriorly by an upward pull on the pubis, an oblique pull in an upward and posterior direction on the anterior iliac crest, or a downward pull posteriorly on the ischium. The muscles or parts of muscles that are aligned in these directions of pull are the Rectus abdominis, the lateral fibers of the External oblique, and the hip extensors. These muscles may act to tilt the pelvis posteriorly whether the subject is standing erect or lying supine. However, in the supine position, during double leg lowering, the hip extensors are not in a position to assist in maintaining the flexion of the lumbar spine and the posterior pelvic tilt. Consequently, the Rectus abdominis and External oblique muscles assume the major role in the effort to maintain the position of the low back and pelvis during the leg-lowering movement.

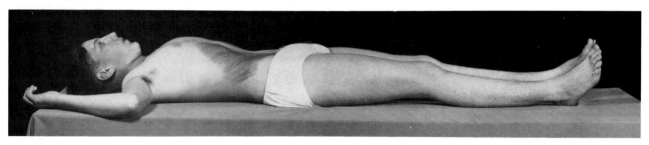

The lateral fibers of the External oblique act to tilt the pelvis posteriorly and may do so with little or no assistance from the Rectus abdominis.

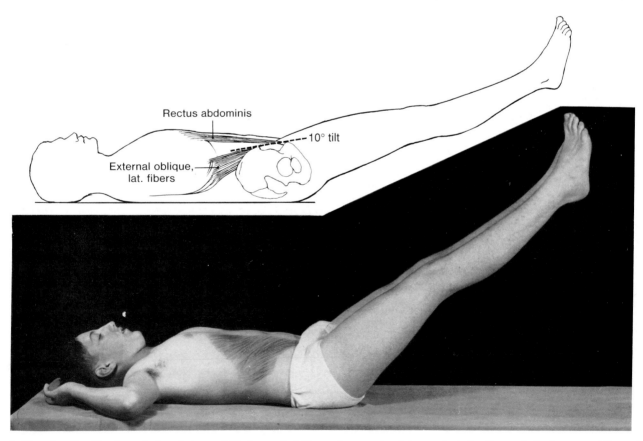

Action by the Rectus abdominis and External oblique is required to maintain the pelvis in a position of posterior tilt and the low back flat on the table as legs are raised or lowered.

A subject with *marked weakness of abdominal muscles* and *strong hip flexors* can hold the extended extremities in flexion on the pelvis and lower them slowly but the low back arches, increasingly, as the legs approach the horizontal. The force exerted by the weight of the extremities, and by the hip flexors holding the extremities in flexion on the pelvis, pulls the pelvis in anterior tilt overcoming the force of the weak abdominal muscles that are attempting to pull in the direction of posterior tilt.

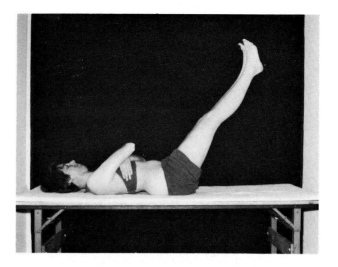

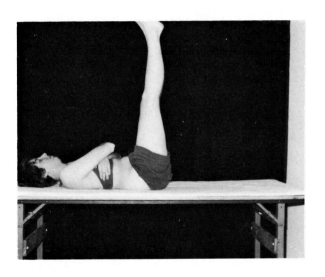

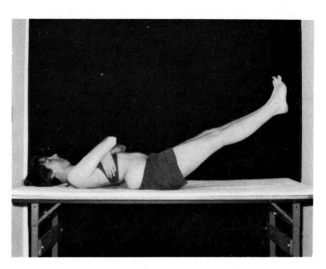

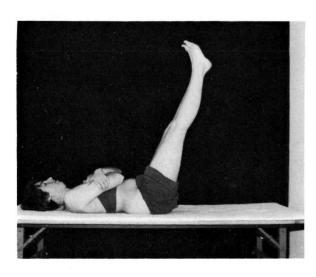

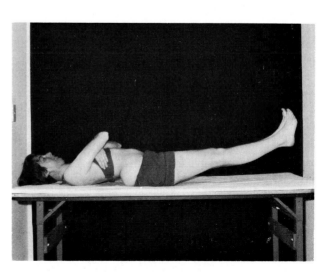

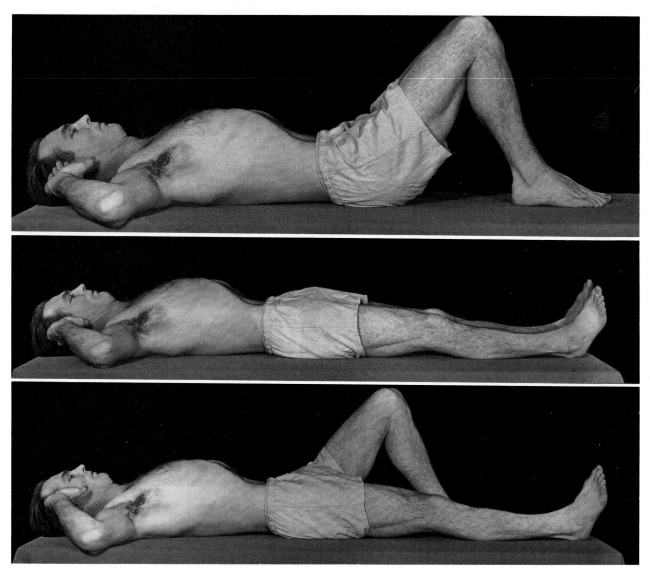

Posterior pelvic tilt and leg-sliding exercise done correctly to exercise the External oblique.

The lower abdomen is pulled up and in, and the pelvis is tilted posteriorly to flatten the low back on the table by action of the External oblique, especially the posterior lateral fibers. The subject should be taught to palpate the lateral fibers of the oblique to ensure their action and should avoid using the Gluteus maximus to tilt the pelvis when doing this exercise.

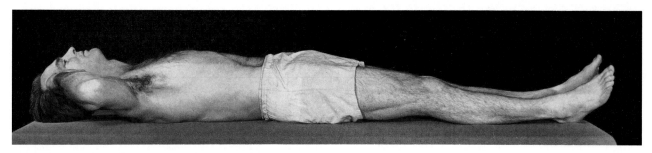

Pelvic tilt may be done with the Rectus abdominis, but should not be done in this manner when emphasis is on strengthening the External oblique.

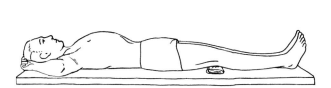

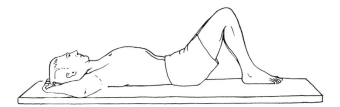

Posterior Pelvic Tilt: In the back-lying position, with hands up beside the head, tilt the pelvis to flatten the low back on the table by *pulling up and in* with the muscles in the lower abdomen. *Do not* tilt the pelvis by contracting the Gluteal (buttock) muscles.

Without depressing the rib cage, hold the low back flat and breathe in and out easily, relaxing the upper abdominal muscles. There should be good chest expansion during the inspiration but the low back should not arch upward from the table to raise the chest and make it appear like chest expansion. Hold the position several seconds, then relax. Repeat the exercise several times. (See photographs on facing page.) When standing, try to carry over the feeling of holding the lower abdomen up and in. See wall-sitting and wall-standing exercises on pp. 68 and 118.

Posterior Pelvic Tilt and Leg Sliding: In the back-lying position, bend the knees and place the feet flat on the table. With hands up beside the head, tilt the pelvis to flatten the low back on the table by *pulling up and in* with the muscles in the lower abdomen. *Do not* perform the pelvic tilt by pushing with the feet and rocking back on the buttocks.

Hold the back flat and slide the heels along the table. Straighten the legs as far as possible with the back held flat. Keeping the back flat, return the knees to bent position, *sliding one back at a time.* Try to breathe in and out about three times while the feet slide down and return to bent position. Repeat several times. (See photographs on facing page.)

Note: Hip flexor exercise is held to a minimum by not lifting legs or feet from the table.

TEMPORARY USE OF KNEE-BENT POSITION

When one-joint hip flexors are short, they hold the pelvis in anterior tilt and the low back in hyperextension when standing or when supine with legs extended. From this position, it is difficult, if not impossible, to do posterior pelvic tilt exercises to strengthen abdominal muscles. Since the head and shoulder raising movement involves a simultaneous posterior pelvic tilt, there is interference with this exercise also.

As an effort is made to tilt the pelvis, the short hip flexors become taut and prevent the movement. To release this restraint and make it easier to tilt the pelvis, the knee-bent position has been widely advocated.

This position, obviously, gives in to the short, tight hip flexors. It also makes it relatively easy to perform the tilt, oftentimes merely by pressing the feet against the table in order to "rock the pelvis back." With shortness of hip flexors, the hips and knees should be bent, but *only as much as is needed*, to allow the pelvis to tilt back. This position should be maintained *passively* by using a large enough roll or pillow under the knees. From this position the pelvic tilt and trunk curl exercises may be done to strengthen abdominal muscles.

Although bending the hips and knees initially is needed and justified, the *position should not be continued indefinitely*. The extent and duration of modifying the exercise become important. The goals set should be based on the desired end result and exercises should be directed toward attaining it. A desired end result in standing is the ability to maintain good alignment of the pelvis with the legs straight, i.e., the hip joints and knee joints in good alignment. Working toward this goal in exercise is accomplished by minimizing and gradually decreasing the amount of hip flexion permitted by the knee-bent position.

Tilting the pelvis posteriorly with the legs extended as much as possible moves the pelvis in the direction of elongating hip flexors while strengthening abdominals. Although this movement is not sufficient to stretch the hip flexors, it helps establish the pattern of muscle action necessary when attempting to correct a faulty lordotic posture in standing. Concurrently with doing proper abdominal exercise, the hip flexors should be stretched so that in time the individual will be capable of doing the posterior tilt with legs extended. (See pp. 53, 118, and 352.)

159

External Oblique in Relation to Posture

The muscles that hold the pelvis in posterior tilt during leg lowering are chiefly the Rectus abdominis and External oblique. In *many* instances, abdominal strength is normal on the trunk-raising test, but the muscles grade very weak on the leg-lowering test. Since the Rectus must be strong in order to do the trunk curl, the inability to keep the low back flat during the leg lowering cannot be attributed to that muscle. It is logical to attribute the lack of strength to the External oblique not to the Rectus. Furthermore, the postural deviations that exist in persons who show weakness on the leg-lowering test are associated with elongation of the External oblique.

There are two types of posture that exhibit this weakness: 1) Anterior tilt (lordotic posture) and 2) anterior displacement of the pelvis with posterior displacement of the thorax (sway-back posture). The lateral fibers of the External oblique extend diagonally from posterolateral rib cage to anterolateral pelvis. By this line of pull, they are in a position to help maintain good alignment of the thorax in relation to the pelvis, or to restore the alignment when there is displacement. (See accompanying photographs.)

The difference in grades between the trunk-raising test and the leg-lowering test is often very marked. Examination frequently reveals leg-lowering grades of only fair (5) to fair + (6) in persons who can perform many curled trunk sit-ups. It becomes very clear in such situations that the trunk-raising exercise does not improve the ability to hold the low back flat during leg lowering. Indeed, it appears that repeated and persistent trunk flexion exercises may contribute to continued weakness of the lateral fibers of the External oblique. (See p. 153.)

The type of postural deviation that occurs depends to a great extent on associated muscle weakness. In the anterior tilt, *lordotic posture,* there is often *hip flexor tightness* along with the abdominal weakness; in the *sway-back posture* there is *hip flexor weakness,* specifically, Iliopsoas.

The type of exercise indicated for strengthening the obliques depends upon what other muscles are involved and what postural problems are associated with the weakness. The manner in which movements are combined in exercises determines whether they will be therapeutic for the individual. For example, alternate leg raising along with pelvic tilt exercises would be contraindicated in cases of hip flexor shortness, but would be indicated in cases of hip flexor weakness.

To correct anterior pelvic tilt, posterior pelvic tilt exercises are indicated. The movement should be done by the External obliques, not by the Rectus nor by the hip extensors. The effort must be made to pull upward and inward with the abdominal muscles, making them very firm, particularly in the area of the lateral External oblique fibers. (See p. 158.)

To exercise the External oblique in cases of a sway-back posture the same effort should be made to pull upward and inward with the lower abdominal muscles but the pelvic tilt is not emphasized. In this type of faulty posture, there is already a posterior pelvic tilt along with the hip flexor weakness. Contracting the lateral fibers of the External oblique in standing must be accompanied by *straightening, not flexing,* the upper back as the muscles act to shift the thorax forward and the pelvis back by the diagonal line of pull. Properly done, this movement brings the chest up and forward and restores the normal anterior curve in the low back. (See below.)

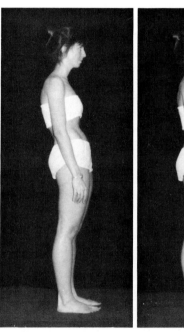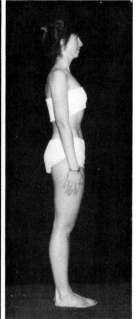

When properly done the wall-sitting and the wall-standing exercises (pp. 68 and 117) stress the use of the muscles of the lower abdomen and lateral fibers of the External oblique.

Such expressions as "make the lower abdomen cave in," or "hide the tummy under the chest," or in the vernacular of the military, "suck in your gut," are all used to try to encourage the subject to exert strong effort in the exercise.

Proper exercise of abdominal muscles should be a part of preventive medicine and physical fitness programs. Good strength in these muscles is essential to the maintenance of good posture, but caution should be taken to avoid overdoing both the trunk curl and the pelvic tilt exercises. *The normal anterior curve in the low back should not be obliterated in the standing posture.*

Length of Oblique Abdominal Muscles in Relation to Posture

Note the similarity between the lordotic and the sway-back curves in the back. Without careful analysis of the differences in plumb alignment and pelvic tilt, the sway-back curve might be referred to as a lordosis, which it is not.

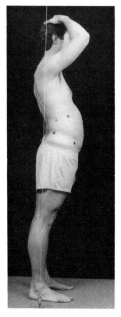

Lordosis Posture: Pelvis is in anterior tilt.

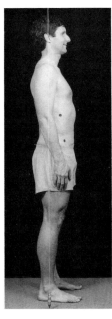

Good Postural Alignment: Pelvis is in neutral position.

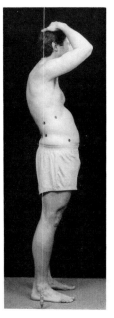

Sway-Back Posture: Pelvis is in posterior tilt.

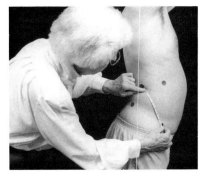

Dots representing the External oblique are 7 inches apart with the subject in a lordotic posture.

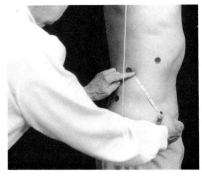

Dots representing the External oblique, are 6 inches apart with the subject in good alignment.

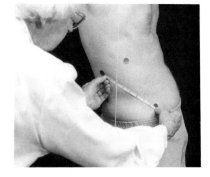

Dots representing the External oblique are 7-1/2 inches apart with the subject in sway-back posture.

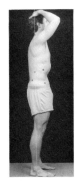

Flat-Back Posture: Often the External oblique is strong in this type posture.

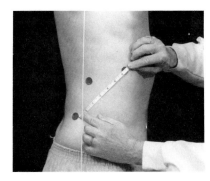

Dots representing the Internal oblique are 6 inches apart with the subject in good alignment.

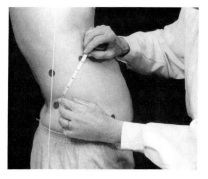

Dots representing the Internal oblique are 5 inches apart with the subject in sway-back posture.

Anterior Trunk Flexors: Upper Abdominal Muscle Test

ANALYSIS OF THE TRUNK-RAISING MOVEMENT

Preliminary to doing this test, test the flexibility of the back so that restriction of motion is not interpreted as muscle weakness.

The trunk-raising movement, properly done as a test, consists of two parts: Spine flexion (trunk curl), and hip flexion (sit-up).

During the *trunk curl phase*, the abdominal muscles contract and shorten, flexing the spine. The upper back rounds, the low back flattens, and the *pelvis tilts posteriorly*. At the completion of the curl, the spine is fully flexed with the low back and pelvis still flat on the table. The abdominal muscles act to flex the spine only. During this phase, heels should remain in contact with the table.

The trunk curl is followed by the *hip flexion phase* during which the hip flexors contract and shorten lifting the trunk and pelvis up from the table by flexion at the hip joints, pulling the pelvis in the direction of *anterior tilt*. Since abdominal muscles do not cross the hip joints, they cannot assist in the sit-up movement but, if strong enough, they continue to hold the trunk curled.

The hip flexion phase is included in the test because it provides resistance against the abdominal muscles. The crucial point in the test is the moment that movement enters the hip flexion phase.

It is at this point that, for some, the feet may start to come up from the table and may be held down if the force exerted by the extended lower extremities does not counterbalance the force exerted by the flexed trunk. If the feet are held down, attention must be focused on whether the trunk maintains the curl, because it is at this point that the strong resistance offered by the hip flexors can overcome the ability of the abdominals to maintain the curl. If this occurs, the pelvis will quickly tilt anteriorly, the back will arch, and the subject will continue the sit-up movement with the feet stabilized.

TEST FOR UPPER ABDOMINAL MUSCLES

Patient: Supine, legs extended. If hip flexor muscles are short and prevent posterior pelvic tilt with flattening of the lumbar spine, place a roll under the knees to *passively* flex the hips enough to allow the back to flatten. (Arm positions are described below under *Grading*.)

Fixation: None necessary during the *initial phase* of the test (i.e., the trunk curl) in which the spine is flexed and the thorax and pelvis are approximated. *Do not hold the feet down* during the trunk curl phase. Stabilization of the feet will allow hip flexors to initiate trunk raising by flexing the pelvis on the thighs.

Test Movement: Have the subject do a trunk curl *slowly*, completing spine flexion (thereby completing the range of motion that can be performed by the abdominal muscles). Without interrupting the movement, the subject continues on into the hip flexion phase (the sit-up) for the purpose of obtaining *strong resistance* against the abdominal muscles in order to obtain an adequate strength test.

Resistance: During the trunk curl phase, resistance is offered by the weight of the head, upper trunk, and arms which are placed in various positions for purposes of grading. However, the *resistance offered by the weight of the head, shoulders, and arms (placed in various positions to increase resistance) is not sufficient to provide an adequate test for strength of the abdominal muscles.*

The hip flexion phase provides strong resistance against the abdominals because the hip flexors pull strongly downward on the pelvis as the abdominals work to hold the pelvis in the direction of posterior tilt. (See facing page.)

Grading: (See facing page.)

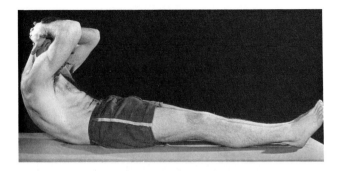

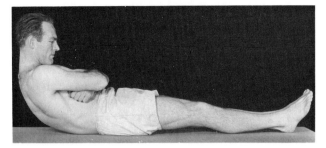

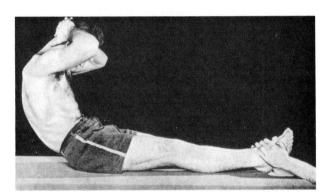

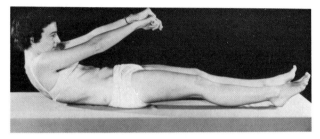

Good (8) grade. With arms folded across the chest, the subject is able to flex the vertebral columm and *keep it flexed while entering the hip-flexion phase and coming to a sitting position.*

Normal (10) grade:* With hands clasped behind the head, the subject is able to flex the vertebral column (top figure), and *keep it flexed while entering the hip-flexion phase and coming to a sitting position* (bottom figure). Feet may be held down during the hip-flexion phase, if necessary, but close observation is required to be sure that the subject maintains the flexion of the trunk.

Because many people are able to do the curled-trunk sit-up with hands clasped behind the head, it is usually permissible to have a subject place the hands in this position, initially, and attempt to perform the test. However, if there is concern about the difficulty of the test, start with the arms reaching forward, progress to placing arms folded across the chest, and then to hands behind the head.

Fair + (6) grade. With arms extended forward, the subject is able to flex the vertebral column and *keep it flexed while entering the hip-flexion phase and coming to a sitting position.*

Fair (5) grade. With arms extended forward, the subject is able to flex the vertebral column, but is unable to maintain the flexion when attempting to enter the hip-flexion phase.

See p. 176 for tests and grades in cases of marked weakness of anterior trunk muscles.

*See numerical equivalents for word symbols used in grading, p. 188; and *Key to Muscle Grading*, p. 189.

Effect of Holding Feet Down During Trunk Raising Forward

The center of gravity of the body is generally given as being at approximately the level of the first sacral segment, and this point is above the hip joint. If half the body weight is above the center of gravity, then more than half the body weight is above the hip joint. (Basmajian states that the lower extremities constitute about one third of the body weight (32).) For most people, this means that the force exerted by the trunk in supine position is greater than that exerted by both lower extremities. *Usually*, double leg raising (with knees straight) can be initiated without overbalancing the weight of the trunk in the supine position. *Seldom* can the straight trunk or hyperextended trunk (see facing page) be raised from supine toward a sitting position without some outside force being applied (such as pressure downward on the feet) in addition to that exerted by the extended extremities.

On the other hand, if the trunk curls sufficiently as the trunk raising is started, the center of gravity of the body moves downward toward, or below, the hip joints. As this occurs, the curled trunk can be raised in flexion toward the thighs without having the feet held down. Most adolescents (especially those in whom the legs are long in relation to the trunk) and most adult females can perform the sit-up with legs extended and without the feet being held down. In contrast, many men may need to have some added force applied (usually very little) at the point where the trunk curl is completed and the hip flexion phase begins.

For the curled-trunk sit-up to be used as a test of abdominal muscle strength, it must be made certain that the ability to curl the trunk is being measured. The trunk curl must precede the hip flexion phase in the trunk-raising movement. When the feet are not held down, the pelvis tilts posteriorly as the head and shoulders are raised in initiating the trunk curl. With feet held down, the hip flexors are given fixation and the trunk raising can immediately become an arched-back sit-up with flexion at the hip joints. Hence, *to help ensure that the test determines the ability to curl the trunk before the hip flexion phase starts, the feet must not be held down during the trunk flexion phase.*

The question is frequently asked whether holding the feet down causes any problem *if abdominal strength is normal*. The answer is that it might not if one is performing only a few sit-ups, but it can make a great deal of difference if many repetitions are performed. One or two curled-trunk sit-ups, properly done, determines normal strength. It does not determine endurance. An individual may grade normal, and perform several sit-ups properly. With repeated sit-ups, the abdominal muscles may fatigue and the person may "slip into" doing an arched-back sit-up. This situation arises frequently because abdominal muscles do not have the endurance exhibited by hip flexors.

The transition to an arched-back sit-up could and would go undetected if the feet were held down from the beginning of the sit-up. However, if the feet were not held down during the initial spine flexion phase, the inability to curl the trunk would become obvious as fatigue sets in. One might find that an individual could do as many as 100 sit-ups with the feet held down, yet no more than five if the feet were not held down. This would indicate that the trunk-raising became an arched-back sit-up after the first five.

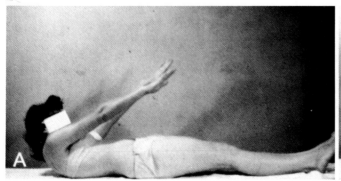

The above photograph shows an individual with marked abdominal muscle weakness who, with arms in a relatively easy (grade of 6 or fair +) test position, is unable to flex the lumbar spine and complete the sit-up when feet are not held down.

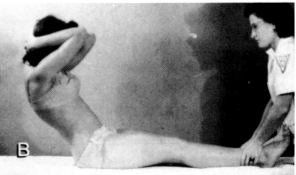

The above photograph shows the same individual as in Figure A who, with arms in 10 or normal grade test position is able to perform the sit-up by hip flexor action because the feet are held down. As a test this latter measures only hip flexor strength.

Abdominal Muscle Weakness: Sit-Up with Low Back Hyperextended

When abdominal muscles are too weak to curl the trunk, the hip flexors tilt the pelvis forward and hyperextend the low back as they raise the trunk to a sitting position. Some people cannot do the sit-up unless the feet are held down *from the start*.

Usually these are the people who have marked weakness of the abdominal muscles. They should practice the trunk curl only and *avoid* doing the sit-up in the manner illustrated here.

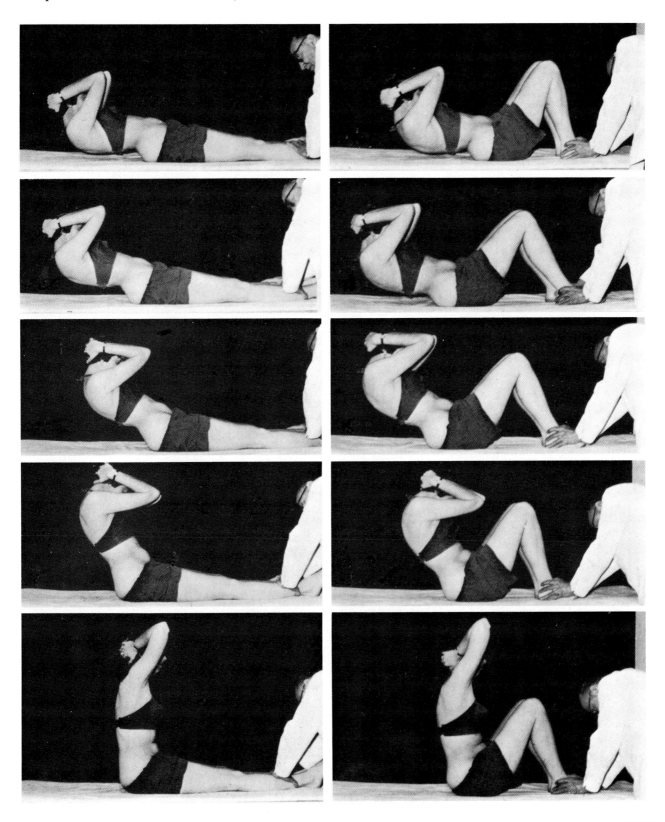

For purposes of strengthening those abdominal muscles that show weakness on the trunk-raising test, it is desirable, in most instances, to have the subject perform only the trunk curl part of the movement. Doing so provides the advantage of exercising the abdominal muscles without strong hip flexor exercise. In addition, according to Nachemson and Elfstron, there is less intradiscal pressure when doing only the trunk curl as compared to completing the sit-up (33).

When the subject can perform the curl to completion of spine flexion, the resistance may be increased by folding forearms across the chest and completing the curl; later more resistance can be added by placing hands behind the head and completing the curl. At each stage, work for some endurance, i.e., completion of curl, holding it for several seconds, and repeating about ten times.

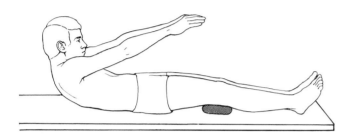

Abdominal Exercise: Trunk curl. In the back-lying position, place a small roll under the knees. Tilt the pelvis to flatten the low back on the table by pulling up and in with muscles of the lower abdomen. With arms extended forward, raise the head and shoulders upward from the table. Raise the upper trunk as high as the back will bend, but *do not try to come to a sitting position.*

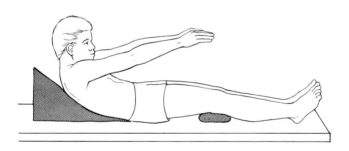

Abdominal Exercise: Assisted trunk curl. When the abdominal muscles are very weak and the subject cannot lift the shoulders upward from the table, modify the above exercise by placing a wedge-shaped pillow (or the equivalent) under the head and shoulders. This position will enable the subject to exercise within a short range. As the ability to hold the completed curl improves, use a smaller pillow and have subject flex to completion of the curl.

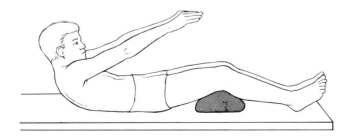

Abdominal Exercise: Modified when hip flexors are short. When the hip flexor muscles are short and restrict the posterior pelvic tilt movement, modify the above trunk curl exercise by *temporarily* placing a pillow under the knees to passively flex the hips. (See explanation p. 159.)

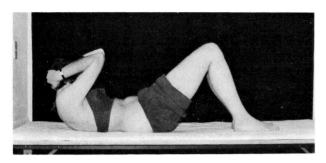

The subject in the above photograph with arms in 10 or normal grade test position, and with knees flexed, can flex the vertebral column but cannot raise the trunk any higher from the table than illustrated.

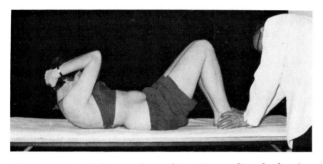

With feet held down, the subject immediately begins the hip flexion phase and can continue to a full sitting position, as seen in the series of photographs of this same individual on p. 165.

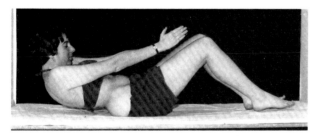

In this illustration, the subject is making an effort to sit up with the arms in an easy test position, feet not held down. It is obvious that she goes immediately into the hip flexion phase. Legs tend to extend in an effort to move the center of gravity of the lower extremities more distally and offset the force exerted by the trunk. The same problems exist with respect to the stabilization of the feet whether knees are extended or flexed.

The ability to do a curled-trunk sit-up should be considered a normal accomplishment. People should be able to get up easily from a supine position without having to roll over on the side or push themselves up with their arms. When there is weakness in either or both of the muscle groups involved in the curled-trunk sit-up (namely, abdominal and hip flexor muscles) efforts should be made to correct the weakness and restore the ability to perform the movement correctly. While hip flexors may exhibit some weakness associated with postural problems, it is rarely to the degree that it interferes with performing the sit-up (hip flexion) movement. The problem in performing the trunk curl is due to weakness of abdominal muscles. Using the sit-up exercise to try to correct the abdominal weakness is a mistake because, when marked weakness exists, the hip flexors initiate and perform the movement with the low back hyperextended.

For many years, sit-ups were done most frequently with the legs extended. In recent years, emphasis has been placed on doing the exercise in the knee-bent position which automatically flexes the hips in the supine position. *The sit-up, whether legs are straight or bent, is a strong hip flexor exercise*, the difference being in the *arc* of hip-joint motion through which the hip flexors act. With legs extended, they act through an arc from zero to about 80°; with hips and knees flexed, from about 50° (the starting position) to completion of range at 125° flexion for a total of about 75°.

Ironically, the knee-bent sit-up has been advocated as a means of minimizing the action of the hip flexors. The idea has persisted for many years, both among professional and lay people, that having the hips and knees bent in the back-lying position would put the hip flexors "on a slack" and would rule out or eliminate the action of the hip flexors while doing the sit-up; and that in this position the sit-up would be performed by abdominal muscles. *These ideas are not based on facts; they are false and misleading.* The abdominal muscles can only curl the trunk and cannot perform the hip flexion part (which is the major part) of the trunk-raising movement. Furthermore, the Iliacus is a one-joint muscle which is expected to complete the movement of hip flexion and, as such, is not put on a slack. The two-joint Rectus femoris is not put on a slack because it is lengthened over the knee joint while it is shortened over the hip joint. *Except for the Sartorius to some extent, other hip flexors are not put on a slack in the knee-bent position.*

Sit-Up Exercises: Indications and Contraindications

If hip flexors are not short, an individual, when starting the trunk raising with legs extended, will curl the trunk and the low back will flatten before starting the hip flexion phase. The danger of hyperextension will occur only if the abdominals are too weak to maintain the curl—a reason not to continue into the sit-up.

The real problem in doing sit-ups with legs extended compared to the apparent advantage of flexing the hips and knees stems from dealing with many subjects who have short hip flexors. In the supine position, the person with short hip flexors will lie with the low back hyperextended (arched forward). The hazard of doing the sit-up from this position is that the hip flexors will further hyperextend the low back, causing a stress on the low back while doing the exercise, and will increase the tendency toward a lordotic posture in standing. The knee-bent position, on the other hand, releases the downward pull by the short hip flexors, allowing the pelvis to tilt posteriorly and the low back to flatten, thereby relieving strain on the low back.

Instead of recognizing and treating the problem of the short hip flexors, the "solution" has been to "give in" to them by flexing the hips and knees. But there are problems that arise from this solution. The same hazard of coming up with the low back hyperextended can occur with knees bent, and does occur when the abdominal muscles are too weak to curl the trunk. (See p. 165.) In trying to come up, the subject requires more pressure than usual to hold the feet down, or more extension of the legs, or is aided by performing the movement quickly with added momentum. Sometimes it is advocated (inadvisedly) that the arms be placed overhead and brought quickly forward to help in performing the sit-up. This added momentum enables the subject to do the sit-up, but the low back is hyperextended causing strain on the abdominal muscles as well as stress on the low back.

The sit-up is a strong hip flexor exercise whether knees are bent or legs are extended. The hip joint moves to completion of hip joint flexion with hips and knees bent making this type of sit-up more conducive to the development of shortness in the Iliopsoas than the sit-up with knees and hips extended. (As illustrated on pages 171 and 170, the hip joint moves to an angle of 55° for the former, and to an angle of 100° for the latter.)

While normal flexibility of the back is a desirable feature, excessive flexibility is not. Hazards of doing the knee-bent sit-up also relate to the danger of hyperflexion of the trunk (spine curving convexly backward). With the body in the anatomical position or supine with legs extended, the center of gravity is slightly anterior to the first or second sacral segment. With hips and knees bent, the center of gravity moves cranially (toward the head). *The lower extremities exert less force in counter-balancing the trunk during the sit-up with hips and knees bent than with legs extended.* There are two alternatives in accomplishing the sit-up from this knee-bent position: Outside pressure must be exerted to hold the feet down (more than is required for those few who need it with the legs extended), or the trunk must curl excessively to move the center of gravity downward. This excessive flexion is portrayed as an exaggerated thoracic curve (marked rounding of the upper back) and/or as abnormal flexion involving the thoracolumbar area (roundness extending into the low back area). The latter is accentuated when the knee-bent sit-up is done without the feet being held down and with heels close to the buttocks.

The people most in danger of being adversely affected by repeated sit-ups with the knees bent are children and youths because they start with more flexibility than adults. Those adults who have low back pain that is associated with excessive low back flexibility also may be affected adversely by this exercise. An interesting phenomenon that occurs in some subjects who have done a great number of knee-bent sit-ups is that they show excessive flexion in sitting or in forward bending, but a lordosis in standing.

It is unfortunate that the ability to do a certain number of sit-ups, *regardless of how they are performed*, is used as a measure of physical fitness. Coupled with push-ups, these two exercises probably are stressed more than any others in fitness programs. (See pp. 7 and 8.) Done to excess, these exercises tend to increase or produce postural faults.

When, how, and to what extent the knee-bent position should be used is discussed on p. 159.

Joint and Muscle Analysis of Curled-Trunk Sit-Up

AN ANALYSIS OF MOVEMENTS AND MUSCLE ACTIONS DURING A CURLED-TRUNK SIT-UP

The illustrations on pp. 170 and 171 show the various stages of movement of the spine and hip joints that occur during a curled-trunk sit-up. On p. 172–174, the illustrations are repeated and the accompanying text describes the associated muscle actions.

Outlines of the basic features have been made from photographs. Drawings of the femur and pelvis, and a dotted line representing part of the vertebral column have been added. The solid line from the anterior-superior spine to the symphysis pubis is the line of reference for the pelvis. A dotted line parallel to the solid line has been drawn through the pelvis to the hip joint and continues as a reference line through the femur to indicate the angle of the hip joint, i.e., the angle of flexion, at the various stages of movement.

Specific degrees, based on the average normal ranges of motion presented here and in *Chapter 2*, are used to help explain the movements that occur. Because of individual variations with respect to ranges of motion of the spine and hip joints, there will be variations in the manner in which subjects perform these movements.

For this particular analysis, it is assumed that the abdominal and erector spinae muscles, as well as the hip flexor and extensor muscles, are normal in length and strength and that the spine and hip joints permit normal range of motion.

Normal hip joint extension is given as 10°. From the standpoint of stability in standing, it is desirable to have a few degrees of extension; it is not desirable to have more than a few degrees. In the upright or supine position with hips and knees extended, a posterior pelvic tilt of 10° results in 10° of hip joint extension. It occurs because the pelvis is tilted posteriorly toward the back of the thigh instead of the thigh being moved posteriorly toward the pelvis. Flattening the lumbar spine accompanies the posterior pelvic tilt. Flexion to the point of straightening or flattening the low back is considered normal flexion on the basis that it is an acceptable and desirable range of motion.

With the knee flexed, the hip joint can flex approximately 125° from the zero position to an acute angle of approximately 55° between the femur and the pelvis. With the knee extended (as in the straight-leg-raising test for Hamstring length) the leg can be raised approximately 80° from the table. The equivalent of this is a trunk-raising movement, with legs extended, in which the pelvis is flexed toward the thighs through a range of approximately 80° from the table.

For convenience in measuring joint motion, the trend is to use the *anatomical position as zero*. Thus, the straight position of the hip joint is considered to be zero position. However, it is necessary to adhere to *geometric terms* when describing angles and the number of degrees in angles.

On pp. 170 and 171, the right-hand column under "Hip Joint" refers to the angle of flexion anteriorly between the reference line through the pelvis and the line through the femur, and degrees are expressed in geometric terms. Changes in the angle of flexion represent corresponding changes in the length of hip flexors.

The second column from the right under "Hip Joint" lists the number of degrees from anatomical position through which the hip joint has moved, first in extension, then in flexion.

Movements during a Curled-Trunk Sit-up with Legs Extended

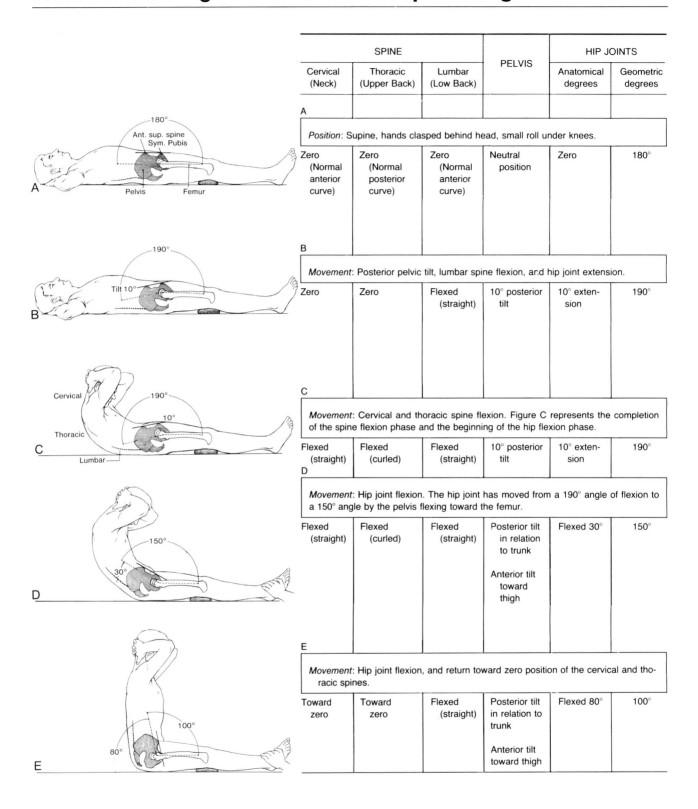

	SPINE			PELVIS	HIP JOINTS	
	Cervical (Neck)	Thoracic (Upper Back)	Lumbar (Low Back)		Anatomical degrees	Geometric degrees
A						
Position: Supine, hands clasped behind head, small roll under knees.						
	Zero (Normal anterior curve)	Zero (Normal posterior curve)	Zero (Normal anterior curve)	Neutral position	Zero	180°
B						
Movement: Posterior pelvic tilt, lumbar spine flexion, and hip joint extension.						
	Zero	Zero	Flexed (straight)	10° posterior tilt	10° extension	190°
C						
Movement: Cervical and thoracic spine flexion. Figure C represents the completion of the spine flexion phase and the beginning of the hip flexion phase.						
	Flexed (straight)	Flexed (curled)	Flexed (straight)	10° posterior tilt	10° extension	190°
D						
Movement: Hip joint flexion. The hip joint has moved from a 190° angle of flexion to a 150° angle by the pelvis flexing toward the femur.						
	Flexed (straight)	Flexed (curled)	Flexed (straight)	Posterior tilt in relation to trunk Anterior tilt toward thigh	Flexed 30°	150°
E						
Movement: Hip joint flexion, and return toward zero position of the cervical and thoracic spines.						
	Toward zero	Toward zero	Flexed (straight)	Posterior tilt in relation to trunk Anterior tilt toward thigh	Flexed 80°	100°

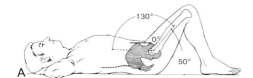

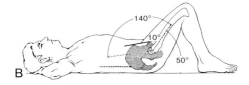

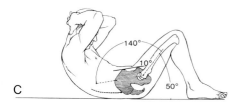

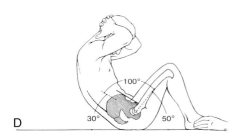

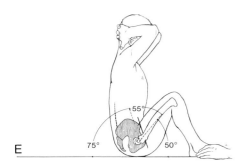

	SPINE			PELVIS	HIP JOINTS	
	Cervical (Neck)	Thoracic (Upper Back)	Lumbar (Low Back)		Anatomical degrees	Geometric degrees
A						
Position: Supine, hands clasped behind head, knees bent.						
	Zero (Normal anterior curve)	Zero (Normal posterior curve)	Zero (Normal anterior curve)	Neutral position	50°	130°
B						
Movement: Lumbar spine flexion and 10° decrease in hip joint flexion by virtue of posterior pelvic tilt.						
	Zero	Zero	Flexed (straight)	10° posterior tilt	50° flexion of thigh	140°
C						
Movement: Cervical and thoracic spine flexion. Figure C represents completion of the spine flexion and the beginning of the flexion of the pelvis toward the flexed thigh.						
	Flexed (straight)	Flexed (curled)	Flexed (straight)	10° posterior tilt	50° flexion of thigh	140°
D						
Movement: Hip joint flexion. The hip joint has moved from a 140° angle of flexion to a 100° angle by the pelvis flexing toward the femur.						
	Flexed (straight)	Flexed (curled)	Flexed (straight)	Posterior tilt in relation to trunk Anterior tilt toward thigh	80° (50° thigh + 30° pelvis)	100°
E						
Movement: Hip joint flexion, and a return toward zero position of the cervical and thoracic spines. On the basis of 125° being complete flexion, the hip joint has reached the position of complete flexion.						
	Toward zero	Toward zero	Flexed (straight)	Posterior tilt in relation to trunk Anterior tilt toward thigh	125° (50° thigh + 75° pelvis)	55°

Abdominal and Hip Flexor Muscles during a Curled-Trunk Sit-Up

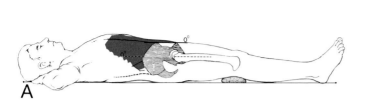

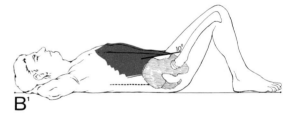

ZERO POSITION OF SPINE, PELVIS AND HIP JOINTS

Figures A and A[1] may be regarded as hypothetical starting positions. In reality, especially with knees bent, the low back tends to flatten (i.e., the lumbar spine flexes) when a normally flexible individual assumes the supine position.

In Figure A, the length of the hip flexors corresponds with the zero anatomical position of the hip joints.

ZERO POSITION OF SPINE AND PELVIS, FLEXION OF HIP JOINTS

In Figure A[1], because of the flexed position of the hips, the one-joint hip flexors are shorter in length than in Figure A. In relation to its overall length, the Iliacus is at about 40% of its range of motion which is within the middle third of the overall range.

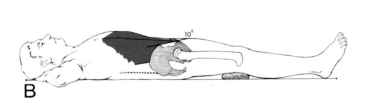

POSTERIOR PELVIC TILT, LUMBAR SPINE FLEXION, AND HIP JOINT EXTENSION

Figures B and B[1] represent a stage of movement in which the pelvis is tilted posteriorly prior to beginning the trunk raising. (Note the 10° posterior pelvic tilt.) In testing, this movement often is performed as a separate stage to ensure lumbar spine flexion.

When the posterior tilt is not done as a separate movement, as in Figures B and B[1], it occurs simultaneously with the beginning phase of trunk raising (i.e., the trunk-curl phase) *unless* abdominal muscles are extremely weak or hip flexors are so short they prevent posterior tilt when supine with legs extended.

In Figure B, the hip flexors have lengthened, and the one-joint hip flexors (chiefly the Iliacus) have reached the limit of length permitted by the hip joint extension. At this length they help stabilize the pelvis by restraining further posterior pelvic tilt.

POSTERIOR PELVIC TILT, LUMBAR SPINE FLEXION, AND HIP JOINT FLEXION

In Figure B[1], the hip flexor length is slightly more than in Figure A[1] because the pelvis has tilted posteriorly 10° away from the femur. Posterior pelvic tilt exercises are frequently used with the intention of strengthening the abdominal muscles. Too often the tilt is done without any benefit to the abdominals. The subject performs the movement by contracting the buttocks muscles (hip extensors) and, in the case of the knee-bent position, by pushing with the feet to help "rock" the pelvis back into posterior tilt.

To ensure that the pelvic tilt is performed by the abdominal muscles, there must be an upward-inward pull by these muscles with the front and sides of the lower abdomen becoming very firm. (See p. 158.)

It is necessary to discourage use of the buttocks muscles in order to force action by the abdominals when performing the posterior pelvic tilt.

Abdominal and Hip Flexor Muscles during a Curled-Trunk Sit-Up

SPINE FLEXION PHASE (TRUNK CURL) COMPLETED

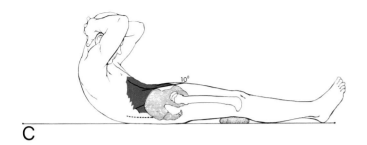

C

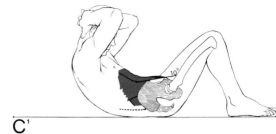

C¹

In Figures C and C¹, the neck (cervical spine), the upper back (thoracic spine), and the low back (lumbar spine) are flexed. The low back remained in the same degree of flexion as in Figures B and B¹ where it reached maximum flexion for this subject.

In Figures C and C¹, the abdominal muscles have shortened to their fullest extent with the completion of spine flexion. In Figure C, the hip flexors have remained lengthened to the same extent as in Figure B.

In Figure C¹, the one-joint hip flexors have not reached the limit of their length and, therefore, do not act passively to restrain posterior tilt. The hip flexors contract to stabilize the pelvis, and, on palpation of the superficial hip flexors, there is evidence of firm contraction as the subject *begins* to lift the head and shoulders from the table.

HIP FLEXION PHASE (SIT-UP) INITIATED

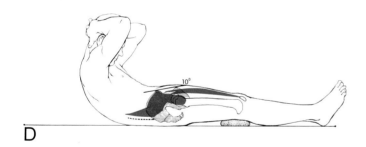

D

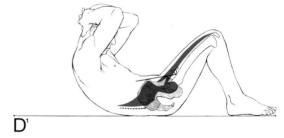

D¹

With flexion of the spine complete (as in Figures C, C¹, D and D¹), no further movement in the direction of coming to a sitting position can occur except by flexion of the hip joints.

Since abdominal muscles do not cross the hip joint, these muscles cannot assist in the movement of hip flexion.

From a supine position, hip flexion can be performed only by the hip flexors acting to bring the pelvis in flexion toward the thighs.

Figures D and D¹ represent the beginning of the sit-up phase as well as the end of the trunk curl phase.

HIP FLEXION PHASE (SIT-UP) CONTINUED

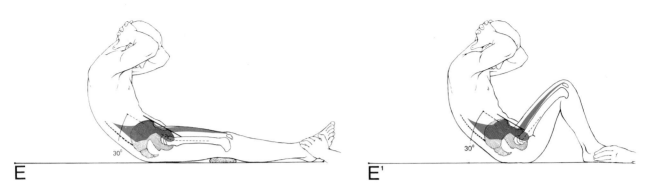

E

E¹

Figures E and E¹ show a point in the arc of movement between the completed trunk curl (as seen in C, C¹, D and D¹) and the full sit-up. The abdominal muscles maintain the trunk in flexion, and the hip flexors have lifted the flexed trunk upward toward the sitting position through an arc of about 30° from the table.

When it is necessary, the feet *may* be held down at the initiation of, and during, the hip flexion phase. (See p. 164.) Prior to the hip flexion phase, the feet must not be held down.

HIP FLEXION PHASE (SIT-UP) COMPLETED

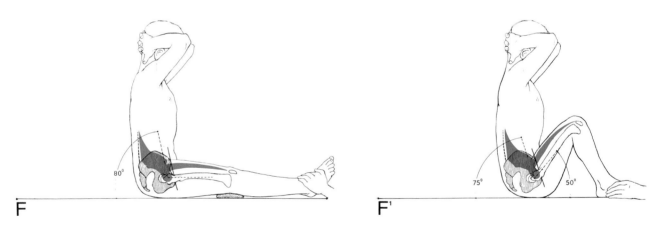

F

F¹

In Figures F and F¹, as the subjects reach the sitting position, the cervical and thoracic spines are no longer fully flexed, and the abdominal muscles relax to some extent.

In Figure F, the hip flexors have moved the pelvis in flexion toward the thigh, completing an arc of about 80° from the table. In this position, with knees extended, and lumbar spine flexed, the hip joint is as fully flexed as the range of normal Hamstring length permits. The lumbar spine remains flexed because moving from the flexed position of the low back to the zero position (normal anterior curve) would require that the pelvis be tilted 10° more in flexion toward the thigh and the Hamstring length does not permit it.

In Figure F¹, the hip flexors have moved the pelvis in flexion toward the thigh through an arc of about 75° from the table. The lumbar spine remains in flexion because the hip joint has already reached the 125° of full flexion. Further flexion of the hip joints by tilting the pelvis forward (and bringing the low back into normal anterior curve) could be done only if the flexion of the thigh were decreased by moving the heels farther from the buttocks in this sitting position.

When marked weakness and imbalance exist in abdominal muscles it is possible, to some extent, to determine the imbalance by observing the deviations of the umbilicus. The umbilicus will deviate toward a strong or away from a weak segment. If, for example, three segments, the left External and both left and right Internal obliques, are equally strong and there is a marked weakness of the right External, the umbilicus will deviate decidedly toward the left Internal. This happens not because the left Internal is the strongest, but because it has no opposition in the right External. This shows deviation away from a weak segment.

On the other hand, deviation may mean that there is one strong segment and that the other three are weak, and the deviation will be toward the strongest segment. The relative strengths must then be determined by palpation, and by the extent to which the umbilicus deviates during the performance of localized test movements.

There are times when the umbilicus deviates, not because of active muscle contraction, but because of a stretching of the muscle. The examiner must be sure the muscles being tested are actively contracting before deviations of the umbilicus can be used as indicative of strength or weakness.

To obtain true deviations, the abdominal muscles should first be in a relaxed position. The knees may be bent sufficiently to relax the back flat on the table. Then the patient may be asked to attempt head raising or tilting the pelvis posteriorly (even though the back is already flat). If resistive arm and leg movements are used in testing, they should be started from this relaxed position also. Movements should be such that they produce actual shortening of the muscle. When weakness is very apparent, the initial test should be a mild active movement, with resistance gradually applied. It should be noted, first, to what extent the muscle can approximate its origin and insertion; and second, how much pressure can be added before the pull "breaks" and the muscle starts to stretch.

An individual unfamiliar with the examination of abdominal muscles may find it very difficult to be sure of the deviations of the umbilicus. If a tape or cord is held transversely, then diagonally, over the umbilicus as the test movements are performed, the direction of the deviation can be determined more readily. The umbilicus may deviate up or down from the transverse tape showing uneven pull of upper and lower Rectus. If it also shows a deviation from the tape held diagonally over the umbilicus, it will exhibit an imbalance between the obliques.

Lines made with ink or skin pencil on the anterior iliac crests, the costal margins, just above the pubis, and below the sternum may be an aid to the examiner. As the test movement is done, the tape is held from umbilicus to the various marks. Actual shortening or stretch of the segments can be detected as a movement is attempted.

ARM MOVEMENTS USED IN TESTING ABDOMINAL MUSCLES

Arm movements are performed against resistance or held against pressure when used in abdominal muscle testing because unresisted arm movements do not demand appreciable action of trunk muscles for fixation.

Normally an upward movement of the arms in the forward plane requires fixation by back muscles; a downward movement in the forward plane requires fixation by abdominal muscles. When abdominal weakness exists, however, fixation for the downward pull or push of the arm may be provided by the back muscles. For example, if a patient is placed in a supine position and given resistance to a downward pull of both arms, normal abdominal muscles will contract to fix the thorax firmly toward the pelvis. However, if extensive abdominal weakness is present, the back will arch from the table, and the thorax will pull away from the pelvis until it is firmly fixed by extension of the thoracic spine. The arching of the back stretches the abdominal muscles, and they may become taut and feel firm on palpation. The examiner must be careful not to mistake this tautness for the firmness that accompanies contraction of the muscles.

In cross-sectional or diagonal arm movements, if the abdominal muscles are normal, the External oblique on the same side as the arm and the Internal oblique on the opposite side contract to fix the thorax to the pelvis. If cross-section weakness exists in that line of pull, the opposite oblique muscles may act to give fixation. The examiner should understand these substitute actions in order to do an accurate examination.

Objective grading of the anterolateral abdominal muscles is not difficult when strength is fair (5), and above. Below fair (5), it is more difficult to grade accurately. The tests and grades described here furnish guidelines for grading the weak muscles.

When marked imbalance exists in the abdominal muscles, one must observe the deviations of the umbilicus (see previous page) and rely on palpation for grading.

Preliminary to doing the tests listed below, it is necessary to test the strength of the anterior neck muscles.

ANTERIOR ABDOMINAL MUSCLES, MAINLY RECTUS ABDOMINIS

Fair – (4): In supine position with knees slightly flexed (rolled towel under knees), the patient is able to tilt the pelvis posteriorly and keep the pelvis and thorax approximated as the head is raised from the table.

Poor (2): In the same position as above the patient is able to tilt the pelvis posteriorly, but as the head is raised the abdominal muscles cannot hold against that resistance anteriorly, and the thorax moves away from the pelvis.

T or trace: In the supine position, when patient attempts to depress the chest or tilt the pelvis posteriorly, a contraction can be felt in the anterior abdominal muscles, but there is no approximation of the pelvis and thorax.

OBLIQUE ABDOMINAL MUSCLES

Fair – (4): In the supine position with the examiner giving moderate resistance against a diagonally downward pull of the arm, the cross-sectional pull of the oblique abdominal muscles will be very firm on palpation, and will pull the costal margin toward the opposite iliac crest. If the arm is weak, pushing the shoulder forward in a diagonal direction toward the opposite hip and holding against pressure may be substituted for the arm movement.

In the supine position with one leg held straight in approximately 60° hip flexion, the examiner applies moderate pressure against the thigh in a downward-outward direction. The strength of oblique muscles should be sufficient to pull the iliac crest toward the opposite costal margin. (This test can be used only if hip flexor strength is good.)

Poor (2): The patient is able to approximate the iliac crest toward the opposite costal margin.

T or trace: A contraction can be felt in the oblique muscle when the patient makes an effort to pull the costal margin toward the opposite iliac crest, i.e., a slight lateral shift of thorax over pelvis, but there will be no approximation of these parts.

LATERAL TRUNK MUSCLES

Fair – (4): In side-lying, there will be firm fixation and approximation of the rib cage and iliac crest laterally during active leg abduction, and arm adduction against resistance.

Poor (2): In the supine position, the patient is able to approximate the iliac crest and rib cage laterally as an effort is made to elevate the pelvis laterally or adduct the arm against resistance.

T or trace: In the supine position, a contraction can be felt in the lateral abdominal muscles as an effort is made to elevate the pelvis laterally or adduct the arm against resistance, but there is no approximation of thorax and lateral iliac crest.

RECORDING GRADES OF ABDOMINAL MUSCLE STRENGTH

Abdominal muscle grades are recorded in two different ways, depending on the amount of strength.

When strength is 5 or fair or better in the trunk-raising and leg-lowering tests, it is usually sufficient to grade and record on the basis of these tests, figure A. Intrinsic imbalance between parts of the Rectus or the obliques seldom necessitates grading parts separately if these tests show a grade of fair (5) or better.

When marked weakness or imbalance exists, it is necessary to indicate findings in relation to specific muscles (figure B).

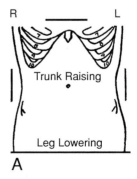

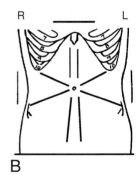

A

B

Lower Extremity Strength Tests

MUSCLE STRENGTH TESTING

This chapter includes principles involved in manual muscle strength testing, definitions of terms used in describing the test procedures, a detailed discussion of grading, and a discussion about the dual use of the word "normal" in grading and in interpretation of grades.

Manual testing is an important tool in the diagnosis, prognosis, and treatment of musculoskeletal disorders. Diagnostic manual muscle testing requires the best possible differentiation of muscle actions.

A few muscles can be *isolated* because no other muscles cross the joint to assist in the movement. These muscles are: Flexor digitorum profundus, Flexor pollicis longus, Flexor digitorum longus, and Flexor hallucis longus. Other muscles are differentiated as follows:

> A one-joint muscle from a two-joint (or multi-joint) muscle.
> A one-joint muscle from another one-joint muscle.
> A multi-joint muscle from another multi-joint muscle.
> A part of a fan-shaped muscle from another part of the muscle.

In order to differentiate, it is necessary to understand the differences between one-joint and two-joint muscles. The following **principles** apply:

> A normal one-joint muscle possesses sufficient contractility to shorten through the full range of motion afforded by the joint. It can exert a strong, effective force in its most shortened position which is at completion of joint range. The **optimal test position for a one-joint muscle** is at completion of range of motion.

> A normal two-joint muscle does *not* possess sufficient contractility to shorten through the full range of motion afforded by both joints simultaneously. It exerts a strong, effective force within the mid-range of its overall length (i.e., the mid-range of the length-tension curve). The **optimal test position for a two-joint muscle** is within the mid-range of its overall length.

> A **one-joint muscle** can be differentiated from a two-joint muscle that crosses over the same joint by shortening the two-joint muscle and making it ineffective.

If actively shortened as far as possible, or if passively placed in a shortened position, the two-joint muscle becomes incapable of assisting with further movement although more range of joint motion exists. Example: Subject prone with knee flexed to shorten Hamstrings during test for Glu-teus maximus. This principle that a two-joint muscle can be made ineffective must be applied judiciously. The two-joint muscle may cramp if strong pressure is applied when it is in this shortened position. For example, it is not uncommon for the Hamstrings to cramp during the Gluteus maximus test.

In muscle testing and exercises, the expression *put the muscle on a slack* or *make the muscle slack* is used to describe a muscle in a shortened position in which it is incapable of developing enough tension to exert an effective force. Within this context, the word slack has the same meaning as **actively insufficient** as described by O'Connell and Gardner:

> If a muscle which crosses two or more joints produces simultaneous movement at all of the joints that it crosses, it soon reaches a length at which it can no longer generate a useful amount of force. Under these conditions the muscle is said to be *actively insufficient*. An example of such insufficiency occurs when one tries to achieve full hip extension with maximal knee flexion. The two-joint hamstrings are incapable of shortening sufficiently to produce a complete range of motion of both joints simultaneously (34).

The words slack and actively insufficient, as described here, apply to muscles that cross two or more joints, but not to one-joint muscles *intact* in the body. If both the one-joint and multi-joint muscles were made ineffective by being placed in a shortened position, the action of the one-joint muscle could not be differentiated from that of the multi-joint muscle.

When **testing a two-joint muscle,** it must be elongated over one joint in order to shorten over the other joint. For example, when testing the strength of finger flexors, the wrist is extended to elongate the flexors over the wrist joint while they shorten over the finger joints. If the wrist is allowed to flex as the fingers flex, strength of finger flexion is greatly diminished and a true measure of strength cannot be obtained. If an attempt is made to hold against strong pressure in this fully shortened position, the flexors will start to cramp. The position of maximal shortening of the flexors must be avoided.

When differentiating **a one-joint muscle from another one-joint muscle** that has some actions which are similar and some that are different, distinction must be made on the basis of the actions that are different. Both the Rhomboids and Trapezius adduct and elevate the scapula, but the Rhomboids downwardly rotate and the Trapezius upwardly rotates. Consequently, the scapula must be in *upward rotation* and adduction in order to obtain a test of the Trapezius, and in *downward rotation* and adduction to obtain a test of the Rhomboids.

Differentiating a **multi-joint muscle from another multi-joint muscle** requires precise positioning of the joints to restrict certain action. For example, the Flexor digitorum superficialis can be distinguished from the Flexor digitorum profundus by testing for strength of proximal interphalangeal joint flexion (action by Superficialis) with the distal interphalangeal joints remaining extended (not permitting action by the Profundus).

Differentiating **parts of a fan-shaped muscle** can be done by precision in positioning and by correct application of pressure. For example, the upper part of the Pectoralis major can be differentiated from the lower part by placing the arm in horizontal adduction and applying pressure in the direction of horizontal abduction. Testing the lower part requires positioning the arm in a diagonal position and applying pressure in a diagonally opposite direction.

The credibility of manual muscle testing depends upon the examiner's accuracy in testing which, in turn, depends upon adhering to the basic principles and to rules of procedure.

BASIC RULES OF PROCEDURE THAT APPLY TO MUSCLE STRENGTH TESTING

Place subject in a position that offers the best fixation of the body as a whole (usually supine, prone, or side-lying).

Stabilize the part proximal to the tested part or, as in the case of the hand, adjacent to the tested part. Stabilization is necessary for specificity in testing.

Place the part to be tested in precise antigravity test position, whenever it is appropriate, to help elicit the desired muscle action and aid in grading.

Use test movement in the horizontal plane when testing muscles that are too weak to function against gravity. Use test movement in antigravity positions for most trunk muscles and certain extremity muscles in which body weight offers sufficient resistance.

Apply pressure directly opposite the line of pull of the muscle or muscle segment being tested. Like the antigravity position, the direction of pressure helps elicit the desired muscle action.

Apply pressure gradually, but not too slowly, allowing the subject to "get set and hold." Apply uniform pressure, avoiding localized pressure that can cause discomfort.

Use a long lever whenever possible, unless contraindicated. The length of the lever is determined by the location of the pressure along the lever arm. Better discrimination of strength for purposes of grading is obtained through use of the long lever.

Use a short lever if intervening muscles do not provide sufficient fixation for use of a long lever.

By the action of some muscles to *safeguard* others, nature has provided a mechanism to protect multi-joint muscles from overshortening when contracting, and to protect multi-joint antagonists from being overlengthened. This natural safeguarding mechanism is employed in manual muscle testing of multi-joint muscles. To prevent the contracting muscle (the agonist) from becoming too short and thereby ineffective, it must be elongated over one or more joints while being shortened over another joint or joints.

An example of safeguarding action is illustrated by the action of wrist extensors during finger flexion. The Extensor carpi radialis longus and brevis and the Extensor carpi ulnaris hold the wrist in extension, thereby elongating the finger flexors over the wrist joint while they shorten over the finger joints. At the same time, this position of the wrist prevents overstretching the Extensor digitorum, the tendons of which pass over the wrist and all the finger joints.

This safeguarding action is found in numerous places in the body. It is nature's way of establishing a position of strength. In order for the Biceps to completely flex the elbow joint against strong resistance, the muscle must be elongated over the shoulder joint. This is accomplished naturally by the shoulder extensors extending this joint during strong elbow flexion. In the lower extremity, full knee flexion against strong resistance is accomplished in a position of hip and knee flexion. Hip flexors hold the hip in flexion in order to elongate the Hamstrings over the hip joint if full knee flexion is to be held against strong resistance.

The close relationship of muscles determines their action in substitution, assistance, and stabilization during tests of individual muscles. The grouping of muscles according to joint action, as seen in the charts on pp. 232–233 and 296–297, has been done to aid the examiner in understanding the allied actions of muscles.

Although most muscle testing is applied to patients with varying degrees of weakness or paralysis, the authors have chosen to use normal subjects to show normal muscle function, and the contour and location of muscles in test action.

The order in which muscles are tested is largely a matter of choice but generally arranged to avoid frequent and unnecessary changes of position for the subject. Muscles that are closely related in position or action tend to appear in sequence in order to distinguish test differences. As a general rule, length testing precedes strength testing. When the specific order of tests is important, it is so indicated in the text.

TERMS USED IN THE DESCRIPTION OF MUSCLE STRENGTH TESTS

Descriptions of the muscle tests in *Chapters 6, 7, and 8* are presented under headings of *Patient, Fixation, Test,* and *Pressure.* Each of these topics is discussed in detail in order to point out its particular significance in relation to accurate muscle testing.

Patient

In the description of each muscle test, this heading is followed by the position in which the patient is placed in order to accomplish the desired test. The position is important in relation to the test in two respects: 1) Insofar as practical, the position of the body should permit function against gravity for all muscles in which gravity is a factor in grading, and 2) the body should be placed in such a position that parts not being tested will remain as stable as possible. (This point is discussed further under *fixation.)*

In all muscle testing, the comfort of the patient and the intelligent handling of affected muscles are important factors. There are instances when the comfort of the patient or the condition of the affected muscles necessitates some modification of the test position. Insisting on an antigravity position may result in absurd positioning of a patient. Side-lying, which offers the best test position for several muscles, may be uncomfortable and result in strain of other muscles.

Fixation

This heading refers to the firmness or stability of the body or body part, necessary to insure an accurate test of a muscle or muscle group. Stabilization (holding steady or holding down), support (holding up), and counterpressure (equal and opposite pressure) are all included under fixation which implies holding firm. Fixation will be influenced by the firmness of the table, body weight, and, in some tests, by muscles that furnish fixation.

Adequate fixation depends to a great extent on the firmness of the *examining table,* which offers much of the necessary support. Testing and grading of strength will not be accurate if the table on which the patient lies has a thick soft pad or soft mattress that gives as the examiner applies pressure.

Body weight may furnish the necessary fixation. Because the weight of the body is an important factor in offering stability, the *horizontal position,* whether supine, prone, or side-lying, offers the best fixation for most tests. In the extremities, the part proximal to the tested part must be stable.

The *examiner* may stabilize the proximal part in tests of finger, wrist, toe, and foot muscles, but in other tests the body weight should help to stabilize the proximal part. In some instances the examiner may offer fixation in addition to the weight of the proximal part. There may be a need to hold a part firmly down on the table so that the pressure applied on the distal part, plus the weight of that part, does not displace the weight of the proximal part. In rotation tests it is necessary for the examiner to apply counterpressure to ensure exact test performance. (See pp. 217, 219, 280, and 281.)

In some tests, *muscles* furnish fixation. The muscles that furnish fixation do not cross the same joint(s) as the muscle being tested. The muscles that stabilize the scapula during arm movements and the pelvis during leg movements are referred to as fixation muscles. They do not enter directly into the test movement but do stabilize the movable scapula to the trunk, or the pelvis to the thorax, and make it possible for the tested muscle to have a firm origin from which to pull. In the same way, anterior abdominal muscles fix the thorax to the pelvis as anterior neck flexors act to lift the head forward in flexion from a supine position. (See p. 141 regarding action of opposite hip flexors in stabilizing the pelvis during hip extension.)

Muscles that have an antagonistic action give fixation by preventing excessive joint movement. This principle is illustrated by the fixation provided by the Lumbricales and Interossei in restricting hyperextension at the metacarpophalangeal joint during finger extension. In the presence of weak Lumbricales and Interossei, the pull of a strong Extensor digitorum results in hyperextension of these joints and passive flexion of the interphalangeal joints. This hyperextension does not occur and the fingers can be extended normally if the examiner prevents hyperextension of the metacarpophalangeal joints by fixation equivalent to that of the Lumbricales and Interossei. (See bottom of p. 250.)

When the fixation muscles are too weak or too strong, the examiner can simulate the normal stabilization by assisting or restricting movement of the part. The examiner must be able to differentiate between the normal action of these muscles in fixation and the abnormal actions that occur when substitution or muscle imbalance is present.

Test

This heading is followed by a description of the *test position* in which the part is placed by the examiner, and held (if possible) by the patient. It is the position used for the purpose of evaluating strength.

The *optimal test position* for one-joint muscles is at completion of range of motion; for two-joint muscles, it is a position within the mid-range of the overall length of the muscle. The photographs of the muscle tests in this and the next chapter show the test position for the muscles.

Test position (as opposed to test movement) offers the advantages of precision in positioning and accuracy in testing. In addition, the examiner determines immediately whether any limitation of motion exists by moving the part through the existing range of motion to test position.

The use of test position enables the examiner to detect substitution movements. When muscle weakness exists, other muscles immediately substitute in an attempt to hold a position resembling the test position. The visible shift from test position indicates a substitution movement.

Placing the part in test position also expedites grading the muscle strength. As the effort is made to hold test position, the ability or inability to hold the position against gravity is at once established. If the position is held, the examiner then applies pressure to grade above fair; if it fails to hold, the examiner tests for strength below fair. (See *Key to Muscle Grading,* p. 189.)

Test Movement

Test movement is a movement of the part in a specified direction and through a specific arc of motion. For strength tests of extremity muscles, it is used in testing muscles that are too weak to act against gravity (i.e., muscles that grade in the range of poor). Test movement is also used when testing the following muscles: trunk lateral flexors, upper abdominal flexors, back extensors, and Quadratus lumborum, Serratus anterior test in standing, Sartorius, Popliteus, and Gastrocnemius. When test movement is used in strength testing to ascertain the ability of the muscle to move through a specific arc of motion, the *grading* of strength must be done in optimal test position for purpose of standardization. (See discussion under *Grading*, pp. 184–188.)

Test movement may be used for certain muscles such as those that cross hinge joints, but it is not practical when a test requires a combination of two or more joint positions or movements. It is difficult for a patient to assume the exact position through verbal instruction or through imitating a movement demonstrated by the examiner. For accurate testing, the examiner should place the part precisely in the desired test position.

In muscle testing, weakness must be distinguished from restriction of range of motion. Frequently a muscle cannot complete the normal range of joint motion. It may be that the muscle is too weak to complete the movement; or it may be that the range of motion is restricted due to shortness of muscles, capsule, or ligamentous structures. The examiner should passively carry the part through the range of motion to determine whether any restriction exists. If no restriction is present, failure to hold the test position may be interpreted as weakness unless joint or tendon laxity is present.

In testing one-joint muscles in which the ability to hold at completion of motion is expected, the examiner must distinguish between muscle weakness and tendon insufficiency. For example, Quadriceps may be strong but unable to fully extend the knee because the patellar tendon or Quadriceps tendon has been stretched.

Muscle examinations should take into account such superimposed factors as relaxed, unstable joints. The degree of actual muscle weakness is difficult to judge in such cases. From the standpoint of function, the muscle is weak and should be so graded. But when the muscle exhibits a strong contraction, it is important to recognize this fact as potential for improvement. In a muscle that fails to function because of joint instability rather than weakness of the muscle itself, it is important that treatment be directed to correcting the joint problem and relieving strain on the muscle. Instances are not uncommon in which the Deltoid muscle shows a "fullness" of contraction throughout the muscle belly, and yet cannot begin to lift the weight of the arm. Such a muscle should be protected from strain by application of an adequate support with the express purpose of allowing the joint structures to shorten to their normal position. The failure to distinguish between real and apparent muscle weakness resulting from joint instability may deprive a patient of adequate follow-up treatment.

Pressure and Resistance

Pressure is used throughout this text to denote the external force applied by the examiner to determine the strength of the muscle holding in test position.

Resistance is a force tending to hinder motion, and is applied by the examiner or by gravity (or by both) during certain strength tests in which test movement is used. (See *Test Movement,* on facing page.)

The placement, the direction, and the amount of pressure are important factors when testing for strength above the grade of fair.

In the description of the muscle tests, pressure is specified as against and in the direction of. *Against* refers to the position of the examiner's hand in relation to the patient; *in the direction of* describes the direction of the force that is applied directly opposite the line of pull of the muscle or its tendon.

In some of the illustrations of muscle tests, the examiner's hand has been held extended for the purpose of indicating, photographically, that the direction of pressure is perpendicular to the palmar surface of the hand. Pressure should be applied in the direction indicated; it is not intended that an extended hand position be imitated during actual muscle testing.

Just as the direction of the pressure is an important part of accurate test performance, the *amount* of pressure is the determining factor in grading above fair. (See *Grading,* p. 185. for further discussion related to amount of pressure.)

The *place* at which pressure is applied depends upon muscle insertions, strength of intervening muscles, and leverage. As a general rule, pressure is applied near the distal end of the part on which the muscle is inserted. For example, pressure is applied near the distal end of the forearm during the Biceps test. Exceptions to the general rule occur when pressure on the bone of insertion does not provide adequate leverage to obtain discrimination for grading.

The length of the lever and the amount of pressure are closely related with respect to grading above fair. The use of a long lever makes it possible to apply slight, moderate, or strong pressure when testing for strength. Applying strong pressure on the scapula (the bone of insertion) when testing middle Trapezius may result in the *appearance* of normal strength. If tested using the arm as a lever, the muscle may only hold against slight pressure and grade no more than fair +. When testing strong muscles like hip abductors, it is necessary to use a long lever, i.e., placing pressure just proximal to the ankle. To avoid strain on the anteromedial area of the knee joint, adductors are tested using a shorter lever, i.e., just above the knee.

The principle of leverage must be utilized in muscle testing. Test results might be more indicative of the lack of strength of the examiner than of the patient, if the examiner did not have the advantage of leverage.

Pressure must be *applied gradually* in order to determine the degree of strength in muscles above fair. The patient must be allowed to *get set and hold* the test position against the examiner's pressure. The examiner cannot gauge the degree of strength unless pressure is applied gradually because slight pressure applied suddenly can "break" the pull of a strong muscle. Grading strength involves a subjective evaluation based on the amount of pressure applied. Differences in strength are so apparent, however, that an observer, who understands grading, can estimate the strength with a high degree of accuracy while watching the examiner apply pressure.

Weakness, Shortness, and Contracture

Included with the descriptions of the muscles in this text is a discussion of the loss of movement or the position of deformity that results from muscle weakness or muscle shortness. **Weakness** is used as an overall term covering a range of strength from zero to fair in non-weight-bearing muscles, but may be inclusive of fair + in weight-bearing muscles.

Weakness will result in loss of movement if the muscle cannot contract sufficiently to move the part through partial or complete range of motion. A contracture or shortness will result in loss of motion if the muscle cannot be elongated through its full range of motion. **Contracture** refers to a degree of shortness that results in a marked loss of range of motion, and **shortness** refers to a degree of shortness that results in slight to moderate loss of range of motion.

A fixed deformity usually does not exist as a result of weakness unless contractures develop in the stronger opponents. In the wrist, for example, a fixed deformity will not develop as a result of wrist extensor weakness unless the opposing flexors contract to hold the position of wrist flexion.

A state of **muscle imbalance** exists when a muscle is weak and its antagonist is strong. The stronger of the two opponents tends to shorten, and the weaker one tends to elongate. Either weakness or shortness can cause faulty alignment. Weakness *permits* a position of deformity; shortness *creates* a position of deformity.

In some parts of the body, positions of deformity may develop as a result of weakness even though the opposing muscles do not become contracted. Gravity and body weight exist as the opposing force. A kyphotic position of the upper back may result from weakness of the upper back muscles whether or not the anterior trunk muscles become contracted. A position of pronation of the foot may exist if the inverters are weak because the body weight in standing will distort the bony alignment. If opposing peroneal muscles become contracted, a fixed deformity will result.

The word **tight** has two meanings. It may be used interchangeably with the word **short,** or it may be used to mean **taut** in which case it may be applied to either a short or a stretched muscle. On palpation, Hamstrings that are *short* and drawn taut will feel tight. Hamstrings that are *stretched* and drawn taut will also feel tight. From the standpoint of prescribing treatment, it is very important to recognize the difference between stretched muscles and shortened muscles. In addition, some muscles are short and remain in what appears to be a state of semicontraction. On palpation, they feel firm or even rigid without being drawn taut. For example, posterior neck and upper Trapezius muscles often are tight in people with bad posture of upper back, head, and shoulders.

Substitution

When a muscle or muscle group attempts to compensate for the lack of function of a weak or paralyzed muscle, the result is a substitution movement. Muscles that normally act together in movements may act in substitution. These include fixation muscles, agonists, and antagonists.

Substitution by *fixation muscles* occurs specifically in relation to movements of the shoulder joint and hip joint. Muscles that move the scapula may produce a secondary movement of the arm; muscles that move the pelvis may produce a secondary movement of the thigh. These substitution movements appear similar to, but are not actually, movements of the shoulder or hip joint.

True abduction of the hip joint is accomplished by hip abductors with normal fixation by the lateral trunk muscles. When hip abductors are weak, apparent abduction may occur by the substitution action of lateral trunk muscles. The pelvis is hiked up laterally and the leg is raised from the table but there is no true hip joint abduction. (See pp. 145 and 223.)

Antagonists may produce movements similar to test movements. If finger flexors are weak, action of the wrist extensors may produce passive finger flexion by the tension placed on flexor tendons.

Substitution by other *agonists* results in either: 1) a movement of the part in the direction of the stronger agonist; or 2) a shift of the body in such a way so as to favor the pull of that agonist. For example, during the Gluteus medius test in side-lying, the thigh will tend to flex if the Tensor fasciae latae is attempting to substitute for the Gluteus medius; or the trunk may rotate back so that the Tensor fasciae latae can hold a position that appears to be the desired test position.

When there is restriction of joint motion due to contracted muscles, a movement to relieve tension of a tight muscle may appear similar to a movement of substitution. (See discussion of substitution under *Note* in Hamstring test, p. 210.)

For accurate muscle examinations, no substitutions should be permitted. The position or movement described as the test should be done without shifting the body or turning the part. Such secondary movements allow other muscles to substitute for the weak or paralyzed muscle.

An experienced examiner, who is aware of the ease with which normal muscles perform the tests, will readily detect substitutions. When test position is employed instead of test movement, even an inexperienced examiner can detect the sudden shift of the body or of the part that results from the effort to compensate for the muscle weakness.

GRADING

Grades are an expression of an examiner's assessment of the strength or weakness of a muscle or muscle group. In manual muscle testing, grading is based on a system in which the ability to hold the tested part in a given position against gravity establishes a grade referred to as *fair* or the numerical equivalent (depending upon the symbols of grading being used). The grade of fair is the most objective grade because the pull of gravity is a constant factor.

For grades above fair, pressure is applied in addition to the resistance offered by gravity. A *break test* is a muscle strength test to determine the maximal effort exerted by a subject who is performing an isometric contraction as the examiner applies a *gradual* build-up of pressure to the point that the effort by the subject is overcome. It is used in determining grades of fair + through good +.

No effort is made to break the subject's hold if the examiner has determined that the strength is normal; to continue exerting force to make the muscle yield by performing a break test is unnecessary and may be injurious.

The *symbols* used in grading vary and include the use of words, letters, numbers, or other signs. To avoid listing the equivalents each time reference is made to a grade, the word symbols are used in the descriptions of grades below. (See *Key to Grading Symbols*, p. 188.)

Gravity is a form of resistance basic to manual muscle testing, and is used in tests of trunk, neck, and extremity muscles. However, it is a factor in only about 60% of the extremity muscles. It is not required in tests of finger and toe muscles because the weight of the part is so small in comparison with the strength of the muscle that the effect of gravity on the part is negligible. Supination and pronation of the forearm are movements of rotation in which the effect of gravity is not a significant factor.

Testing muscles that are very weak involves *movements in the horizontal plane* in which the resistance by gravity is decreased. To avoid the terms "gravity-lessened," "gravity-decreased," or "gravity-minimized" the text and the *Key to Muscle Grading* (p. 189) will refer to "movements in the horizontal plane."

Detailed grading of muscle strength is more important in relation to prognosis than to diagnosis. The extent of involvement may be determined by such simple grading as zero, weak, normal. On the other hand, more precise grading helps establish the rate and degree of return of muscle strength, and is useful in determining a prognosis. A muscle might appear "weak" for months, while the record shows that it has progressed from poor − to fair during that period.

Accuracy in grading depends upon many factors: the stable position of the patient, the fixation of the part proximal to the tested part, the precision of the test position, and the direction and amount of pressure. The amount of pressure varies according to the age and size of the patient, the part being tested, and the leverage. If one extremity is unaffected, the examiner may use the strength in the unaffected extremity as an index to the patient's normal strength when testing the affected extremity.

An examiner must build a basis for comparison of test results through experience in muscle testing. Such experience is necessary on both paralytic and normal individuals. For many, experience in muscle testing has been limited to examination of patients with disease or injury. The result is that their idea of normal strength tends to be a measure of what appears to be good functional recovery following weakness.

The authors recommend that an examiner make an effort to test individuals of various ages, both male and female, and those with good posture as well as those with faulty posture. If it is not possible to examine a large number of normal individuals, an effort should be made to examine the trunk and unaffected extremities in cases involving only one or two extremities.

Testing and grading procedures are modified in the examination of infants and children to the age of 5 or 6. The ability to determine a child's muscle strength up to the grade of fair is usually not difficult, but grading above fair depends on the cooperation of the child in holding against resistance or pressure. Young children seldom cooperate in strong test movements. Very often tests must be recorded as "apparently normal" which indicates that strength may be normal, although one cannot be sure.

Grades Above Fair

Standardization of muscle testing techniques related to grading strength above fair requires that there be *a specific place in the arc of motion* where the part is held by the subject as manual pressure is applied.

Muscle strength is not constant throughout the range of motion and in manual muscle testing it is not practical to try to grade the strength at various points in the arc of motion. The place in the arc used as the *position for grading* is determined, chiefly, on the basis of whether the muscle is a one-joint or a multi-joint muscle.

The position for a *one-joint muscle* is at completion of the range of joint motion. From a clinical standpoint, it appears that a one-joint muscle reaches peak performance at completion of range of motion when the muscle is most fully shortened. From the standpoint of function, it is advisable and necessary that testing determine the ability of one-joint muscles to hold against strong pressure at completion of range of motion.

In keeping with the principle of the length-tension curve, a *two-joint muscle* reaches peak performance at a point within the mid-range of the overall length of the muscle. The muscle strength diminishes as the muscle shortens beyond that range to reach a point of becoming ineffective. The precise position of the joint where pressure is applied depends upon the position of the other joint or joints over which the muscle crosses. The position can be standardized except in instances when it is necessary to modify the test position.

Whether the part is placed in test position or actively moves to that position, grading above fair is determined by the ability to hold *in* test position.

If *test position* is used, the part is placed in the specific position by the examiner and pressure is applied. If *test movement* is used, the movement must proceed to the same place in the arc of motion as that established as test position if there is to be standardization of testing techniques and grading. For this reason, the movement factor is omitted in the *Key to Muscle Grading* when defining grades above fair.

Normal Grade

The grade of *normal* means that the muscle can hold the test position against strong pressure. It is not intended to indicate the maximum strength of the subject but, rather, the maximum pressure that the examiner applies to obtain what might be termed a "full" strength of the muscle. In terms of judgment, it might be described as strength that is adequate for ordinary functional activities. To become competent in judging this full strength, an examiner should test normal individuals of various ages and sizes.

Good Grade

The grade of *good* means that the muscle can hold the test position against moderate pressure.

Fair Grade

The grade of *fair* indicates that a muscle can hold the part in test position against the resistance of

gravity but cannot hold if even slight pressure is added. In tests such as Triceps and Quadriceps, the examiner should avoid a "locked" position of the joint that could give undue advantage to a muscle that was slightly less than fair in strength.

It is in the area of the fair grade that the question arises about whether the strength to hold the test position is equivalent to the strength required to move through range of motion to the test position. There are some exceptions, but the general rule is that the test movement can be performed if the test position can be held.

In some muscle tests, the bone on which the muscle is inserted moves from a position of suspension in the vertical plane toward the horizontal plane. The Quadriceps, Deltoid, and hip rotators tested in the sitting position, and the Triceps and shoulder rotators tested in the prone position compose this group. The leverage exerted by the weight of the part increases as the part moves toward completion of arc, and the muscle strength required to hold the test position against gravity usually is sufficient to perform the test movement against gravity.

In a few tests, the bone on which the muscle is inserted moves from a horizontal position toward a vertical position and less strength is required to hold the test position than to perform the test movement. This occurs during tests of Hamstrings when tested by knee flexion in the prone position; and of the elbow flexors tested in the supine position.

Fair Minus Grade in Antigravity Position

The *fair –* grade is visible to the examiner or an observer as a *very gradual release* from the antigravity test position. It may be described by such phrases as "it sags slowly from test position," "it almost holds test position," or "it does not quite hold test position." It is an acceptably objective grade.

Poor Grade

See discussion on p. 187.

Trace Grade

A grade of *trace* means that a feeble contraction can be felt in a muscle that can be palpated, or the tendon becomes slightly prominent, but there is no visible movement of the part. Trace grades can be determined in almost any position.

When testing muscles that are very weak, the examiner usually moves the part into test position, trying to help the patient feel the movement in order to elicit a muscle response. The examiner should be sure that the movement starts from a relaxed position. If the part is carried to the beginning of the range of motion and slight tension put on the muscle, there may be a rebound or springing back which can be confused with active movement.

Zero Grade

The grade of *zero* means that there is no evidence of any muscle contraction.

Poor Grade

The ability to move through a partial arc of motion in the horizontal plane is graded *poor minus*. The grade of *poor* means that the muscle is capable of completing range of motion in the horizontal plane. The grade of *poor plus* denotes the ability to move in the horizontal plane to completion of range of motion against resistance, or to hold the completed position against pressure. It also means that the muscle is capable of moving through a partial arc of motion in the antigravity position.

The ranges of strength within the grade of poor are significant enough to deserve these sub-classifications for purposes of more definitive grading. The ability to perform full range of motion in the horizontal plane is not close to the ability to perform the test against gravity for most muscles, notably those of the hip joint. Adding pressure or resistance to the element of movement in the horizontal plane provides the added force that approaches that of gravity in the antigravity position.

Hip abductors, for example, may complete the movement of abduction in a supine position (i.e., horizontal plane) which would give a grade of poor. As strength improves, the patient can hold against more and more pressure in the abducted position, or can move to the abducted position against increasingly greater resistance. Experience will disclose the amount of pressure or resistance that must be applied in the supine position in order to exhibit strength that approaches the ability to perform to completion of range in the antigravity position. With hip abductors it requires that the muscles tolerate moderate to strong resistance or pressure in the supine position before being able to hold for a fair grade in the antigravity position.

It is important to record the important changes in strength that occur during the time that it takes to move from the grade of poor − to poor and to poor +.

Testing for the various grades of poor is *justified, and meaningful* when used appropriately. In the rehabilitation of persons with severe neuromuscular and musculoskeletal involvement, the minute but visible changes that show improvement are very important. Maintaining a record of these significant changes, however slight, is important to the morale and the continuing motivation of the patient, and is necessary in determining progress. In the broad scope of rehabilitation, these small changes at one end of the spectrum can be more significant than the 10, 20, 30 (or more) pounds of force that can be gained by a recovering athlete at the other end of the spectrum.

After all that explanation, it may also be said that the overall grade of poor can be "assumed" without unnecessary changes of position required for the tests in the horizontal plane. If it has been determined that the muscle does not grade a fair − by the test in the antigravity position, but does grade more than a trace (which can be established in almost any position), the overall grade of poor exists without any further testing.

There are instances in which assuming the grade of poor may be justified: if there is no need for more specific grading than normal, good, fair, poor, and trace; or if the patient has extensive weakness and is easily fatigued; or if the condition is longstanding with no appreciable change.

Establishing the grade of poor often requires that the patient be moved from one position to another. In practice, frequent change of the patient's position or repetition of the test in various positions is fatiguing to the patient and time-consuming for the examiner. It is also possible that the patients with the most weakness would be subjected to the most changes of position. Patients should not be subjected to unnecessary procedures in examination if the results obtained are not meaningful.

Tests in the horizontal plane include several variables. The partial range of motion for the poor − grade is not specific. Since there is no indication of where in the arc of motion the partial range should be, it may be at the beginning of the range, within the mid-range, or near the end of the range of motion.

With respect to partial arc of motion in antigravity position for a poor + grade, it may mean starting from the suspended (vertical) position for Quadriceps. For Hamstrings, it may mean that in the prone position the subject can flex the last few degrees required to bring the leg to the vertical position.

When testing hip extensors or hip flexors in side-lying, a horizontal movement through the range of motion furnishes a means of obtaining an objective grade of poor. However, the surface of the table may be smooth or rough, changing the amount of friction and resistance considerably. The strength of hip adductors (if the underneath leg is being tested) may make a material difference in results of the flexor and extensor tests. If the adductors are paralyzed, the full weight of the extremity will rest on the table and make flexion and extension difficult. If the adductor muscles are strong they will tend to raise the extremity so the full weight does not rest on the table, thereby reducing the friction, and the flexion and extension movements will be made easier.

GRADING SYMBOLS

Robert W. Lovett, M.D., introduced a method of testing and grading muscle strength, using gravity as resistance (35). A description of the Lovett system was published in 1932 and listed the following definitions:

Gone—no contraction felt.
Trace—muscle can be felt to tighten, but cannot produce movement.
Poor—produces movement with gravity eliminated, but cannot function against gravity.
Fair—can raise part against gravity.
Good—can raise part against outside resistance as well as against gravity.
Normal—can overcome a greater amount of resistance than a good muscle

While symbols may vary, the movement and weight factors set forth by Lovett form the basis of most present-day muscle testing. The Kendalls introduced the 0 to 100% scale of grading in order to use numbers for computing the amount of change in muscle strength when doing research with patients recovering from poliomyelitis. They had used the word and letter symbols prior to using numerals and, for the most part, it was possible to translate grades from one scale to the other.

The authors of this text believe that it is in the best interest of those who engage in manual muscle testing that an effort be made to standardize as much as possible the descriptions of the tests and the symbols used. There is increasing use of numerals, and such use is needed for research that involves muscle test grades.

The *Key to Muscle Grading* on the following page is basically the same as the Lovett system with added definitions for the minus and plus grades. The poor+ grade provides for movement in the horizontal plane and for partial arc against gravity. Both methods for grading poor+ are in common use.

In this text the percent sign has been dropped, normal– grade has been eliminated, and the scale changed to 0 to 10. Leaving zero as 0 and trace as T, the word and letter symbols translate directly as indicated by the *Key to Grading Symbols* below. As noted in the *Key to Muscle Grading*, there is no movement involved with the 0 and T grades, and the numerals 1 to 10 refer to Test Movement and Test Position grades.

The scale of 0 to 10 consists of whole numbers, and does not involve the use of fractions or decimals. If computations were to be made using the scale of 5, the minus and plus symbols would translate as indicated below.

Key To Grading Symbols

Normal	N	10	5	(5)	(5.0)	+ + + +
Good +	G+	9	4+	(4 1/2)	(4.5)	
Good	G	8	4	(4)	(4.0)	+ + +
Good –	G–	7	4–	(3 2/3)	(3.66)	
Fair +	F+	6	3+	(3 1/3)	(3.33)	
Fair	F	5	3	3	(3.0)	+ +
Fair –	F–	4	3–	(2 2/3)	(2.66)	
Poor +	P+	3	2+	(2 1/3)	(2.33)	
Poor	P	2	2	(2)	(2.0)	+
Poor –	P–	1	2–	(1 1/2)	(1.5)	
Trace	T	T	1	(1)	(1.0)	
Zero	0	0	0	(0)	(0.0)	0

	Function of the Muscle	Grade Symbols		
No Movement	No contraction felt in the muscle	Zero	0	0
	Tendon becomes prominent or feeble contraction felt in the muscle, but no visible movement of the part	Trace	T	T
Test Movement	**MOVEMENT IN HORIZONTAL PLANE**			
	Moves through partial range of motion	Poor −	P −	1
	Moves through complete range of motion	Poor	P	2
	Moves to completion of range against resistance _or_ Moves to completion of range and holds against pressure **ANTIGRAVITY POSITION** Moves through partial range of motion	Poor +	P +	3
Test Position	_Gradual_ release from test position	Fair −	F −	4
	Holds test position (no added pressure)	Fair	F	5
	Holds test position against slight pressure	Fair +	F +	6
	Holds test position against slight to moderate pressure	Good −	G −	7
	Holds test position against moderate pressure	Good	G	8
	Holds test position against moderate to strong pressure	Good +	G +	9
	Holds test position against strong pressure	Normal	N	10

Comparison of grading symbols

0-10	0-5
0	0
T	1
1 2 3 4	2
5	3
6 7 8 9	4
10	5

Use of the Word "Normal" in Relation to Muscle Grading

The word normal has a variety of meanings. It may mean average, typical, natural, or standard. As used in various methods of grading, it has been defined as that degree of strength which will perform a movement against gravity and hold against strong resistance. By virtue of this definition the word normal has been used as a *standard*.

If one adheres to the usage in this sense, then a grade of poor will be recorded for a small child who cannot lift his head in flexion from a supine position. Knowing that it is natural for small children to exhibit weakness of the anterior neck muscles, an examiner might say this child's neck is normal, using normal in the sense that it is *natural*. Upon administering a leg-lowering test for abdominal strength in a large group of adolescent children, and finding that a grade of fair + or good — is average strength for the group, one might say this grade of strength is normal for this age. Thus we have three different uses of the word normal applied rather freely in muscle testing: as standard, as natural, and as average.

Since normal is defined as a standard when used in the scale of grading, grades of strength should relate to that standard and appropriate terms other than normal should be used in interpretations.

One of the advantages of the use of numerical grades is that it leaves the term "normal" free for use in interpretation of grades. In the following discussion it will be employed in this manner.

Since most grades are based on adult standards, it is necessary to acknowledge when a grade less than the standard is normal for children of a given age. This is particularly true with respect to the strength of the anterior neck and anterior abdominal muscles. The size of the head and trunk in relation to the lower extremities, as well as the long span and normal protrusion of the abdominal wall affect the relative strength of these muscles. Anterior neck muscles may grade about poor + in a 3-year-old child, about fair in a 5-year-old, and gradually increase up to the standard of performance for adults by as early as 10 or 12 years of age. Many adults will exhibit no more than fair + strength, but this need not be interpreted as neurogenic because it is usually found to be associated with faulty posture of the head and upper back.

The prime example of a standard that is an infant accomplishment instead of an adult one is that of toe flexor strength. In general, children have more strength in their toe flexors than adults. It is not uncommon to find that women, who have worn high heels and rather narrow-toed shoes, have weakness of toe flexors in which the grade is no more than fair —. With the standard being the ability to flex the toes and hold against strong resistance or pressure, the adult must be graded against that standard, but this weakness of toe flexors should not be interpreted as normal for age. One becomes so accustomed to toe flexor weakness among adults that it might be assumed that a degree of weakness is normal in the sense that normal is average. Marked weakness of toe flexors is almost invariably associated with some degree of disability of the foot and the word normal should not apply to such weakness, unless one is ready to accept the disability as normal.

The toe flexor weakness represents a loss of strength from childhood to adulthood and should be regarded as an unnatural, *acquired* weakness. This type of weakness may be present in other muscles as a result of stretch and strain associated with occupational or recreational activities, or faulty posture. Acquired weakness usually does not drop below the grade of fair, but fair and fair + grades of strength might be interpreted as neurogenic if one were not aware that such degrees of weakness can result from stretch and strain of the muscles.

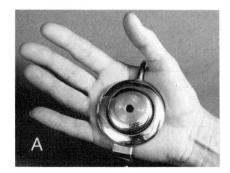 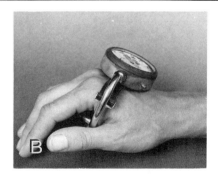

In 1941, a hand-held device was designed (by the senior author of this text) to measure the force applied by the examiner during manual muscle testing. Figure A shows the pressure-sensitive pad in the palm of the hand from which force was transmitted to the gauge on the dorsum of the hand, figure B. (See also *Historical Note*, p. 6.)

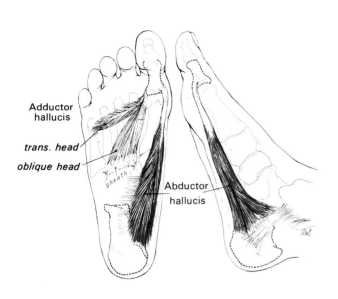

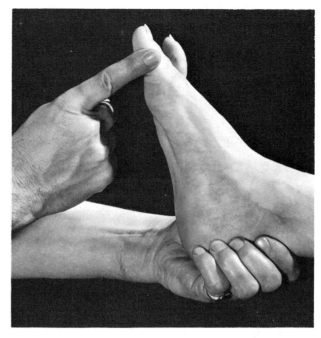

ABDUCTOR HALLUCIS

Origin: Medial process of tuberosity of calcaneus, flexor retinaculum, plantar aponeurosis, and adjacent intermuscular septum.

Insertion: Medial side of base of proximal phalanx of great toe. Some fibers are attached to the medial sesamoid bone, and a tendinous slip may extend to the base of the proximal phalanx of the great toe.

Action: Abducts and assists in flexion of the metatarsophalangeal joint of the great toe, and assists with adduction of the forefoot.

Nerve: Tibial, L4, **5**, S1.

Patient: Supine or sitting.

Fixation: The examiner grips the heel firmly.

Test: If possible, abduction of the big toe from the axial line of the foot. This is difficult for the average individual, and the action may be demonstrated by having the patient pull the forefoot in adduction against pressure by the examiner.

Pressure: Against the medial side of the first metatarsal and proximal phalanx. The muscle can be palpated and often seen along the medial border of the foot.

Weakness: Allows forefoot valgus, hallux valgus, and medial displacement of the navicular.

Contracture: Pulls the foot into forefoot varus with the big toe abducted.

ADDUCTOR HALLUCIS

Origin: *Oblique head* from bases of second, third, and fourth metatarsal bones, and sheath of tendon of Peroneus longus. *Transverse head* from plantar metatarsophalangeal ligaments of third, fourth, and fifth digits and deep transverse metatarsal ligament.

Insertion: Lateral side of base of proximal phalanx of great toe.

Action: Adducts and assists in flexing the metatarsophalangeal joint of the great toe.

Nerve: Tibial, S1, 2.

Contracture: Adduction deformity of great toe (hallux valgus).

Note: NO TEST ILLUSTRATED

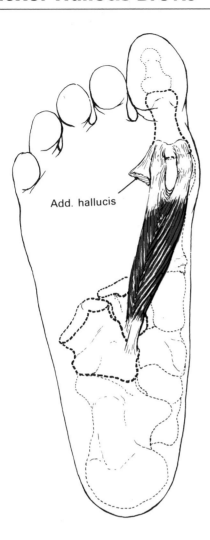

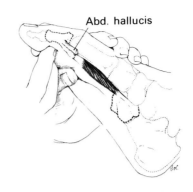

Abd. hallucis

Add. hallucis

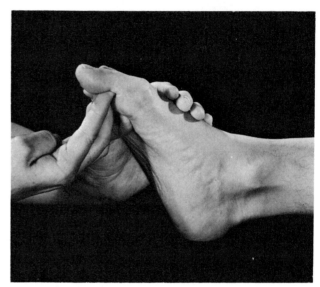

Origin: Medial part of plantar surface of cuboid bone, adjacent part of lateral cuneiform bone, and from prolongation of tendon of Tibialis posterior.

Insertion: Medial and lateral sides of base of proximal phalanx of great toe.

Action: Flexes the metatarsophalangeal joint of the great toe.

Nerve: Tibial L4, **5**, S1.

Patient: Supine or sitting.

Fixation: The examiner stabilizes the foot proximal to the metatarsophalangeal joint, and maintains a neutral position of the foot and ankle. (Plantar flexion of the foot may cause restriction of the test movement by the tension of the opposing long toe extensor muscles.)

Test: Flexion of the metatarsophalangeal joint of the great toe.

Pressure: Against the plantar surface of the proximal phalanx in the direction of extension.

Note: When the Flexor hallucis longus is paralyzed and the brevis is active, the action of the brevis is clear because the toe flexes at the metatarsophalangeal joint without any flexion of the interphalangeal joint. When the Flexor hallucis brevis is paralyzed and the longus is active, the metatarsophalangeal joint hyperextends, and the interphalangeal joint flexes.

Weakness: Allows hammer toe position of great toe. Lessens stability of the longitudinal arch.

Contracture: The proximal phalanx is held in flexion.

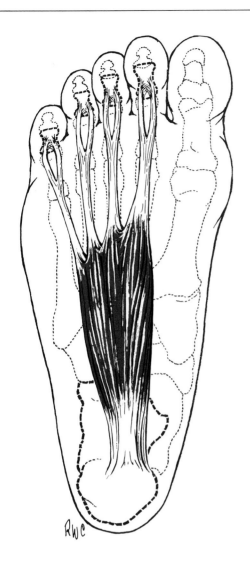

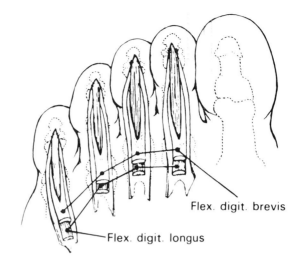

Flex. digit. brevis

Flex. digit. longus

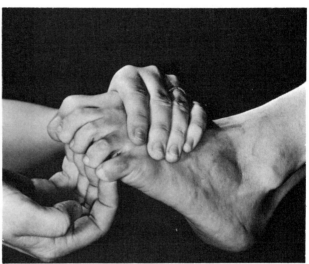

Origin: Medial process of tuberosity of calcaneus, central part of plantar aponeurosis, and adjacent intermuscular septa.

Insertion: Middle phalanx of second through fifth digits.

Action: Flexes the proximal interphalangeal joints, and assists in flexion of the metatarsophalangeal joints of the second through fifth digits.

Nerve: Tibial, L4, **5**, S1.

Patient: Supine or sitting.

Fixation: The examiner stabilizes the proximal phalanges, and maintains a neutral position of the foot and ankle. If the Gastrocnemius and Soleus are paralyzed, the examiner must stabilize the calcaneus, which is the bone of origin, during the toe flexor test.

Test: Flexion of the proximal interphalangeal joints of the second, third, fourth, and fifth digits.

Pressure: Against the plantar surface of the middle phalanx of the four toes in the direction of extension.

Note: When the Flexor digitorum longus is paralyzed and the brevis is active, the toes flex at the middle phalanx while the distal phalanx remains extended.

Weakness: The ability to flex the proximal interphalangeal joints of the four lateral toes is decreased, and the muscular support of the longitudinal and transverse arches is diminished.

Contracture: Restriction of extension of the toes. The middle phalanges flex, and there is a tendency toward a cavus if the Gastrocnemius and Soleus are weak.

Note: Testing for strength of Flexor digitorum brevis is important in cases of longitudinal arch strain. Often, a point of acute tenderness is found at the origin of this muscle on the calcaneus.

Flexor Hallucis Longus

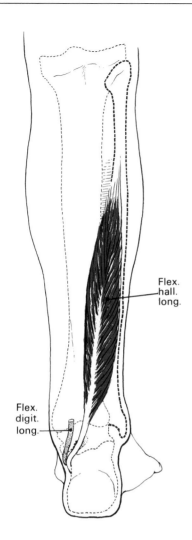

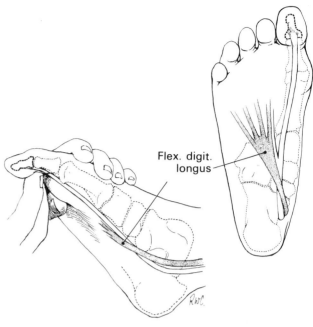

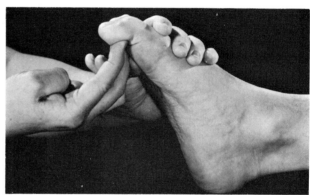

Origin: Posterior surface of distal two thirds of fibula, interosseus membrane, and adjacent intermuscular septa and fascia.

Insertion: Base of distal phalanx of great toe, plantar surface.

Note: The Flexor hallucis longus is connected to the Flexor digitorum longus by a strong tendinous slip.

Action: Flexes the interphalangeal joint of the great toe, and assists in flexion of the metatarsophalangeal joint, plantar flexion of the ankle joint, and inversion of the foot.

Nerve: Tibial, L5, S1, 2.

Patient: Supine or sitting.

Fixation: The examiner stabilizes the metatarsophalangeal joint in neutral position and maintains the ankle joint approximately midway between dorsal and plantar flexion. (Full dorsiflexion may produce passive flexion of the interphalangeal joint, and full plantar flexion would allow the muscle to shorten too much to exert its maximum force.) If the Flexor hallucis brevis is very strong and the Flexor hallucis longus weak, it is necessary to restrict the tendency for the metatarsophalangeal joint to flex by holding the proximal phalanx in slight extension.

Test: Flexion of the interphalangeal joint of the great toe.

Pressure: Against the plantar surface of the distal phalanx in the direction of extension.

Weakness: Results in tendency toward hyperextension of interphalangeal joint and hammer-toe deformity of great toe. Decreases the strength of inversion of the foot and plantar flexion of the ankle. In weight bearing, permits a tendency toward a pronation of the foot.

Contracture: Claw-toe deformity of great toe.

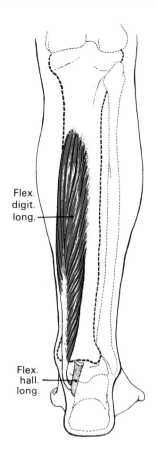

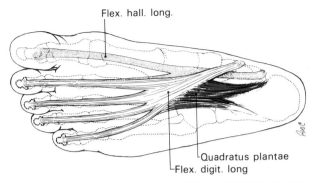

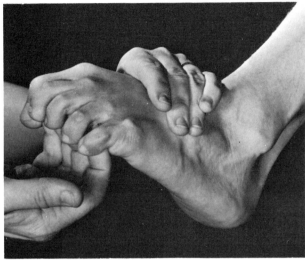

FLEXOR DIGITORUM LONGUS

Origin: Middle three fifths of posterior surface of body of tibia, and from fascia covering the Tibialis posterior.

Insertion: Bases of distal phalanges of second through fifth digits.

Action: Flexes proximal and distal interphalangeal and metatarsophalangeal joints of the second through fifth digits. Assists in plantar flexion of the ankle joint and inversion of the foot.

Nerve: Tibial, L5, S1, (2).

Patient: Supine or sitting. In the presence of Gastrocnemius tightness, the knee should be flexed to permit a neutral position of the foot.

Fixation: The examiner stabilizes the metatarsals and maintains a neutral position of the foot and ankle.

Test: Flexion of the distal interphalangeal joints of the second, third, fourth, and fifth digits. The Flexor digitorum is assisted by Quadratus plantae.

Pressure: Against the plantar surface of the distal phalanges of the four toes in the direction of extension.

Weakness: Results in tendency toward hyperextension of distal interphalangeal joints of the four toes. Decreases the ability to invert the foot and plantar flex the ankle. In weight bearing, weakness permits a tendency toward a pronation of the foot.

Contracture: Flexion deformity of distal phalanges of four lateral toes, with restriction of dorsiflexion and eversion of foot.

QUADRATUS PLANTAE (FLEXOR ACCESSORIUS)

Origin of Medial Head: Medial surface of calcaneus, and medial border of long plantar ligament.

Origin of Lateral Head: Lateral border of plantar surface of calcaneus, and lateral border of long plantar ligament.

Insertion: Lateral margin, and dorsal and plantar surfaces of tendon of Flexor digitorum longus.

Action: Modifies the line of pull of the Flexor digitorum longus tendons, and assists in flexing the second through fifth digits.

Nerve: Tibial, S1, 2.

Note: NO TEST ILLUSTRATED

Lumbricales and Interossei

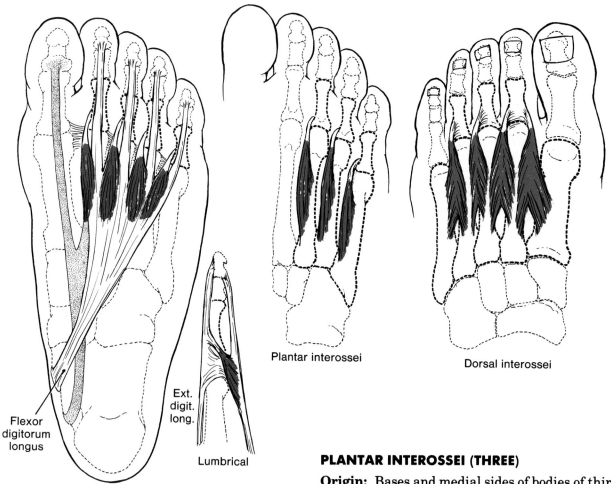

Flexor digitorum longus

Ext. digit. long.

Lumbrical

Lumbricales

Plantar interossei

Dorsal interossei

LUMBRICALES

Origin: First from medial side of first Flexor digitorum longus tendon, second from adjacent sides of first and second Flexor digitorum longus tendons, third from adjacent sides of second and third Flexor digitorum longus tendons, fourth from adjacent sides of third and fourth Flexor digitorum longus tendons.

Insertions: Medial side of proximal phalanx and dorsal expansion of the Extensor digitorum longus tendon of the second through fifth digits.

Action: Flexes the metatarsophalangeal joints and assists in extending the interphalangeal joints of the second through fifth digits.

Nerve to Lumbricalis I: Tibial, L4, **5,** S1.

Nerve to Lumbricales II, III, IV: Tibial, L (4), (5), S1, 2.

PLANTAR INTEROSSEI (THREE)

Origin: Bases and medial sides of bodies of third, fourth, and fifth metatarsal bones.

Insertion: Medial sides of bases of proximal phalanges of same digit.

Action: Adduct the third, fourth, and fifth digits toward the axial line through the second digit. Assist in flexion of the metatarsophalangeal joints, and may assist in extension of interphalangeal joints of third, fourth, and fifth digit.

Nerve: Tibial, S1, 2.

DORSAL INTEROSSEI (FOUR)

Origin: Each by two heads from adjacent sides of the metatarsal bones.

Insertions: Side of proximal phalanx and capsule of metatarsophalangeal joint. First, to medial side of second digit; other three to lateral sides of second, third, and fourth digits.

Action: Abducts the second, third, and fourth digits from the axial line through the second digit. Assists in flexion of the metatarsophalangeal joints, and may assist in extension of interphalangeal joints of second, third, and fourth digits.

Nerve: Tibial, S1, 2.

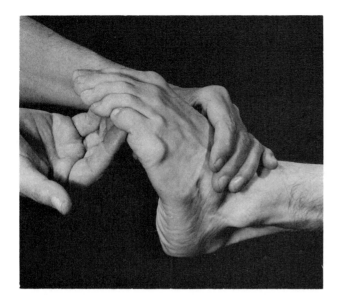 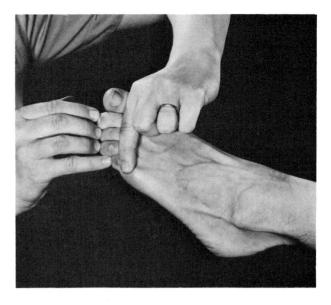

Patient: Supine or sitting.

Fixation: Examiner stabilizes the midtarsal region and maintains a neutral position of the foot and ankle.

Test: Flexion of the metatarsophalangeal joints of the second, third, fourth, and fifth digits with an effort to avoid flexion of the interphalangeal joints.

Pressure: Against the plantar surface of the proximal phalanges of the four lateral toes.

Weakness: When these muscles are weak, and the Flexor digitorum longus is active, hyperextension occurs at the metatarsophalangeal joints. The distal joints flex causing a hammer toe position of the four lateral toes. Muscular support of the transverse arch is decreased.

Patient: Supine or sitting.

Fixation: The examiner stabilizes the metatarsophalangeal joints, and maintains the foot and ankle in approximately 20° to 30° plantar flexion.

Test: Extension of the interphalangeal joints of the four lateral toes. (A separate test for the adduction and abduction actions of the interossei is not practical since most individuals cannot perform these movements of the toes.)

Pressure: Against the dorsal surface of the distal phalanges, in the direction of flexion.

Note: Testing for strength of Lumbricales is important in cases of hammer toes and of metatarsal arch strain.

DEFORMITIES OF THE FOOT AND ANKLE

In the following list, foot deformities are defined in terms of the positions of the involved joints. In severe deformities the position of the joint is beyond the normal range of joint motion.

Talipes valgus: Foot everted and accompanied by flattening of the longitudinal arch.

Talipes varus: Foot inverted and accompanied by an increase in the height of the longitudinal arch.

Talipes equinus: Ankle joint plantar flexed.

Talipes equinovalgus: Ankle joint plantar flexed and foot everted.

Talipes equinovarus: Ankle joint plantar flexed and foot inverted. (Club foot.)

Talipes calcaneus: Ankle joint dorsiflexed.

Talipes calcaneovalgus: Ankle joint dorsiflexed and foot everted.

Talipes calcaneovarus: Ankle joint dorsiflexed and foot inverted.

Talipes cavus: Ankle joint dorsiflexed, forefoot plantar flexed, resulting in a high longitudinal arch. With the change in position of the calcaneus, the posterior prominence of the heel tends to be obliterated, and weight bearing on the calcaneus shifts posteriorly.

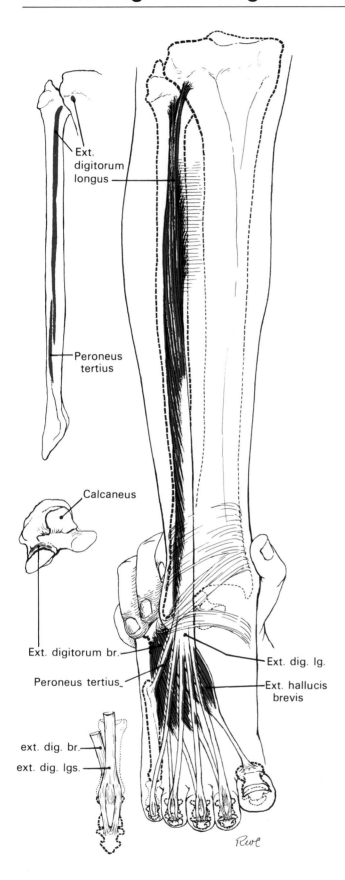

EXTENSOR DIGITORUM LONGUS

Origin: Lateral condyle of tibia, proximal three fourths of anterior surface of body of fibula, proximal part of interosseus membrane, adjacent intermuscular septa, and deep fascia.

Insertion: By four tendons to the second through fifth digits. Each tendon forms an expansion on the dorsal surface of the toe, and divides into an intermediate slip attached to base of middle phalanx and into two lateral slips attached to base of distal phalanx.

Action: Extends the metatarsophalangeal joints and assists in extending the interphalangeal joints of the second through fifth digits. Assists in dorsiflexion of the ankle joint and eversion of the foot.

Nerve: Peroneal, **L4, 5, S1.**

EXTENSOR DIGITORUM BREVIS

Origin: Distal part of superior and lateral surfaces of calcaneus, lateral talocalcaneal ligament, and apex of inferior extensor retinaculum.

Insertion: By four tendons to first through fourth digits. The most medial slip, also known as the Extensor hallucis brevis, inserts into dorsal surface of base of proximal phalanx of great toe. Other three tendons join lateral sides of tendons of Extensor digitorum longus to second, third, and fourth digits.

Action: Extends the metatarsophalangeal joints of the first through fourth digits, and assists in extending the interphalangeal joints of second, third, and fourth digits.

Nerve: Deep peroneal, **L4, 5, S1.**

Note: Since the Extensor digitorum brevis tendons fuse with the tendons of the Extensor longus to the second, third, and fourth digits, the brevis as well as the longus will extend all joints of these toes. Without an Extensor longus, however, there will be no extension of the fifth digit at the metatarsophalangeal joint. To differentiate, palpate the tendon of the longus and the belly of the brevis; and try to detect any difference in movement of the toes.

PERONEUS TERTIUS

Origin: Distal one third of anterior surface of fibula, interosseus membrane and adjacent intermuscular septum.

Insertion: Dorsal surface, base of fifth metatarsal.

Action: Dorsiflexes ankle joint and everts foot.

Nerve: Deep peroneal, **L4, 5, S1.**

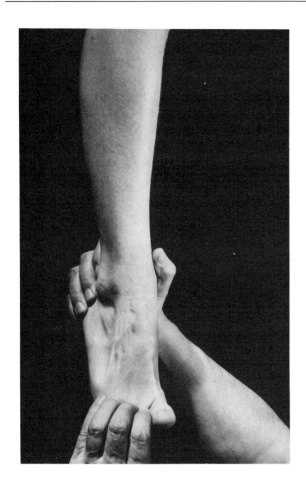 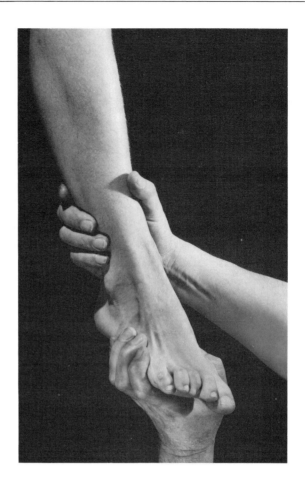

EXTENSOR DIGITORUM LONGUS AND BREVIS

Patient: Supine or sitting.

Fixation: The examiner stabilizes the foot in slight plantar flexion.

Test: Extension of all joints of the second, third, fourth, and fifth digits.

Pressure: Against the dorsal surface of the toes in the direction of flexion.

Weakness: Allows a tendency toward drop-foot and forefoot varus. Diminishes the ability to dorsiflex the ankle joint and evert the foot. In many cases of flat feet (collapse of the long arch) there is an accompanying weakness of toe extensors.

Contracture: Hyperextension of metatarsophalangeal joints.

PERONEUS TERTIUS

Patient: Supine or sitting.

Fixation: The examiner supports the leg above the ankle joint.

Test: Dorsiflexion of the ankle joint, with eversion of the foot.

Note: The Peroneus tertius is assisted in this test by the Extensor digitorum longus of which it is a part.

Pressure: Against the lateral side, dorsal surface of the foot in the direction of plantar flexion and inversion.

Weakness: Decreases the ability to evert the foot and dorsiflex the ankle joint.

Contracture: Dorsiflexion of the ankle joint and eversion of the foot.

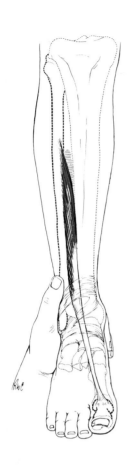

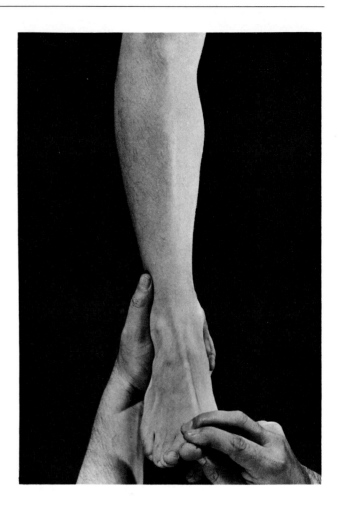

EXTENSOR HALLUCIS LONGUS

Origin: Middle two quarters of anterior surface of fibula and adjacent interosseous membrane.

Insertion: Base of distal phalanx of great toe.

Action: Extends the metatarsophalangeal and interphalangeal joints of the great toe. Assists in inversion of the foot and dorsiflexion of the ankle joint.

Nerve: Deep peroneal, L4, **5**, S1.

EXTENSOR HALLUCIS BREVIS (MEDIAL SLIP of EXTENSOR DIGITORUM BREVIS)

Origin: Distal part of superior and lateral surfaces of calcaneus, lateral talocalcaneal ligament, and apex of inferior extensor retinaculum. (See p. 198.)

Insertion: Dorsal surface of base of proximal phalanx of great toe.

Action: Extends the metatarsophalangeal joint of great toe.

Nerve: Deep peroneal L4, **5**, S1.

Patient: Supine or sitting.

Fixation: The examiner stabilizes the foot in slight plantar flexion.

Test: Extension of metatarsophalangeal and interphalangeal joints of the great toe.

Pressure: Against the dorsal surface of the distal and proximal phalanges of the great toe in the direction of flexion.

Weakness: Decreases the ability to extend the great toe, and allows a position of flexion. The ability to dorsiflex the ankle joint is decreased.

Contracture: Extension of the great toe, with the head of the first metatarsal driven downward.

Note: The paralysis of an Extensor hallucis brevis (first slip of the Extensor digitorum brevis) cannot be determined accurately in the presence of a strong Extensor hallucis longus. However, in paralysis of the longus the action of the brevis is clear. The distal phalanx does not extend, and the proximal phalanx extends in the direction of adduction (toward the axial line of the foot).

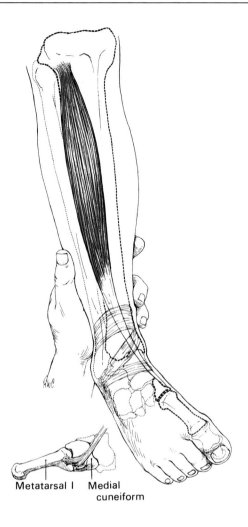

Metatarsal I Medial
cuneiform

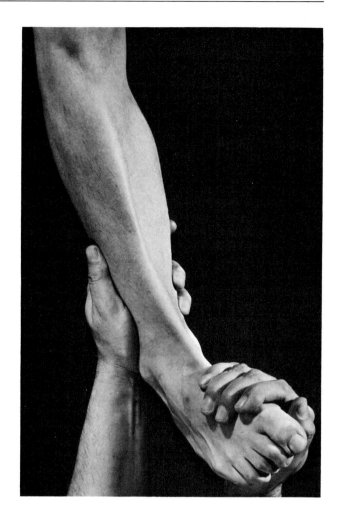

Origin: Lateral condyle and proximal one half of lateral surface of tibia, interosseus membrane, deep fascia, and lateral intermuscular septum.

Insertion: Medial and plantar surface of medial cuneiform bone, base of first metatarsal bone.

Action: Dorsiflexes the ankle joint and assists in inversion of the foot.

Nerve: Deep peroneal, L4, **5,** S1.

Patient: Supine or sitting (with knee flexed if any Gastrocnemius tightness is present).

Fixation: The examiner supports the leg just above the ankle joint.

Test: Dorsiflexion of the ankle joint and inversion of the foot, without extension of the great toe.

Pressure: Against the medial side, dorsal surface of the foot, in the direction of plantar flexion of the ankle joint and eversion of the foot.

Weakness: Decreases the ability to dorsiflex the ankle joint and allows a tendency toward eversion of the foot. This may be seen as a partial drop-foot and tendency toward pronation.

Contracture: Dorsiflexion of ankle joint with inversion of the foot, that is, calcaneovarus position of the foot.

Note: Although Tibialis anterior weakness may be found in conjunction with a pronated foot, such weakness is seldom found in a congenital flatfoot.

Tibialis Posterior

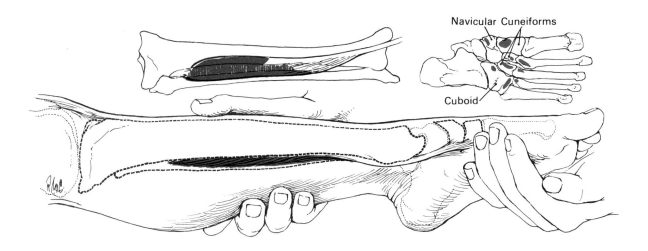

Navicular Cuneiforms

Cuboid

Origin: Most of interosseus membrane, lateral portion of posterior surface of tibia, proximal two thirds of medial surface of fibula, adjacent intermuscular septa, and deep fascia.

Nerve: Tibial L(4), **5,** S1.

Insertion: Tuberosity of navicular bone and by fibrous expansions to the sustentaculum tali, three cuneiforms, cuboid, and bases of second, third, and fourth metatarsal bones.

Action: Inverts the foot and assists in plantar flexion of the ankle joint.

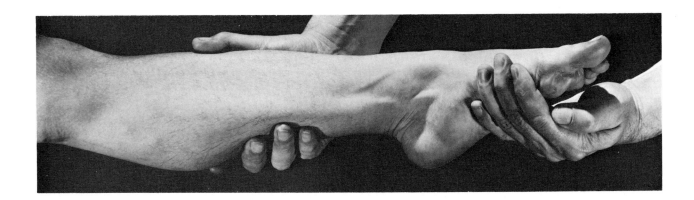

Patient: Supine with extremity in lateral rotation.

Fixation: The examiner supports the leg above the ankle joint.

Test: Inversion of the foot with plantar flexion of the ankle joint.

Pressure: Against the medial side and plantar surface of the foot, in the direction of dorsiflexion of the ankle joint and eversion of the foot.

Note: If the Flexor hallucis longus and Flexor digitorum longus are being substituted for the Tibialis posterior, the toes will be strongly flexed as pressure is applied.

Weakness: Decreases the ability to invert the foot and plantar flex the ankle joint. Results in pronation of the foot and decreased support of the longitudinal arch. Interferes with the ability to rise on toes, and inclines toward what is commonly called a Gastrocnemius limp.

Contracture: Equinovarus position in non-weight bearing, and a supinated position of the heel with forefoot varus in weight bearing.

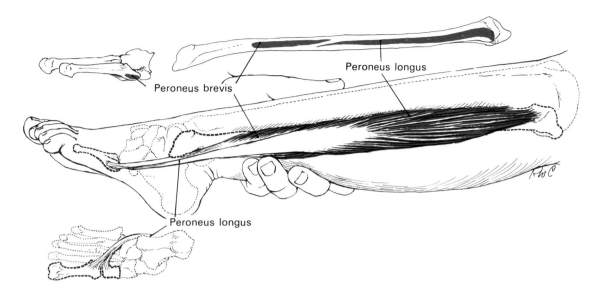

Peroneus brevis

Peroneus longus

Peroneus longus

PERONEUS LONGUS

Origin: Lateral condyle of tibia, head and proximal two thirds of lateral surface of fibula, intermuscular septa, and adjacent deep fascia.

Insertion: Lateral side of base of first metatarsal and of medial cuneiform bone.

Action: Everts foot, assists in plantar flexion of ankle joint, and depresses head of first metatarsal.

Nerve: Superficial peroneal, L4, **5, S1.**

PERONEUS BREVIS

Origin: Distal two thirds of lateral surface of fibula and adjacent intermuscular septa.

Insertion: Tuberosity at base of fifth metatarsal bone, lateral side.

Action: Everts foot, and assists in plantar flexion of ankle.

Nerve: Superficial peroneal, L4, **5, S1.**

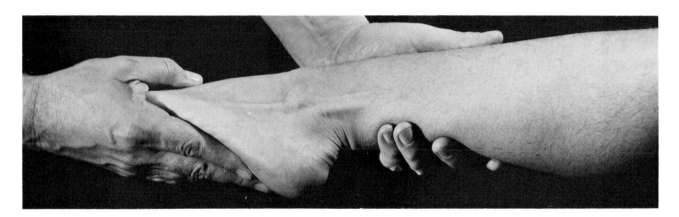

Patient: Supine with extremity medially rotated, or sidelying (on opposite side).

Fixation: The examiner supports the leg above the ankle joint.

Test: Eversion of the foot with plantar flexion of the ankle joint.

Pressure: Against the lateral border and sole of the foot in the direction of inversion of the foot and dorsiflexion of the ankle joint.

Weakness: Decreases the strength of eversion of the foot and plantar flexion of the ankle joint. Allows a varus position of the foot and lessens the ability to rise on the toes. Lateral stability of the ankle is decreased.

Contracture: Results in an everted or valgus position of the foot.

Note: In weight bearing, with a strong pull on its insertion at the base of the first metatarsal, the Peroneus longus causes the head of the first metatarsal to be pressed downward into the supporting surface.

Soleus

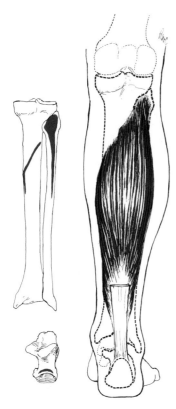

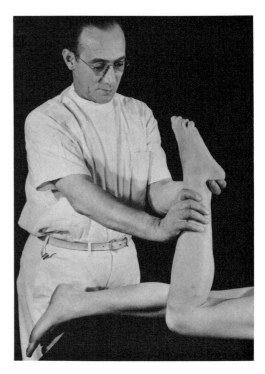

Origin: Posterior surfaces of head of fibula and proximal one third of its body, soleal line and middle one third of medial border of tibia, and tendinous arch between tibia and fibula.

Insertion: With tendon of Gastrocnemius into posterior surface of calcaneus.

Action: Plantar flexes the ankle joint.

Nerve: Tibial, L5, S1, 2.

Patient: Prone with the knee flexed at least 90°.

Fixation: The examiner supports the leg proximal to the ankle.

Test: Plantar flexion of the ankle joint without inversion or eversion of the foot.

Pressure: Against the calcaneus (as illustrated) pulling the heel in a caudal direction (i.e., in the direction of dorsiflexing the ankle). When there is marked weakness, the patient may not be able to hold against pressure at the heel. When weakness is not marked, more leverage is necessary and is obtained by applying pressure simultaneously against the sole of the foot. (See p. 206).

Note: Inversion of the foot shows substitution by Tibialis posterior and toe flexors. Eversion shows substitution by the Peroneals. Extension of the knee is evidence of attempting to assist with Gastrocnemius, that is, the Gastrocnemius is at a disadvantage with the knee flexed 90° or more, and, to bring it into a stronger action, the patient will attempt to extend the knee.

Weakness: Permits a calcaneus position of the foot and predisposes toward a cavus. Results in inability to rise on toes. In standing, the insertion of the Soleus muscle on the calcaneus becomes the fixed point for action of this muscle in maintaining normal alignment of the leg in relation to the foot. The deviation that results from weakness of the Soleus may appear as a slight knee flexion fault in posture, but more often results in an anterior displacement of the body weight from the normal plumb line distribution, as seen when the plumb line is hung slightly anterior to the outer malleolus.

A nonparalytic type of weakness may result from sudden trauma to the muscle as in landing from a jump in a position of ankle dorsiflexion and knee flexion; or gradual trauma from repeated deep knee bending in which the ankle is fully dorsiflexed. The Gastrocnemius escapes the stretch because of the knee flexion.

Contracture: Equinus position of the foot both in weight bearing and non-weight bearing.

Shortness: A tendency toward hyperextension of the knee in the standing position. When walking barefoot the shortness is compensated for by toeing out, thereby transferring the weight from posterolateral heel to anteromedial forefoot. In shoes with heels, the shortness may go unnoticed.

Note: This test is important in examination of cases in which there is a deviation of the body forward from the plumb line. It is also advisable to test this muscle in cases in which there is an increase in the height of the longitudinal arch.

204

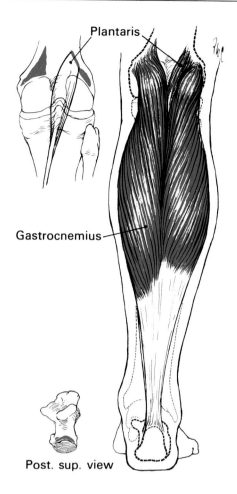

Plantaris

Gastrocnemius

Post. sup. view

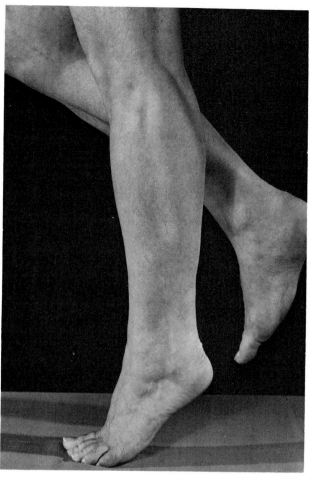

GASTROCNEMIUS

Origin of Medial Head: Proximal and posterior part of medial condyle and adjacent part of femur, capsule of knee joint.

Origin of Lateral Head: Lateral condyle and posterior surface of femur, capsule of knee joint.

Insertion: Middle part of posterior surface of calcaneus.

Nerve: Tibial, S1, 2.

PLANTARIS

Origin: Distal part of lateral supracondylar line of femur and adjacent part of its popliteal surface, oblique popliteal ligament of knee joint.

Insertion: Posterior part of calcaneus.

Nerve: Tibial, L4, 5, S1, (2).

Action: The Gastrocnemius and the Plantaris plantar flex the ankle joint and assist in flexion of the knee joint.

ANKLE PLANTAR FLEXORS

Patient: Standing. (Patient may steady himself with a hand on the table, but should not take any weight on the hand.)

Test Movement: Patient rises on toes, pushing the body weight directly upward.

Resistance: Body weight.

Note: Inclining the body forward and flexing the knee is evidence of weakness; the patient dorsi-flexes the ankle joint attempting to clear the heel from the floor by tension of the plantar flexors as the body weight is thrown forward.

Shortness: Shortness of the Gastrocnemius and Soleus muscles tends to develop among women who constantly wear high-heeled shoes.

Muscles that Act in Plantar Flexion:

Soleus Gastrocnemius Plantaris	Ankle joint plantar flexors. (Tendo calcaneus group)
Tibialis posterior Peroneus longus Peroneus brevis	Forefoot, and ankle joint plantar flexors.
Flexor hallucis longus Flexor digit. longus	Toe, forefoot, and ankle joint plantar flexors.

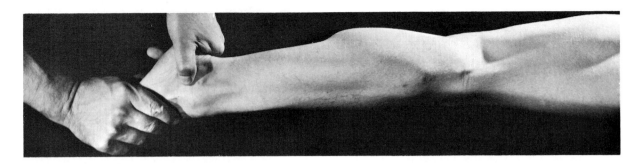

Patient: Prone with knee extended, and the foot projecting over the end of the table.

Fixation: The weight of the extremity resting on a firm table should be sufficient fixation of the part.

Test: Plantar flexion of the foot with emphasis on pulling the heel upward more than pushing the forefoot downward. This test movement does not attempt to isolate the Gastrocnemius action from other plantar flexors, but the presence or absence of a Gastrocnemius can be determined by careful observation during the test.

Pressure: For maximum pressure in this position, it is necessary to apply pressure against the forefoot as well as against the calcaneus. If the muscle is very weak, pressure against the calcaneus is sufficient.

The Gastrocnemius usually can be seen and always can be palpated if it is contracting during the plantar flexion test. Movements of the toes and forefoot should be observed carefully during the test to detect substitutions. The patient may be able to flex the anterior part of the foot by toe flexors, Tibialis posterior, and Peroneus longus without a direct upward pull on the heel by the Tendo calcaneus. If the Gastrocnemius and Soleus are weak, the heel will be *pushed* up secondary to flexion of the anterior part of the foot rather than *pulled* up simultaneously with the flexion of the forepart of the foot. If pressure is applied to the heel rather than to the ball of the foot, it is possible to isolate, partially, the combined action of the Gastrocnemius and Soleus from the other plantar flexors. Movement of the foot toward eversion or inversion will show imbalance in opposing lateral and medial muscles and, if pronounced, will show an attempt to substitute the Peroneals or Tibialis posterior for the Gastrocnemius and Soleus.

Action of the Gastrocnemius often can be demonstrated in the knee flexion test when the Hamstrings are weak. In the prone position with the knee fully extended, the patient is asked to bend the knee against resistance. If the Gastrocnemius is strong, there will be plantar flexion at the ankle as the Gastrocnemius acts to *initiate* knee flexion, followed by ankle dorsiflexion as the knee flexes.

Weakness: Permits a calcaneus position of the foot if the Gastrocnemius and Soleus are weak. In standing, results in hyperextension of the knee and inability to rise on toes. In walking, the inability to transfer weight normally results in a "Gastrocnemius limp."

Contracture: Equinus position of the foot and flexion of the knee.

Shortness: Restriction of dorsiflexion of the ankle when the knee is extended, and restriction of knee extension when the ankle is dorsiflexed. During stance phase in walking, shortness limits the normal dorsiflexion of the ankle joint and the subject toes out during the transfer of weight from heel to forefoot.

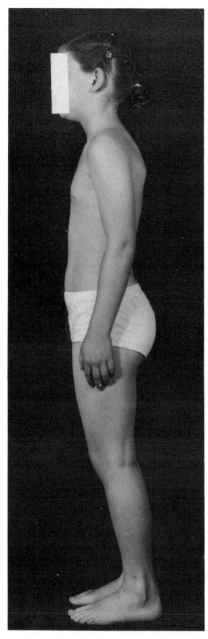 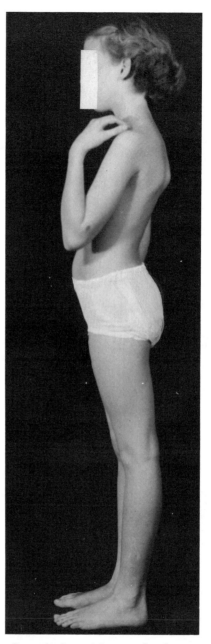

In standing, the knee joints tend to *flex* and the ankle joints dorsiflex if the *Soleus* muscles are weak.

In standing, the knee joints tend to *hyperextend* and the ankle joints plantar flex if the *Gastrocnemius* muscles are weak.

Because the Soleus acts to plantar flex the foot, in standing it acts to hold the leg back in normal alignment with foot. With *weakness* of the muscle, the ankle joint dorsiflexes. In standing, this generally is accompanied by some knee flexion or may be accompanied by a forward inclination of the body as a whole from the ankles up. A *strong* Soleus may help compensate for a weak Quadriceps by pulling the leg back, thus passively extending the knee.

Unlike the Soleus, the Gastrocnemius passes over the knee joint. It is a flexor of the knee joint and as such is a stabilizer in helping to prevent hyperextension. While the action of the Gastrocnemius is the same as the Soleus on the ankle joint, and conceivably weakness could result in the same change of alignment as does weakness of the Soleus, this does not occur. Instead, with Gastrocnemius weakness, the knee tends to hyperextend in standing.

Medial Hamstrings: Semitendinosus and Semimembranosus

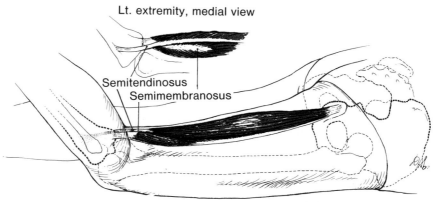

Lt. extremity, medial view

Semitendinosus
Semimembranosus

Rt. extremity, posterolateral view

SEMITENDINOSUS

Origin: Tuberosity of ischium by tendon common with long head of Biceps femoris.

Insertion: Proximal part of medial surface of body of tibia, and deep fascia of leg.

Action: Flexes and medially rotates the knee joint. Extends and assists in medial rotation of the hip joint.

Nerve: Sciatic (tibial branch), L4, **5**, S1, **2**.

SEMIMEMBRANOSUS

Origin: Tuberosity of ischium, proximal and lateral to Biceps femoris and Semitendinosus.

Insertion: Posteromedial aspect of medial condyle of tibia.

Action: Flexes and medially rotates the knee joint. Extends and assists in medial rotation of the hip joint.

Nerve: Sciatic (tibial branch), L4, **5**, S1, 2.

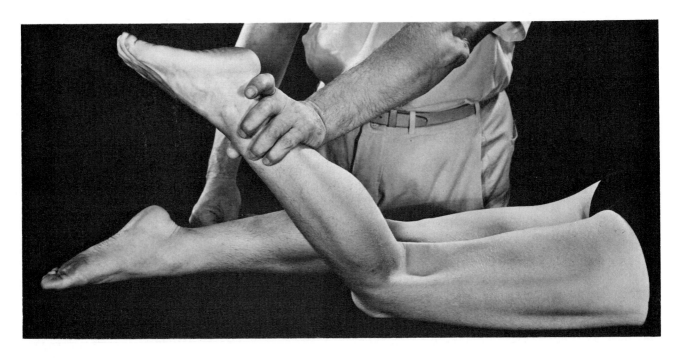

Patient: Prone.

Fixation: The examiner should hold the thigh down firmly on the table. (To avoid covering the muscle belly of the medial Hamstrings, fixation is not illustrated.)

Test: Flexion of the knee between 50° and 70° with the thigh in medial rotation, and the leg medially rotated on the thigh.

Pressure: Against the leg proximal to the ankle in the direction of knee extension. Do not apply pressure against the rotation component.

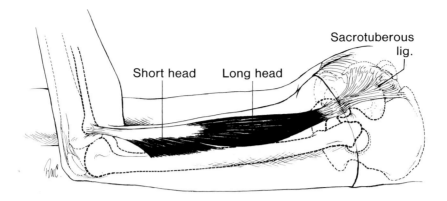

Origin of Long Head: Distal part of sacrotuberous ligament, and posterior part of tuberosity of ischium.

Origin of Short Head: Lateral lip of linea aspera, proximal two thirds of supracondylar line, and lateral intermuscular septum.

Insertion: Lateral side of head of fibula, lateral condyle of tibia, deep fascia on lateral side of leg.

Action: The long and short heads of the Biceps femoris flex and laterally rotate the knee joint. In addition, the long head extends and assists in lateral rotation of the hip joint.

Nerve to Long Head: Sciatic (tibial branch), L5, S1, 2, 3.

Nerve to Short Head: Sciatic (peroneal branch), L5, S1, 2.

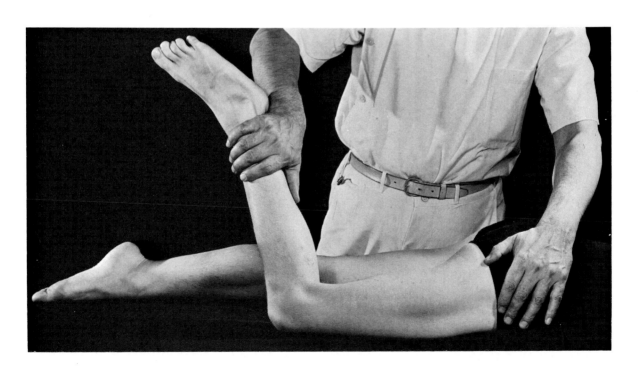

Patient: Prone.

Fixation: The examiner should hold the thigh firmly down on the table. (Not illustrated in order to avoid covering the muscles.)

Test: Flexion of the knee between 50° and 70° with the thigh in slight lateral rotation, and the leg in slight lateral rotation on the thigh.

Pressure: Against the leg proximal to the ankle in the direction of knee extension. Do not apply pressure against the rotation component.

209

Weakness: Slight weakness of either the medial or lateral Hamstrings is first noted by the subject's inability to maintain the rotation when asked to hold the test position. Weakness of both the medial and lateral Hamstrings permits hyperextension of the knee. When this weakness is bilateral, the pelvis may tilt anteriorly and the lumbar spine may assume a lordotic position. If the weakness is unilateral, a pelvic rotation may result. Weakness of lateral Hamstrings causes a tendency toward loss of lateral stability of the knee, allowing a thrust in the direction of bowleg position in weight-bearing. Weakness of medial Hamstrings decreases the medial stability of the knee joint, and permits a knock-knee position with a tendency toward lateral rotation of the leg on the femur.

Contracture: Contracture of both the medial and lateral Hamstrings results in a position of knee flexion, and, if the contracture is extreme, it will be accompanied by a posterior tilting of the pelvis and a flattening of the lumbar spine.

Shortness: Restriction of knee extension when the hip is flexed, or restriction of hip flexion when the knee is extended. Shortness of Hamstrings *does not cause* a posterior pelvic tilt, but a posterior pelvic tilt and a flattening of the lumbar spine often are seen in subjects who have Hamstring shortness.

Note: Ordinarily, the hip flexors act to *safeguard* the Hamstrings during knee flexion. Do not expect the subject to hold full knee flexion nor to hold against the same amount of pressure with the hip extended in the prone position that could be resisted with a hip flexed in sitting. The frequent occurrence of muscle cramping during the Hamstring test results from the muscle being in too short a position and attempting to hold against strong pressure. To test Hamstrings in full knee flexion, the hip must be flexed to take up some of the slack. However, there will be assistance from the Sartorius in both hip and knee flexion when Hamstrings are tested with the hip flexed.

Weakness of Popliteus and Gastrocnemius may interfere with initiating knee flexion. Substitution of Sartorius action will appear in the form of hip flexion as knee flexion is *initiated*. A short Rectus femoris, limiting knee flexion range of motion, will cause hip flexion as the knee flexion motion is *completed*. (Hip flexion in the prone position is seen as an anterior tilt of the pelvis with lumbar spine hyperextension.) Assistance from the Gastrocnemius in flexing the knee will be seen as an effort to *dorsiflex* the ankle, elongating the Gastrocnemius over the ankle to make it more effective in knee flexion.

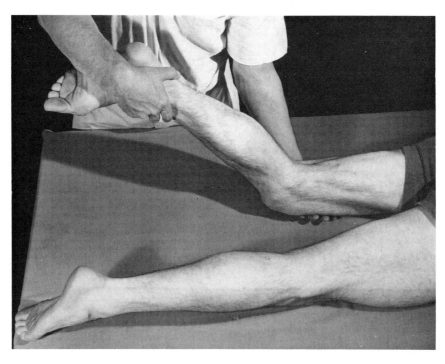

The action of the Gracilis as a knee flexor is illustrated by this figure. It is brought into action by the test position and pressure as used for the medial Hamstrings. The Gracilis has its origin on the pubis, and the medial Hamstrings arise from the ischium.

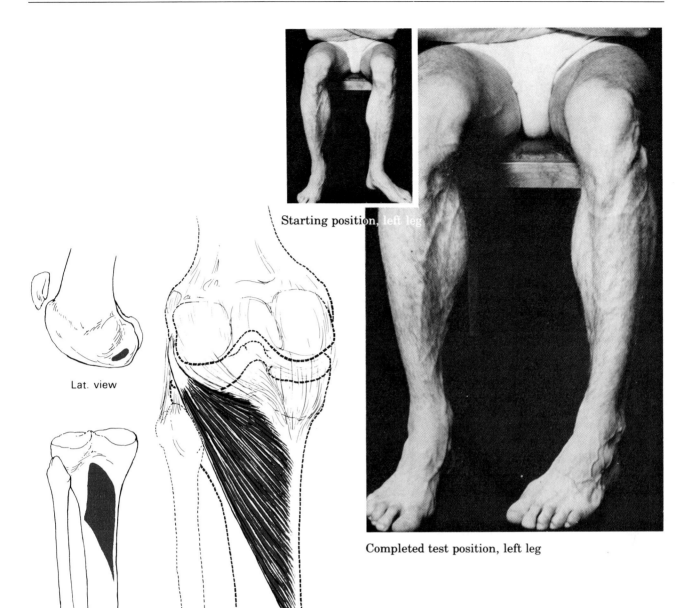

Starting position, left leg

Completed test position, left leg

Lat. view

Post. view

Origin: Anterior part of groove on lateral condyle of femur, and oblique popliteal ligament of knee joint.

Insertion: Triangular area proximal to soleal line on posterior surface of tibia, and fascia covering the muscle.

Action: In non-weight bearing (that is, *with the origin fixed*) the Popliteus medially rotates the tibia on the femur and flexes the knee joint. In weight bearing (that is, *with the insertion fixed*), it laterally rotates the femur on the tibia and flexes the knee joint. This muscle helps to reinforce the posterior ligaments of the knee joint.

Nerve: Tibial L4, 5, S1.

Patient: Sitting with knee flexed at right angle and with leg in lateral rotation of tibia on femur.

Fixation: None necessary.

Test Movement: Medial rotation of the tibia on the femur.

Pressure: Seldom is resistance or pressure applied since the movement is not used as a test for the purpose of grading Popliteus, but merely to indicate whether the muscle is active or not.

Weakness: May result in hyperextension of the knee and lateral rotation of the leg on the thigh. A Popliteus weakness is usually found in instances of imbalance between the lateral and medial Hamstrings in which the medial Hamstrings are weak and the lateral are strong.

Shortness: Results in slight flexion of the knee and medial rotation of the leg on the thigh.

211

Quadriceps Femoris

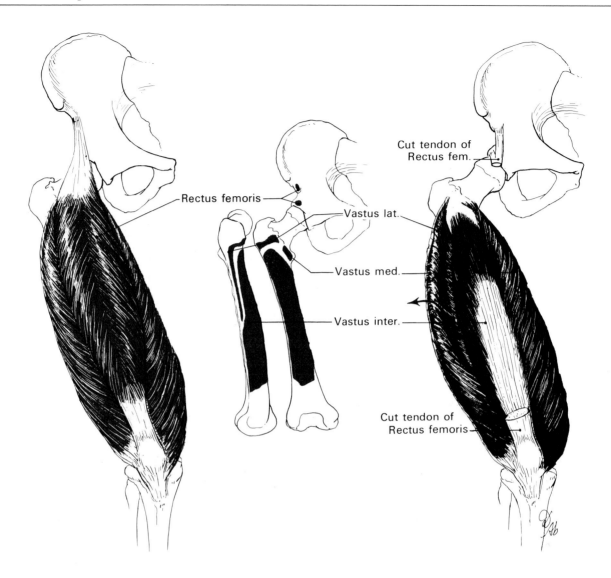

Origin of Rectus Femoris: *Straight head* from anterior inferior iliac spine. *Reflected head* from groove above rim of acetabulum.

Origin of Vastus Lateralis: Proximal part of intertrochanteric line, anterior and inferior borders of greater trochanter, lateral lip of gluteal tuberosity, proximal one half of lateral lip of linea aspera, and lateral intermuscular septum.

Origin of Vastus Intermedius: Anterior and lateral surfaces of proximal two thirds of body of femur, distal one half of linea aspera, and lateral intermuscular septum.

Origin of Vastus Medialis: Distal one half of intertrochanteric line, medial lip of linea aspera, proximal part of medial supracondylar line, tendons of Adductor longus and Adductor magnus, and medial intermuscular septum.

Insertion: Proximal border of patella and through patellar ligament to tuberosity of tibia.

Action: The Quadriceps extends the knee joint, and the Rectus femoris portion flexes the hip joint.

Nerve: Femoral, L2, 3, 4.

The *Articularis genus* is a small muscle which may be blended with the Vastus intermedius, but usually is distinct from it. (Not shown in drawing.)

Origin: Anterior surface of distal part of body of femur.

Insertion: Proximal part of synovial membrane of knee joint.

Action: Draws articular capsule proximally.

Nerve: Branch of nerve to Vastus intermedius.

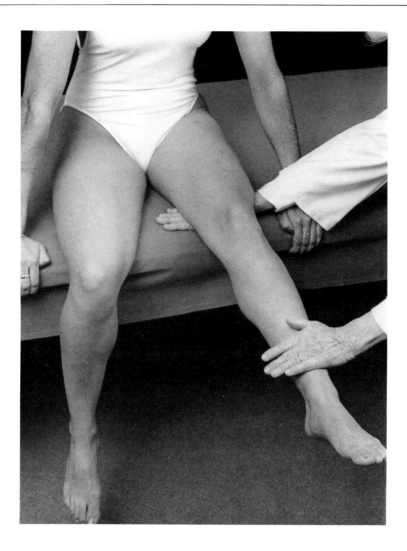

Patient: Sitting with knees over side of table, holding on to table.

Fixation: The examiner may hold the thigh firmly down on the table, or, because the weight of the trunk is usually sufficient to stabilize the patient during this test, the examiner may put a hand under the distal end of the thigh to cushion that part against table pressure.

Test: Extension of the knee joint without rotation of the thigh.

Pressure: Against the leg above the ankle, in the direction of flexion.

Note: Inclining the body backward may be evidence of an attempt to release Hamstring tension when those muscles are contracted. When the Tensor fasciae latae is being substituted for the Quadriceps, it medially rotates the thigh and exerts a stronger pull if the hip is extended. If the Rectus femoris is the strongest part of the Quad-riceps the patient will lean backward to extend the hip thereby obtaining maximum action of the Rectus femoris.

Weakness: Interferes with the function of stair climbing or walking up an incline, as well as getting up and down from a sitting position. The weakness results in knee hyperextension, not in the sense that such weakness permits a posterior knee position, but in the sense that walking with a weak Quadriceps requires that the patient lock the knee joint by slight hyperextension. Continuous thrust in the direction of hyperextension in growing children may result in a very marked degree of deformity.

Contracture: Knee extension.

Shortness: Restriction of knee flexion. A shortness of the Rectus femoris part of the Quadriceps results in restriction of knee flexion when the hip is extended, or restriction of hip extension when the knee is flexed. (See test, pp. 34 and 35.)

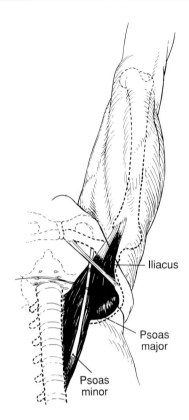

Iliacus

Psoas major

Psoas minor

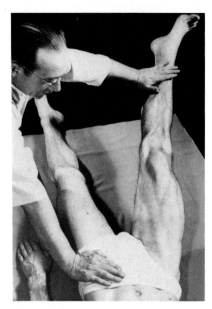

PSOAS MAJOR

Origin: Ventral surfaces of transverse processes of all lumbar vertebrae, sides of bodies and corresponding intervertebral discs of the last thoracic and all lumbar vertebrae and membranous arches that extend over the sides of the bodies of the lumbar vertebrae.

Insertion: Lesser trochanter of femur.

Nerve: Lumbar plexus, L1, **2, 3,** 4.

ILIACUS

Origin: Superior two thirds of iliac fossa, internal lip of iliac crest, iliolumbar and ventral sacroiliac ligaments and ala of sacrum.

Insertion: Lateral side of tendon of Psoas major, and just distal to the lesser trochanter.

Nerve: Femoral, L(1), **2, 3,** 4.

ILIOPSOAS

Action: *With the origin fixed,* the Iliopsoas flexes the hip joint by flexing the femur on the trunk as in supine alternate leg raising, and may assist in lateral rotation and abduction of the hip joint. *With the insertion fixed* and acting bilaterally, the Iliopsoas flexes the hip joint by flexing the trunk on the femur as in the sit-up from supine position. The Psoas major, acting bilaterally with the insertion fixed, will increase the lumbar lordosis; acting unilaterally, assists in lateral flexion of the trunk toward the same side.

ILIOPSOAS (WITH EMPHASIS ON PSOAS MAJOR)

Patient: Supine.

Fixation: The examiner stabilizes the opposite iliac crest. The Quadriceps stabilize the knee in extension.

Test: Hip flexion in a position of slight abduction and slight lateral rotation. The muscle is not seen in the photograph because it lies deep beneath the Sartorius, the femoral nerve, and the blood vessels contained in the femoral sheath.

Pressure: Against the anteromedial aspect of the leg in the direction of extension and slight abduction, directly opposite the line of pull of the Psoas major from the origin on the lumbar spine to the insertion on the lesser trochanter of the femur.

Weakness and Contracture: See Hip flexors, p. 215. Weakness tends to be *bilateral* in cases of lumbar kyphosis and sway-back posture, and *unilateral* in cases of lumbar scoliosis.

PSOAS MINOR

This muscle is not a lower extremity muscle because it does not cross the hip joint. It is relatively unimportant, and only present in about 40% of the population.

Origin: Sides of bodies of 12th thoracic and first lumbar vertebrae and from the intervertebral disc between them.

Insertion: Iliopectineal eminence, arcuate line of ilium, and iliac fascia.

Action: Flexion of pelvis on lumbar spine and vice versa.

Nerve: Lumbar plexus, L1, **2.**

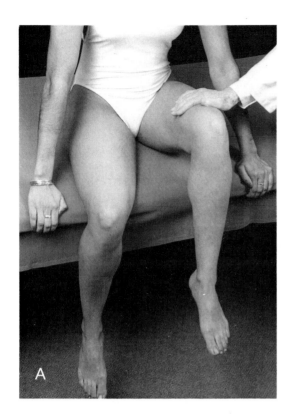

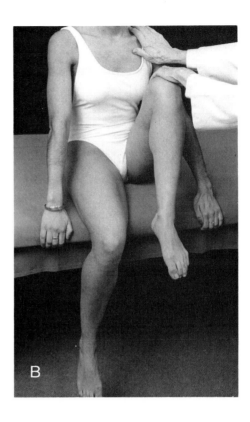

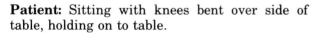

Patient: Sitting with knees bent over side of table, holding on to table.

Fixation: The weight of the trunk may be sufficient to stabilize the patient during this test but holding on to the table gives added stability. If the trunk is weak, place the patient supine during the test.

Test for Hip Flexors as a Group: (Figure A) Hip flexion with the knee flexed, raising the thigh a few inches from the table.

Pressure: Against the anterior thigh in the direction of extension.

Test for Iliopsoas: (Figure B) Full hip flexion with knee flexed. This test places emphasis on the one-joint hip flexor by requiring completion of the arc of motion. The grade is based on the ability to hold the completed position. With weakness of the Iliopsoas, the fully flexed position cannot be held against resistance, but as the thigh drops to the position assumed in the group test, the strength may grade normal. This test is used to confirm the findings in the supine test described on the facing page.

Pressure. One hand against the anterior shoulder area gives counterpressure, and the other applies pressure against the thigh in the direction of hip extension.

Note: Lateral rotation with abduction of the thigh as pressure is applied generally is evidence of Sartorius strength, or that the Tensor fasciae latae is too weak to counteract the pull of the Sartorius. Medial rotation of the thigh shows the Tensor fasciae latae stronger than the Sartorius. If adductors are primarily responsible for the flexion, the thigh will be adducted as it is flexed. If the anterior abdominals do not fix the pelvis to the trunk, the pelvis will flex on the thighs, and the hip flexors may hold against strong resistance but not at maximum height.

Weakness: Decreases the ability to flex the hip joint and results in marked disability in stair-climbing or walking up an incline, getting up from a reclining position, and bringing the trunk forward in the sitting position preliminary to rising from a chair. In marked weakness, walking is difficult because the leg must be brought forward by *pelvic motion* (produced by anterior or lateral abdominal muscle action) rather than by hip flexion. The effect of hip flexor weakness on posture is seen on pp. 85, 87, and 354.

Contracture: Bilaterally, hip flexion deformity with increased lumbar lordosis. (See p. 80, figure A.) Unilaterally, hip position of flexion, abduction and lateral rotation.

Shortness: In the standing position, shortness of the hip flexors is seen as a lumbar lordosis with an anterior pelvic tilt.

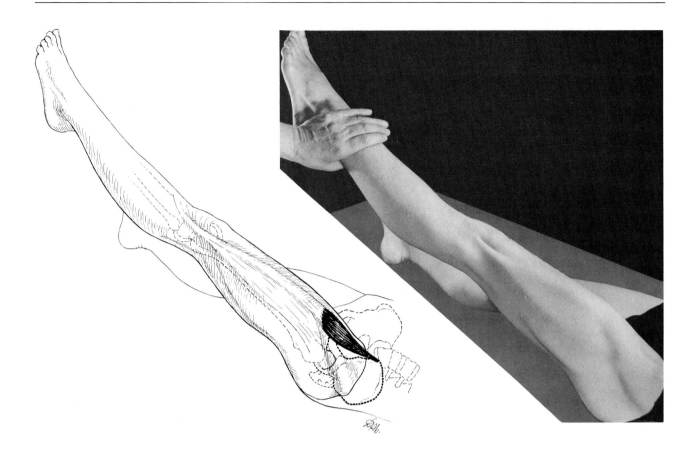

Origin: Anterior part of external lip of iliac crest, outer surface of anterior superior iliac spine, and deep surface of fascia lata.

Insertion: Into iliotibial tract of fascia lata at junction of proximal and middle thirds of thigh.

Action: Flexes, medially rotates, and abducts the hip joint; tenses the fascia lata; and may assist in knee extension. (See p. 58.)

Nerve: Superior gluteal, L4, 5, S1.

Shortness: The effect of shortness of the Tensor fasciae latae in standing depends upon whether the tightness is bilateral or unilateral. If bilateral, there is an anterior pelvic tilt, and sometimes bilateral knock-knee. If unilateral, the abductors of the hip and fascia lata are tight along with the Tensor fasciae latae and there is an associated lateral pelvic tilt, low on the side of tightness. The knee on that side will tend toward a knock-knee position. If the Tensor fasciae latae and other hip flexor muscles are tight, there is an anterior pelvic tilt and a medial rotation of the femur, as indicated by the position of the patella.

Patient: Supine.

Fixation: The patient may hold on to the table. Quadriceps action is necessary to hold the knee extended. Usually no fixation is necessary by the examiner, but if there is instability and the patient has difficulty in maintaining the pelvis firmly on the table, then one hand of the examiner should support the pelvis anteriorly on the opposite side.

Test: Abduction, flexion and medial rotation of the hip with the knee extended.

Pressure: Against the leg in the direction of extension and adduction. Do not apply pressure against the rotation component.

Weakness: Moderate weakness is evident immediately by the failure to maintain the medially rotated test position. In standing, there is a thrust in the direction of a bowleg position, and the extremity tends to rotate laterally from the hip.

Contracture: Hip flexion and knock-knee position. In a supine or standing position, the pelvis will be anteriorly tilted if the legs are brought into adduction.

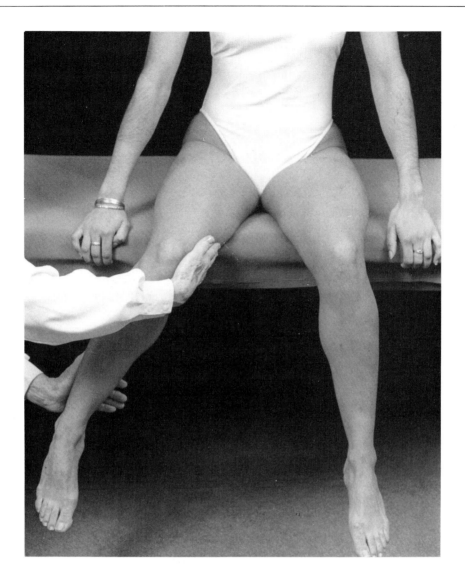

The medial rotators of the hip joint consist of the Tensor fasciae latae, Gluteus minimus, and Gluteus medius (anterior fibers).

Patient: Sitting on table with knees bent over side of table, holding on to table.

Fixation: The weight of the trunk stabilizes the patient during this test. Stabilization is also given in the form of counterpressure as described below under *Pressure.*

Test: Medial rotation of the thigh, with the leg in position of completion of outward arc of motion.

Pressure: Counterpressure is applied by one hand of the examiner at the medial side of the lower end of the thigh. The other hand of the examiner applies pressure to the lateral side of the leg above the ankle, pushing the leg inward in an effort to rotate the thigh laterally.

Weakness: Results in lateral rotation of the lower extremity in standing and walking.

Contracture: Medial rotation of the hip, with in-toeing and a tendency toward knock-knee in weight bearing.

Shortness: Inability to laterally rotate the thigh through full range of motion. Inability to sit in a cross-legged position (tailor fashion).

Note: If the rotator test is done in a supine position, the pelvis will tend to tilt anteriorly if much pressure is applied, but this is not a substitution movement. Due to its attachments, the Tensor fasciae latae, when contracting to maximum, pulls forward on the pelvis as it medially rotates the thigh.

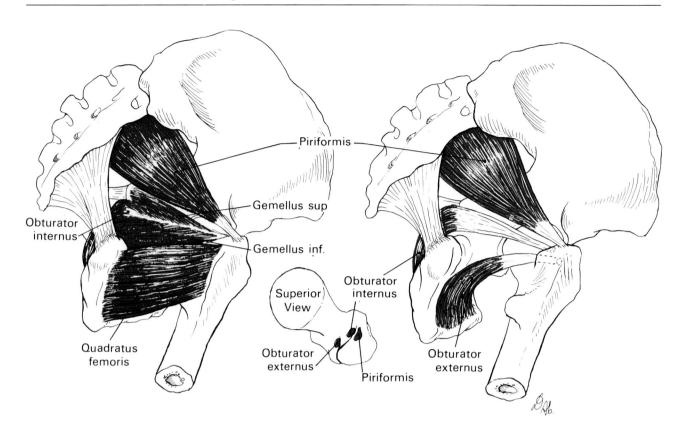

PIRIFORMIS

Origin: Pelvic surface of sacrum between (and lateral to) 1, 2, 3, and 4 pelvic sacral foramina, margin of greater sciatic foramen, and pelvic surface of sacrotuberous ligament.

Insertion: Superior border of greater trochanter of femur.

Nerve: Sacral plexus, L(5), S1, 2.

QUADRATUS FEMORIS

Origin: Proximal part of lateral border of tuberosity of ischium.

Insertion: Proximal part of quadrate line extending distally from intertrochanteric crest.

Nerve: Sacral plexus, L4, 5, S1, (2).

OBTURATOR INTERNUS

Origin: Internal or pelvic surface of obturator membrane and margin of obturator foramen, and pelvic surface of ischium posterior and proximal to obturator foramen, and, to a slight extent, from the obturator fascia.

Insertion: Medial surface of greater trochanter of femur proximal to trochanteric fossa.

Nerve: Sacral plexus, L5, S1, 2.

OBTURATOR EXTERNUS

Origin: Rami of pubis and ischium, and external surface of obturator membrane.

Insertion: Trochanteric fossa of femur.

Nerve: Obturator, L3, 4.

GEMELLUS SUPERIOR

Origin: External surface of spine of ischium.

Insertion: With tendon of Obturator internus into medial surface of greater trochanter of femur.

Nerve: Sacral plexus, L5, S1, 2.

GEMELLUS INFERIOR

Origin: Proximal part of tuberosity of ischium.

Insertion: With tendon of Obturator internus into medial surface of greater trochanter of femur.

Nerve: Sacral plexus, L4, 5, S1, (2).

Action: All of the above muscles laterally rotate the hip joint. In addition, the Obturator externus may assist in adduction of the hip joint, and the Piriformis, Obturator internus and Gemelli may assist in abduction when the hip is flexed. The Piriformis may assist in extension.

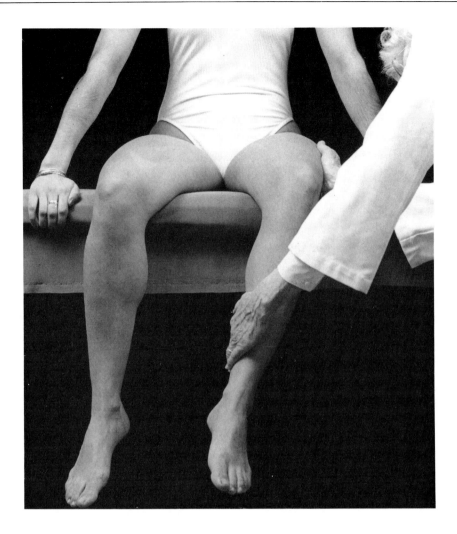

Patient: Sitting on table with knees bent over side of table, holding onto table.

Fixation: The weight of the trunk stabilizes the patient during this test. Stabilization is also given in the form of counterpressure as described below under *Pressure.*

Test: Lateral rotation of the thigh, with the leg in position of completion of the inward arc of motion.

Pressure: Counterpressure is applied by one hand of the examiner at the lateral side of the lower end of the thigh. The other hand of the examiner applies pressure to the medial side of the leg above the ankle, pushing the leg outward in an effort to rotate the thigh medially.

Weakness: Usually, medial rotation of the femur accompanied by pronation of the foot, and a tendency toward knock-knee position.

Contracture: Lateral rotation of the thigh, usually in an abducted position.

Shortness: The range of medial rotation of the hip will be limited. (Frequently there is excessive range of lateral rotation.) In the standing posture, there is a lateral rotation of the femur and out-toeing.

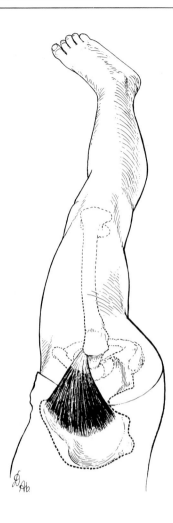

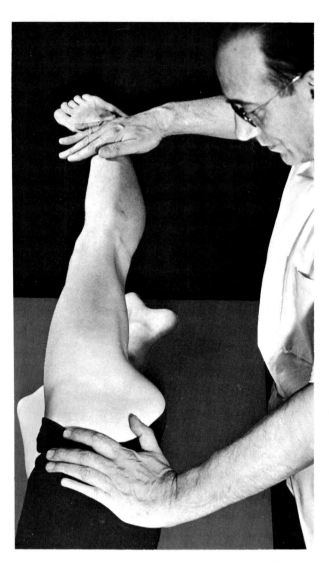

Origin: External surface of ilium between anterior and inferior gluteal lines, and margin of greater sciatic notch.

Insertion: Anterior border of greater trochanter of femur, and hip joint capsule.

Action: Abducts, medially rotates, and may assist in flexion of the hip joint.

Nerve: Superior gluteal, L4, 5, S1.

Patient: Side-lying.

Fixation: The examiner stabilizes the pelvis. (See Note under photograph.)

Test: Abduction of the hip in a position neutral between flexion and extension, and neutral in regard to rotation.

Pressure: Against the leg in the direction of adduction and very slight extension.

Weakness: Lessens the strength of medial rotation and abduction of the hip joint.

Contracture and Shortness: Abduction and medial rotation of the thigh. In standing, lateral pelvic tilt, low on the side of shortness, plus medial rotation of femur.

Note: In tests of the Gluteus minimus and medius, or the abductors as a group, the stabilization of the pelvis is necessary but often difficult. It requires a strong fixation by many trunk muscles, aided by stabilization on the part of the examiner. The flexion of the hip and knee of the underneath leg aids in stabilizing the pelvis against anterior or posterior tilt. The examiner's hand attempts to stabilize the pelvis to prevent the tendency to roll forward or backward, the tendency to tilt anteriorly or posteriorly, and, if possible, any unnecessary hiking or dropping of the pelvis laterally. Any one of these six shifts in position of the pelvis may result primarily from trunk weakness, or such shifts may indicate an attempt to substitute anterior or posterior hip joint muscles or lateral abdominals in the movement of leg abduction. When the trunk muscles are strong, it is not too difficult to maintain good stabilization of the pelvis; but when trunk muscles are weak, the examiner may need the assistance of a second person to hold the pelvis steady.

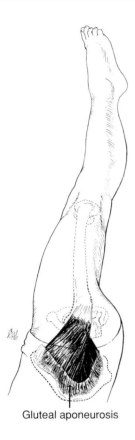

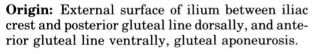

Gluteal aponeurosis

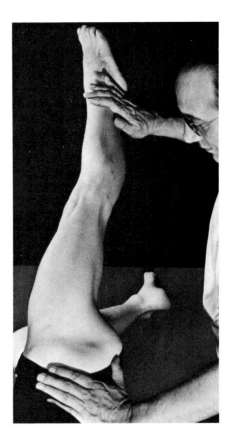

Origin: External surface of ilium between iliac crest and posterior gluteal line dorsally, and anterior gluteal line ventrally, gluteal aponeurosis.

Insertion: Oblique ridge on lateral surface of greater trochanter of femur.

Action: Abducts the hip joint. The anterior fibers medially rotate and may assist in flexion of the hip joint; the posterior fibers laterally rotate and may assist in extension.

Nerve: Superior gluteal, L4, 5, S1.

Patient: Side-lying with underneath leg flexed at hip and knee, and *pelvis rotated slightly forward* to place the posterior Gluteus medius in an antigravity position.

Fixation: The muscles of the trunk and the examiner stabilize the pelvis. (See *Note* on facing page.)

Test (emphasis on posterior portion): Abduction of hip with slight extension and slight external rotation. Knee is maintained in extension. *Differentiating the posterior Gluteus medius is very important. Hip abductors, tested as a group, may be normal in strength while a precise test of the Gluteus medius may reveal appreciable weakness.*

When external rotation of the hip joint is limited, *do not* allow the pelvis to rotate backward in order to obtain the *appearance* of hip joint external rotation. With backward rotation of the pelvis, the

Tensor fasciae latae and Gluteus minimus become active in abduction. Even though pressure may be applied properly in the right direction against the Gluteus medius, the specificity of the test is greatly diminished. Weakness of the Gluteus medius may become apparent immediately by the subject's inability to hold the precise test position, by the tendency for the muscle to cramp, or by an attempt to rotate the pelvis backward in order to substitute with the Tensor fasciae latae and the Gluteus minimus.

Pressure: Against the leg, near the ankle, in the direction of adduction and slight flexion; do not apply pressure against the rotation component. The pressure is applied against the leg for the purpose of obtaining a long lever. To determine normal strength, strong force is needed and can be obtained by the examiner with the added advantage of a long lever. There is relatively little danger of injuring the lateral knee joint because it is reinforced by the strong iliotibial tract. (See p. 216.)

Weakness: See the following two pages regarding weakness of the Gluteus medius and abductors.

Contracture and Shortness: An abduction deformity that, in standing, may be seen as a lateral pelvic tilt low on the side of tightness, along with some abduction of the extremity.

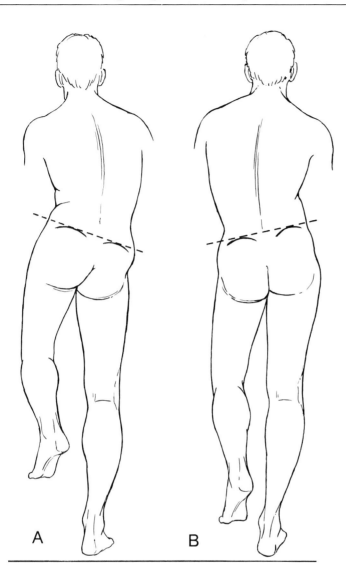
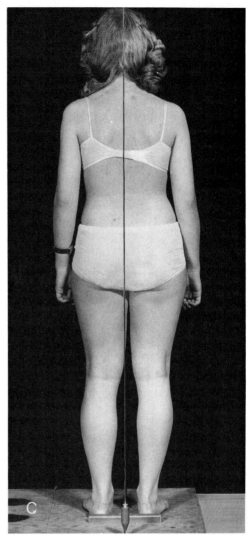

When body weight is supported, alternately, on one leg as in walking, the body must be stabilized on the weight-bearing leg during each step. By reverse action (i.e., origin pulled toward insertion), strong hip abductors can stabilize the pelvis on the femur in hip joint *abduction,* as seen in figure A above. The lateral trunk flexors on the left act, also, by pulling upward on the pelvis.

Figure B shows a position of hip joint *adduction* that results when hip abductors are too weak to stabilize the pelvis on the femur. The pelvis drops downward on the opposite side. Strong lateral trunk flexors on the left cannot raise the pelvis on that side, in standing, without the opposite abductors providing a counter pull on the right.

Figure B also illustrates the test used to elicit the *Trendelenburg sign.* Originally, the test was used in the diagnosis of a congenital dislocated hip. The *Trendelenburg gait* is one in which the affected hip goes into hip joint adduction during each weight-bearing phase of the gait. The femur rides upward because the acetabulum is too shallow to support the head of the femur. If the problem is bilateral, there is a waddling gait.

Figure C illustrates a relaxed postural position in an individual who has mild weakness of the right hip abductors. The Gluteus medius is the chief abductor, and a test which emphasizes the posterior Gluteus medius often demonstrates more weakness than the test for hip abductors as a group. Often this weakness of the Gluteus medius is found in association with other weaknesses present in the handedness patterns. (See pp. 89 and 90.)

Testing the strength of the Gluteus medius is important in cases of pain in the region of this muscle, and in cases of low back pain associated with lateral pelvic tilt.

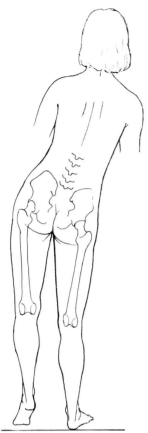

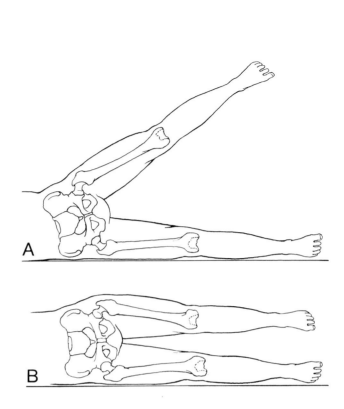

Paralysis or Marked Weakness of Right Gluteus Medius: When there is paralysis or marked weakness of the Gluteus medius, there will be a Gluteus medius limp in walking. This consists of displacement of the trunk laterally toward the side of weakness, shifting the center of gravity in such a way that the body can be balanced over the extremity with minimal muscular support at the hip joint.

Hip Joint Abduction: *Actual* abduction of the hip joint is accomplished by the hip abductors with normal fixation by the lateral trunk muscles, as shown in figure A. *Apparent* abduction may occur, when hip abductors are weak, by substitution action of the lateral trunk muscles. The leg drops into adduction, the pelvis is hiked up laterally, and the leg is raised upward from the table, as shown in figure B.

EXERCISES AND PRECAUTIONS

The normal range of hip joint abduction is approximately 45°, and adduction about 10°. When abductors are too weak to raise the leg in abduction against gravity in a side-lying position, exercises in that position should be *avoided*. A subject can learn to substitute by hiking the pelvis up laterally and bringing the leg into *apparent* abduction, but doing so actually *stretches and strains* the abductors rather than shortening and strengthening them. Substitution can take place in the supine position also, but it can be prevented

and an *appropriate exercise* can be done in the supine position.

On a table or firm bed, the *unaffected leg* is moved in abduction to completion of range of motion. This position will block any effort to hike the pelvis up on the *affected* side, thereby preventing substitution. Movement of the thigh in abduction will require true hip joint motion—not just a sideways movement of the extremity. Whatever assistance is appropriate may be used: Manually assist, or assist with some apparatus or adaptive measures such as smooth or powdered board or roller skate.

Apparent Leg Length Discrepancy Due to Muscle Imbalance

Without any actual difference in leg length, there is an appearance of a longer leg on the high side when the pelvis is tilted laterally. In the right photograph below, the appearance has been created by displacing the pelvis laterally. (The feet were anchored to the floor.)

If tightness develops in the Tensor fasciae latae and Iliotibial band on one side, the pelvis will be tilted down on that side. If there is Gluteus medius weakness on one side, the pelvis will ride higher on the side of the weakness.

The habit of standing with weight mainly on one leg and the pelvis swayed sideways weakens the abductors, especially the Gluteus medius on that side. If tightness of the Tensor fasciae latae on one side and weakness of the Gluteus medius on the other is mild, treatment may be as simple as breaking the habit and standing evenly on both legs. If the imbalance is more marked, treatment may involve stretching of the tight Tensor fasciae latae and Iliotibial band and use of a lift on the low side. The lift will help stretch the tight Tensor and relieve strain on the opposite Gluteus medius. (For a detailed discussion, see p. 60.)

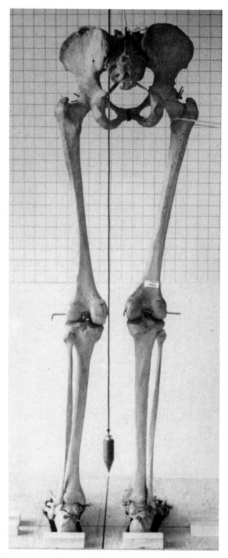

Legs are equal in length.
Pelvis is level.
Both hip joints are neutral between adduction and abduction.
Length of abductors is equal.

As pelvis sways sideways the pelvis is higher on the right.
The right hip joint is adducted.
The left hip joint is abducted.
The right hip abductors are elongated.
The left hip abductors and fascia lata are in a shortened position.

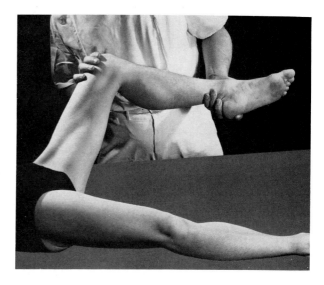

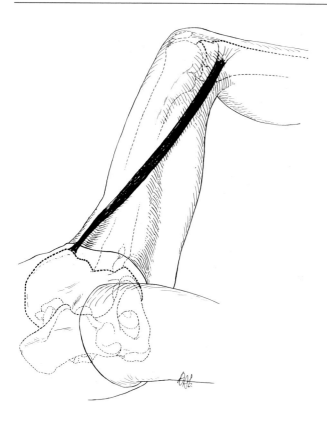

Origin: Anterior superior iliac spine and superior half of notch just distal to spine.

Insertion: Proximal part of medial surface of tibia near anterior border.

Action: Flexes, laterally rotates, and abducts the hip joint. Flexes and assists in medial rotation of the knee joint.

Nerve: Femoral, L2, 3, (4).

Patient: Supine.

Fixation: None necessary on the part of the examiner. The patient may hold on to the table.

Test Movement: Lateral rotation, abduction, and flexion of the thigh, with flexion of the knee.

Resistance: Against the anterolateral surface of the lower thigh, in the direction of hip extension, adduction and medial rotation, and against the leg in the direction of knee extension. The examiner's hands are in position to resist the lateral rotation of the hip joint by pressure and counterpressure (in the same way as described under hip lateral rotator test, p. 219.) The examiner must resist the multiple action test movement by a combined resistance movement.

Weakness: Decreases strength of hip flexion, abduction, and lateral rotation. Contributes to anteromedial instability of the knee joint.

Contracture: Flexion, abduction, and lateral rotation deformity of the hip, with flexion of the knee.

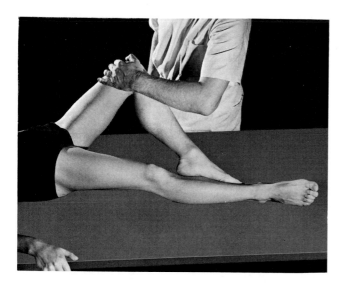

ERROR IN TESTING SARTORIUS

The position of the leg, as illustrated in the accompanying photograph, resembles the Sartorius test position in its flexion, abduction, and lateral rotation. However, the ability to hold this position is essentially a function of the hip adductors and requires little assistance from the Sartorius.

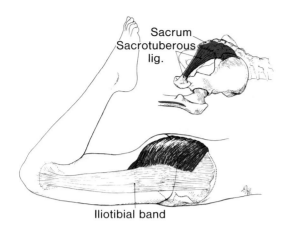

Sacrum
Sacrotuberous lig.

Iliotibial band

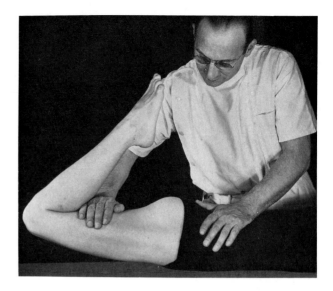

Origin: Posterior gluteal line of ilium and portion of bone superior and posterior to it, posterior surface of lower part of sacrum, side of coccyx, aponeurosis of erector spinae, sacrotuberous ligament, and gluteal aponeurosis.

Insertion: Larger proximal portion and superficial fibers of distal portion of muscle into iliotibial tract of fascia lata. Deep fibers of distal portion into gluteal tuberosity of femur.

Action: Extends, laterally rotates, and lower fibers assist in adduction of the hip joint. The upper fibers assist in abduction. Through its insertion into the iliotibial tract, helps to stabilize the knee in extension.

Nerve: Inferior gluteal L5, S1, 2.

Patient: Prone with knee flexed 90° or more. (The more the knee is flexed, the less the hip will extend, due to restricting tension of the Rectus femoris anteriorly.)

Fixation: Posteriorly, the back muscles, laterally, the lateral abdominal muscles, and, anteriorly, the *opposite* hip flexors fix the pelvis to the trunk.

Test: Hip extension with knee flexed.

Pressure: Against the lower part of the posterior thigh in the direction of hip flexion.

Weakness: Bilateral marked weakness of the Gluteus maximus makes walking extremely difficult, and necessitates the aid of crutches. The individual bears weight on the extremity in a position of posterolateral displacement of the trunk over the femur. Raising the trunk from a forward-bent position requires the action of the Gluteus maximus, and in cases of weakness patients must push themselves to an upright position by using their arms.

Note: Testing for strength of the Gluteus maximus is of particular importance as a preliminary test to examining strength of back extensors (see p. 140), and in cases of coccyalgia (see p. 359).

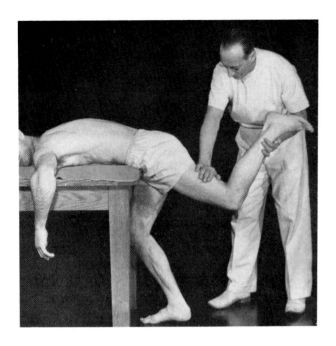

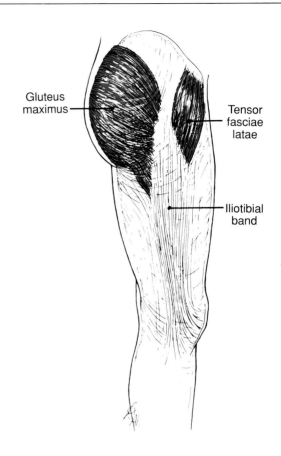

Gluteus maximus

Tensor fasciae latae

Iliotibial band

MODIFIED TEST

When back extensor muscles are weak or hip flexor muscles tight, it is often necessary to modify the Gluteus maximus test. The above figure shows the modified test.

Patient: Trunk prone on table, legs hanging over the end of the table.

Fixation: The patient usually needs to hold on to the table when pressure is applied.

Test: Extension of the hip: 1) with the knee passively flexed by the examiner, as illustrated, or 2) with the knee extended, permitting Hamstring assistance.

Pressure: This test presents a rather difficult problem in regard to application of pressure. If the Gluteus maximus is to be isolated as much as possible from the Hamstrings, it requires that knee flexion be maintained by the examiner, otherwise the Hamstrings will unavoidably act in maintaining the antigravity knee flexion. Trying to maintain knee flexion passively and apply pressure to the thigh makes it difficult to obtain an accurate test.

If this test is used because of marked hip flexor tightness, it may be impractical to flex the knee, thereby increasing the Rectus femoris tension over the hip joint.

The extensive deep fascia which covers the gluteal region and the thigh like a sleeve is called the fascia lata. It is attached proximally to the external lip of the iliac crest, the sacrum and coccyx, the sacrotuberous ligament, the ischial tuberosity, the ischiopubic rami, and the inguinal ligament. Distally it is attached to the patella, the tibial condyles, and the head of the fibula. The fascia on the medial aspect of the thigh is thin while that on the lateral side is very dense, especially the portion between the tubercle of the iliac crest and the lateral condyle of the tibia, designated as the Iliotibial band. Upon reaching the borders of the Tensor fasciae latae and the Gluteus maximus, the fascia lata divides and invests both the superficial and deep surfaces of these muscles. In addition, both the Tensor fasciae latae and three fourths of the Gluteus maximus insert into the iliotibial band so that its distal extent serves as a conjoint tendon of these muscles. This structural arrangement permits both muscles to influence the stability of the extended knee joint.

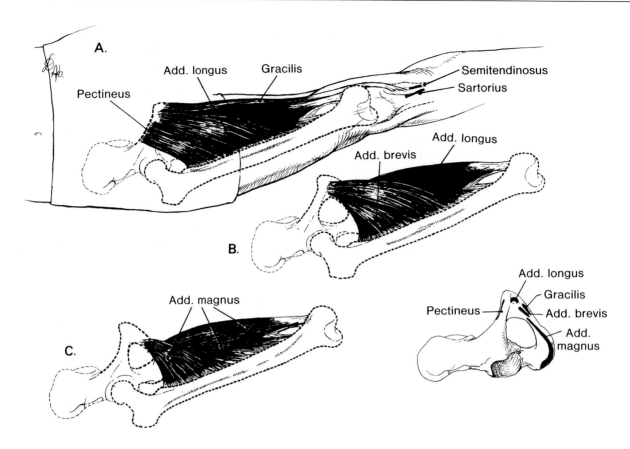

Stippled lines indicate muscle attachments located on posterior surface of femur.

PECTINEUS

Origin: Surface of superior ramus of pubis ventral to pecten between iliopectineal eminence and pubic tubercle.

Insertion: Pectineal line of femur.

Nerve: Femoral and Obturator, L2, 3, 4.

ADDUCTOR MAGNUS

Origin: Inferior pubic ramus, ramus of ischium (anterior fibers), and ischial tuberosity (posterior fibers).

Insertion: Medial to gluteal tuberosity, middle of linea aspera, medial supracondylar line, and adductor tubercle of medial condyle of femur.

Nerve: Obturator, L2, **3, 4,** and Sciatic, L4, 5, S1.

GRACILIS

Origin: Inferior half of symphysis pubis and medial margin of inferior ramus of pubic bone.

Insertion: Medial surface of body of tibia, distal to condyle, proximal to insertion of Semitendinosus, and lateral to insertion of Sartorius.

Nerve: Obturator, L2, **3, 4.**

ADDUCTOR BREVIS

Origin: Outer surface of inferior ramus of pubis.

Insertion: Distal two thirds of pectineal line, and proximal half of medial lip of linea aspera.

Nerve: Obturator, L2, 3, 4.

ADDUCTOR LONGUS

Origin: Anterior surface of pubis at junction of crest and symphysis.

Insertion: Middle one third of medial lip of linea aspera.

Nerve: Obturator L2, 3, 4.

Action: All the above adduct the hip joint. In addition, the Pectineus, Adductor brevis, and Adductor longus flex the hip joint. The anterior fibers of the Adductor magnus which arise from the rami of the pubis and ischium may assist in flexion, while the posterior fibers that arise from the ischial tuberosity may assist in extension. The Gracilis, in addition to adducting the hip joint, flexes and medially rotates the knee joint. (See p. 230 for discussion of rotation action on the hip joint.)

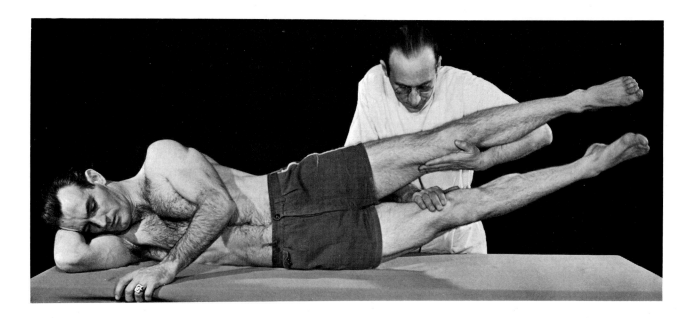

Patient: Lying on right side to test right (and vice versa), body in straight line, with lower extremities and lumbar spine straight.

Fixation: The examiner holds the upper leg in abduction. The patient should hold on to the table for stability.

Test: Adduction of the underneath extremity upward from the table without rotation, flexion, or extension of the hip, or tilting of the pelvis.

Pressure: Against the medial aspect of the distal end of the thigh in the direction of abduction (downward toward the table). Pressure is applied at a point above the knee to avoid strain of the tibial collateral ligament.

Note: Forward rotation of the pelvis with extension of the hip joint shows attempt to hold with lower fibers of Gluteus maximus. Anterior tilting of the pelvis, or flexion of the hip joint (with backward rotation of the pelvis on upper side), allows substitution by the hip flexors.

Adductor longus, Adductor brevis, and Pectineus aid in hip flexion. If the side-lying position is maintained and the hip tends to flex as the thigh is adducted during the test, it is not necessarily evidence of substitution but merely evidence that the adductors that flex the hip are doing more than the rest of the adductors that assist in this movement, or that hip extensors are not helping to maintain the thigh in neutral position.

Contracture: Hip adduction deformity. In standing, the position is one of lateral pelvic tilt, with the pelvis so high on the side of contracture, that it becomes necessary to plantar flex the foot on the same side, holding it in equinus in order for the toes to touch the floor. As an alternative, if the foot is placed flat on the floor, the opposite extremity must be either flexed at the hip and knee, or abducted to compensate for the apparent shortness on the adducted side.

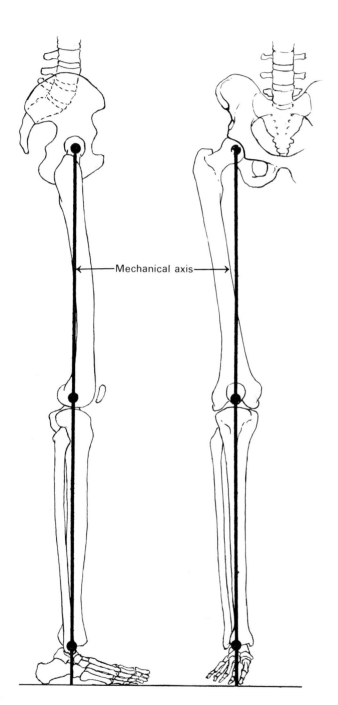

Mechanical axis

The following brief discussion about the rotator action of the adductors is not an attempt to solve the controversy that appears to exist but, rather, to present some of the reasons why a controversy exists.

On the accompanying illustration, it is important to note that in anatomical position, and from anterior view, the femur extends obliquely with the distal end more medial than the proximal. From lateral view, the shaft of the femur is convexly curved in an anterior direction. The *anatomical axis* of the femur extends longitudinally along the shaft. If rotation of the hip took place about this axis, there would be no doubt that the adductors, attached as they are posteriorly along the linea aspera, would be lateral rotators.

However, rotation of the hip joint does not occur about the anatomical axis of the femur, but rather about the *mechanical axis*, which passes from the center of the hip joint to the center of the knee joint and is at the intersection of the two planes represented by the solid black lines in the accompanying figure.

The muscles or major portions of muscles that insert on the part of the femur that is anterior to the mechanical axis will act as medial rotators of the femur. (See lateral view.) On the other hand, the muscles or major portions of the muscles that insert on the part of the femur posterior to the mechanical axis will act as lateral rotators.

When the position of the extremity in relation to the pelvis changes from that illustrated as the anatomical position, the actions of the muscles change. Thus, if the femur is medially rotated, a larger portion of the shaft comes to lie anterior to the mechanical axis with the result that more of the adductor insertions will be anterior to the axis and, therefore, will act as medial rotators. With increased lateral rotation, more of the adductors will act as lateral rotators.

Besides the change that occurs with movement, there are normal variations of bone structure of the femur that tend to make variable the rotator action of the adductors.

Chart for Analysis of Muscle Imbalance: Lower Extremity

Name:..Date: 1st. Ex.-.....................2nd. Ex.-.........................

Diagnosis:...Onset:.........................Exam. of..............extremity

		2nd EX.	1st. EX.	1st. EX.	2nd. EX.		
	ILIOPSOAS SARTORIUS TENSOR FAS. LAT. RECTUS FEMORIS } HIP FLEXORS					GLUTEUS MAXIMUS	
	HIP ADDUCTORS					GLUTEUS MEDIUS	
						GLUTEUS MINIMUS	
						TENSOR FASCIAE LATAE	
	HIP LATERAL ROTATORS					HIP MEDIAL ROTATORS	
	QUADRICEPS					MEDIAL HAMSTRINGS LATERAL	
	TIBIALIS ANTERIOR					SOLEUS	
						GASTROCNEMIUS & SOLEUS	
						PERONEUS LONGUS & BREVIS	
	TIBIALIS POSTERIOR					PERONEUS TERTIUS	
	FLEXOR DIGITORUM LONGUS	1 2 3 4				1 DISTAL INTER-PHALANGEAL 2 JOINT EXTENSORS 3 4	
	FLEXOR DIGITORUM BREVIS	1 2 3 4				1 PROXIMAL INTER- 2 PHALANGEAL 3 JOINT EXTENSORS 4	
	LUMBRICALES & INTEROSSEI	1 2 3 4				1 2 EXT. DIGITORUM LONGUS 3 & BREVIS 4	
	FLEXOR HALLUCIS LONGUS					EXTENSOR HALLUCIS LONGUS & BREVIS	
	FLEXOR HALLUCIS BREVIS						
	ABDUCTOR HALLUCIS					ADDUCTOR HALLUCIS	

231

Chart of Lower Extremity Muscles

Listed According to Spinal Segment Innervation and Grouped According to Joint Action

Spinal Segment

Lumb. 1	2	3	4	5	Sac. 1	2	3	Muscle	HIP Flexion	Adduction	Med. Rotat.	Abduction	Lat. Rotat.	Extension	KNEE Extension	In flexion Lat. Rotat.	In flexion Med. Rotat.
1	2	3	4					Psoas major	Psoas maj.			Psoas maj.	Psoas maj.				
(1)	2	3	4					Iliacus	Iliacus			Iliacus	Iliacus				
	2	3	(4)					Sartorius	Sartorius			Sartorius	Sartorius				Sartorius
	2	3	4					Pectineus	Pectineus	Pectineus							
	2	3	4					Adductor long.	Add. long.	Add. long.	Add. long.						
	2	3	4					Adductor brev.	Add. brev.	Add. brev.	Add. brev.						
	2	3	4					Gracilis		Gracilis							Gracilis
	2	3	4					Quadriceps	Rect. fem.						Quadriceps		
	2	3	4					Add. mag. (ant.)	Add. m. (ant.)	Add. mag.							
		3	4					Obturator ext.		Obt. ext.			Obt. ext.				
			4	5	1			Add. mag. (post.)		Add. mag.				Ad. m. post.			
			4	5	1			Tibialis ant.									
			4	5	1			Ten. fas. lat.	Tensor f.l.		Tensor f.l.	Tensor f.l.			Tensor f.l.		
			4	5	1			Gluteus minimus	Glut. min.		Glut. min.	Glut. min.					
			4	5	1			Gluteus medius	G. med., ant.		G. med., ant.	Glut. med.	G. med., post.	G. med., post.			
			4	5	1			Popliteus									Popliteus
			4	5	1			Ext. dig. long.									
			4	5	1			Peroneus tertius									
			4	5	1			Ext. hall. long.									
			4	5	1			Ext. dig. brev.									
			4	5	1			Flex. dig. brev.									
			4	5	1			Flex. hall. brev.									
			4	5	1			Lumbricalis I									
			4	5	1			Abductor hall.									
			4	5	1			Peroneus longus									
			4	5	1			Peroneus brevis									
			(4)	5	1			Tibialis post.									
			4	5	1	(2)		Gemelli inferior				Gem. inf.	Gem. inf.				
			4	5	1	(2)		Quadratus fem.					Quadratus f.				
			4	5	1	(2)		Plantaris									
			4	5	1	2		Semimembranosus		Semimemb.				Semimemb.			Semimemb.
			4	5	1	2		Semitendinosus		Semitend.				Semitend.			Semitend.
				5	1	(2)		Flex. dig. long.									
				5	1	2		Gluteus maximus	G. max., low.			G. max., upp.	Glut. max.	Glut. max.			
				5	1	2		Biceps, short h.								Bic., s.h.	
				5	1	2		Flex. hall. long.									
				5	1	2		Soleus									
				(5)	1	2		Piriformis				Piriformis	Piriformis	Piriformis			
				5	1	2		Gemelli superior				Gem. sup.	Gem. sup.				
				5	1	2		Obturator int.				Obt. int.	Obt. int.				
				5	1	2	3	Biceps, long h.					Biceps l.h.	Biceps l.h.		Bic., l.h.	
			(4)	(5)	1	2		Lumb. II, III, IV									
					1	2		Gastrocnemius									
					1	2		Dorsal inteross.									
					1	2		Plantar inteross.									
					1	2		Abd. dig. min.									
					1	2		Adductor hall.									

Listed According to Spinal Segment Innervation and Grouped According to Joint Action (*Continued*)

KNEE Flexion	Dorsiflex.	Plant flex.	Eversion	Inversion	MTP Extension	MTP Flexion	MTP Abduction	MTP Adduction	Digs. 2–5 Prox. Interphal. Jts. Extension	Flexion	Digs. 1–5 Distal Interphal. Jts. Extension	Flexion
Sartorius												
Gracilis												
	Tib. ant.			Tib. ant.								
Popliteus												
	Ext. d. long.		Ext. d. long.		(2-5 dig.) Ext. d. long				(2-5 dig.) Ext. d. long		(2-5 dig.) Ext. d. long	
	Peroneus t.		Peroneus t.									
	Ext. hall. l.			Ext. hall. l.	Ext. hall. l.				▨	▨	Ext. hall. l.	
					(1-4 dig.) Ext. dig. br.				(1-4 dig.) Ext. dig. br.		(1-4 dig.) Ext. dig. br.	
						(2-5 dig.) Flex. dig. br.				(2-5 dig.) Flex. dig. br.		
						Flex. hall. br.			▨	▨		
						2nd dig. Lumb. I			(2nd dig.) Lumb. I		(2nd dig.) Lumb. I	
						Abd. hall.	Abd. hall.		▨	▨		
		Peroneus l.		Peroneus l.								
		Peroneus b.		Peroneus b.								
		Tib. post.		Tib. post.								
Plantaris		Plantaris										
Semimemb.												
Semitend.												
		Flex. dig. l.		Flex. dig. l.		(2-5 dig.) Flex. dig. l.				(2-5 dig.) Flex. dig. l.		(2-5 dig.) Flex. dig. l.
Bic., s.h.												
		Flex. hall. l.		Flex. hall. l.		Flex. hall. l.			▨	▨		Flex. hall. l.
		Soleus										
Bic., l.h.												
					(3-5 dig.) Lumb. II-IV				(3-5 dig.) Lumb. II-IV		(3-5 dig.) Lumb. II-IV	
Gastroc.		Gastroc.										
					(2-4 dig.) Dor. int.	(2-4 dig.) Dor. int.			(2-4 dig.) Dor. int.		(2-4 dig.) Dor. int.	
					(3-5 dig.) Plant. int.			(3-5 dg.) Plant. int.	(3-5 dig.) Plant. int.		(3-5 dig.) Plant. int.	
							Abd. d. min.					
						Add. hall.		Add. hall.	▨	▨		

Neck, Trunk, and Lower Extremity Muscle Chart

PATIENT'S NAME   CLINIC No.

LEFT   RIGHT

					EXAMINER DATE							
					Neck flexors							
					Neck extensors							
					Back extensors							
					Quadratus lumborum							
					Rectus abdominis							
					External oblique							
					Internal oblique							
					Lateral abdominals							
					Gluteus maximus							
					Gluteus medius							
					Hip abductors							
					Hip adductors							
					Hip medial rotators							
					Hip lateral rotators							
					Hip flexors							
					Tensor fasciae latae							
					Sartorius							
					Medial hamstrings							
					Lateral hamstrings							
					Quadriceps							
					Gastrocnemius							
					Soleus							
					Peroneus longus							
					Peroneus brevis							
					Peroneus tertius							
					Tibialis posterior							
					Tibialis anterior							
					Extensor hallucis longus							
					Flexor hallucis longus							
					Flexor hallucis brevis							
					1 Extensor digitorum longus 1							
					2 Extensor digitorum longus 2							
					3 Extensor digitorum longus 3							
					4 Extensor digitorum longus 4							
					1 Extensor digitorum brevis 1							
					2 Extensor digitorum brevis 2							
					3 Extensor digitorum brevis 3							
					4 Extensor digitorum brevis 4							
					1 Flexor digitorum longus 1							
					2 Flexor digitorum longus 2							
					3 Flexor digitorum longus 3							
					4 Flexor digitorum longus 4							
					1 Flexor digitorum brevis 1							
					2 Flexor digitorum brevis 2							
					3 Flexor digitorum brevis 3							
					4 Flexor digitorum brevis 4							
					1 Lumbricalis 1							
					2 Lumbricalis 2							
					3 Lumbricalis 3							
					4 Lumbricalis 4							
					Leg length							
					Thigh circumference							
					Calf circumference							

NOTES:

chapter 8

Upper Extremity and Shoulder Girdle Strength Tests

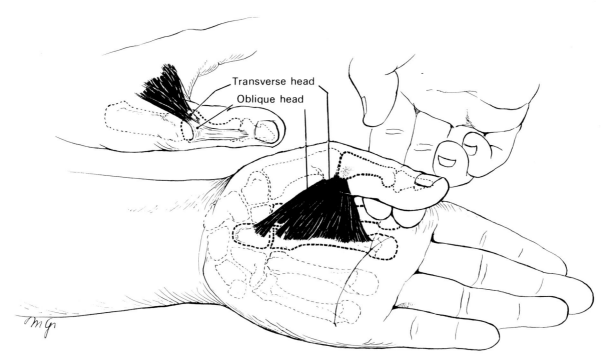

Origin of Oblique Fibers: Capitate bone, and bases of second and third metacarpal bones.

Origin of Transverse Fibers: Palmar surface of third metacarpal bone.

Insertion: Transverse head into ulnar side of base of proximal phalanx of thumb, and oblique head into extensor expansion.

Action: Adducts the carpometacarpal joint, and adducts and assists in flexion of the metacarpophalangeal joint, so that the thumb moves toward the plane of the palm. Aids in opposition of the thumb toward the little finger. By virtue of the attachment of the oblique fibers into the extensor expansion, may assist in extending the interphalangeal joint.

Nerve: Ulnar, C8, **T1.**

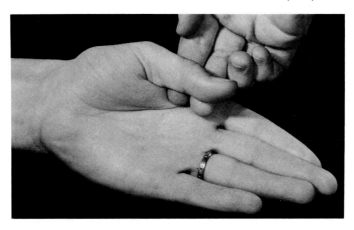

Patient: Sitting or supine.

Fixation: The hand may be stabilized by the examiner, or rest on the table for support (as illustrated).

Test: Adduction of the thumb toward the palm.

Pressure: Against the medial surface of the thumb in the direction of abduction away from palm.

Weakness: Results in inability to clench the thumb firmly over the closed fist.

Contracture: Adduction deformity of the thumb.

Note: A test that is frequently used to determine the strength of the Adductor pollicis is the ability to hold a piece of paper between the thumb and second metacarpal. In an individual with a well-developed Adductor, the bulk of the muscle itself prevents close approximation of these parts.

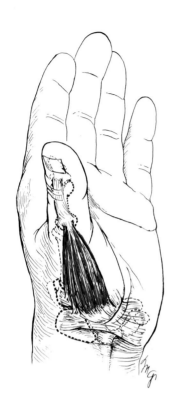

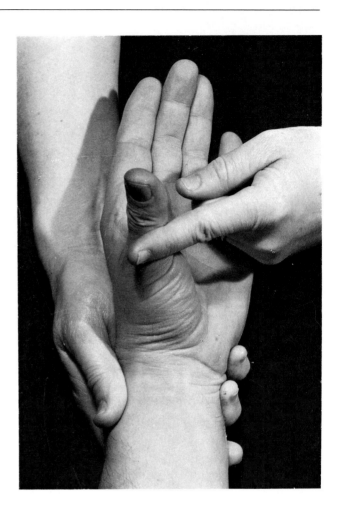

Origin: Flexor retinaculum, tubercle of trapezium bone, and tubercle of scaphoid bone.

Insertion: Base of proximal phalanx of thumb, radial side, and extensor expansion.

Action: Abducts the carpometacarpal and metacarpophalangeal joints of the thumb in a ventral direction perpendicular to the plane of the palm. By virtue of its attachment into the dorsal extensor expansion, extends the interphalangeal joint of the thumb. Assists in opposition, and may assist in flexion and medial rotation of the metacarpophalangeal joint.

Nerve: Median, C6, 7, 8, T1.

Patient: Sitting or supine.

Fixation: The examiner stabilizes the hand.

Test: Abduction of the thumb ventralward from the palm.

Pressure: Against the proximal phalanx in the direction of adduction toward the palm.

Weakness: Decreases the ability to abduct the thumb, making it difficult to grasp a large object. An adduction deformity of the thumb may result from marked weakness.

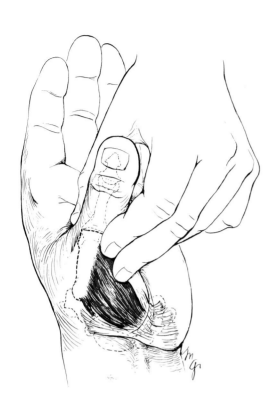

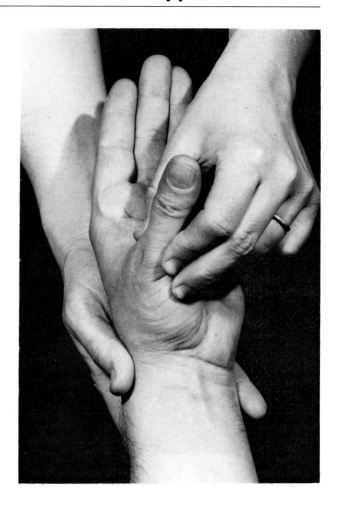

Origin: Flexor retinaculum and tubercle of trapezium bone.

Insertion: Entire length of first metacarpal bone, radial side.

Action: Opposes (i.e., flexes and abducts with slight medial rotation) the carpometacarpal joint of the thumb, placing the thumb in a position so that, by flexion of the metacarpophalangeal joint, it can oppose the fingers. For true opposition of the thumb and little finger, the *pads* of these digits come in contact. Bringing the tips of these digits together can be done without Opponens action.

Nerve: Median, C6, 7, 8, T1.

Patient: Sitting or supine.

Fixation: The examiner stabilizes the hand.

Test: Flexion, abduction, and slight medial rotation of the metacarpal bone so that the thumbnail shows in palmar view.

Pressure: Against the metacarpal bone in the direction of extension and adduction with lateral rotation.

Weakness: Results in a flattening of the thenar eminence, extension and adduction of the first metacarpal, and difficulty in holding a pencil for writing, or in grasping objects firmly between the thumb and fingers.

Note: The attachment of the Palmaris longus and the Opponens pollicis to the flexor retinaculum accounts for the fact that the Palmaris longus contracts during the Opponens test.

Flexor Pollicis Longus

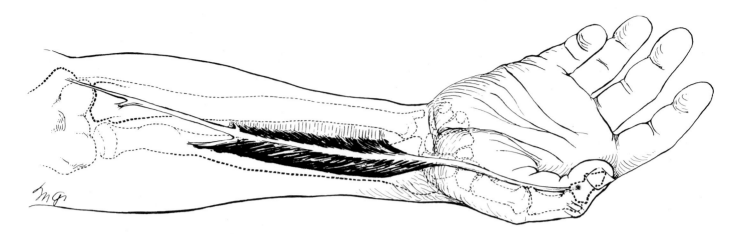

Origin: Anterior surface of body of radius below tuberosity, interosseus membrane, medial border of coronoid process of ulna, and/or medial epicondyle of humerus.

Insertion: Base of distal phalanx of thumb, palmar surface.

Action: Flexes the interphalangeal joint of the thumb, assists in flexion of the metacarpophalangeal and carpometacarpal joints, and may assist in flexion of the wrist.

Nerve: Median, C(6), 7, **8**, T1.

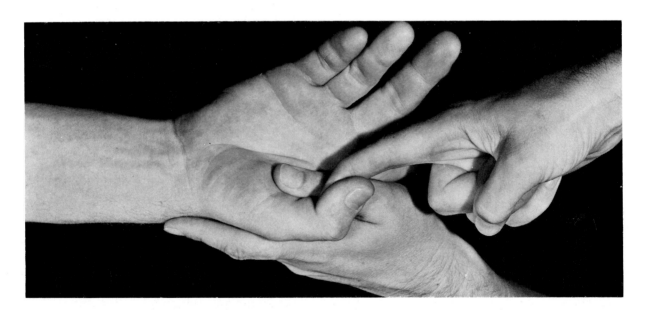

Patient: Sitting or supine.

Fixation: The hand may rest on the table for support (as illustrated) with the examiner stabilizing the metacarpal bone and proximal phalanx of the thumb in extension; or the hand may rest on its ulnar side with the wrist in slight extension and the examiner stabilizing the proximal phalanx of the thumb in extension.

Test: Flexion of the interphalangeal joint of the thumb.

Pressure: Against the palmar surface of the distal phalanx in the direction of extension.

Weakness: Decreases the ability to flex the distal phalanx, making it difficult to hold a pencil for writing or to pick up minute objects between the thumb and fingers. Marked weakness may result in a hyperextension deformity of the interphalangeal joint.

Contracture: Flexion deformity of interphalangeal joint.

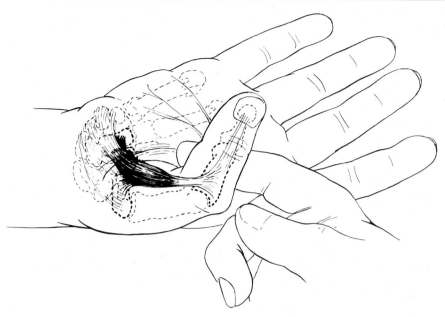

Origin of Superficial Head: Flexor retinaculum and trapezium bone.

Origin of Deep Head: Trapezoid and capitate bones.

Insertion: Base of proximal phalanx of thumb, radial side, and extensor expansion.

Action: Flexes the metacarpophalangeal and carpometacarpal joints of the thumb, and assists in opposition of the thumb toward the little finger. By virtue of its attachment into the dorsal extensor expansion, may extend the interphalangeal joint.

Nerve to Superficial Head: Median, C6, 7, 8, T1.

Nerve to Deep Head: Ulnar, C8, T1.

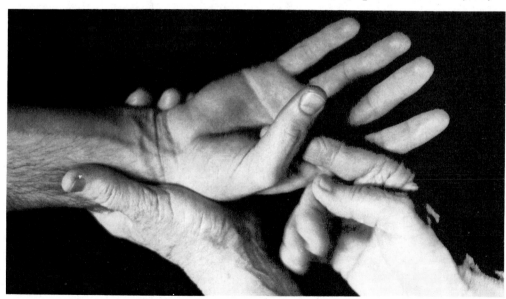

Patient: Sitting or supine.

Fixation: The examiner stabilizes the hand.

Test: Flexion of the metacarpophalangeal joint of the thumb without flexion of the interphalangeal joint.

Pressure: Against the palmar surface of the proximal phalanx in the direction of extension.

Weakness: Decreases the ability to flex the metacarpophalangeal joint making it difficult to grip objects firmly between the thumb and fingers. Marked weakness may result in a hyperextension deformity of the metacarpophalangeal joint.

Contracture: Flexion deformity of the metacarpophalangeal joint.

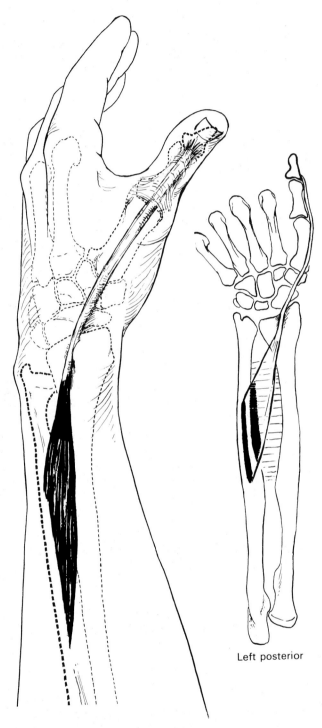

Left posterior

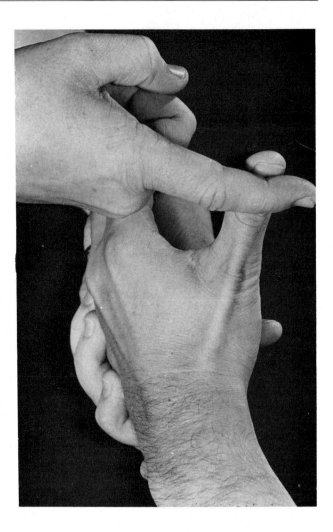

Origin: Middle one third of posterior surface of ulna distal to origin of Abductor pollicis longus, and interosseus membrane.

Insertion: Base of distal phalanx of thumb, dorsal surface.

Action: Extends the interphalangeal joint and assists in extension of the metacarpophalangeal and carpometacarpal joints of the thumb. Assists in abduction and extension of the wrist.

Nerve: Radial, C6, **7, 8**.

Patient: Sitting or supine.

Fixation: The examiner stabilizes the hand and gives counterpressure against the palmar surface of the first metacarpal and proximal phalanx.

Test: Extension of the interphalangeal joint of the thumb.

Pressure: Against the dorsal surface of the interphalangeal joint of the thumb in the direction of flexion.

Weakness: Decreases the ability to extend the interphalangeal joint, and may result in a flexion deformity of that joint.

Note: In a radial nerve lesion, the interphalangeal joint of the thumb may be extended by the action of the Abductor pollicis brevis, the Flexor pollicis brevis, the oblique fibers of the Adductor pollicis, or by the first Palmar interosseus by virtue of their insertions into the extensor expansion of the thumb. Interphalangeal joint extension in an otherwise complete radial nerve lesion should not be interpreted as regeneration or partial involvement if only this one action is observed.

147-157
I

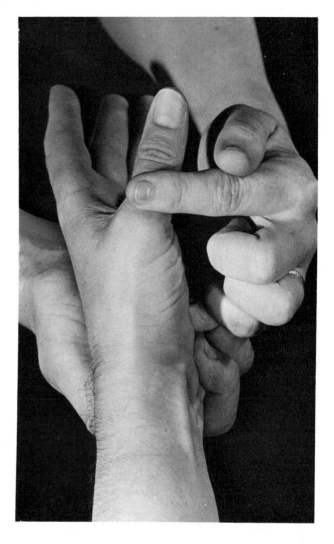

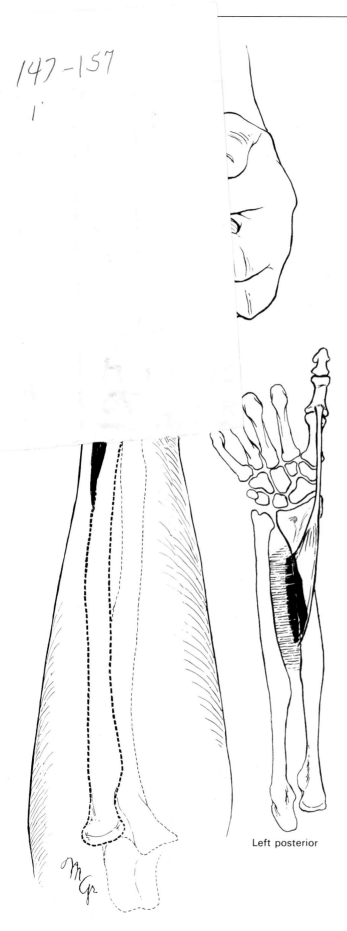

Left posterior

Origin: Posterior surface of body of radius distal to origin of Abductor pollicis longus, and interosseus membrane.

Insertion: Base of proximal phalanx of thumb, dorsal surface.

Action: Extends the metacarpophalangeal joint of the thumb, extends and abducts the carpometacarpal joint, and assists in abduction (radial deviation) of the wrist.

Nerve: Radial, C6, **7**, **8**.

Patient: Sitting or supine.

Fixation: The examiner stabilizes the wrist.

Test: Extension of the metacarpophalangeal joint of the thumb

Pressure: Against the dorsal surface of the proximal phalanx in the direction of flexion.

Weakness: Decreases the ability to extend the metacarpophalangeal joint, and may result in a position of flexion of that joint.

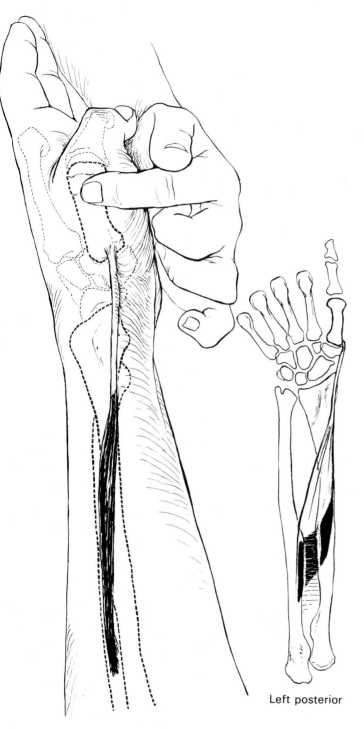

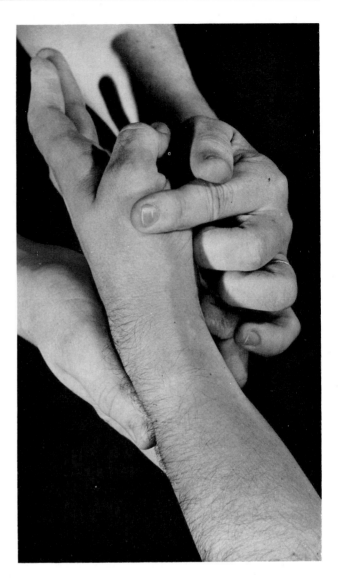

Left posterior

Origin: Posterior surface of body of ulna distal to origin of Supinator, interosseus membrane, and posterior surface of middle one third of body of radius.

Insertion: Base of first metacarpal bone, radial side.

Action: Abducts and extends the carpometacarpal joint of the thumb; abducts (radial deviation) and assists in flexing the wrist.

Nerve: Radial, C6, **7**, **8**.

Patient: Sitting or supine.

Fixation: The examiner stabilizes the wrist.

Test: Abduction and slight extension of the first metacarpal bone.

Pressure: Against the lateral surface of the distal end of the first metacarpal in the direction of adduction and flexion.

Weakness: Decreases the ability to abduct the first metacarpal, and the ability to abduct the wrist.

Contracture: Abducted and slightly extended position of the first metacarpal with slight radial deviation of the hand.

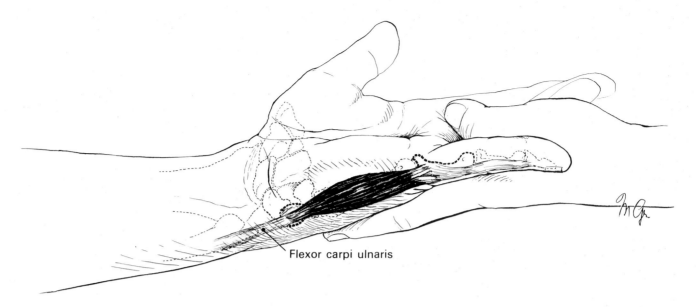

Flexor carpi ulnaris

Origin: Tendon of Flexor carpi ulnaris and pisiform bone.

Insertion: By two slips: one into base of proximal phalanx of little finger, ulnar side; the second, into the ulnar border of the extensor expansion.

Action: Abducts, assists in opposition, and may assist in flexion of the metacarpophalangeal joint of the little finger; by virtue of insertion into the extensor expansion, may assist in extension of interphalangeal joints.

Nerve: Ulnar, C(7), **8**, T1.

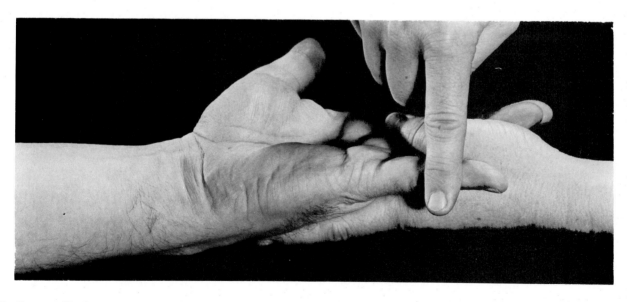

Patient: Sitting or supine.

Fixation: The hand may be stabilized by the examiner or rest on the table for support.

Test: Abduction of the little finger.

Pressure: Against the ulnar side of the little finger in the direction of adduction toward the midline of the hand.

Weakness: Decreases the ability to abduct the little finger, and results in adduction of this digit.

Note: One should be consistent in the placing of pressure in all finger abduction and adduction tests. Pressure against the sides of the middle phalanges seems most appropriate for all these tests.

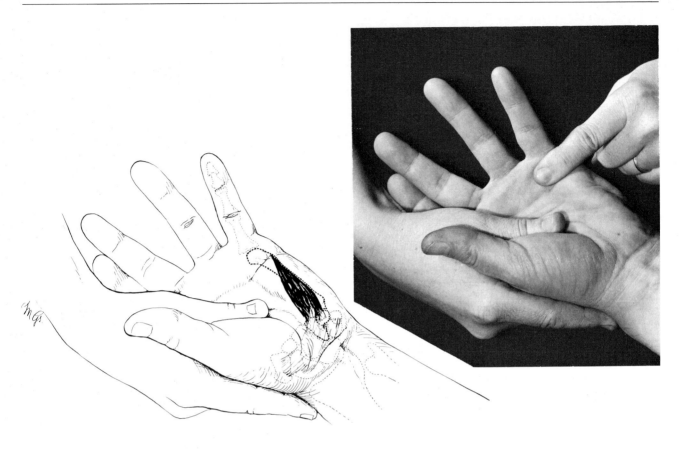

Origin: Hook of hamate bone, and flexor retinaculum.

Insertion: Entire length of fifth metacarpal bone, ulnar side.

Action: Opposes (i.e., flexes with slight rotation) the carpometacarpal joint of the little finger, lifting the ulnar border of the hand into a position so that the metacarpophalangeal flexors can oppose the little finger to the thumb. (See p. 19.) Helps to cup the palm of the hand.

Nerve: Ulnar, C(7), **8, T1**.

Patient: Sitting or supine.

Fixation: The hand may be stabilized by the examiner or rest on the table for support. The first metacarpal is held firmly by the examiner.

Test: Opposition of the fifth metacarpal toward the first.

Pressure: Against the palmar surface along the fifth metacarpal in the direction of flattening the palm of the hand. The one-finger pressure was used in the illustration to avoid obscuring the belly of the muscle, but usually the thumb is used to apply pressure along the fifth metacarpal.

Weakness: Results in a flattening of the palm and makes it difficult, if not impossible, to oppose the little finger to the thumb.

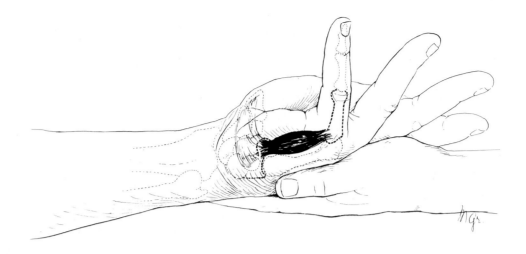

Origin: Hook of hamate bone, and flexor retinaculum.

Insertion: Base of proximal phalanx of little finger, ulnar side.

Action: Flexes the metacarpophalangeal joint of the little finger and assists in opposition of the little finger toward the thumb.

Nerve: Ulnar, C(7), **8**, T1.

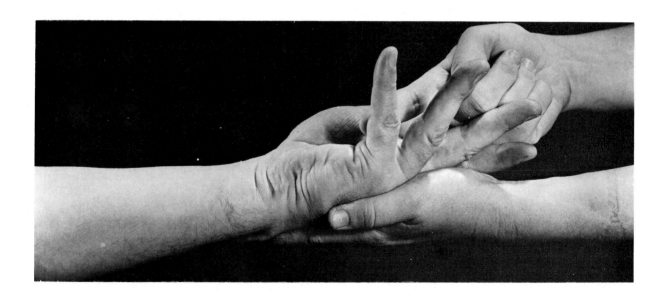

Patient: Sitting or supine.

Fixation: The hand may rest on the table for support, or be stabilized by the examiner.

Test: Flexion of the metacarpophalangeal joint with interphalangeal joints extended.

Pressure: Against the palmar surface of the proximal phalanx in the direction of extension.

Weakness: Decreases the ability to flex the little finger and oppose it toward the thumb.

Dorsal Interossei

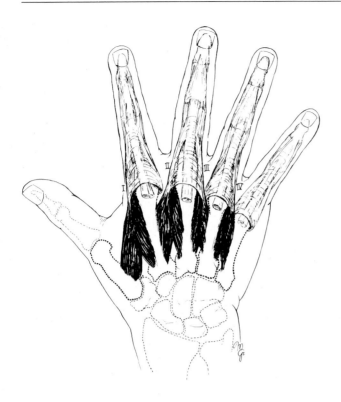

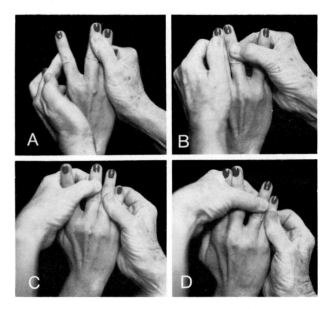

Origins:

First, lateral head: Proximal one half of ulnar border of first metacarpal bone.

First, medial head: Radial border of second metacarpal bone.

Second, third, and fourth: Adjacent sides of metacarpal bones in each interspace.

Insertions: Into extensor expansion and to base of proximal phalanx as follows:

First: Radial side of index finger, chiefly to base of proximal phalanx.

Second: Radial side of middle finger.

Third: Ulnar side of middle finger, chiefly into extensor expansion.

Fourth: Ulnar side of ring finger.

Action: Abducts the index, middle, and ring fingers from the axial line through the third digit. Assists in flexion of metacarpophalangeal joints and extension of interphalangeal joints of the same fingers. The first assists in adduction of the thumb.

Nerve: Ulnar, C8, T1.

Patient: Sitting or supine.

Fixation: In general, stabilization of adjacent digits, to give fixation of digit toward which finger is moved, and to prevent assistance from digit on other side.

Test, and Pressure or Traction (against middle phalanx):

First: (Figure A) Abduction of index finger toward thumb. Pressure against radial side of index finger in direction of middle finger.

Second: (Figure B) Abduction of middle finger toward index finger. Hold middle finger and pull in direction of ring finger.

Third: (Figure C) Abduction of middle finger toward ring finger. Hold middle finger and pull in direction of index finger.

Fourth: (Figure D) Abduction of ring finger toward little finger. Hold ring finger and pull in direction of middle finger.

Weakness: Decreases the ability to abduct the index, middle, and ring fingers. Decreases the strength of extension of the interphalangeal joints and flexion of the metacarpophalangeal joints of index, middle, and ring fingers.

Contracture: Abduction of index and ring fingers.

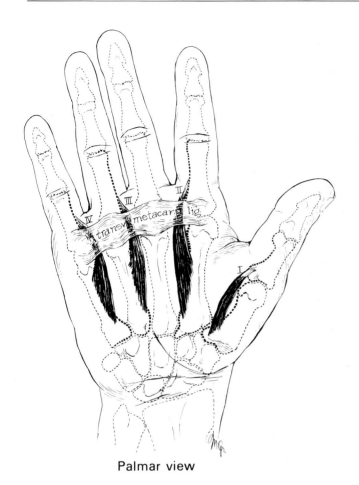

Palmar view

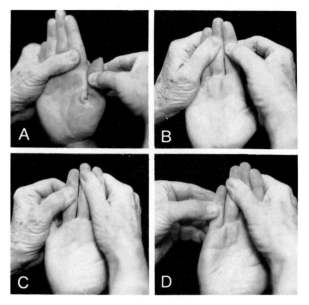

Origins:

First: Base of first metacarpal bone, ulnar side.

Second: Length of second metacarpal bone, ulnar side.

Third: Length of fourth metacarpal bone, radial side.

Fourth: Length of fifth metacarpal bone, radial side.

Insertions: Chiefly, into the extensor expansion of the respective digit, with possible attachment to base of proximal phalanx as follows:

First: Ulnar side of thumb.

Second: Ulnar side of index finger.

Third: Radial side of ring finger.

Fourth: Radial side of little finger.

Action: Adduct the thumb, index, ring, and little finger toward the axial line through the third digit. Assist in flexion of metacarpophalangeal joints, and extension of interphalangeal joints of the three fingers.

Nerve: Ulnar, C8, T1.

Patient: Sitting or supine.

Fixation: In general, stabilization of adjacent digits, to give fixation of digit toward which finger is moved, and to prevent assistance from digit on other side.

Test and Traction (against middle phalanx):

First: (Figure A) Adduction of thumb toward index finger (acting with Adductor pollicis and first Dorsal interosseus). Hold thumb and pull in radial direction.

Second: (Figure B) Adduction of index finger toward middle finger. Hold index finger and pull in direction of thumb.

Third: (Figure C) Adduction of ring finger toward middle finger. Hold ring finger and pull in direction of little finger.

Fourth: (Figure D) Adduction of little finger toward ring finger. Hold little finger and pull in ulnar direction.

Weakness: Decreases ability to adduct thumb, index, ring, and little fingers. Decreases strength in flexion of metacarpophalangeal joints and extension of interphalangeal joints of the index, ring, and little fingers.

Contracture: Fingers held in adduction. May result from wearing a cast with fingers in adduction.

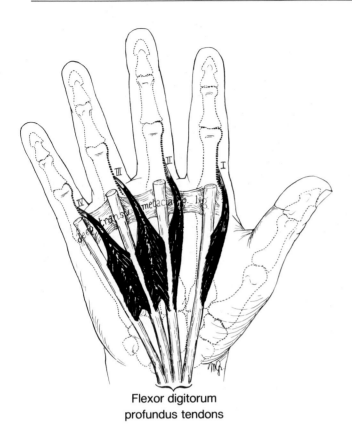

Flexor digitorum
profundus tendons

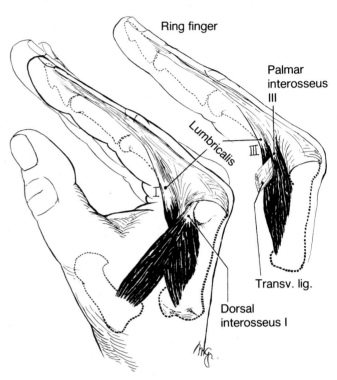

Origin of First and Second: Radial surface of Flexor profundus tendons of index and middle fingers, respectively.

Origin of Third: Adjacent sides of Flexor profundus tendons of middle and ring fingers.

Origin of Fourth: Adjacent sides of Flexor profundus tendons of ring and little fingers.

Insertion: Into the radial border of the extensor expansion on the dorsum of the respective digits.

Action: Extend the interphalangeal joints and simultaneously flex the metacarpophalangeal joints of the second through fifth digits. The Lumbricales also extend the interphalangeal joints when the metacarpophalangeal joints are extended. As the fingers are extended at all joints, the Flexor digitorum profundus tendons offer a form of passive resistance to this movement. Since the Lumbricales are attached to the Flexor profundus tendons, they can diminish this resistive tension by contracting and pulling these tendons distally, and this release of tension decreases the contractile force needed by the muscles that extend the finger joints.

Nerve to Lumbricales I, II: Median, C(6), 7, **8**, **T1**.

Nerve to Lumbricales III, IV: Ulnar, C(7), **8**, **T1**.

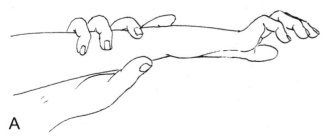

A

Hyperextension of the metacarpophalangeal joints due to weakness of the Lumbricales and Interossei prevents normal function of the Extensor digitorum in extending the interphalangeal joints, as seen in figure A.

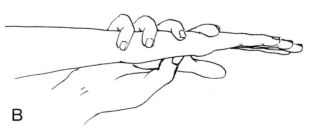

B

When the examiner offers fixation that normally is afforded by the Lumbricales and Interossei, a strong Extensor digitorum will extend the fingers, as in figure B.

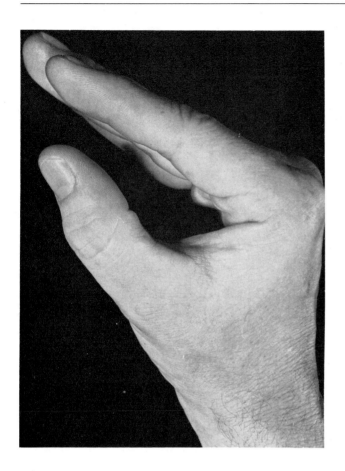

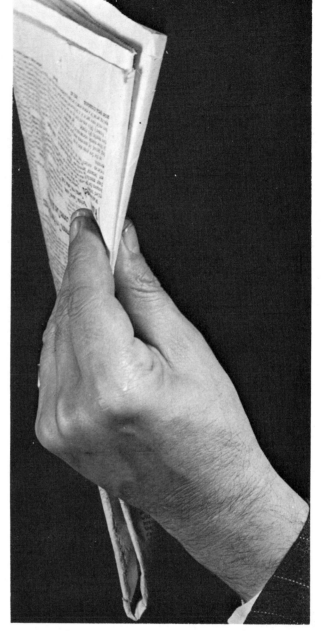

LUMBRICALES AND INTEROSSEI

Patient: Sitting or supine.

Fixation: The examiner stabilizes the wrist in slight extension if there is any weakness of wrist muscles.

Test: Extension of interphalangeal joints with simultaneous flexion of metacarpophalangeal joints.

Pressure: First, against the dorsal surface of the middle and distal phalanges in the direction of flexion; and second, against the palmar surface of the proximal phalanges in the direction of extension. Pressure is not illustrated in the photograph because it is *applied in two stages*, not both simultaneously.

Weakness: Results in claw-hand deformity.

Contracture: Metacarpophalangeal joint flexion with interphalangeal joint extension.

Shortness: See following page.

An important function of the Lumbricales and Interossei is illustrated by the above photograph. With marked weakness or paralysis of these muscles an individual cannot hold a newspaper or a book upright in one hand. The complaint by a patient that a newspaper could not be held in one hand was a clue to this type of weakness.

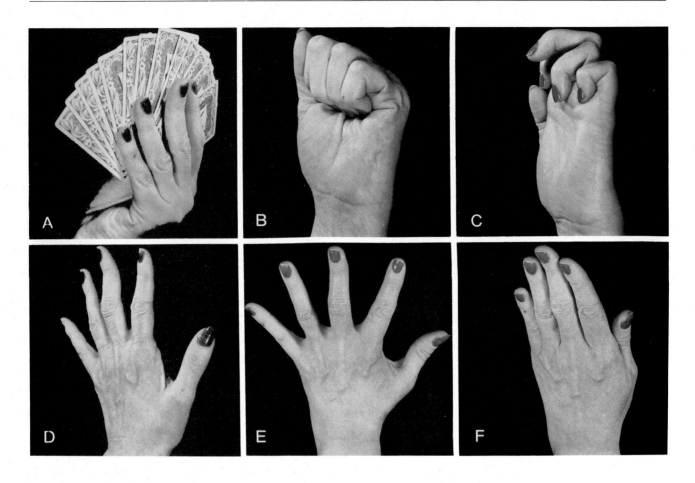

SHORTNESS OF THE INTRINSIC MUSCLES OF THE HAND

The case, illustrated by the above photographs, was that of a middle-aged woman whose complaint was that her middle finger occasionally pained rather severely and there was a constant tight, "drawing" feeling along the sides of this finger. She did not feel that the pain was actually in the joints of the finger. A medical checkup had revealed no arthritis. This person was an avid card player, and the condition was present in the left hand which was the hand in which she held her cards.

Figure A shows the position of the subject's hand in holding a hand of cards. This position is one of strong Lumbrical and Interosseus action. Just as in holding a newspaper, the middle finger is the one which strongly opposes the thumb.

On testing for length of the intrinsic muscles there was evidence of shortness chiefly in the muscles in the middle finger.

The patient could close the fingers to make a fist as in B. This was possible although some shortness existed in the Lumbricales and Inter-ossei because the muscles were being elongated over the interphalangeal joints only, not over the metacarpophalangeal joints.

The patient could extend the fingers as in D. This was possible because the muscles were being elongated over the metacarpophalangeal joints only, not over the interphalangeal joints. (The distal phalanx of the middle finger, which opposes the thumb in holding the cards, is in slight hyperextension.)

When attempting to close the hand into a claw-hand position C, the shortness became apparent. In closing the fingers into this position, the Lumbricales and Interossei must elongate over all three joints at the same time. The middle finger shows the greatest limitation. The ring finger shows slight limitation which is demonstrated by the lack of distal joint flexion as well as by decreased hyperextension of the metacarpophalangeal joint.

The fact that the fingers could be spread apart as in E, and closed sideways as in F, suggests that the shortness may have been in the Lumbricales more than in the Interossei.

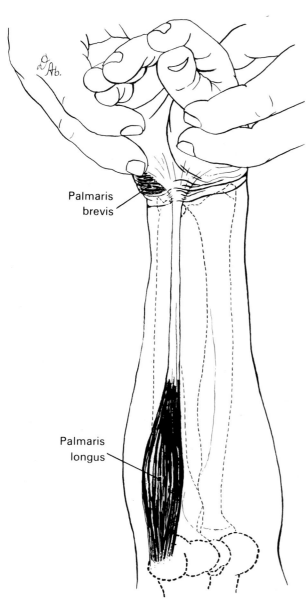

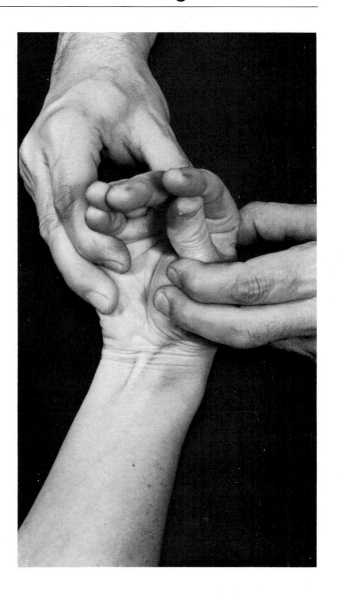

Palmaris brevis

Palmaris longus

PALMARIS LONGUS

Origin: Common flexor tendon from medial epicondyle of humerus, and deep antebrachial fascia.

Insertion: Flexor retinaculum, and palmar aponeurosis.

Action: Tenses the palmar fascia, flexes the wrist, and may assist in flexion of the elbow.

Nerve: Median, C(6), **7**, **8**, T1.

PALMARIS BREVIS

Origin: Ulnar border of palmar aponeurosis and palmar surface of flexor retinaculum.

Insertion: Skin on ulnar border of hand.

Action: Corrugates the skin on ulnar side of hand.

Nerve: Ulnar, C(7), **8**, T1.

PALMARIS LONGUS

Patient: Sitting or supine.

Fixation: The forearm rests on the table for support, in a position of supination.

Test: Tensing of the palmar fascia by strongly cupping the palm of the hand, and flexion of the wrist.

Pressure: Against the thenar and hypothenar eminences in the direction of the flattening the palm of the hand, and against the hand in the direction of extending the wrist.

Weakness: Decreases the ability to cup the palm of the hand. Strength of wrist flexion is diminished.

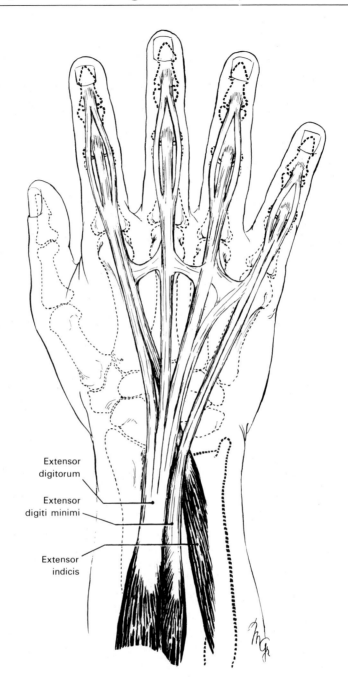

Extensor
digitorum

Extensor
digiti minimi

Extensor
indicis

EXTENSOR INDICIS

Origin: Posterior surface of body of ulna distal to origin of Extensor pollicis longus, and interosseus membrane.

Insertion: Into extensor expansion of index finger with Extensor digitorum longus tendon.

Action: Extends the metacarpophalangeal joint and, in conjunction with the Lumbricalis and Interossei, extends the interphalangeal joints of the index finger. May assist in adduction of the index finger.

Nerve: Radial, C6, **7, 8**.

EXTENSOR DIGITI MINIMI

Origin: Common extensor tendon from lateral epicondyle of humerus, and deep antebrachial fascia.

Insertion: Into extensor expansion of little finger with Extensor digitorum tendon.

Action: Extends the metacarpophalangeal joint and, in conjunction with the Lumbricalis and Interosseus, extends the interphalangeal joints of the little finger. Assists in abduction of the little finger.

Nerve: Radial, C6, **7, 8**.

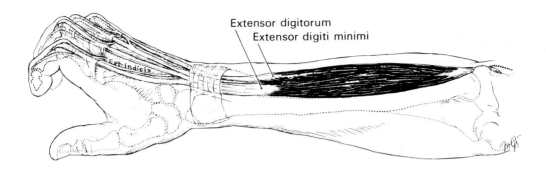

Extensor digitorum
Extensor digiti minimi

Ext. indicis

Origin: Common extensor tendon from lateral epicondyle of humerus, and deep antebrachial fascia.

Insertion: By four tendons, each penetrating a membranous expansion on the dorsum of the second to fifth digits and dividing over the proximal phalanx into a medial and two lateral bands. The medial band inserts into the base of the middle phalanx while the lateral bands reunite over the middle phalanx and insert into the base of the distal phalanx.

Action: Extends the metacarpophalangeal joints and, in conjunction with the Lumbricales and Interossei, extends the interphalangeal joints of the second through fifth digits. Assists in abduction of the index, ring, and little fingers; and assists in extension and abduction of the wrist.

Nerve: Radial, C**6, 7, 8**.

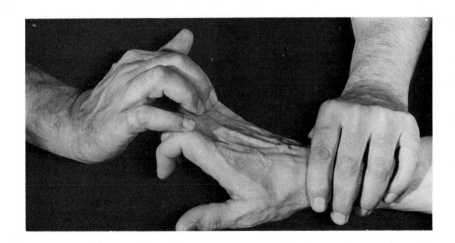

Patient: Sitting or supine.

Fixation: The examiner stabilizes the wrist, avoiding full extension.

Test: Extension of the metacarpophalangeal joints of the second through fifth digits, with interphalangeal joints relaxed.

Pressure: Against the dorsal surfaces of the proximal phalanges in the direction of flexion.

Weakness: Decreases the ability to extend the metacarpophalangeal joints of the second through fifth digits, and may result in a position of flexion of these joints. Strength of wrist extension is diminished.

Contracture: Hyperextension deformity of the metacarpophalangeal joints.

Shortness: Hyperextension of the metacarpophalangeal joints if the wrist is flexed, or extension of the wrist if the metacarpophalangeal joints are flexed.

Flexor Digitorum Superficialis

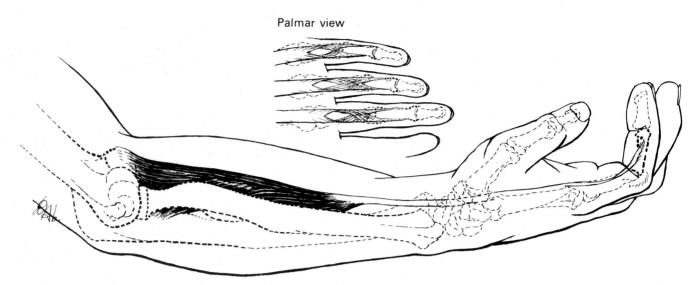

Palmar view

Origin of Humeral Head: Common flexor tendon from medial epicondyle of humerus, ulnar collateral ligament of elbow joint, and deep antebrachial fascia.

Origin of Ulnar Head: Medial side of coronoid process.

Origin of Radial Head: Oblique line of radius.

Insertion: By four tendons into sides of middle phalanges of second through fifth digits.

Action: Flexes the proximal interphalangeal joints of second through fifth digits, assists in flexion of the metacarpophalangeal joints and in flexion of the wrist.

Nerve: Median, C**7, 8**, T**1**.

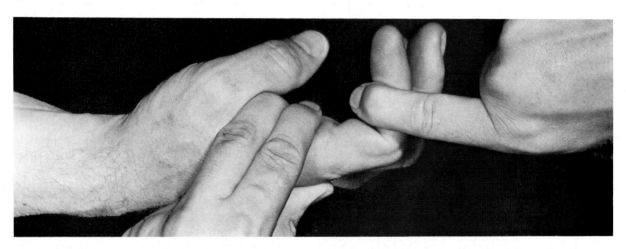

Patient: Sitting or supine.

Fixation: The examiner stabilizes the metacarpophalangeal joint, with the wrist in neutral position or in slight extension.

Test: Flexion of the proximal interphalangeal joint with the distal interphalangeal joint extended, of the second, third, fourth and fifth digits (see **Note**). Each finger is tested as illustrated for the index finger.

Pressure: Against the palmar surface of the middle phalanx in the direction of extension.

Weakness: Decreases the strength of the grip and of wrist flexion. Interferes with finger function in such activities as typing, piano playing, and playing some stringed instruments in which the proximal interphalangeal joint is flexed while the distal joint is extended. Weakness causes loss of joint stability at the proximal interphalangeal joints of the fingers so that in finger extension these joints hyperextend.

Contracture: Flexion deformity of the middle phalanges of the fingers.

Shortness: Flexion of the middle phalanges of the fingers if the wrist is extended, or flexion of the wrist if the fingers are extended.

Note: It appears to be the exception rather than the rule to obtain isolated Flexor superficialis action in the fifth digit.

Palmar view

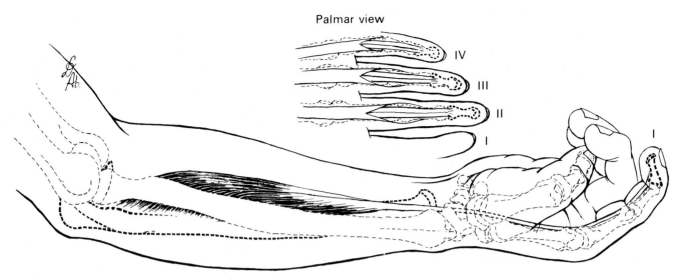

Origin: Anterior and medial surfaces of proximal three fourths of ulna, interosseus membrane, and deep antebrachial fascia.

Insertion: By four tendons into bases of distal phalanges, anterior surface.

Action: Flexes distal interphalangeal joints of index, middle, ring, and little fingers, and assists in flexion of proximal interphalangeal and metacarpophalangeal joints; may assist in flexion of the wrist.

Nerve to Profundus I and II: Median, C7, **8,** T1.

Nerve to Profundus III and IV: Ulnar, C7, **8,** T1.

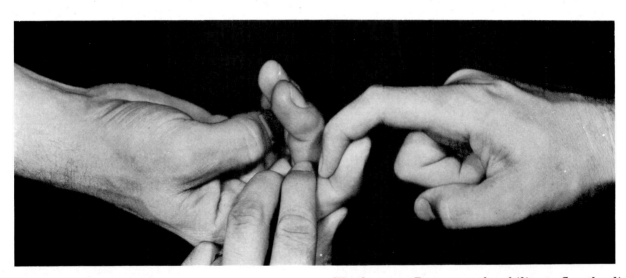

Patient: Sitting or supine.

Fixation: With the wrist in slight extension, the examiner stabilizes the proximal and middle phalanges.

Test: Flexion of the distal interphalangeal joint of the second, third, fourth, and fifth digits. Each finger is tested as illustrated above for the index finger.

Pressure: Against the palmar surface of the distal phalanx in the direction of extension.

Weakness: Decreases the ability to flex the distal joints of the fingers in direct proportion to the extent of weakness since this is the only muscle that flexes the distal interphalangeal joints. Flexion strength of the proximal interphalangeal, metacarpophalangeal, and wrist joints may be diminished.

Contracture: Flexion deformity of the distal phalanges of the fingers.

Shortness: Flexion of the fingers if the wrist is extended, or flexion of the wrist if the fingers are extended.

Flexor Carpi Radialis

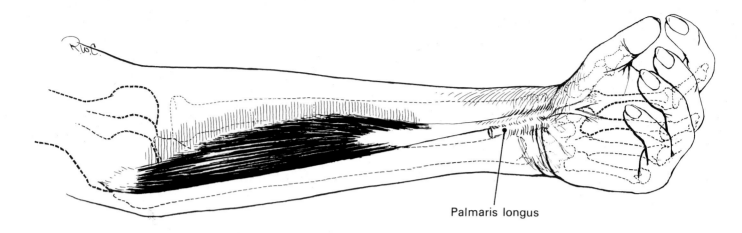

Palmaris longus

Origin: Common flexor tendon from medial epicondyle of humerus, and deep antebrachial fascia. (Fascia indicated by parallel lines.)

Insertion: Base of second metacarpal bone and a slip to base of third metacarpal bone.

Action: Flexes and abducts the wrist, and may assist in pronation of the forearm and flexion of the elbow.

Nerve: Median, C**6**, **7**, 8.

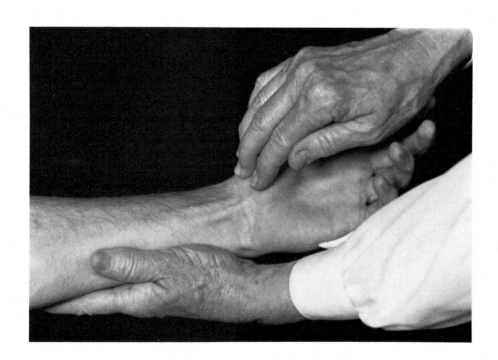

Patient: Sitting or supine.

Fixation: The forearm is in slightly less than full supination and rests on the table for support or is supported by the examiner.

Test: Flexion of the wrist toward the radial side. (See **Note** under **Flexor carpi ulnaris.**)

Pressure: Against the thenar eminence in the direction of extension toward the ulnar side.

Weakness: Decreases the strength of wrist flexion, and pronation strength may be diminished. Allows an ulnar deviation of the hand.

Contracture: Wrist flexion toward the radial side.

Note: The Palmaris longus cannot be ruled out in this test.

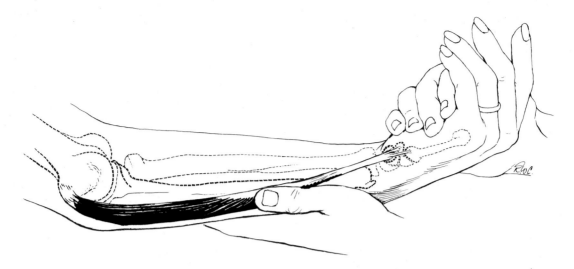

Origin of the Humeral Head: Common flexor tendon from medial epicondyle of humerus.

Origin of Ulnar Head: By aponeurosis from the medial margin of olecranon, proximal two thirds of posterior border of ulna, and from the deep antebrachial fascia.

Insertion: Pisiform bone and, by ligaments, to hamate and fifth metacarpal bones.

Action: Flexes and adducts the wrist, and may assist in flexion of the elbow.

Nerve: Ulnar, C7, **8**, T1.

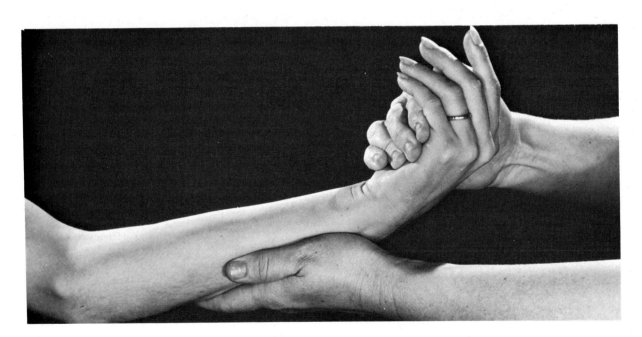

Patient: Sitting or supine.

Fixation: The forearm is in full supination and rests on the table for support or is supported by the examiner.

Test: Flexion of the wrist toward the ulnar side.

Pressure: Against the hypothenar eminence in the direction of extension toward the radial side.

Weakness: Decreases the strength of wrist flexion, and may result in a radial deviation of the hand.

Contracture: Wrist flexion toward the ulnar side.

Note: Normally, fingers will be relaxed when the wrist is flexed. If the fingers actively flex as wrist flexion is initiated, the finger flexors (profundus and superficialis) are attempting to substitute for the wrist flexors.

Extensor Carpi Radialis Longus and Brevis

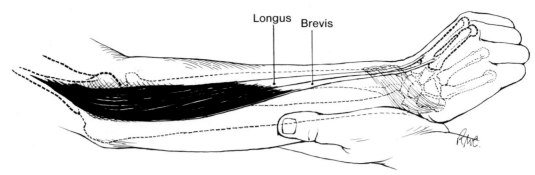

Longus Brevis

EXTENSOR CARPI RADIALIS LONGUS

Origin: Distal one third of lateral supracondylar ridge of humerus, and lateral intermuscular septum.

Insertion: Dorsal surface of base of second metacarpal bone, radial side.

Action: Extends and abducts the wrist, and assists in flexion of the elbow.

Nerve: Radial, C5, **6**, **7**, 8.

EXTENSOR CARPI RADIALIS BREVIS

Origin: Common extensor tendon from lateral epicondyle of humerus, radial collateral ligament of elbow joint, and deep antebrachial fascia.

Insertion: Dorsal surface of base of third metacarpal bone.

Action: Extends and assists in abduction of the wrist.

Nerve: Radial, C **6**, **7**, 8.

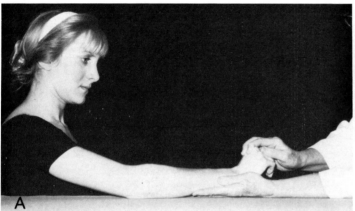

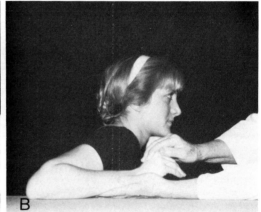

EXTENSOR CARPI RADIALIS LONGUS AND BREVIS

Patient: Sitting with elbow about 30° from zero extension (A).

Fixation: The forearm is in slightly less than full pronation and rests on the table for support.

Test: Extension of the wrist toward the radial side. (Fingers should be allowed to flex as the wrist is extended.)

Pressure: Against the dorsum of the hand along the second and third metacarpal bones in the direction of flexion toward the ulnar side.

Weakness: Decreases the strength of wrist extension, and allows an ulnar deviation of the hand.

Contracture: Wrist extension with radial deviation.

Note: (See note under Extensor carpi ulnaris.)

EXTENSOR CARPI RADIALIS BREVIS

Patient: Sitting with elbow fully flexed (B). (Have subject lean forward to flex elbow.)

Fixation: The forearm is in slightly less than full pronation and rests on the table for support.

Test: Extension of the wrist toward the radial side. Elbow flexion makes the Extensor carpi radialis longus less effective by being in a shortened position.

Pressure: Against the dorsum of the hand along the second and third metacarpal bones in the direction of flexion toward the ulnar side.

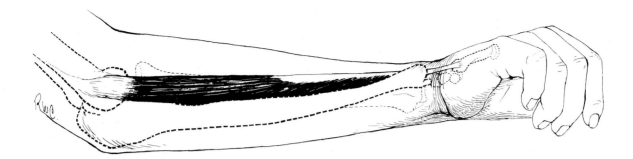

Origin: Common extensor tendon from lateral epicondyle of humerus, by aponeurosis from posterior border of ulna, and deep antebrachial fascia.

Insertion: Base of fifth metacarpal bone, ulnar side.

Action: Extends and adducts the wrist.

Nerve: Radial, C6, **7**, **8**.

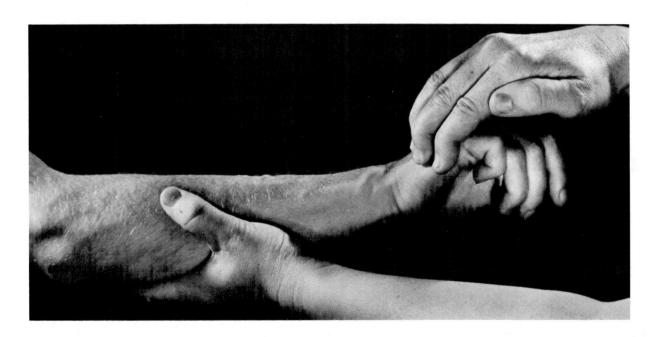

Patient: Sitting or supine.

Fixation: The forearm is in full pronation and rests on the table for support or is supported by the examiner.

Test: Extension of the wrist toward the ulnar side.

Pressure: Against the dorsum of the hand along the fifth metacarpal bone in the direction of flexion toward the radial side.

Weakness: Decreases the strength of wrist extension, and may result in a radial deviation of the hand.

Contracture: Ulnar deviation of the hand with slight extension.

Note: Normally, fingers will be in a position of passive flexion when the wrist is extended. If the fingers actively extend as wrist extension is initiated, the finger extensors (digitorum, indicis, and digiti minimi) are attempting to substitute for the wrist extensors.

Pronator Teres and Pronator Quadratus

PRONATOR TERES

Origin of Humeral Head: Immediately above medial epicondyle of humerus, common flexor tendon, and deep antebrachial fascia.

Origin of Ulnar Head: Medial side of coronoid process of ulna.

Insertion: Middle of lateral surface of radius.

Action: Pronates the forearm and assists in flexing the elbow joint.

Nerve: Median, C**6**, **7**.

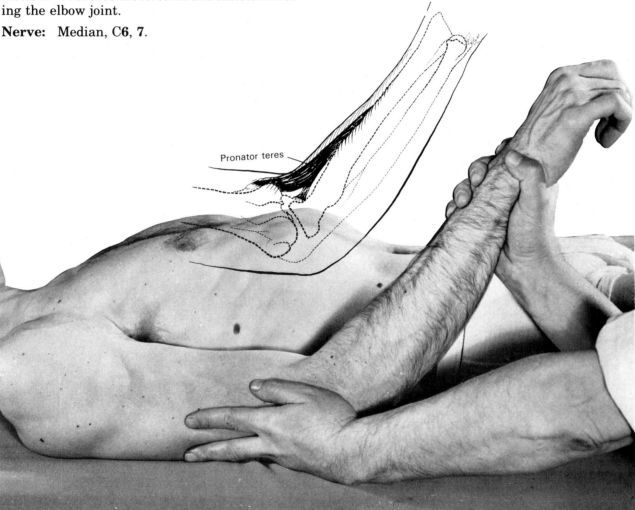

Pronator teres

PRONATORS TERES AND QUADRATUS

Patient: Supine or sitting.

Fixation: The elbow should be held against the patient's side, or be stabilized by the examiner to avoid any shoulder abduction movement.

Test: Pronation of the forearm with the elbow partially flexed.

Pressure: At the lower forearm above the wrist (to avoid twisting the wrist) in the direction of supinating the forearm.

Weakness: Allows a supinated position of the forearm; interferes with many everyday functions such as turning a doorknob, using a knife to cut meats, or turning the hand downward in picking up a cup or other object.

Contracture: With the forearm held in a position of pronation, there is a marked interference with many normal functions of the hand and forearm that require moving from pronation to supination.

Origin: Medial side, anterior surface of distal one fourth of ulna.

Insertion: Lateral side, anterior surface of distal one fourth of radius.

Action: Pronates the forearm.

Nerve: Median, C7, **8**, T1.

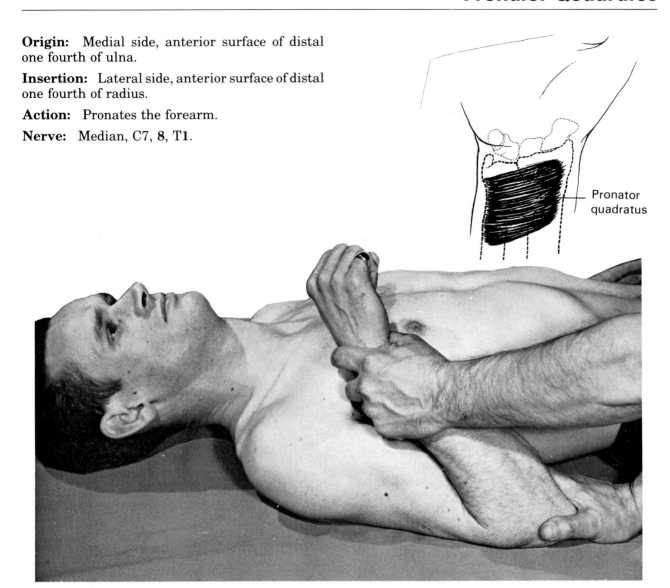

Pronator quadratus

Patient: Supine or sitting.

Fixation: The elbow should be held against the patient's side (by either the patient or the examiner) to avoid shoulder abduction.

Test: Pronation of the forearm with the elbow completely flexed in order to make the humeral

head of the Pronator teres less effective by being in a shortened position.

Pressure: At the lower forearm above the wrist (to avoid twisting the wrist) in the direction of supinating the forearm.

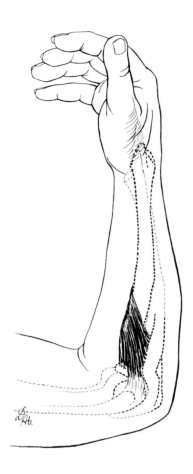

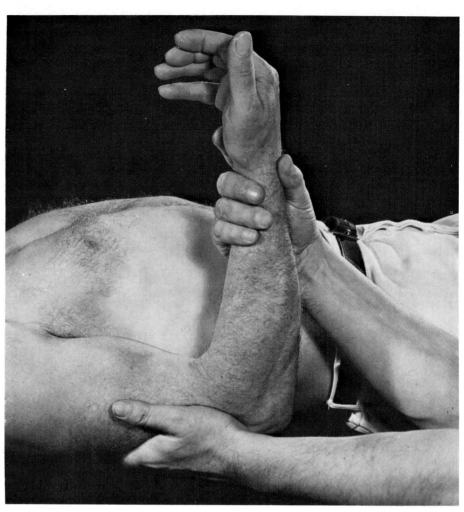

SUPINATOR

Origin: Lateral epicondyle of humerus, radial collateral ligament of elbow joint, annular ligament of radius, and supinator crest of ulna.

Insertion: Lateral surface of upper one third of body of radius covering part of anterior and posterior surfaces.

Action: Supinates the forearm.

Nerve: Radial, C5, **6**, (7).

SUPINATOR AND BICEPS

Patient: Supine.

Fixation: The elbow should be held against the patient's side to avoid shoulder movement.

Test: Supination of the forearm with elbow at right angle or slightly below.

Pressure: At the distal end of the forearm above the wrist (to avoid twisting the wrist) in the direction of pronating the forearm.

Weakness: Allows the forearm to remain in a pronated position. Interferes with many functions of the extremity, particularly those involved in feeding oneself.

Contracture: Elbow flexion with forearm supination. Results in marked interference with functions of the extremity that involve the change from supinated to pronated position of the forearm.

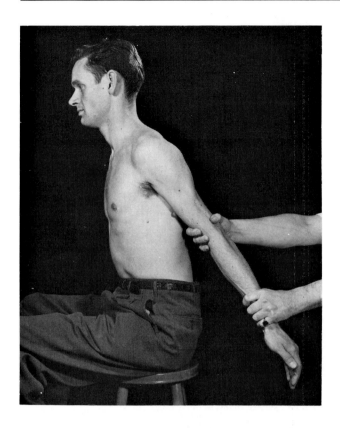

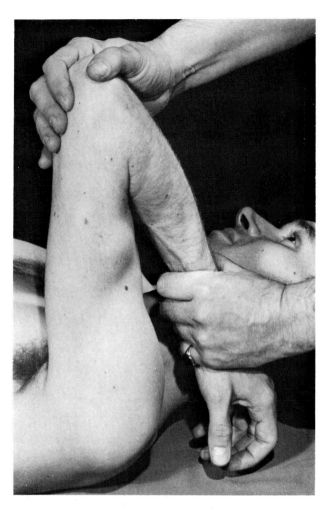

SUPINATOR

(Tested with Biceps elongated.)

Patient: Sitting or standing.

Fixation: The examiner holds the shoulder and elbow in extension.

Test: Supination of the forearm.

Pressure: At the distal end of the forearm above the wrist, in the direction of pronation. The subject may attempt to rotate the humerus laterally to make it appear that the forearm remains in supination as pressure is applied and the forearm starts to pronate.

SUPINATOR

(Tested with Biceps in shortened position.)

Patient: Supine.

Fixation: The examiner holds the shoulder in flexion with the elbow completely flexed. It is usually advisable to have the subject close the fingers in order to keep them from touching the table, which may be done in an effort to brace the forearm in test position.

Test: Supination of the forearm.

Pressure: At the distal end of the forearm above the wrist in the direction of pronation. Care should be taken to *avoid* maximum pressure because, as strong pressure is applied, the Biceps comes into action and, in this shortened position, goes into a cramp. A severe cramp may leave the muscle sore for several days. This test should be used merely as a differential diagnostic aid.

Note: In a radial nerve lesion involving the supinator, the test position cannot be maintained. The forearm will fail to hold the fully supinated position even though the Biceps is normal.

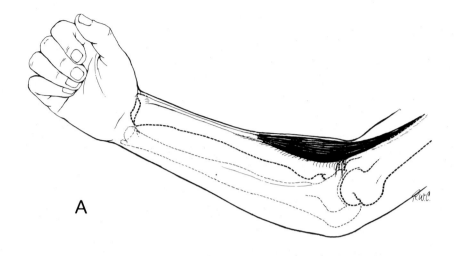

A

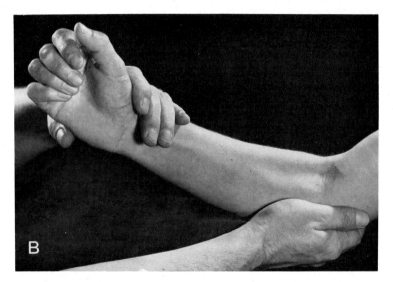

B

Origin: Proximal two thirds of lateral supracondylar ridge of humerus, and lateral intermuscular septum.

Insertion: Lateral side of base of styloid process of radius.

Action: Flexes the elbow joint, and assists in pronating and supinating the forearm when these movements are resisted.

Nerve: Radial: C**5, 6**.

Patient: Supine or sitting.

Fixation: The examiner places one hand under the elbow to cushion it from table pressure.

Test: Flexion of the elbow with the forearm neutral between pronation and supination. The belly of the brachioradialis (visible in B) must be seen and felt during this test because the movement can be produced by other muscles which flex the elbow.

Pressure: Against the lower forearm in the direction of extension.

Weakness: Decreases the strength of elbow flexion and of resisted supination or pronation to midline.

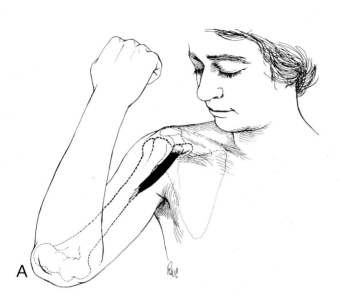

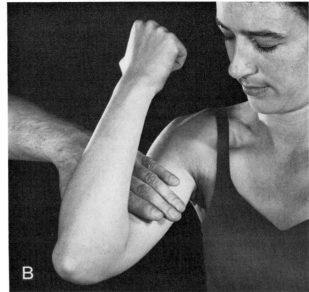

Origin: Apex of coracoid process of scapula.

Insertion: Medial surface of middle of shaft of humerus, opposite deltoid tuberosity.

Action: Flexes and adducts the shoulder joint.

Nerve: Musculocutaneous, C**6, 7**.

Patient: Sitting or supine.

Fixation: If trunk is stable, no fixation by examiner should be necessary.

Test: Shoulder flexion in lateral rotation with the elbow completely flexed and forearm supinated. Assistance from the biceps in shoulder flex-ion is decreased in this test position because the complete elbow flexion and forearm supination place the muscle in too short a position to be effective in shoulder flexion.

Pressure: Against the anteromedial surface of the lower third of the humerus in the direction of extension and slight abduction (B).

Weakness: Decreases the strength of shoulder flexion particularly in movements that involve complete elbow flexion and supination, for example, combing the hair.

Shortness: The coracoid process is depressed anteriorly when the arm is down at the side.

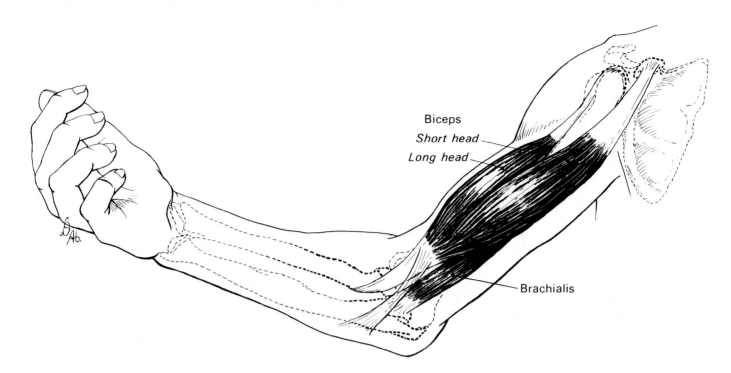

Biceps
Short head
Long head

Brachialis

BICEPS BRACHII

Origin of Short Head: Apex of coracoid process of scapula.

Origin of Long Head: Supraglenoid tubercle of scapula.

Insertion: Tuberosity of radius, and aponeurosis of Biceps brachii (lacertus fibrosus).

Action: Flexes the shoulder joint, and the long head may assist with abduction if the humerus is laterally rotated. *With the origin fixed,* flexes the elbow joint moving the forearm toward the humerus, and supinates the forearm. *With the insertion fixed,* flexes the elbow joint moving the humerus toward the forearm as in pull-up or chinning exercises.

Nerve: Musculocutaneous, C**5, 6**.

BRACHIALIS

Origin: Distal one half of anterior surface of humerus, and medial and lateral intermuscular septa.

Insertion: Tuberosity and coronoid process of ulna.

Action: *With the origin fixed,* flexes the elbow joint moving the forearm toward the humerus. *With the insertion fixed,* flexes the elbow joint moving the humerus toward the forearm as in pull-up or chinning exercises.

Nerve: Musculocutaneous, and small branch from radial, C**5, 6**.

Patient: Supine or sitting.

Fixation: The examiner places one hand under the elbow to cushion it from table pressure.

Test: Elbow flexion slightly less than or at right angle, with forearm in supination.

Pressure: Against the lower forearm in the direction of extension.

Weakness: Decreases the ability to flex the forearm against gravity. There is marked interference with such daily activities as feeding oneself or combing the hair.

Contracture: Flexion deformity of the elbow.

Note: If the Biceps and Brachialis are weak as in a musculocutaneous lesion, the patient will pronate the forearm before flexing the elbow using Brachioradialis, Extensor carpi radialis longus, Pronator teres, and wrist flexors.

The lower figure on the facing page illustrates that, against resistance, the Biceps acts in flexion even though the forearm is in pronation. Since the Brachialis is inserted on the ulna, the position of the forearm, whether in supination or pronation, does not affect the action of this muscle in elbow flexion. The Brachioradialis appears to have a slightly stronger action in the pronated position of the forearm in the elbow flexion test than in the supinated position, although its strongest action in flexion is with the forearm in midposition.

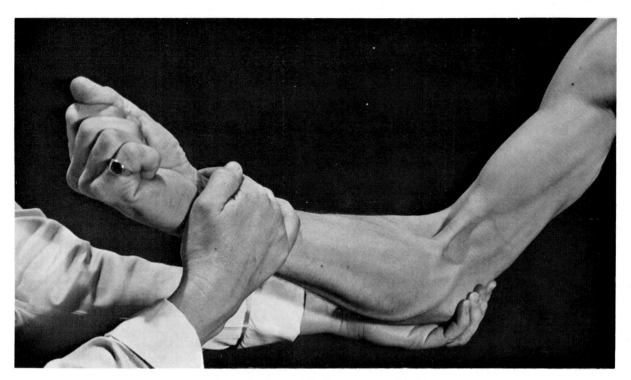

Elbow flexion with forearm supinated.

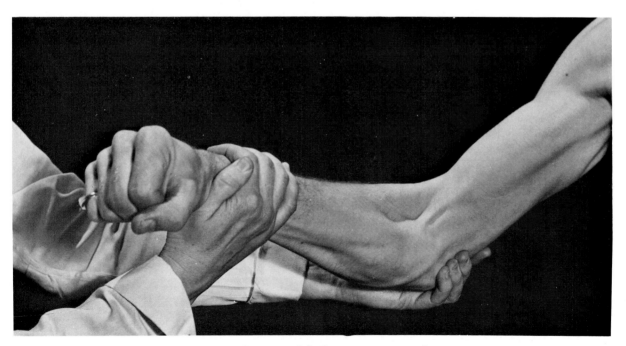

Elbow flexion with forearm pronated.

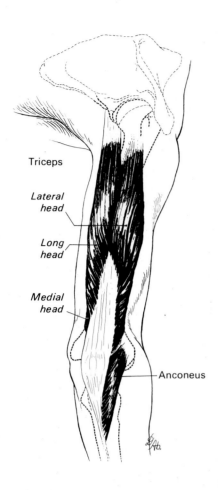

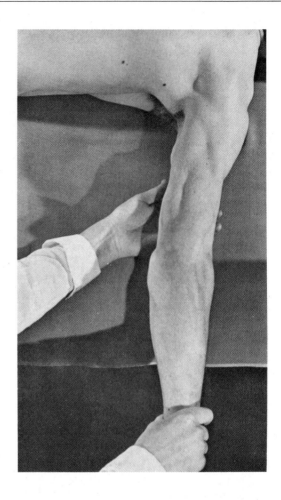

TRICEPS BRACHII

Origin of Long Head: Infraglenoid tubercle of scapula.

Origin of Lateral Head: Lateral and posterior surfaces of proximal one half of body of humerus, and lateral intermuscular septum.

Origin of Medial Head: Distal two thirds of medial and posterior surfaces of humerus below the radial groove, and from medial intermuscular septum.

Insertion: Posterior surface of olecranon process of ulna and antebrachial fascia.

Action: Extends the elbow joint. In addition, the long head assists in adduction and extension of the shoulder joint.

Nerve: Radial, C6, **7**, **8**, T1.

ANCONEUS

Origin: Lateral epicondyle of humerus, posterior surface.

Insertion: Lateral side of olecranon process, and upper one fourth of posterior surface of body of ulna.

Action: Extends the elbow joint, and may stabilize the ulna during pronation and supination.

Nerve: Radial, C**7**, **8**.

TRICEPS BRACHII AND ANCONEUS

Patient: Prone.

Fixation: The shoulder is at 90° abduction, neutral with regard to rotation, and with the arm supported between the shoulder and the elbow by the table. The examiner places one hand under the arm near the elbow to cushion the arm from table pressure.

Test: Extension of the elbow joint (to slightly less than full extension).

Pressure: Against the forearm in the direction of flexion.

TRICEPS BRACHII AND ANCONEUS

Patient: Supine.

Fixation: The shoulder is at approximately 90° flexion, with the arm supported in a position perpendicular to the table.

Test: Extension of the elbow (to slightly less than full extension).

Pressure: Against the forearm in the direction of flexion.

Weakness: Results in the inability to extend the forearm against gravity. There is interference with everyday functions which involve elbow extension as in reaching upward toward a high shelf. There is loss of ability to throw objects or push with the extended elbow. An individual is handicapped in using crutches or a cane because of inability to extend the elbow and transfer weight to the hand.

Contracture: Extension deformity of the elbow. Marked interference with everyday functions that involve elbow flexion.

Note: When the shoulder is horizontally abducted (see facing page), the long head of the Triceps is shortened over both the shoulder and elbow joints. When the shoulder is flexed (horizontally adducted), the long head of the Triceps is shortened over the elbow joint while elongated over the shoulder joint. Because of this two-joint action of the long head, it is made less effective in the prone position by being shortened over both joints, with the result that *the Triceps withstands less pressure when tested in the prone position than in the supine position.*

While the Triceps and Anconeus act together in extending the elbow joint, it may be useful to differentiate these two muscles. Since the belly of the Anconeus muscle is below the elbow joint, it can be distinguished from the Triceps by palpation. The branch of the radial nerve to the Anconeus arises near the midhumeral level and is quite long. It is possible for a lesion to involve only this branch leaving the Triceps unaffected. Paralysis of the Anconeus reduces the strength of elbow extension. One may find that a grade of good elbow extension strength is actually the result of a normal Triceps and a zero Anconeus.

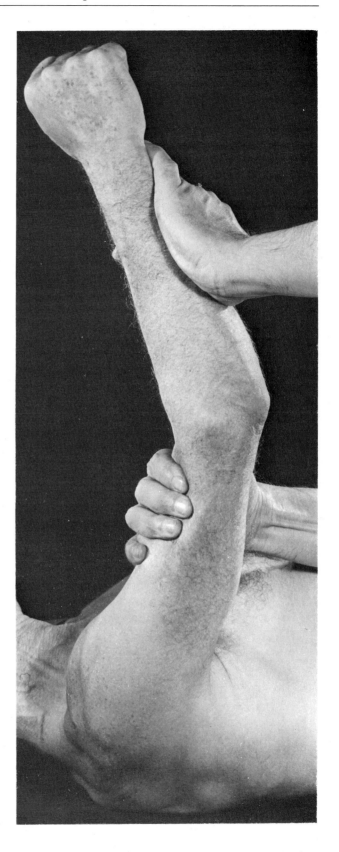

Supraspinatus

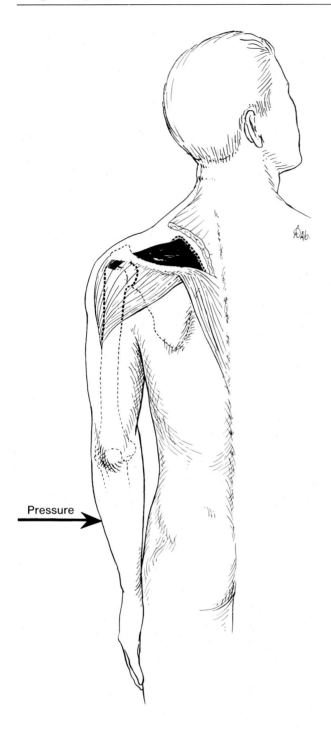

Origin: Medial two thirds of supraspinous fossa of scapula.

Insertion: Superior facet of greater tubercle of humerus, and shoulder joint capsule.

Action: Abducts the shoulder joint, and stabilizes the head of the humerus in the glenoid cavity during movements of this joint.

Nerve: Suprascapular, C4, **5, 6.**

Patient: Sitting or standing with arm at side, head and neck extended and laterally flexed to same side and the face rotated toward the opposite side.

Fixation: None necessary since maximum pressure is not required.

Note: No effort is made to distinguish the Supraspinatus from the Deltoid in the strength test for the purpose of grading since these muscles act simultaneously in abducting the shoulder. However, the Supraspinatus can be palpated to determine whether it is active.

Since the Supraspinatus is completely covered by the upper and middle fibers of the Trapezius, to palpate this muscle the Trapezius should be as relaxed as possible. This is accomplished by extending and laterally flexing the head and neck so that the face is rotated toward the opposite side, as illustrated; and by testing the activity of the Supraspinatus at the beginning of the abduction movement when the activity of the Trapezius is at a low level. The Deltoid and the Supraspinatus act together in initiating abduction, and this test is not to be construed to mean that the Supraspinatus is responsible for the first few degrees of abduction.

Test: Initiation of abduction of the humerus.

Pressure: Against the forearm in the direction of adduction.

Weakness: The tendon of the Supraspinatus is firmly attached to the superior surface of the capsule of the shoulder joint. Weakness of the muscle or a rupture of the tendon decreases shoulder joint stability, allowing the head of the humerus to alter its relationship with the glenoid cavity.

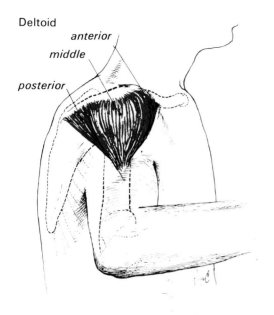

Deltoid
  anterior
  middle
  posterior

Superior View

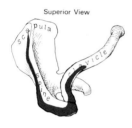

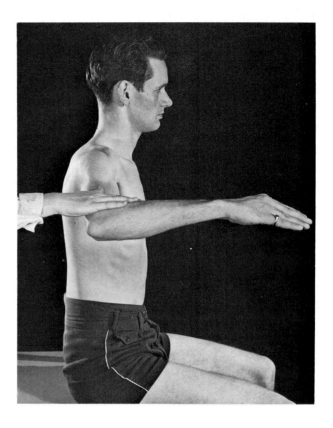

DELTOID

Origin of Anterior Fibers: Anterior border, superior surface, lateral one third of clavicle.

Origin of Middle Fibers: Lateral margin and superior surface of acromion.

Origin of Posterior Fibers: Inferior lip of posterior border of spine of scapula.

Insertion: Deltoid tuberosity of humerus.

Action: Abduction of the shoulder joint, performed chiefly by the middle fibers with stabilization by the anterior and posterior fibers. In addition, the anterior fibers flex and, in the supine position, medially rotate the shoulder joint; the posterior fibers extend and, in the prone position, laterally rotate.

Nerve: Axillary, C5, **6**.

Patient: Sitting.

Fixation: The position of the trunk in relation to the arm in this test is such that a stable trunk will need no further stabilization by the examiner. If the scapular fixation muscles are weak, the examiner must stabilize the scapula.

Test: Shoulder abduction without rotation. When placing the shoulder in test position, the elbow should be flexed to indicate the neutral position of rotation, but may be extended after the shoulder position is established in order to use the extended extremity for a longer lever. The examiner should be consistent in the technique for subsequent tests.

Pressure: Against the dorsal surface of the distal end of the humerus if the elbow is flexed, or against the forearm if the elbow is extended.

Weakness: Results in the inability to lift the arm in abduction against gravity. In the presence of paralysis of the entire Deltoid and Supraspinatus, the humerus tends to subluxate downward if the arm remains unsupported in a hanging position. The capsule of the shoulder joint permits almost an inch of separation of the head of the humerus from the glenoid cavity. In cases of axillary nerve involvement in which the Deltoid is weak while the Supraspinatus is not affected, the relaxation of the joint is not as marked, but tends to progress if the Deltoid strength does not return.

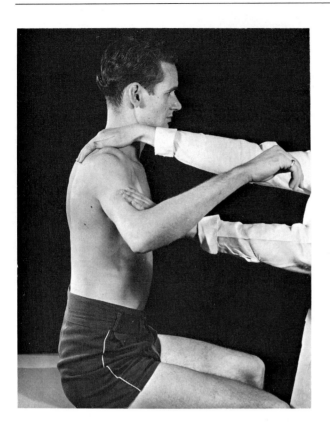 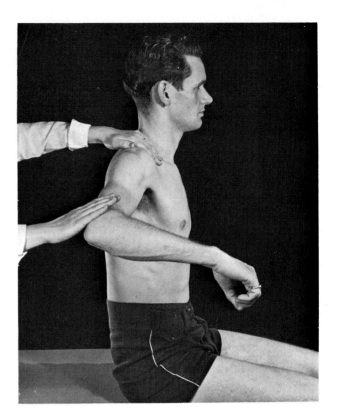

ANTERIOR DELTOID

Patient: Sitting.

Fixation: If scapular fixation muscles are weak, the scapula must be stabilized by the examiner. As pressure is applied on the arm, counterpressure is applied posteriorly to the shoulder girdle.

Test: Shoulder abduction in slight flexion, with the humerus in slight lateral rotation. In the erect sitting position it is necessary to place the humerus in slight lateral rotation to increase the effect of gravity on the anterior fibers. (The anatomical action of the anterior Deltoid, which entails slight medial rotation, is part of the test of the anterior Deltoid in the supine position.) (See facing page.)

Pressure: Against the anteromedial surface of the arm in the direction of adduction and slight extension.

POSTERIOR DELTOID

Patient: Sitting.

Fixation: If scapular fixation muscles are weak, the scapula must be stabilized by the examiner. As pressure is applied on the arm, counterpressure is applied anteriorly on the shoulder girdle.

Test: Shoulder abduction in slight extension, with the humerus in slight medial rotation. In the erect sitting position it is necessary to place the humerus in slight medial rotation in order to have the posterior fibers in an antigravity position. (The anatomical action of the posterior Deltoid, which entails slight lateral rotation, is part of the test of the posterior Deltoid in the prone position.) (See facing page.)

Pressure: Against the posterolateral surface of the arm above the elbow in the direction of adduction and slight flexion.

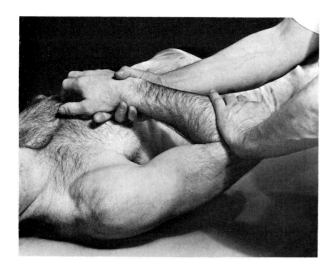

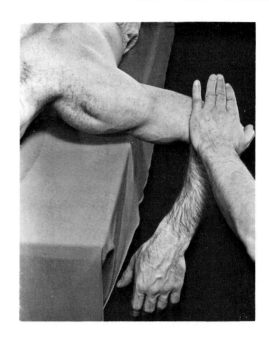

ANTERIOR DELTOID

Patient: Supine.

Fixation: The Trapezius and Serratus anterior should stabilize the scapula in all the Deltoid tests, and if these muscles are weak the examiner should stabilize the scapula.

Test: Shoulder abduction in the position of slight flexion and medial rotation. One hand of the examiner is placed under the patient's wrist to make sure that the elbow is not lifted by reverse action of the wrist extensors which may occur if the patient is allowed to press the hand down on the chest.

Pressure: Against the anterior surface of the arm just above the elbow, in the direction of adduction toward the side of the body.

POSTERIOR DELTOID

Patient: Prone.

Fixation: The scapula must be held stable by scapular muscles or by the examiner.

Test: Horizontal abduction of the shoulder with slight lateral rotation.

Pressure: Against the posterolateral surface of the arm in a direction obliquely downward midway between adduction and horizontal adduction.

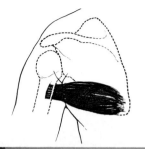

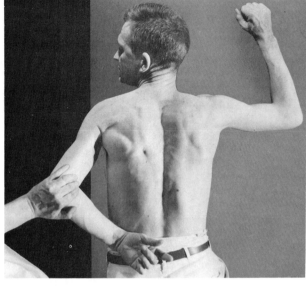

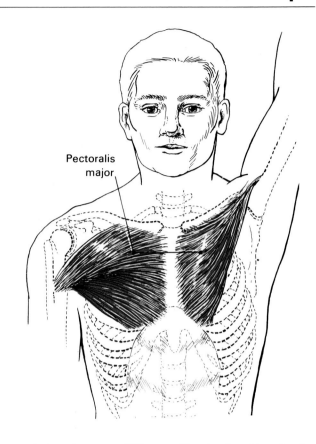

Pectoralis major

Origin: Dorsal surfaces of inferior angle and lower third of lateral border of scapula.

Insertion: Crest of lesser tubercle of humerus.

Action: Medially rotates, adducts, and extends the shoulder joint.

Nerve: Lower subscapular, C5, **6**, 7.

Patient: Prone.

Fixation: Usually none is necessary because the weight of the trunk is sufficient fixation. If necessary, the opposite shoulder may be held down on the table.

Test: Extension and adduction of the humerus in the medially rotated position, with the hand resting on the posterior iliac crest.

Pressure: Against the arm above the elbow in the direction of abduction and flexion.

Weakness: Diminishes the strength of medial rotation, adduction and extension of the humerus.

Shortness: Prevents full range of lateral rotation and abduction of the humerus. With tightness of the Teres major the scapula will begin to rotate laterally almost simultaneously with flexion or abduction. Scapular movements that accompany shoulder flexion and abduction are influenced by the degree of muscle shortness of the Teres major and Subscapularis.

Origin of Upper Fibers (Clavicular Portion): Anterior surface of sternal one half of clavicle.

Origin of Lower Fibers (Sternocostal Portion): Anterior surface of sternum, cartilages of first six or seven ribs, and aponeurosis of the External oblique.

Insertion of Upper and Lower Fibers: Crest of greater tubercle of humerus. Upper fibers are more anterior and caudal on the crest than the lower fibers which twist on themselves and are more posterior and cranial.

Action of Muscle as a Whole: *With the origin fixed,* it adducts and medially rotates the humerus. With the *insertion fixed,* the Pectoralis major may assist in elevating the thorax as in forced inspiration. In crutch-walking or in parallel-bar work, it will assist in supporting the weight of the body.

Action of Upper Fibers: Flex and medially rotate the shoulder joint, and horizontally adduct the humerus toward the opposite shoulder.

Nerve to Upper Fibers: Lateral Pectoral C5, **6**, 7.

Action of Lower Fibers: Depress the shoulder girdle by virtue of attachment on the humerus, and obliquely adduct the humerus toward the opposite iliac crest.

Nerves to Lower Fibers: Lateral and medial pectoral, C6, **7**, 8, T1.

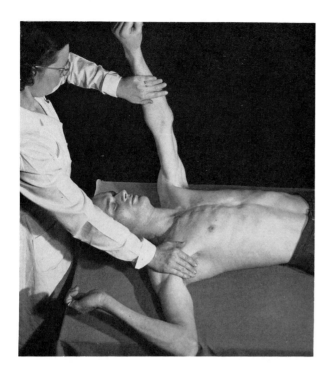

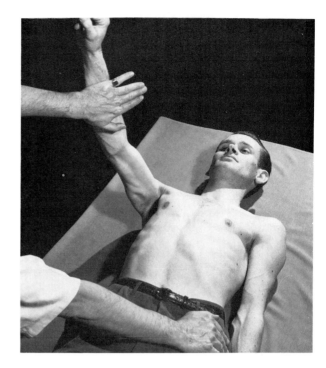

Patient: Supine.

Fixation: The examiner holds the opposite shoulder firmly on the table. The Triceps maintains the elbow in extension.

Test: Starting with the elbow extended, and the shoulder in 90° flexion and slight medial rotation, the humerus is horizontally adducted toward the sternal end of the clavicle.

Pressure: Against the forearm in the direction of horizontal abduction.

Weakness: Decreases the ability to draw the arm in horizontal adduction across the chest, making it difficult to touch the hand to the opposite shoulder. Decreases strength of shoulder flexion and medial rotation.

Shortness: The range of motion in horizontal abduction and lateral rotation of the shoulder is decreased. A shortness of the Pectoralis major holds the humerus in medial rotation and adduction, and, secondarily results in abduction of the scapula from the spine.

Note: The authors have seen one patient with rupture and another with weakness of the lower part of the Pectoralis major resulting from arm wrestling. The arm was in a position of lateral rotation and abduction when a forceful effort was made to medially rotate and adduct it.

Patient: Supine.

Fixation: The examiner places one hand on opposite iliac crest to hold the pelvis firmly on the table. The anterior parts of the External and Internal oblique muscles stabilize the thorax on the pelvis. In cases of abdominal weakness, the thorax instead of the pelvis, must be stabilized. The Triceps maintains the elbow in extension.

Test: Starting with the elbow extended, and the shoulder in flexion and slight medial rotation, adduction of the arm obliquely toward the opposite iliac crest.

Pressure: Against the forearm obliquely in a lateral and cranial direction.

Weakness: Decreases the strength of adduction obliquely toward the opposite hip. There is a loss of continuity of muscle action from the Pectoralis major to External oblique and Internal oblique on the opposite side with the result that chopping or striking movements are difficult. From a supine position, if the subject's arm is placed diagonally overhead, it will be difficult to lift the arm from the table. The subject will also have difficulty holding any large or heavy object in both hands at or near waist level.

Shortness: There is a forward depression of the shoulder girdle by the pull of the Pectoralis major on the humerus that often accompanies the pull of a tight Pectoralis minor on the scapula. Flexion and abduction ranges of motion overhead are limited.

Pectoralis Minor

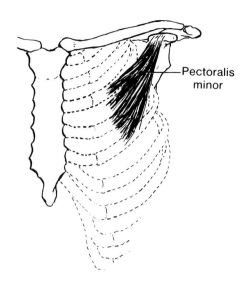

Pectoralis minor

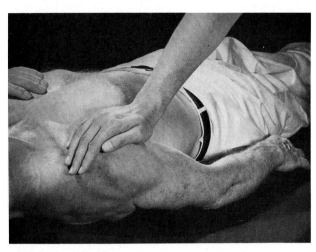

Origin: Superior margins, outer surfaces of third, fourth, and fifth ribs near the cartilages; and from fascia over corresponding intercostal muscles.

Insertion: Medial border, superior surface of coracoid process of scapula.

Action: *With the origin fixed,* tilts the scapula anteriorly, i.e., rotates the scapula about a coronal axis so that the coracoid process moves anteriorly and caudally, while the inferior angle moves posteriorly and medially. With the scapula stabilized *to fix the insertion,* the Pectoralis minor assists in forced inspiration.

Nerve: Medial pectoral with fibers from a communicating branch of the lateral pectoral, C(6), **7, 8,** T1. (For explanation, see p. 405.)

TEST FOR SHORTNESS OF PECTORALIS MINOR

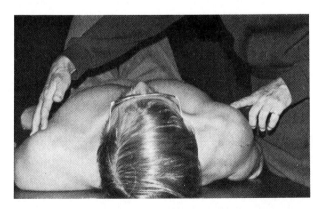

Left, normal length; right, short, holding shoulder forward.

Patient: Supine.

Fixation: None by the examiner unless the abdominal muscles are weak, in which case the rib cage on the same side should be held firmly down.

Test: Forward thrust of the shoulder with the arm at the side. The subject must exert no downward pressure on the hand to force the shoulder forward. (If necessary raise the subject's hand and elbow off the table.)

Pressure: Against the anterior aspect of the shoulder downward toward the table.

Weakness: Strong extension of the humerus is dependent upon fixation of the scapula by the Rhomboids and Levator scapulae posteriorly and the Pectoralis minor anteriorly. With weakness of the Pectoralis minor, the strength of arm extension is diminished.

With the scapula stabilized in a position of good alignment, the Pectoralis minor acts as an accessory muscle of inspiration. Weakness of this muscle will increase respiratory difficulty in patients already suffering from involvement of respiratory muscles.

Contracture: With the origin of this muscle on the ribs and the insertion on the coracoid process of the scapula, a contracture of this muscle tends to depress the coracoid process of the scapula forward and downward. Such muscle contracture is an important contributing factor in many cases of arm pain. With the cords of the brachial plexus and the axillary blood vessels lying between the coracoid process and rib cage, contracture of the Pectoralis minor may produce an impingement on these large vessels and nerves.

A contracted Pectoralis minor restricts flexion of the shoulder joint by limiting scapular rotation and preventing the glenoid cavity from attaining the cranial orientation necessary for complete flexion of the joint.

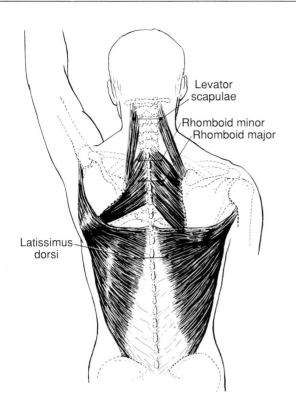

Origin: Spinous processes of last six thoracic vertebrae, last three or four ribs, through the thoracolumbar fascia from the lumbar and sacral vertebrae and posterior one third of external lip of iliac crest, a slip from the inferior angle of the scapula.

Insertion: Intertubercular groove of humerus.

Action: *With the origin fixed,* medially rotates, adducts, and extends the shoulder joint. By continued action, depresses the shoulder girdle, and assists in lateral flexion of the trunk. (See p. 144.) *With the insertion fixed,* assists in tilting the pelvis anteriorly and laterally. Acting bilaterally, this muscle assists in hyperextending the spine and anteriorly tilting the pelvis, or in flexing the spine, depending upon its relation to the axes of motion.

This muscle is important in relation to movements such as climbing, walking with crutches, or hoisting the body up on parallel bars, in which the muscles act to lift the body toward the fixed arms. The strength of the Latissimus dorsi is a factor in such forceful arm movements as swimming, rowing, and chopping. All adductors and medial rotators act in these strong movements but the Latissimus dorsi may be of major importance.

The Latissimus dorsi may act as an accessory muscle of respiration.

Nerve: Thoracodorsal, C6, **7, 8**.

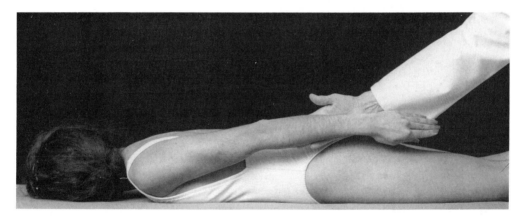

Patient: Prone.

Fixation: One hand of the examiner may apply counter-pressure laterally on pelvis.

Test: Adduction of the arm, with extension, in the medially rotated position.

Pressure: Against the forearm in the direction of abduction and slight flexion of the arm.

Weakness: Weakness interferes with activities that involve adduction of the arm toward the body or the body toward the arm. The strength of lateral trunk flexion is diminished.

Shortness: Results in a limitation of elevation of the arm in flexion or abduction. Tends to depress the shoulder girdle down and forward. In a right C-curve of the spine, the lateral fibers of the left Latissimus dorsi usually are shortened. The anterior fibers are shortened bilaterally in a marked kyphosis.

Shortness of the Latissimus dorsi may be found in individuals who have walked with crutches for a prolonged period of time, as, for example, the paraplegic who uses a swing-through gait.

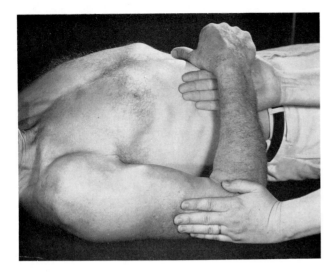

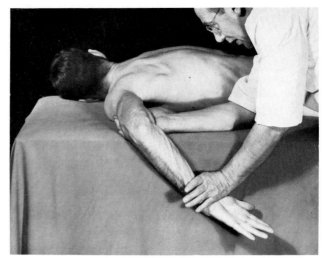

The chief muscles acting in this shoulder medial rotation test are Latissimus dorsi, Pectoralis major, Subscapularis, and Teres major.

Patient: Supine.

Fixation: Counterpressure is applied by the examiner against the outer aspect of the distal end of the humerus in order to ensure a rotation motion.

Test: Medial rotation of the humerus with arm at side and elbow held at right angle.

Pressure: Using the forearm as a lever, pressure is applied in the direction of laterally rotating the humerus.

Note: For the purpose of objectively grading a weak medial rotator group against gravity, the test in the prone position (see above right) is preferred over the test in supine position. For a maximum strength test, the test in supine position is preferred because less scapular fixation is required.

Patient: Prone.

Fixation: The arm rests on the table. The examiner's hand, near the elbow, cushions against table pressure and stabilizes the humerus to ensure a rotation action by preventing any adduction or abduction. The Rhomboids give fixation of the scapula.

Test: Medial rotation of the humerus with the elbow held at right angle.

Pressure: Using the forearm as a lever, pressure is applied in the direction of laterally rotating the humerus.

Weakness: Inasmuch as the medial rotators are also strong adductors, the ability to perform both medial rotation and adduction is decreased.

Shortness: Range of shoulder flexion overhead and lateral rotation are limited.

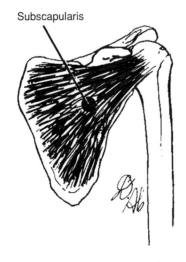

Subscapularis

SUBSCAPULARIS

Origin: Subscapular fossa of scapula.

Insertion: Lesser tubercle of humerus and shoulder joint capsule.

Action: Medially rotates the shoulder joint, and stabilizes the head of the humerus in the glenoid cavity during movements of this joint.

Nerve: Upper and lower subscapular, C5, **6**, 7.

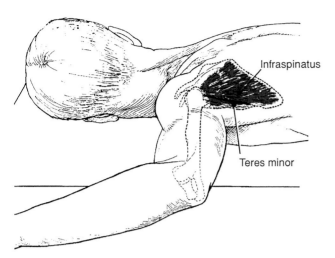

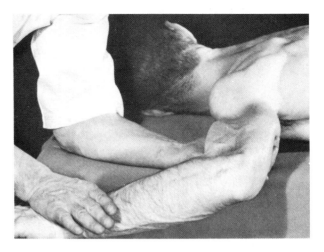

INFRASPINATUS

Origin: Medial two thirds of infraspinous fossa of scapula.

Insertion: Middle facet of greater tubercle of humerus, and shoulder joint capsule.

Action: Laterally rotates the shoulder joint and stabilizes the head of the humerus in the glenoid cavity during movements of this joint.

Nerve: Suprascapular, C(4), **5**, **6**.

TERES MINOR

Origin: Upper two thirds, dorsal surface of lateral border of scapula.

Insertion: Lowest facet of greater tubercle of humerus, and shoulder joint capsule.

Action: Laterally rotates the shoulder joint, and stabilizes the head of the humerus in the glenoid cavity during movements of this joint.

Nerve: Axillary, C**5**, **6**.

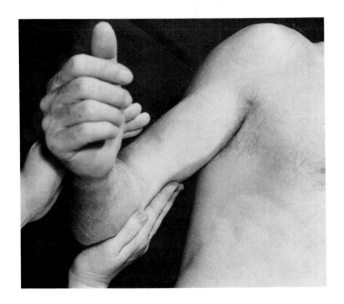

Patient: Prone.

Fixation: The arm rests on the table. The examiner places one hand under the arm near the elbow and stabilizes the humerus to ensure a rotation action by preventing adduction or abduction motion. The examiner's hand cushions against the table pressure. This test requires strong fixation by the scapular muscles, particularly the middle and lower Trapezius, and in using this test one must observe whether the lateral rotators of the scapula or the lateral rotators of the shoulder break when pressure is applied.

Test: Lateral rotation of the humerus with the elbow held at right angle.

Pressure: Using the forearm as a lever, pressure is applied in the direction of medially rotating the humerus.

Patient: Supine.

Fixation: Counterpressure is applied by the examiner against the inner aspect of the distal end of the humerus in order to ensure a rotation motion.

Test: Lateral rotation of the humerus with the elbow held at right angle.

Pressure: Using the forearm as a lever, pressure is applied in the direction of medially rotating the humerus.

Weakness: The humerus assumes a position of medial rotation. Lateral rotation, in antigravity positions, is difficult or impossible.

For the purpose of objectively grading a weak lateral rotator group against gravity and for palpation of the rotator muscles, the test in prone position is preferred over the Teres minor and Infraspinatus test in supine position. For action of these two rotators without much assistance from the posterior Deltoid, and without the necessity of maximal Trapezius fixation, the test in supine position is preferred.

Rhomboids, Levator Scapulae, and Trapezius

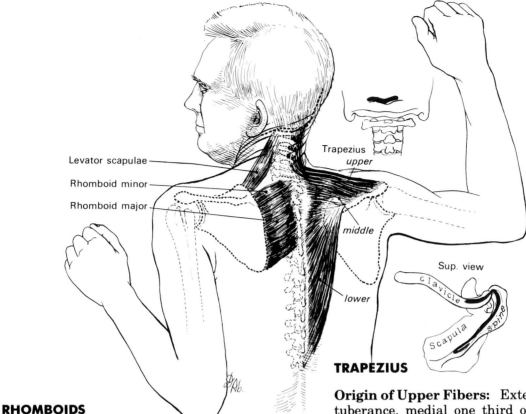

Levator scapulae
Rhomboid minor
Rhomboid major

Trapezius
upper

middle

lower

Sup. view
clavicle
spine
Scapula

RHOMBOIDS

Origin of Major: Spinous processes of second through fifth thoracic vertebrae.

Insertion of Major: By fibrous attachment to medial border of scapula between spine and inferior angle.

Origin of Minor: Ligamentum nuchae, spinous processes of seventh cervical and first thoracic vertebrae.

Insertion of Minor: Medial border at root of spine of scapula.

Action: Adduct and elevate the scapula, and rotate it so the glenoid cavity faces caudally.

Nerve: Dorsal scapular, C4, **5**.

LEVATOR SCAPULAE

Origin: Transverse processes of first four cervical vertebrae.

Insertion: Medial border of scapula between superior angle and root of spine.

Action: *With the origin fixed,* elevates the scapula and assists in rotation so the glenoid cavity faces caudally. *With the insertion fixed,* and acting *unilaterally,* laterally flexes the cervical vertebrae and rotates toward the same side. Acting *bilaterally,* the Levator scapulae may assist in extension of the cervical spine.

Nerve: Cervical **3, 4** and Dorsal scapular C4, **5**.

TRAPEZIUS

Origin of Upper Fibers: External occipital protuberance, medial one third of superior nuchal line, ligamentum nuchae, and spinous process of seventh cervical vertebra.

Origin of Middle Fibers: Spinous processes of first through fifth thoracic vertebrae.

Origin of Lower Fibers: Spinous processes of sixth through 12th thoracic vertebrae.

Insertion of Upper Fibers: Lateral one third of clavicle and acromion process of scapula.

Insertion of Middle Fibers: Medial margin of acromion and superior lip of spine of scapula.

Insertion of Lower Fibers: Tubercle at apex of spine of scapula.

Action: *With the origin fixed,* adduction of the scapula, performed chiefly by the middle fibers with stabilization by the upper and lower fibers. Rotation of the scapula so the glenoid cavity faces cranially, performed chiefly by the upper and lower fibers with stabilization by the middle fibers. In addition, the upper fibers elevate and the lower fibers depress the scapula. *With the insertion fixed,* and acting *unilaterally,* the upper fibers extend, laterally flex, and rotate the head and joints of the cervical vertebrae so that the face turns toward the opposite side; and acting *bilaterally,* the upper Trapezius extends the neck. The Trapezius also acts as an accessory muscle of respiration.

Nerve: Spinal portion of cranial nerve XI (accessory) and ventral ramus, C2, **3**, **4**.

282

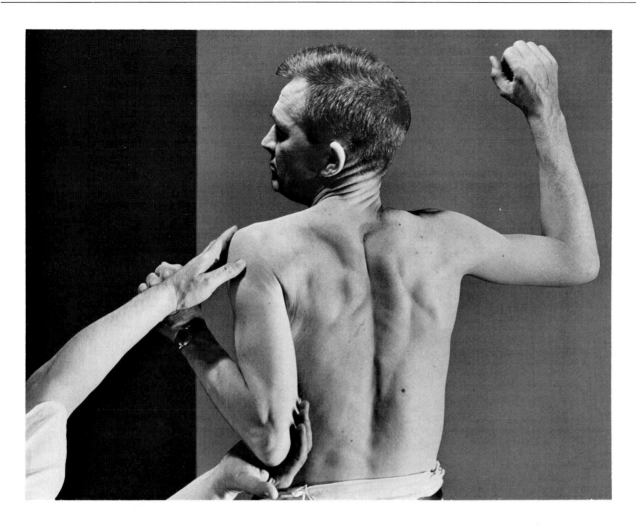

Patient: Prone.

Fixation: None is necessary on the part of the examiner, but it is assumed that the adductors of the shoulder joint have been tested and found to be strong enough to hold the arm for use as a lever in this test.

Test: Adduction and elevation of the scapula with medial rotation of the inferior angle. To obtain this position of the scapula, and to obtain leverage for pressure in the test, the arm is placed in the position as illustrated. With the elbow flexed, the humerus is adducted toward the side of the body in slight extension and slight lateral rotation.

The test is to determine the ability of the Rhomboids to hold the scapula in test position as pressure is applied against the arm. (See alternate test p. 285.)

Pressure: The examiner applies pressure with one hand against the patient's arm in the direction of abducting the scapula and rotating the inferior angle laterally and against the patient's shoulder with the other hand in the direction of depression.

Weakness: The scapula abducts and the inferior angle rotates outward. The strength of adduction and extension of the humerus is diminished by loss of Rhomboid fixation of the scapula. Ordinary function of the arm is affected less by loss of Rhomboids than by loss of either Trapezius or Serratus anterior.

Shortness: The scapula is drawn into a position of adduction and elevation. Shortness tends to accompany paralysis or weakness of the Serratus anterior because the Rhomboids are direct opponents of the Serratus. (See p. 292.)

Modified Test: If the shoulder muscles are weak, the examiner places the scapula in the test position and attempts to abduct, depress, and derotate the scapula.

Note: The accompanying photograph shows the Rhomboids in a state of contraction. (See p. 279, for right Rhomboids in neutral position and left, in elongated position.)

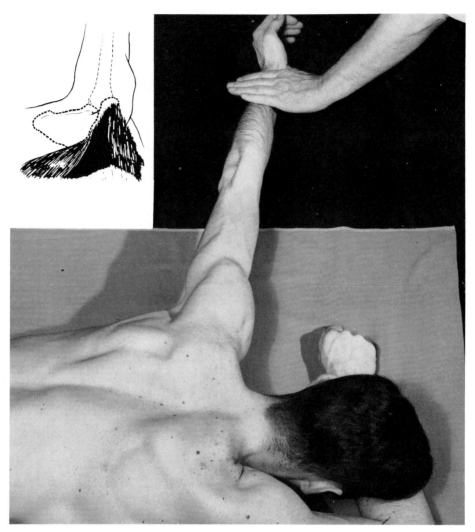

Patient: Prone.

Fixation: The intervening *shoulder joint extensors* (posterior Deltoid, Teres minor, and Infraspinatus, with assistance from middle Deltoid) must give necessary fixation of the humerus to the scapula in order to use the arm as a lever. To a lesser extent, the *elbow extensors* may need to give some fixation of the forearm to the humerus. However, with the shoulder laterally rotated, the elbow is also rotated into a position so that downward pressure on the forearm is exerted against the elbow laterally rather than in the direction of elbow flexion.

The *examiner* gives fixation by placing one hand on the opposite scapular area to prevent trunk rotation (not shown above). (The examiner's hand in the photograph merely indicates the downward direction of pressure.)

Test: Adduction of the scapula with upward rotation (lateral rotation of the inferior angle), and without elevation of the shoulder girdle.

The test position is obtained by placing the shoulder in 90° abduction and in *lateral rotation*

sufficient to bring the scapula into lateral rotation of the inferior angle.

The Teres major is a medial rotator attached along the axillary border of the scapula. Traction on this muscle as the arm is laterally rotated draws the scapula into lateral rotation. The degree of shoulder rotation necessary to produce the effect on the scapula will vary according to the tightness or laxity of the medial rotators. *Usually*, rotation of the arm and hand into a position so that the palm of the hand faces cranially will indicate good positioning of the scapula.

Trapezius and Rhomboids both adduct the scapula, but they differ in their rotation action and differentiating these muscles in testing is based on their rotation actions.

In addition to placing the parts in precise test position, it is necessary to observe the scapula *during the testing* to make sure that rotation is maintained as pressure is applied.

Pressure: Against the forearm in a downward direction toward the table.

Weakness: See p. 287.

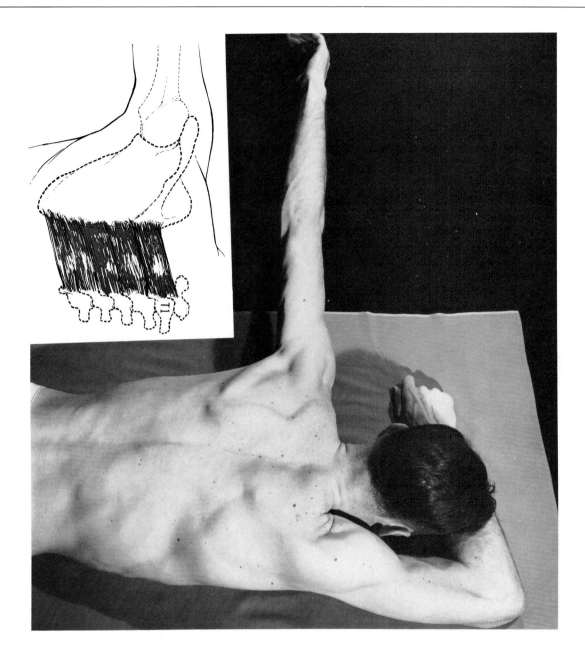

ALTERNATE TEST FOR RHOMBOIDS

If a position of medial rotation of the humerus and elevation of the scapula is permitted in testing the middle Trapezius, it ceases to be a Trapezius test. As seen in this illustration, the humerus is medially rotated, the scapula is elevated, depressed anteriorly, and adducted by Rhomboid action rather than by middle Trapezius action. A comparison of this photograph with the one on the facing page gives an example of what is meant by obtaining the specific action in which a muscle is the prime mover.

The marked difference that often exists between strength of Rhomboids and Trapezius is dramatically demonstrated by careful testing.

Patient: Prone.

Fixation: Same as middle Trapezius except middle Deltoid does not assist as an intervening muscle, and elbow extensors are necessary intervening muscles.

Test: Adduction and elevation of scapula with downward rotation (medial rotation of inferior angle). The position of the scapula is obtained by placing the shoulder in 90° abduction, and in sufficient *medial rotation* to move the scapula into the test position. The palm of the hand faces in a caudal direction.

Pressure: Against the forearm in a downward direction toward the table.

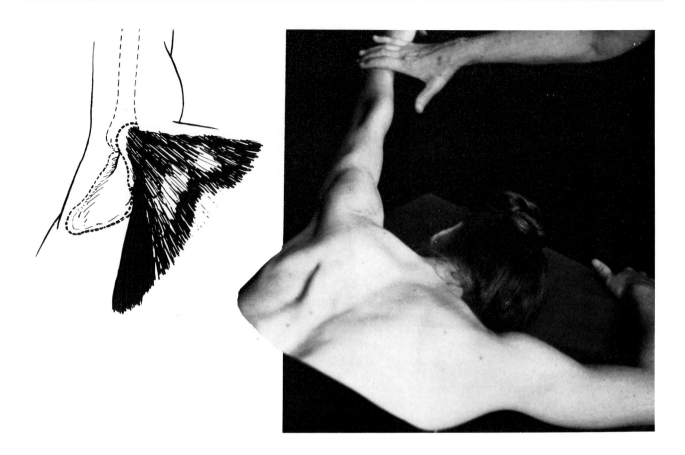

MODIFIED TRAPEZIUS TEST (not illustrated)

For use when posterior shoulder joint muscles are weak.

Patient: Prone with shoulder at edge of table, arm hanging down over side of table.

Fixation: None.

Test: Supporting the weight of the arm, the examiner places the scapula in a position of adduction, with some lateral rotation of the inferior angle, and without elevation of the shoulder girdle.

Pressure: As support of the arm is released, the weight of the suspended arm will exert a force that tends to abduct the scapula. A very weak Trapezius will not hold the scapula adducted against this force. If the Trapezius can hold the scapula in adduction against the weight of the suspended arm, then resist against the middle portion by pressure in the direction of abduction, and against the lower portion by pressure in a diagonal direction toward abduction and elevation. When recording the grade of strength, note that pressure was applied on the scapula because the arm could not be used as a lever.

LOWER TRAPEZIUS TEST

Patient: Prone.

Fixation: The intervening shoulder extensors, particularly the posterior Deltoid must give the necessary fixation of the humerus to the scapula and, to a lesser extent, the elbow extensors need to hold the elbow in extension. (See explanation on p. 284.)

The examiner gives fixation by placing one hand below the scapula on the opposite side (not shown above).

Test: Adduction and depression of the scapula with lateral rotation of the inferior angle. The arm is placed diagonally overhead in line with the lower fibers of the Trapezius. Lateral rotation of the shoulder joint occurs along with elevation so it usually is not necessary to further rotate the shoulder in order to bring the scapula into lateral rotation. (See explanation on previous page.)

Pressure: Against the forearm in a downward direction toward the table.

Note: Tests for lower and middle Trapezius are especially important in examination of cases in which shoulder position is faulty, or in cases of upper back or arm pain.

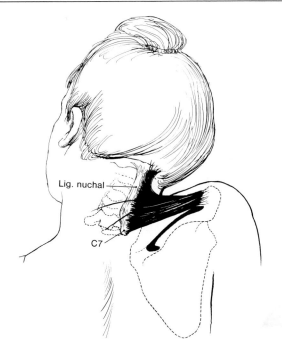

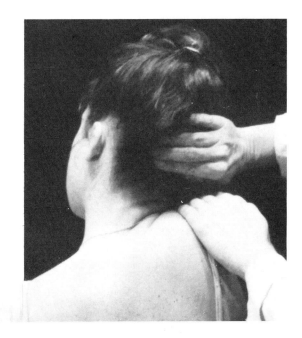

Weakness of Trapezius as a whole: Results in abduction and medial rotation of the scapula with depression of the acromion. Interferes with the ability to raise the arm in abduction overhead. (See p. 293 for posture of shoulder when entire Trapezius is paralyzed.)

Weakness of Lower Trapezius: Allows the scapula to ride upward and tilt forward with depression of the coracoid process. If the upper Trapezius is tight, it helps to pull the scapula upward and acts as an opponent to a weak lower Trapezius.

Weakness of Middle Trapezius: Results in abduction of the scapula and a forward position of the shoulder.

The middle and lower Trapezius reinforce the thoracic spine extensors. Weakness of these fibers of the Trapezius increases the tendency toward a kyphosis.

Weakness of Upper Trapezius: Unilaterally, weakness decreases the ability to approximate the acromion and the occiput; bilaterally, weakness decreases the ability to extend the cervical spine (e.g., to raise the head from a prone position).

Shortness of Upper Trapezius: Results in a position of elevation of the shoulder girdle (commonly seen in prize fighters and swimmers). In a faulty posture with forward head and kyphosis, the cervical spine is in extension and the upper Trapezius muscles are in a shortened position.

Patient: Sitting.

Fixation: None necessary.

Test: Elevation of the acromial end of the clavicle and scapula; posterolateral extension of the neck bringing the occiput toward the elevated shoulder with the face turned in the opposite direction.

The upper Trapezius can be differentiated from other elevators of the scapula because it is the only one that elevates the acromial end of the clavicle and the scapula. It also laterally rotates the scapula as it elevates in contrast to straight elevation that occurs when all elevators contract as in shrugging the shoulders.

Pressure: Against the shoulder in the direction of depression, and against the head in the direction of flexion anterolaterally.

Contracture of Upper Trapezius: Unilateral contracture frequently seen in torticollis cases. For example, the right upper Trapezius is usually contracted along with a contracture of the right Sternocleidomastoid and Scaleni. (See also p. 319.)

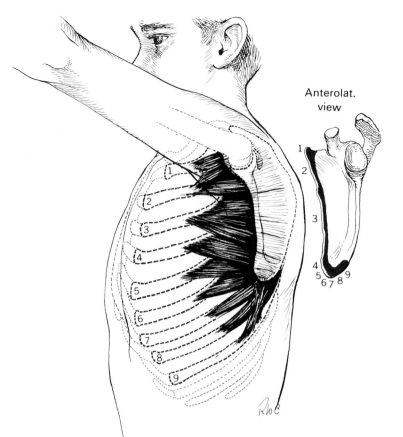

Anterolat. view

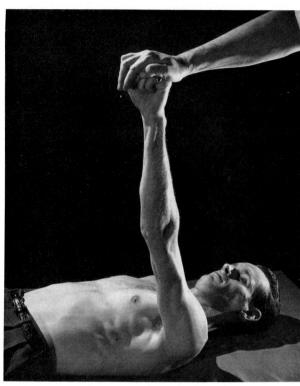

Origin: Outer surfaces and superior borders of upper eight or nine ribs.

Insertion: Costal surface of medial border of scapula.

Action: *With the origin fixed,* abducts the scapula, rotates the inferior angle laterally and the glenoid cavity cranially, and holds the medial border of the scapula firmly against the rib cage. In addition, the lower fibers may depress the scapula, and the upper fibers may elevate it slightly.

Starting from a position with the humerus fixed in flexion and the hands against a wall (see the standing Serratus test, p. 290), the Serratus acts to displace the thorax posteriorly as the effort is made to push the body away from the wall. Another example of this type of action is in a properly executed push-up.

With the scapula stabilized in adduction by the Rhomboids, thereby *fixing the insertion,* the Serratus may act in forced inspiration.

Nerve: Long thoracic, C**5**, **6**, **7**, 8.

Patient: Supine.

Fixation: None necessary unless the shoulder or elbow muscles are weak, in which case the examiner will support the extremity in the perpendicular position as the test is done.

Test: Abduction of the scapula projecting the upper extremity anteriorly (upward from the table). *Movement of the scapula must be observed and the inferior angle palpated to ensure that the scapula is abducting.* Projection of the extremity can be accomplished by the action of the Pectoralis minor (aided by the Levator and Rhomboids) when the Serratus is weak, in which case, the scapula tilts forward at the coracoid process, and the inferior angle moves posteriorly and in the direction of medial rotation. The firm surface of the table supports the scapula so there will be no winging and the pressure against the hand may elicit what appears to be normal strength. Since this type of substitution can occur during this test, the test in sitting as described on the facing page is more accurate and is the *preferred test.*

Pressure: Against the subject's fist, transmitting the pressure downward through the extremity to the scapula in the direction of adducting the scapula. *Slight* pressure may be applied against the lateral border of the scapula as well as against the fist.

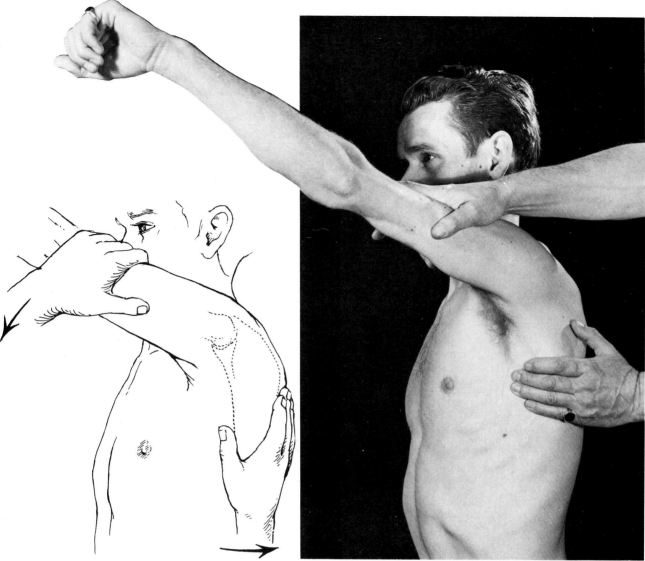

Patient: Sitting.

Fixation: None should be necessary by the examiner if the trunk is stable, but the shoulder flexors must be strong in order to use the arm as a lever in this test. Allow the subject to hold on to the table with one hand.

Test: The ability of the Serratus to stabilize the scapula in a position of abduction and lateral rotation with the arm in a position of approximately 120° to 130° flexion. This test emphasizes the upward rotation action of the Serratus in the abducted position as compared to the emphasis on the abduction action shown in the supine and standing tests.

Pressure: Against the dorsal surface of the arm between shoulder and elbow downward in the direction of extension, and *slight* pressure against the lateral border of the scapula in the direction of rotating the inferior angle medially. The thumb against the lateral border (as in the drawing) acts more to track the movement of the scapula than to offer pressure.

For purposes of photography, the examiner stood behind the subject and applied pressure with the fingertips on the scapula as illustrated. In practice, it is preferable to stand beside the subject and apply pressure as illustrated by the inset. It is not advisable to use a long lever by applying pressure on the forearm or at the wrist because intervening shoulder flexors will often break before the Serratus.

Weakness: Makes it difficult to raise the arm in flexion. Results in winging of the scapula. With marked weakness, the test position cannot be held. With moderate or slight weakness, the scapula cannot hold the position when pressure is applied on the arm. Since the Rhomboids are direct opponents of the Serratus, Rhomboids become shortened in some cases of Serratus weakness. (See also p. 340.)

289

Serratus Anterior

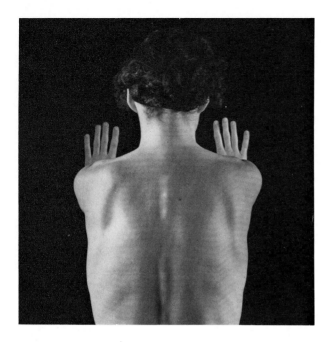

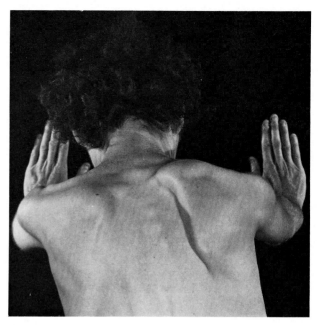

Patient: Standing.

Fixation: None necessary.

Test Movement: Facing a wall and with the elbows straight, the subject places hands against the wall at shoulder level or slightly above. To begin, the thorax is allowed to sag forward so that the scapulae are in a position of some adduction. The subject then pushes hard against the wall, displacing the thorax backward until the scapulae are in a position of abduction.

Resistance: The thorax acts as resistance in this test movement. By fixation of the hands and extended elbows, the scapulae become relatively fixed and the anterolateral rib cage is drawn backward toward the scapulae. (In contrast, the scapula is pulled forward toward the fixed rib cage during the forward thrust of the arm in the supine test shown on p. 288.) Because the resistance of displacing the weight of the thorax makes this a strenuous test, it will differentiate only between strong and weak for purposes of grading.

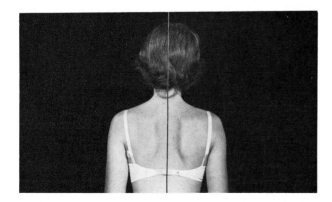

Weakness: Winging of the right scapula as seen in the above photograph.

The accompanying photograph illustrates the posture of the shoulders and scapulae as seen in some cases of mild Serratus weakness. There is slight winging of the scapulae that is readily visible because the upper back is straight. However, one must not assume Serratus weakness on the basis of appearance. When the upper back is straight, the scapulae may be prominent even if the Serratus is normal in strength.

When there is a round upper back, the scapulae will be elevated and adducted by the Rhomboids, which are direct opponents of the Serratus anterior.

Mild Serratus weakness is more prevalent than generally realized, and weakness tends to be more on the left than on the right, regardless of handedness. When weakness exists, it can be aggravated by attempting such strenuous exercises as push-ups.

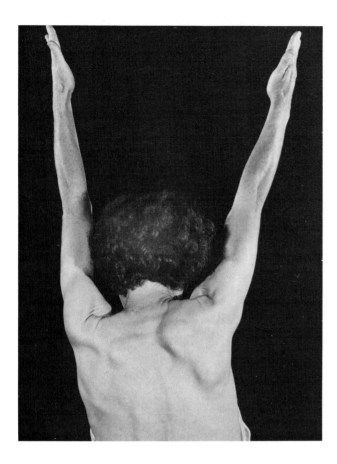

The above photograph shows the extent to which the right arm could be elevated overhead with the subject in standing position. With paralysis of the right Serratus anterior, the arm could not be raised directly forward, and the right scapula could not be abducted nor fully rotated as on the normal left side. The Trapezius compensated to some extent in the rotation of the scapula by the action of the upper and lower fibers which stand out clearly. In repeating the movement five or six times, however, the muscle fatigued and the ability to raise the arm above shoulder level decreased.

In subjects without any paralysis there is wide range of strength in the lower and middle Trapezius. This variation in strength is associated with postural or occupational stress on these muscles. The grade of strength will range from fair to normal. Because of these wide differences there also will be variations in the ability to raise an arm overhead among those who develop marked weakness or isolated paralysis of the Serratus. If an individual already has marked weakness of the Trapezius of a postural or an occupational nature,

and subsequently incurs a Serratus paralysis, that person will not be able to raise the arm overhead as in the accompanying illustration.

The Serratus anterior assists in elevation of the arm in the forward plane by its abduction and upward rotation action. By its abduction action, it moves the arm in an anterior direction (protracts the arm). By its reverse action, during the push-up, it helps move the upper trunk in a posterior direction. When the push-up is properly done, the scapulae abduct as the body is pushed upward. When the scapulae remain in an adducted position during the push-up, the excursion of the trunk movement is not as great as when the scapulae move into abduction.

The senior author of this text has tested the Serratus anterior muscle on hundreds of "normal" individuals. The test in supine position, as traditionally done (see p. 288) *rarely* discloses any weakness. The scapula will not wing because it is supported by the table, and a strong Pectoralis minor tilts the shoulder forward to hold the arm forward in (apparent) test position against pressure. When the same group of individuals is tested with the preferred test (arm in about 120° of flexion), the results are very different.

In groups of about 20 individuals, one or two might be strong on both right and left, and one might be weaker on the right than on the left (regardless of handedness); the rest may be about equally divided between being weaker on the left than on the right, or being bilaterally weak (with some propensity for the left being weaker).

Aside from the usual distribution, it has been necessary, at times, to have a separate category for persons who exhibit good strength through part of the range of motion of abduction but cannot maintain the scapula in full abduction while attempting to support the weight of the arm in flexion. The scapula can be passively brought forward into test position by pulling the arm diagonally up and forward, but it immediately slips back as the subject attempts to hold the arm in test position. This weakness can best be described as a stretch weakness of the Serratus. Stretching that has taken place is graphically illustrated by the photographs on the following page. Invariably, those who fall into the special category are persons who have engaged in doing many push-ups, bench presses, or activities involving strong Rhomboid action. A person may start doing push-ups properly but when the Serratus fatigues the scapulae remain adducted and the push-up is continued by the action of the Pectoralis major and the Triceps, to the detriment of the Serratus.

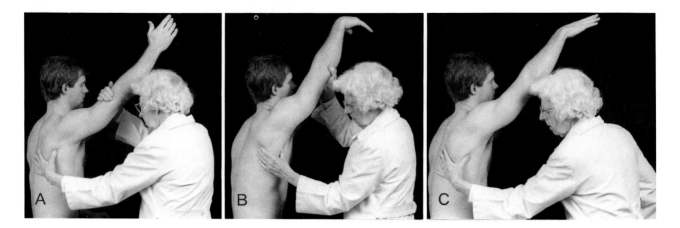

Figure A. When the arm is raised in flexion, in order to position the scapula for the Serratus test, the scapula does not move to the normal position of abduction. (See p. 289.) However, the Serratus tests strong in that position.

Figure B. The scapula can be brought forward to almost normal abduction if the subject relaxes the weight of the arm and allows the examiner to draw the arm diagonally forward into test position.

Figure C. However, the scapula cannot hold the abducted and upwardly rotated position when the examiner releases the arm and the subject attempts to hold it in position.

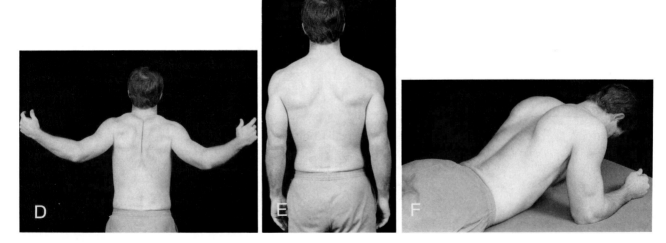

Figure D. This subject, routinely, has performed both bench presses and shoulder adduction exercises, including seated rowing and "bent over rowing" with heavy weights. As seen in the photographs, the Rhomboids have become overdeveloped. The Rhomboids are direct opponents of the Serratus, and this type of exercise is contraindicated in the presence of Serratus weakness.

Figure E. This photograph shows the abnormal position that the scapulae assume at rest.

Figure F. In a prone position, resting on the forearms, there is winging of the scapulae. The Serratus is unable to hold the abducted position against resistance offered by the weight of the trunk in this position.

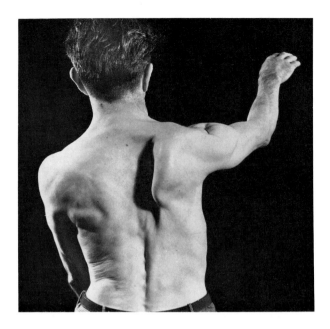

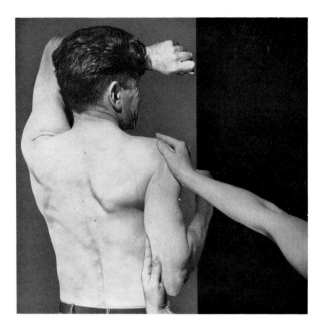

The above photograph shows the subject's inability to raise the arm overhead when both the Serratus and Trapezius are paralyzed. The winging of the medial border of the scapula makes it appear that the Rhomboids were weak, but they were not. (See photo at right.)

The subject in the photograph above is the same as the one at the left, being tested for strength of the Rhomboids. The subject showed good strength in adducting and stabilizing the scapula. If one did not test the Rhomboid but relied on the appearance during the arm raising, one would easily be led to the erroneous conclusion that the Rhomboids were weak.

RIGHT TRAPEZIUS PARALYZED, SERRATUS NORMAL

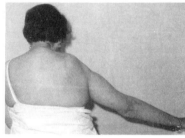 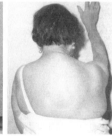

Raising the arm sideways (in the coronal plane) requires *abduction* of the shoulder joint accompanied by upward rotation of the scapula in an *adducted* position. With paralysis of the Trapezius, the scapulae cannot be rotated in the adducted position. Hence, the movement of shoulder abduction is limited as seen in the photograph at left above.

Raising the arm forward (in the sagittal plane) requires that the scapula upwardly rotate in the abducted position. With the Serratus intact, the arm could be raised higher in flexion than in abduction as seen in the photograph at right above.

If the Serratus were weak and the Trapezius strong, the arm could be raised higher in abduction than in flexion.

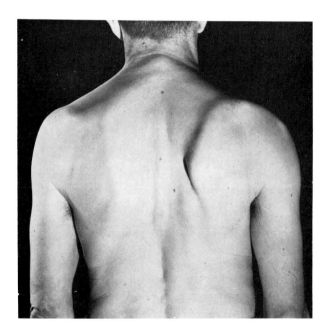

The above photograph shows the abnormal position of the right scapula that results from a paralysis of both the Trapezius and Serratus anterior. The acromial end is abducted and depressed. The inferior angle is rotated medially and elevated.

Scapular Muscle Chart

Scapular Muscles, Listed According to Spinal Segment Innervation and Scapular Movements

Scapular Muscles	Spinal Segment								Elevation	Adduction	Downward or Med. Rotat.	Upward or Lat. Rotat.	Depression	Abduction	Anterior Tilt
	Cervical							Th							
	2	3	4	5	6	7	8	1							
Trapezius	2	**3**	**4**						Upp. Trap.	Trapezius		Trap.	Low. Trap.		
Levator scapulae		3	4	5					Lev. scap.		Lev. scap.				
Rhomboids, mj. & mi.			4	5					Rhomboids	Rhomboids	Rhomboids				
Serratus anterior				5	**6**	**7**	8		Upp. Serratus ant.			Serr. ant.	Low. Serratus ant.	Serr. ant.	
Pectoralis minor					(6)	**7**	**8**	1							Pect. mi.

Shoulder Joint and Scapular Muscles

Muscles acting in combined shoulder joint and scapular movements		
Movement	Shoulder muscles	Scapular muscles
Full flexion (to 180°)	Flexors: Anterior deltoid, Biceps, Pectoralis major, upper, Coracobrachialis Lateral rotators: Infraspinatus, Teres minor, Posterior deltoid	Abductor: Serratus anterior Lateral rotators: Serratus anterior, Trapezius
Full abduction (to 180°)	Abductors: Deltoid, Supraspinatus, Biceps, long head Lateral rotators: Infraspinatus, Teres minor, Posterior deltoid	Adductor: Trapezius, acting to stabilize scapula in adduction Lateral rotators: Trapezius, Serratus anterior
Full extension (to 45°)	Extensors: Posterior deltoid, Teres major, Latissimus dorsi, Triceps, long head	Adductors, medial rotators & elevators: Rhomboids, Levator scapulae Ant. tilt of scapula by: Pectoralis minor
Full adduction to side against resistance	Adductors: Pectoralis major, Teres major, Latissimus dorsi, Triceps, long head	Adductors: Rhomboids, Trapezius

CHART FOR ANALYSIS OF MUSCLE IMBALANCE
UPPER EXTREMITY

me:.. Date: 1st. Ex.-......................... 2nd. Ex.-........................

agnosis:.. Onset:........................... Exam. of.....................extremity

		2nd. EX.	1st. EX.	1st. EX.	2nd. EX.		
	FLEXOR POLLICIS BREVIS					EXTENSOR POLLICIS BREVIS	
	FLEXOR POLLICIS LONGUS					EXTENSOR POLLICIS LONGUS	
	OPPONENS POLLICIS					ADDUCTOR POLLICIS	
	ABDUCTOR POLLICIS LONGUS					1 PALMAR INTEROSSEUS	
	ABDUCTOR POLLICIS BREVIS					1 DORSAL INTER. (THUMB ADD.)	
	PALMAR INTEROSSEUS 2					1 DORSAL INTER. (INDEX ABD.)	
	(DORSAL INTEROSSEUS 3)					2 DORSAL INTEROSSEUS	
	(DORSAL INTEROSSEUS 2)					3 DORSAL INTEROSSEUS	
	PALMAR INTEROSSEUS 3					4 DORSAL INTEROSSEUS	
	PALMAR INTEROSSEUS 4					ABDUCTOR DIGITI MINIMI	
	FLEXOR DIGITORUM PROFUNDUS 1					1	
	2					2 DISTAL INTER-PHALANGEAL	
	3					3 JOINT EXTENSORS	
	4					4	
	FLEXOR DIGITORUM SUPERFICIALIS 1					1	
	2					2 PROXIMAL INTER-PHALANGEAL	
	3					3 JOINT EXTENSORS	
	4					4	
	LUMBRICALES & INTEROSSEI 1					1 EXT. DIGIT. & INDICIS	
	2					2 EXT. DIGIT.	
	3					3 EXT. DIGIT.	
	& FLEXOR DIGITI MINIMI 4					4 EXT. DIGIT. COM. & DIG. MIN.	
	OPPONENS DIGITI MINIMI						
	PALMARIS BREVIS						
	PALMARIS LONGUS					EXTENSOR CARPI RADIALIS LONGUS & BREVIS	
	FLEXOR CARPI ULNARIS						
	FLEXOR CARPI RADIALIS					EXTENSOR CARPI ULNARIS	
	BICEPS ....}SUPINATORS SUPINATOR					PRONATORS{....... QUADRATUS .... TERES	
	BRACHIORADIALIS .....}ELBOW BRACHIALIS ....}FLEXORS BICEPS					ELBOW EXTENSORS{....... TRICEPS .... ANCONEUS	
	CORACOBRACHIALIS						
	ANTERIOR DELTOID						
	MIDDLE DELTOID					LATISSIMUS DORSI	
	POSTERIOR DELTOID					CLAV. PECTORALIS MAJOR	
	SUPRASPINATUS					STER. PECTORALIS MAJOR	
	TERES MINOR & INFRASPINATUS					TERES MAJOR & SUBSCAPULARIS	
	SERRATUS ANTERIOR					RHOMBOIDS & LEV. SCAP.	
	UPPER TRAPEZIUS					LATISSIMUS DORSI	
	MIDDLE TRAPEZIUS					PECTORALIS MAJOR	
	LOWER TRAPEZIUS					PECTORALIS MINOR	

295

Chart of Upper Extremity Muscles

UPPER EXTREMITY MUSCLES, Listed According to Spinal Segment Innervation and Grouped According to Joint Action

Spinal Segment

Cervical 4	5	6	7	8	Th 1	MUSCLE	SHOULDER Abduction	Lat. Rotat.	Flexion	Med. Rotat.	Extension	Adduction	ELBOW Flexion	Extension	FOREARM Supination	Pronation
4	5	6				Supraspinatus	Supraspin.									
(4)	5	6				Infraspinatus		Infraspin.								
	5	6				Teres minor		Teres mi.								
	5	6				Deltoid	Deltoid	Delt., post.	Delt., ant.	Delt., ant.	Delt., post.					
	5	6				Biceps	Biceps, l.h.		Biceps			Biceps, s.h.	Biceps		Biceps	
	5	6				Brachialis							Brachialis			
	5	6				Brachioradialis							Brachiorad.		Brachiorad.	Brachiorad.
	5	6	7			Pectoralis maj., upp.			Pect. mj., u.	Pect. mj., u.		Pect. mj., u.				
	5	6	7			Subscapularis				Subscap.						
	5	6	(7)			Supinator									Supinator	
	5	6	7			Teres major				Teres mj.	Teres mj.	Teres mj.				
	5	6	7	8		Ext. carpi rad. l. & b.							Ext. c. r. l.			
		6	7			Coracobrachialis			Coracobr.			Coracobr.				
		6	7			Pronator teres							Pron. teres			Pron. teres
		6	7	8		Flex. carpi rad.							Fl. c. rad.			Fl. c. rad.
		6	7	8		Latissimus dorsi				Lat. dorsi	Lat. dorsi	Lat. dorsi				
		6	7	8		Ext. digitorum										
		6	7	8		Ext. digit. min.										
		6	7	8		Ext. carpi ulnaris										
		6	7	8		Abd. poll. long.										
		6	7	8		Ext. poll. brev.										
		6	7	8		Ext. poll. long.										
		6	7	8		Ext. indicis										
		6	7	8	1	Pect. maj., lower						Pect. mj., l.				
		6	7	8	1	Triceps					Tri., l.h.	Tri., l.h.		Triceps		
		(6)	7	8	1	Palmaris long.							Palm. l.			
		(6)	7	8	1	Flex. poll. long.										
		(6)	7	8	1	Lumb. I & II										
		6	7	8	1	Abd. poll. brev.										
		6	7	8	1	Opponens poll.										
		6	7	8	1	Flex. poll br. (s. h.)										
			7	8		Anconeus								Anconeus		
			7	8	1	Flex. carpi ulnaris							Fl. c. ul.			
			7	8	1	Flex. digit. super.										
			7	8	1	Flex. digit. prof.										
			7	8	1	Pronator quad.										Pron. quad.
			(7)	8	1	Abd. digiti min.										
			(7)	8	1	Opp. digiti min.										
			(7)	8	1	Flex. digiti min.										
			(7)	8	1	Lumb. III & IV										
				8	1	Dor. interossei										
				8	1	Palm. interossei										
				8	1	Flex. poll. br. (d.h.)										
				8	1	Add. pollicis										

Chart of Upper Extremity Muscles

UPPER EXTREMITY MUSCLES, Listed According to Spinal Segment Innervation and Grouped According to Joint Action (Continued)

WRIST				CARPOMETACARPAL OF THUMB & LITTLE FINGER AND METACARPOPHALANGEAL JOINTS					DIG. 2-5 PROX. INTERPHAL. JTS.		DIG. 1-5 DISTAL INTERPHAL. JTS.	
Extension	Flexion	Abduction	Adduction	Extension	Abduction	Flexion	Opposition	Adduction	Extension	Flexion	Extension	Flexion
Ext. c. r. l & b		Ext. c. r. l & b										
	Fl. c. rad.	Fl. c. rad.										
Ext. dig.		Ext. dig.		Ext. dig.	Ext. dig.				Ext. dig.		Ext. dig.	
				Ext. dig. min.	Ext. dig. min.				Ext. dig. min.		Ext. dig. min.	
Ext. c. ul.			Ext. c. ul.									
	Abd. poll. l.	Abd. poll. l.		Abd. poll. l.	Abd. poll. l.							
	Ext. poll. b.			Ext. poll. b.	Ext. poll. b.							
Ext. poll. l.	Ext. poll. l			Ext. poll. l.							Ext. poll. l.	
				Ext. ind.				Ext. Ind.	Ext. ind.		Ext. ind.	
	Palm. l.											
	Fl. poll. l.					Fl. poll. l.						Fl. poll. l.
						Lumb. I, II			Lumb. I, II		Lumb. I, II	
				Abd. poll. b.	Abd. poll. b.	Abd. poll. b.	Abd. poll. b.				Abd. poll. b.	
							Opp. poll.					
						Fl. poll. b. (s)	Fl. poll. br. (s)				Fl. poll. br. (s)	
	Fl. c. ul.		Fl. c. ul.									
	Fl. dig. sup.					Fl. dig. sup.				Fl. dig. sup.		
	Fl. dig. pro.					Fl. dig. pro.				Fl. dig. pro.		Fl. dig. pro.
				Abd. d. min.	Abd. d. min.	Abd. d. min.			Abd. d. min.		Abd. d. min.	
							Opp. d. min.					
						Fl. d. min.	Fl. d. min.					
						Lumb. II, III			Lumb III, IV		Lumb. III, IV	
					Dor. int.	Dor. int.			Dor. int.		Dor. int.	
						Palm. int.		Palm. int.	Palm. int.		Palm. int.	
						Fl. poll. b. (d)	Fl. poll. b. (d)					
				Add. poll.		Add. poll.	Add. poll.	Add. poll.				

UPPER EXTREMITY MUSCLE CHART

LEFT | | | | | | | | | | | | **RIGHT**

						Examiner Date						
						Trapezius, upper						
						Trapezius, middle						
						Trapezius, lower						
						Serratus anterior						
						Rhomboids						
						Pectoralis minor						
						Pectoralis major						
						Latissimus dorsi						
						Shoulder medial rotators						
						Shoulder lateral rotators						
						Deltoid, anterior						
						Deltoid, middle						
						Deltoid, posterior						
						Biceps						
						Triceps						
						Brachioradialis						
						Supinators						
						Pronators						
						Flexor carpi radialis						
						Flexor carpi ulnaris						
						Extensor carpi radialis						
						Extensor carpi ulnaris						
					1	Flexor digitorum profundus	1					
					2	Flexor digitorum profundus	2					
					3	Flexor digitorum profundus	3					
					4	Flexor digitorum profundus	4					
					1	Flexor digit. superficialis	1					
					2	Flexor digit. superficialis	2					
					3	Flexor digit. superficialis	3					
					4	Flexor digit. superficialis	4					
					1	Extensor digitorum	1					
					2	Extensor digitorum	2					
					3	Extensor digitorum	3					
					4	Extensor digitorum	4					
					1	Lumbricalis	1					
					2	Lumbricalis	2					
					3	Lumbricalis	3					
					4	Lumbricalis	4					
					1	Dorsal interosseus	1					
					2	Dorsal interosseus	2					
					3	Dorsal interosseus	3					
					4	Dorsal interosseus	4					
					1	Palmar interosseus	1					
					2	Palmar interosseus	2					
					3	Palmar interosseus	3					
					4	Palmar interosseus	4					
						Flexor pollicis longus						
						Flexor pollicis brevis						
						Extensor pollicis longus						
						Extensor pollicis brevis						
						Abductor pollicis longus						
						Abductor pollicis brevis						
						Adductor pollicis						
						Opponens pollicis						
						Flexor digiti minimi						
						Abductor digiti minimi						
						Opponens digiti minimi						

NOTES:

chapter 9

Facial, Eye, and Neck Muscles; Muscles of Deglutition; and Respiratory Muscles

Cranial Nerves and Deep Facial Muscles

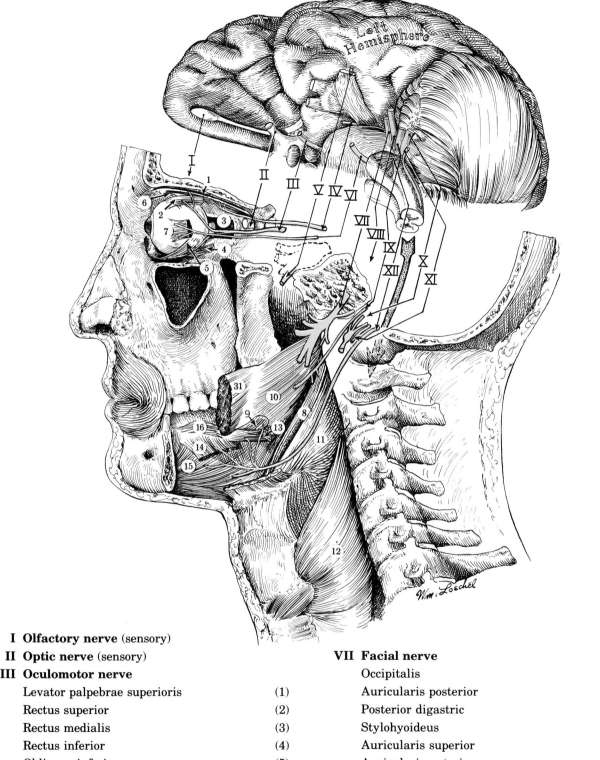

Facial Muscles

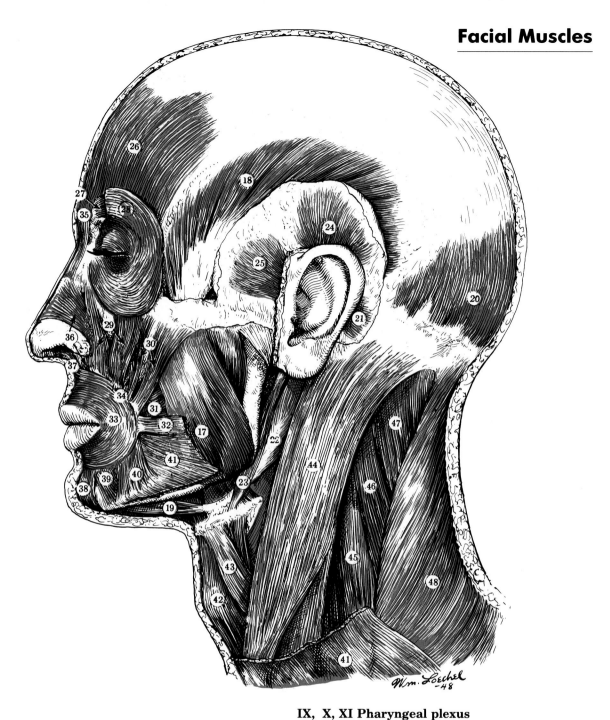

Facial and Eye Muscles Chart

Muscle	Origin	Insertion
Buccinator	Alveolar processes of maxilla, buccinator ridge of mandible, and pterygomandibular ligament	Orbicularis oris at angle of mouth
Corrugator supercilii	Medial end of superciliary arch	Deep surface of skin above middle of orbital arch
Depressor anguli oris	Oblique line of mandible	Angle of mouth, blending with adjacent muscles
Depressor labii inferioris	Oblique line of mandible	Integument of lower lip, blending with Orbicularis oris
Depressor septi nasi	Incisive fossa of maxilla	Ala and septum of nose
Frontalis	Galea aponeurotica	Muscles and skin of eyebrow and root of nose
Levator anguli oris	Canine fossa of maxilla	Angle of the mouth, blending with orbicularis oris
Levator labii superioris	Lower margin or orbit	Orbicularis of upper lip
Levator labii superioris alaeque nasi	Root of nasal process of maxilla	Greater alar cartilage and skin of nose, and lateral part of upper lip
Levator palpebrae superioris	Inferior surface of lesser wing of sphenoid	Skin of eyelid, tarsal plate of upper eyelid, orbital wall, and medial and lateral expansion of aponeurosis of insertion
Masseter	Superficial portion: Zygomatic process of maxilla, and lower border of zygomatic arch	Angle and ramus of mandible
	Profundus portion: Posterior one third of inferior border and medial surface of zygomatic arch	Superior one half of ramus and lateral surface of coronoid process of mandible
Mentalis	Incisive fossa of mandible	Skin of chin
Nasalis, alar portion	Maxilla	Ala of the nose
Nasalis, transverse portion	Above and lateral to incisive fossa of maxilla	By aponeurosis with nasalis on opposite side
Obliquus inferior oculi	Orbital plate of maxilla	Into external part of sclera, between Rectus superior and Rectus lateralis, posterior to equator of eyeball
Obliquus superior oculi	Above medial margin of optic foramen	Into sclera between Rectus superior and Rectus lateralis, posterior to equator of eyeball
Orbicularis oculi	Nasal part of frontal bone, frontal process of maxilla, anterior surface of medial palpebral ligament	Muscle fibers surround the circumference of the orbit, spread downward on the cheek, and blend with adjacent muscular or ligamentous structures

Facial and Eye Muscles Chart

Muscle	Origin	Insertion
Orbicularis oris	Numerous strata of muscular fibers surrounding the orifice of the mouth, derived in part from other facial muscles	Into skin and mucous membrane of lips, blending with other muscles
Platysma	Fascia covering superior portion of Pectoralis major and Deltoid	Lower border of mandible, posterior fibers blending with muscles about angle and lower part of mouth
Procerus	Fascia covering lower part of nasal bone and upper part of lateral nasal cartilage	Into skin over lower part of forehead between eyebrows
Pterygoideus lateralis	Superior head: Lateral surface of great wing of sphenoid, and infratemporal crest Inferior head: Lateral surface of lateral pterygoid plate	Depression, anterior part of condyle of mandible, anterior margin of articular disk of temporomandibular articulation
Pterygoideus medialis	Medial surface of lateral pterygoid plate, pyramidal process of palatine bone, and tuberosity of maxilla	Inferior and posterior part of medial surface of ramus and angle of mandibular foramen
Recti superior, inferior, medialis, and lateralis	Fibrous ring which surrounds superior, medial, and inferior margins of optic foramen	Into sclera, anterior to equator of eyeball at the site implied by each name
Risorius	Fascia over Masseter	Into skin at angle of mouth
Temporalis	Temporal fossa and fascia	Coronoid process and anterior border of ramus of mandible
Zygomaticus major	Zygomatic bone in front of temporal process	Angle of mouth, blending with adjacent muscles
Zygomaticus minor	Malar surface of zygomatic bone	Orbicularis oris of upper lip

Frontalis

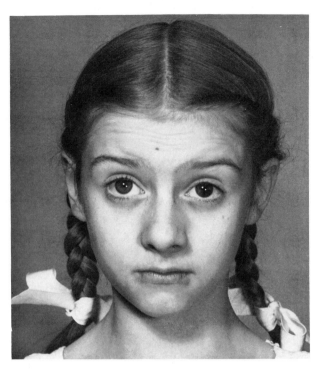

Test: Have the patient raise the eyebrows, wrinkling the forehead as in surprise or fright.

Corrugator Supercilii

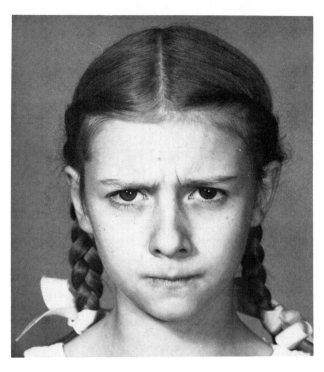

Test: Have the patient draw the eyebrows together as in frowning.

Nasalis, Alar Portion

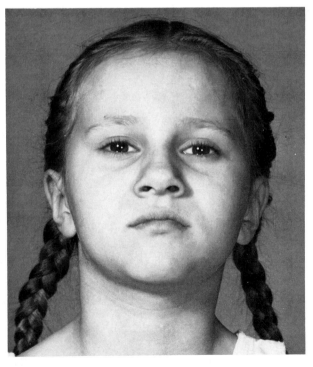

Test: Have the patient widen the apertures of the nostrils as in forced or difficult breathing.

Depressor Septi and Transverse Portion Nasalis

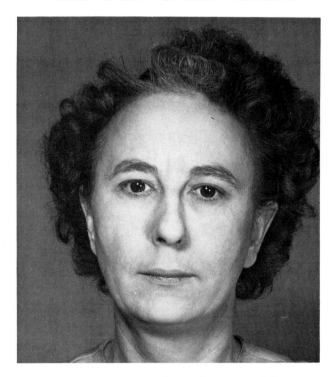

Test: Have the patient draw the point of the nose downward, narrowing the nostrils.

Procerus

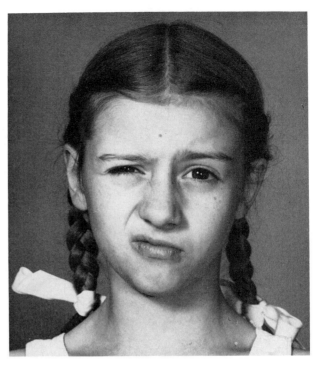

Test: Have the patient pull the skin of the nose upward, forming transverse wrinkles over the bridge of the nose.

Levator Anguli Oris

Test: Have the patient draw the angle of the mouth straight upward, deepening the furrow from the side of the nose to the side of the mouth as in sneering. Suggest that the patient try to show the "eye" (canine) tooth on one side, then the other.

Risorius

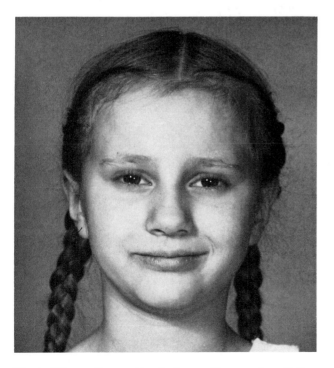

Test: Have the patient draw the angle of the mouth backward.

Zygomaticus Major

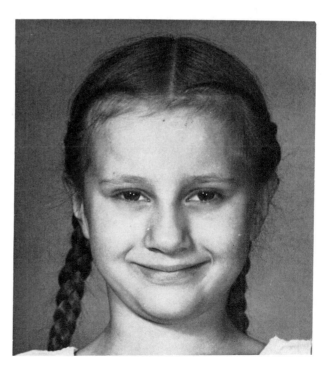

Test: Have the patient draw the angle of the mouth upward and outward as in smiling.

Levator Labii Superioris

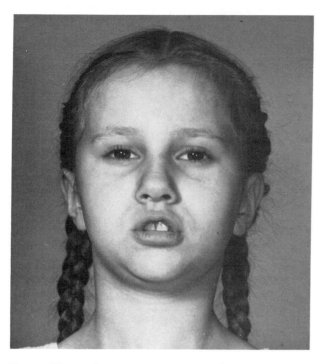

Test: Have the patient raise and protrude the upper lip as if to show the upper gums.

Depressor Labii Inferioris and Platysma

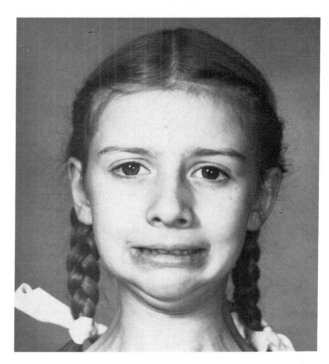

Test: Have the patient draw the lower lip and angle of the mouth downward and outward, tensing the skin over the neck.

Orbicularis Oris

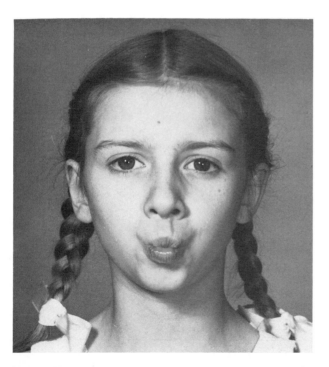

Test: Have the patient close the lips and protrude them forward as in whistling.

Buccinator

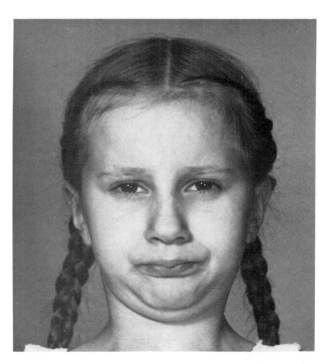

Test: Have the patient press the cheeks firmly against the side teeth, pulling back the angle of the mouth as in blowing a trumpet. (Drawing the chin backward, as seen in this illustration, is not part of the Buccinator action.)

Mentalis

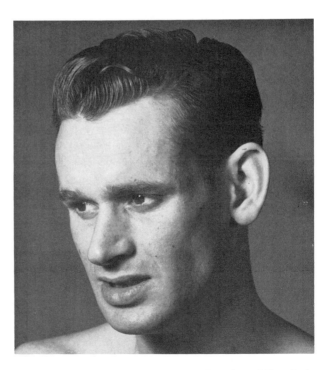

Test: Have the patient raise the skin of the chin. Secondarily, the lower lip will protrude somewhat as in pouting.

Depressor Anguli Oris

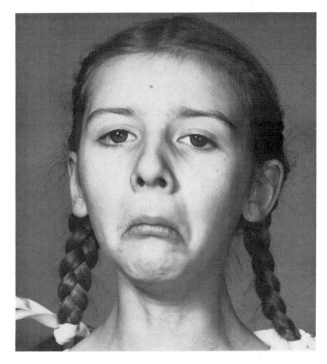

Test: Have the patient draw down the angles of the mouth.

Pterygoideus Medialis and Lateralis

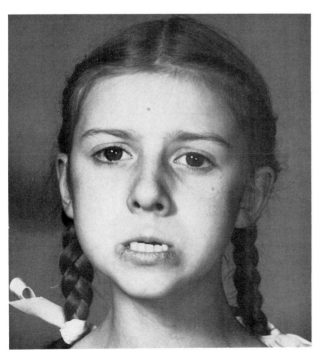

Test: Have the patient protrude the lower jaw.

Temporalis, Masseter, and Pterygoideus Medialis

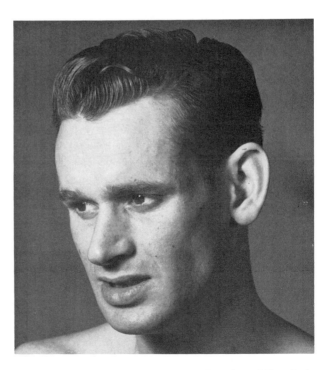

Test: Have the patient bite firmly. (Mouth is slightly open to show that teeth are being clenched.)

Orbicularis Oculi

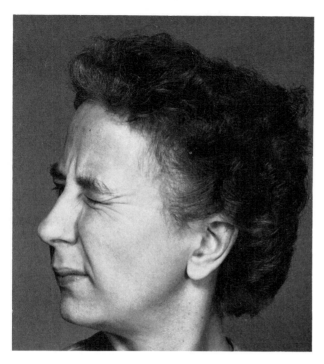

Test orbital part: Have the patient close the eyelid firmly, forming wrinkles radiating from the outer angle.

Test palpebral part: Have the patient close the eyelid gently. (Not illustrated.)

Suprahyoid Muscles

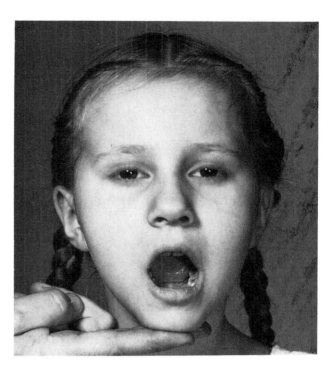

Test: Have the patient depress the lower jaw against resistance. The infrahyoid muscles furnish fixation of the hyoid bone during the action of these muscles. (See p. 320 for origins, insertions, and actions of suprahyoid muscles; and p. 315 for illustration.)

Infrahyoid Muscles

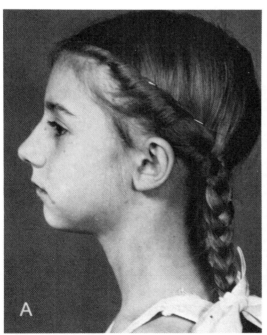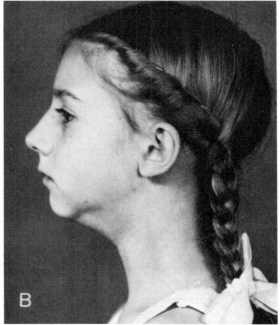

Test: Have the patient depress the hyoid bone (as illustrated). A represents relaxed position; B the test. (See p. 321 for origins, insertions, and actions of infrahyoid muscles; and p. 315 for illustration.)

Rectus Medialis Oculi and Rectus Lateralis Oculi

Levator Palpebrae Superioris et al

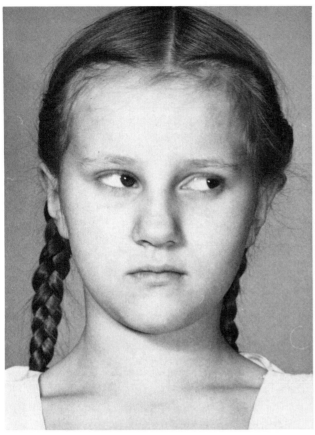

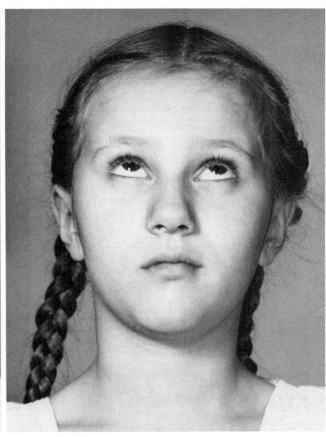

Test Rectus medialis: Have the patient look horizontally inward toward the nose. (Notice right eye in the illustration.)

Test Rectus lateralis: Have the patient look horizontally outward away from the nose. (Notice left eye in the illustration.)

Test Levator palpebrae superioris: Have the patient raise the upper lid.

Test Rectus superior and Obliquus inferior: Have the patient look straight upward toward the brow.

Test Rectus inferior and Obliquus superior: Have patient look straight downward toward the mouth. (Not illustrated.)

Cranial Nerve and Muscle Chart

Name Date

		MUSCLE STRENGTH GRADE	SENSORY OR MOTOR TO:		I Olfactory (S)	II Optic (S)	III Oculomotor (M)	IV Trochlear (M)	V Trigeminal (S & M)	VI Abducens (M)	VII Facial (S & M)	VIII Vestibulocochlear (S)	IX Glossopharyngeal (S & M)	X Vagus (S & M)	XI Accessory (M)	XII Hypoglossal (M)
I	NOSE	S	SENSORY—SMELL		●											
II	EYE	S	SENSORY—SIGHT			●										
	EYELID		LEVATOR PALPEBRAE SUPERIORIS				●									
			RECTUS SUPERIOR				●									
III	EYE		OBLIQUUS INFERIOR				●									
			RECTUS MEDIALIS				●									
			RECTUS INFERIOR				●									
IV	EYE		OBLIQUUS SUPERIOR					●								
	⟶	S	SENSORY—FACE & INT. STRUCTURES OF HEAD						●							
	EAR		TENSOR TYMPANI						●							
	PALATE		TENSOR VELI PALATINI						●							
			MASSETER						●							
	MASTI-		TEMPORALIS						●							
V	CATION		PTERYGOIDEUS MEDIALIS						●							
			PTERYGOIDEUS LATERALIS						●							
	S. HYOID		MYLOHYOIDEUS						●							
			ANTERIOR DIGASTRIC						●							
VI	EYE		RECTUS LATERALIS							●						
	TONGUE	S	SENSORY—TASTE, ANTERIOR ⅔ TONGUE								●					
	⟶	S	SENSORY—EXTERNAL EAR								●					
	EAR		STAPEDIUS								●					
	S. HYOID		POSTERIOR DIGASTRIC								●					
			STYLOHYOIDEUS								●					
	SCALP		OCCIPITALIS								●					
			INTRINSIC EAR MUSCLES	POST. AURICULAR BRANCH							●					
			AURICULARIS POSTERIOR								●					
	EAR		AURICULARIS ANTERIOR								●					
			AURICULARIS SUPERIOR	TEMPORAL BRANCH							●					
	SCALP		FRONTALIS								●					
	EYEBR.		CORRUGATOR SUPERCILII								●					
	EYELID		ORBICULARIS OCULI	TEMP. & ZYGO. BRANCH							●					
VII			PROCERUS								●					
	NOSE		DEP. SEPTI & NAS, TRANS.								●					
			NASALIS, ALAR								●					
			ZYGOMATICUS MAJOR								●					
			LEVATOR LABII SUPERIORIS	BUCCAL BRANCH							●					
			BUCCINATOR								●					
	MOUTH		ORBICULARIS ORIS								●					
			LEVATOR ANGULI ORIS								●					
			RISORIUS								●					
			DEPRESSOR ANGULI ORIS								●					
			DEPRESSOR LABII INFERIORIS	MANDIBULAR BRANCH							●					
	CHIN		MENTALIS								●					
	NECK		PLATYSMA	CERVICAL BRANCH							●					
VIII	EAR	S	SENSORY—HEARING & EQUILIBRIUM									●				
	TONGUE	S	SENSORY—POSTERIOR ⅓ TONGUE										●			
IX		S	SENSORY—PHARYNX, FAUCES, SOFT PALATE										●			
	PHARYNX		STYLOPHARYNGEUS										●			
		—	STRIATED MUSCLES - PHARYNX										●			
	⟶	—	STRIATED MUSCLES—SOFT PALATE, PHARYNX & LARYNX											●		
	⟶	—	INVOLUNTARY MUSCLES—ALIMENTARY TRACT											●		
	⟶	—	INVOLUNTARY MUSCLES—AIR PASSAGES											●		
X	⟶	—	INVOLUNTARY CARDIAC MUSCLE											●		
	⟶	S	SENSORY—AURICULAR											●		
	⟶	S	SENSORY—ALIMENTARY TRACT											●		
	⟶	S	SENSORY—AIR PASSAGES											●		
	⟶	S	SENSORY—ABDOMINAL VISCERA & HEART											●		
	NECK		TRAPEZIUS & STERNOCLEIDOMASTOID												●	
XI	PALATE		LEVATOR VELI PALATINI												●	
	⟶		STRIATED MUSCLES—SOFT PALATE, PHARYNX, & LARYNX												●	
			STYLOGLOSSUS													●
			HYOGLOSSUS													●
XII	TONGUE		GENIOGLOSSUS													●
			TONGUE INTRINSICS													●

SENSORY

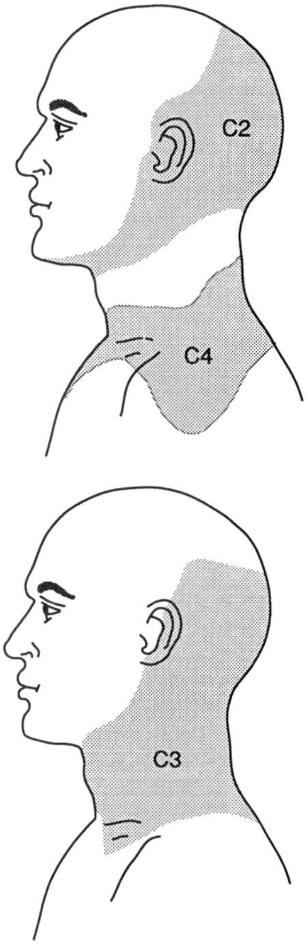
C2
C4
C3

DERMATOMES

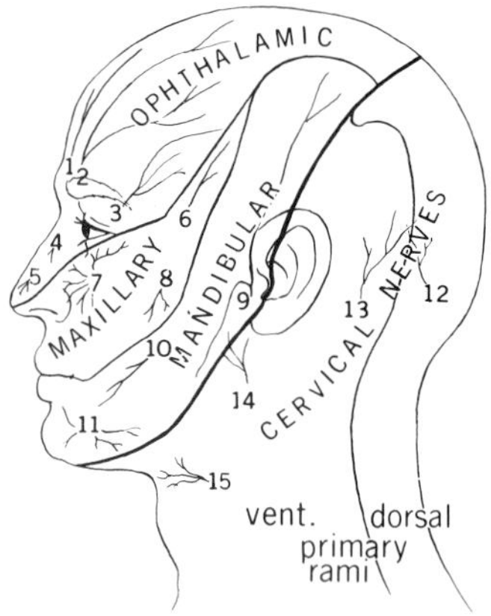
OPHTHALAMIC
MAXILLARY
MANDIBULAR
CERVICAL NERVES
1
2
3
4
5
6
8
9
10
11
12
13
14
15
vent.
dorsal
primary
rami

CUTANEOUS DISTRIBUTION OF CRANIAL NERVES

Ophthalamic
1. Supratrochlear N.
2. Supraorbital N.
3. Lacrimal N.
4. Infratrochlear N.
5. Nasal N.

Maxillary
6. Zygomatico-temporal N.
7. Infraorbital N.
8. Zygomatico-facial N.

Mandibular
9. Auriculotemporal N.
10. Buccal N.
11. Mental N.

Cervical Nerves
12. Greater Occipital N.
13. Lesser Occipital N.
14. Great Auricular N.

Redrawn from *Gray's Anatomy of the Human Body*, 28th ed.

The cranial nerve and muscle chart (p. 310) is designed for use primarily as a reference sheet, and secondarily as a chart to record examination findings for the muscles of expression.

Because of the dual purpose of the chart, it contains some material that would not be included if used only for recording muscle examinations. For example, all the cranial nerves are listed, whether they are sensory, motor or mixed nerves. Some muscles are included that cannot be tested manually either individually or in groups.

On the cranial nerve chart are listed all the cranial nerves with the specific muscles or organs and general regions that they supply. A column is provided at the left of the muscle names in which to record evaluation of strength of those muscles that can be tested. At the right side of the page are drawings of the head showing areas of dermatomes and distribution of the cutaneous nerves.

The illustration on p. 301 shows the superficial musculature. The one on p. 300 is a sagittal section of the skull at about the center of the left orbit except that the complete eyeball is shown. The muscles depicted in this illustration are mainly those of the tongue, the pharyngeal area, and the eyeball.

The left hemisphere of the brain has been reflected upward to show its inferior surface and the cranial nerve roots. Connecting the nerve roots with the corresponding nerve trunks in the lower section of the drawing are lines bearing the numbers of the respective cranial nerves. Nerve roots I, II, and VII, which are sensory, are left white. The motor and mixed nerves are shown in yellow except that only the small motor branch of the fifth is yellow.

On the following pages there appear two charts with recordings of muscle examinations of the facial muscles. In the first case, the onset of the Bell's Palsy was 1 week before the examination date. Three muscles graded zero, ten graded trace, and two graded poor. Three weeks later, the muscles all graded good, and approximately 3 weeks after that, all the muscles graded normal except three that still graded good. This is an example of those facial paralysis cases that make fairly rapid recovery, some within a few days or a week, some, like this case, within a 2-month period.

The second case is one in which there was no evidence of any muscle function except slight action in the Corrugator at the time of the first examination which was 3 weeks after onset. This case showed very little change during the first 3 1/2 months. By the end of 6 months, most of the muscles graded fair or better. By the end of 8 months, there was further improvement and by the end of 9 1/2 months, about one third of the muscles graded fair and all others either good or normal. This case shows the slow but gradual improvement that occurs in some instances.

This second patient was fitted with a very small plastic hook, contoured to fit in the corner of the mouth and attached by means of a rubber band to the sidepiece of the glasses worn by the patient.* She was instructed in giving herself light massage—*upward on the affected side* and *downward* and toward the mouth *on the unaffected side*. At times, transparent scotch tape was used to hold up the side of the mouth and cheek. When she was not using the hook or tape, she was advised to make a habit, when sitting, of resting the right elbow on a table or arm of a chair and placing the right hand with palm under the right chin and fingers along the cheek to hold the right side of the face upward. Also, when speaking, smiling, or laughing, the hand was to be used to push the affected side toward the right and upward to compensate for the weakness, as well as to prevent the unaffected side from distorting the mouth in that direction. She was taught how to exercise the facial muscles by assisting the weak side and restraining the stronger side.

In some cases of facial paralysis, the Orbicular oculi (which closes and squeezes the eye shut) may be slower to respond than some other muscles. During the period of recovery when there is a problem with closing the eye, exercising the Frontalis is discouraged because it acts in opposition to the Orbicularis oculi, i.e., avoid wrinkling the forehead. The reason for this may be illustrated by the following: Lift the eyebrow by contracting the Frontalis. With the fingertips placed just above the eyebrows, keep the eyebrow held upward and 1) try to close the eye; 2) try to squeeze the eye tightly shut. The difficulty in doing both is readily demonstrated.

---

*The sidepiece, or temple, of eyeglasses is the part of the frame that extends from the lens to and over the ear.

Cranial Nerve and Muscle Chart

Name **Case # 1**

Column nerve headers (with S/M type):

S	I Olfactory
S	II Optic
M	III Oculomotor
M	IV Trochlear
S & M	V Trigeminal
M	VI Abducens
S & M	VII Facial
S	VIII Vestibulocochlear
S & M	IX Glossopharyngeal
S & M	X Vagus
M	XI Accessory
M	XII Hypoglossal

SENSORY OR MOTOR TO: **Left**

#	Region	Grade	Sensory or Motor To	Branch	Grade columns	Nerve (●)
I	NOSE	S	SENSORY—SMELL			I Olfactory ●
II	EYE	S	SENSORY—SIGHT			II Optic ●
III	EYELID		LEVATOR PALPEBRAE SUPERIORIS			III Oculomotor ●
III	EYE		RECTUS SUPERIOR			III Oculomotor ●
			OBLIQUUS INFERIOR			III Oculomotor ●
			RECTUS MEDIALIS			III Oculomotor ●
			RECTUS INFERIOR			III Oculomotor ●
IV	EYE		OBLIQUUS SUPERIOR			IV Trochlear ●
V	→	S	SENSORY—FACE & INT. STRUCTURES OF HEAD			V Trigeminal ●
	EAR		TENSOR TYMPANI			V Trigeminal ●
	PALATE		TENSOR VELI PALATINI			V Trigeminal ●
	MASTI-CATION		MASSETER			V Trigeminal ●
			TEMPORALIS			V Trigeminal ●
			PTERYGOIDEUS MEDIALIS			V Trigeminal ●
			PTERYGOIDEUS LATERALIS			V Trigeminal ●
	S. HYOID		MYLOHYOIDEUS			V Trigeminal ●
			ANTERIOR DIGASTRIC			V Trigeminal ●
VI	EYE		RECTUS LATERALIS			VI Abducens ●
VII	TONGUE	S	SENSORY—TASTE, ANTERIOR ⅔ TONGUE			VII Facial ●
	→	S	SENSORY—EXTERNAL EAR			VII Facial ●
	EAR		STAPEDIUS			VII Facial ●
	S. HYOID		POSTERIOR DIGASTRIC			VII Facial ●
			STYLOHYOIDEUS			VII Facial ●
	SCALP		OCCIPITALIS	⎫ POST. AURICULAR BRANCH		VII Facial ●
	EAR		INTRINSIC EAR MUSCLES			VII Facial ●
			AURICULARIS POSTERIOR			VII Facial ●
			AURICULARIS ANTERIOR	⎫ TEMPORAL BRANCH		VII Facial ●
			AURICULARIS SUPERIOR			VII Facial ●
	SCALP	T	FRONTALIS	⎫ TEMP & ZYGO BRANCH	G / N	VII Facial ●
	EYEBR.	T	CORRUGATOR SUPERCILII		G / N	VII Facial ●
	EYELID	P	ORBICULARIS OCULI		G / N	VII Facial ●
	NOSE	P	PROCERUS		G / N	VII Facial ●
		–	DEP. SEPTI & NAS, TRANS		– / –	VII Facial ●
		T	NASALIS, ALAR		G / N	VII Facial ●
	MOUTH		ZYGOMATICUS MAJOR	⎫ BUCCAL BRANCH	G / N	VII Facial ●
			LEVATOR LABII SUPERIORIS		G / N	VII Facial ●
		T	BUCCINATOR		G / N	VII Facial ●
		T	ORBICULARIS ORIS		G / G	VII Facial ●
		T	LEVATOR ANGULI ORIS		G / G	VII Facial ●
		T	RISORIUS		G / N	VII Facial ●
		T	DEPRESSOR ANGULI ORIS	⎫ MANDIBULAR BRANCH	G / N	VII Facial ●
		O	DEPRESSOR LABII INFERIORIS		G / N	VII Facial ●
	CHIN	T	MENTALIS		G / G	VII Facial ●
	NECK	O	PLATYSMA	CERVICAL BRANCH	G / N	VII Facial ●
VIII	EAR	S	SENSORY—HEARING & EQUILIBRIUM			VIII Vestibulocochlear ●
IX	TONGUE	S	SENSORY—POSTERIOR ⅓ TONGUE			IX Glossopharyngeal ●
IX		S	SENSORY—PHARYNX, FAUCES, SOFT PALATE			IX Glossopharyngeal ●
	PHARYNX		STYLOPHARYNGEUS			IX Glossopharyngeal ●
		—	STRIATED MUSCLES - PHARYNX			IX Glossopharyngeal ●
X	→	—	STRIATED MUSCLES—SOFT PALATE, PHARYNX & LARYNX			X Vagus ●
	→	—	INVOLUNTARY MUSCLES—ALIMENTARY TRACT			X Vagus ●
	→	—	INVOLUNTARY MUSCLES—AIR PASSAGES			X Vagus ●
	→	—	INVOLUNTARY CARDIAC MUSCLE			X Vagus ●
	→	S	SENSORY—AURICULAR			X Vagus ●
	→	S	SENSORY—ALIMENTARY TRACT			X Vagus ●
	→	S	SENSORY—AIR PASSAGES			X Vagus ●
	→	S	SENSORY—ABDOMINAL VISCERA & HEART			X Vagus ●
XI	NECK		TRAPEZIUS & STERNOCLEIDOMASTOID			XI Accessory ●
XI	PALATE		LEVATOR VELI PALATINI			XI Accessory ●
	→		STRIATED MUSCLES—SOFT PALATE, PHARYNX, & LARYNX			XI Accessory ●
XII	TONGUE		STYLOGLOSSUS			XII Hypoglossal ●
			HYOGLOSSUS			XII Hypoglossal ●
			GENIOGLOSSUS			XII Hypoglossal ●
			TONGUE INTRINSICS			XII Hypoglossal ●

Muscle strength grade date columns: Feb. 27, Mar. 20, Apr. 13

SENSORY

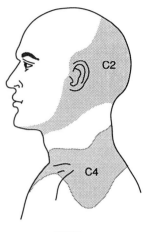

C2
C4

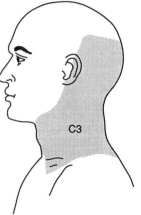

C3

DERMATOMES

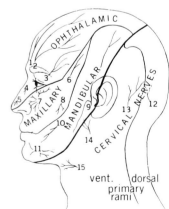

vent. dorsal
primary rami

CUTANEOUS DISTRIBUTION OF CRANIAL NERVES

Ophthalamic
1. Supratrochlear N.
2. Supraorbital N.
3. Lacrimal N.
4. Infratrochlear N.
5. Nasal N.

Maxillary
6. Zygomatico-temporal N.
7. Infraorbital N.
8. Zygomatico-facial N.

Mandibular
9. Auriculotemporal N.
10. Buccal N.
11. Mental N.

Cervical Nerves
12. Greater Occipital N.
13. Lesser Occipital N.
14. Great Auricular N.

Redrawn from *Gray's Anatomy of the Human Body*, 28th ed.

Cranial Nerve and Muscle Chart

Name: **Case # 2** Date: **3 weeks after onset**

Column nerve headers (with Sensory/Motor designation):

I Olfactory	S
II Optic	S
III Oculomotor	M
IV Trochlear	M
V Trigeminal	S & M
VI Abducens	M
VII Facial	S & M
VIII Vestibulocochlear	S
IX Glossopharyngeal	S & M
X Vagus	S & M
XI Accessory	M
XII Hypoglossal	M

The VII (Facial) muscle grade columns are recorded on the following dates: 8-22-61 (= Muscle Strength Grade column), 11-3-61, 12-11-61, 2-28-62, 4-17-62, 6-6-62.

#	Region	Muscle Strength Grade (8-22-61)	Sensory or Motor To — Right	11-3-61	12-11-61	2-28-62	4-17-62	6-6-62	Nerve (dot)
I	NOSE	S	SENSORY—SMELL						I
II	EYE	S	SENSORY—SIGHT						II
III	EYELID		LEVATOR PALPEBRAE SUPERIORIS						III
III	EYE		RECTUS SUPERIOR						III
III	EYE		OBLIQUUS INFERIOR						III
III	EYE		RECTUS MEDIALIS						III
III	EYE		RECTUS INFERIOR						III
IV	EYE		OBLIQUUS SUPERIOR						IV
V	→	S	SENSORY—FACE & INT. STRUCTURES OF HEAD						V
V	EAR		TENSOR TYMPANI						V
V	PALATE		TENSOR VELI PALATINI						V
V	MASTICATION		MASSETER						V
V	MASTICATION		TEMPORALIS						V
V	MASTICATION		PTERYGOIDEUS MEDIALIS						V
V	MASTICATION		PTERYGOIDEUS LATERALIS						V
V	S. HYOID		MYLOHYOIDEUS						V
V	S. HYOID		ANTERIOR DIGASTRIC						V
VI	EYE		RECTUS LATERALIS						VI
VII	TONGUE	S	SENSORY—TASTE, ANTERIOR ⅔ TONGUE						VII
VII	→	S	SENSORY—EXTERNAL EAR						VII
VII	EAR		STAPEDIUS						VII
VII	S. HYOID		POSTERIOR DIGASTRIC						VII
VII	S. HYOID		STYLOHYOIDEUS						VII
VII	SCALP		OCCIPITALIS (POST. AURICULAR BRANCH)						VII
VII			INTRINSIC EAR MUSCLES (POST. AURICULAR BRANCH)						VII
VII	EAR		AURICULARIS POSTERIOR (POST. AURICULAR BRANCH)						VII
VII	EAR		AURICULARIS ANTERIOR						VII
VII	EAR		AURICULARIS SUPERIOR (TEMPORAL BRANCH)						VII
VII	SCALP	O	FRONTALIS (TEMPORAL BRANCH)	T	T	P+	F	F	VII
VII	EYEBR.	P	CORRUGATOR SUPERCILII (TEMP. & ZYGO. BRANCH)	P	–	G–	G	G	VII
VII	EYELID	O	ORBICULARIS OCULI	P–	P	F+	N	N	VII
VII	NOSE	O	PROCERUS	O	P	G–	F	F	VII
VII	NOSE	O	DEP. SEPTI & NAS. TRANS.	–	–	–	–	–	VII
VII	NOSE	O	NASALIS, ALAR	O	?	F	F	F	VII
VII	MOUTH	O	ZYGOMATICUS MAJOR	P–	P	G–	G	G	VII
VII	MOUTH	O	LEVATOR LABII SUPERIORIS (BUCCAL BRANCH)	?	?	F	F	G	VII
VII	MOUTH	O	BUCCINATOR	–	–	F–	F	F	VII
VII	MOUTH	O	ORBICULARIS ORIS	–	T	F	F–	F	VII
VII	MOUTH	O	LEVATOR ANGULI ORIS	T	?	G–	G	G	VII
VII	MOUTH	O	RISORIUS	P–	P	F+	G	G	VII
VII	MOUTH	O	DEPRESSOR ANGULI ORIS	?	–	F	F–	F	VII
VII	MOUTH	O	DEPRESSOR LABII INFERIORIS (MANDIBULAR BRANCH)	?	–	P+	F–	G	VII
VII	CHIN	O	MENTALIS	O	?	F+	G	N	VII
VII	NECK	O	PLATYSMA (CERVICAL BRANCH)	T	–	F+	G	G	VII
VIII	EAR	S	SENSORY—HEARING & EQUILIBRIUM						VIII
IX	TONGUE	S	SENSORY—POSTERIOR ⅓ TONGUE						IX
IX		S	SENSORY—PHARYNX, FAUCES, SOFT PALATE						IX
IX	PHARYNX		STYLOPHARYNGEUS						IX
IX		—	STRIATED MUSCLES - PHARYNX						IX
X	→	—	STRIATED MUSCLES—SOFT PALATE, PHARYNX & LARYNX						X
X	→	—	INVOLUNTARY MUSCLES—ALIMENTARY TRACT						X
X	→	—	INVOLUNTARY MUSCLES—AIR PASSAGES						X
X	→	—	INVOLUNTARY CARDIAC MUSCLE						X
X	→	S	SENSORY—AURICULAR						X
X	→	S	SENSORY—ALIMENTARY TRACT						X
X	→	S	SENSORY—AIR PASSAGES						X
X	→	S	SENSORY—ABDOMINAL VISCERA & HEART						X
XI	NECK		TRAPEZIUS & STERNOCLEIDOMASTOID						XI
XI	PALATE		LEVATOR VELI PALATINI						XI
XI	→		STRIATED MUSCLES—SOFT PALATE, PHARYNX, & LARYNX						XI
XII	TONGUE		STYLOGLOSSUS						XII
XII	TONGUE		HYOGLOSSUS						XII
XII	TONGUE		GENIOGLOSSUS						XII
XII	TONGUE		TONGUE INTRINSICS						XII

SENSORY

Dermatomes illustrated: C2, C3, C4

DERMATOMES

CUTANEOUS DISTRIBUTION OF CRANIAL NERVES

Ophthalmic
1. Supratrochlear N.
2. Supraorbital N.
3. Lacrimal N.
4. Infratrochlear N.
5. Nasal N.

Maxillary
6. Zygomatico-temporal N.
7. Infraorbital N.
8. Zygomatico-facial N.

Mandibular
9. Auriculotemporal N.
10. Buccal N.
11. Mental N.

Cervical Nerves
12. Greater Occipital N.
13. Lesser Occipital N.
14. Great Auricular N.

(head diagram labels: OPHTHALMIC, MAXILLARY, MANDIBULAR, CERVICAL NERVES; vent. / dorsal primary rami)

Redrawn from *Gray's Anatomy of the Human Body*, 28th ed.

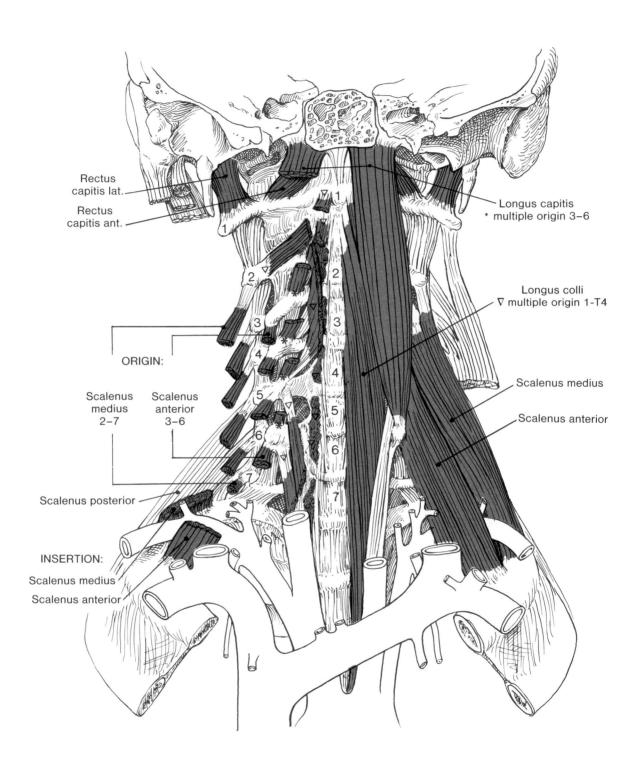

Rectus capitis lat.

Rectus capitis ant.

Longus capitis
* multiple origin 3–6

Longus colli
▽ multiple origin 1-T4

ORIGIN:

Scalenus medius 2–7

Scalenus anterior 3–6

Scalenus medius

Scalenus anterior

Scalenus posterior

INSERTION:

Scalenus medius

Scalenus anterior

Redrawn from Sobotta-Figge (36).

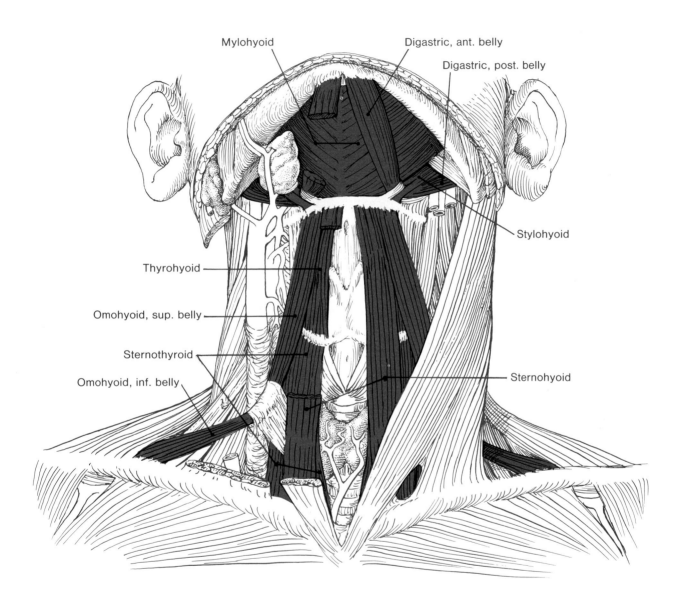

Mylohyoid

Digastric, ant. belly

Digastric, post. belly

Stylohyoid

Thyrohyoid

Omohyoid, sup. belly

Sternothyroid

Omohyoid, inf. belly

Sternohyoid

Redrawn from Sobotta-Figge (36).

Head and Neck Muscles

Muscles	Origin	Insertion
Longus colli[a]	*Superior oblique portion:* Anterior tubercles of transverse processes of third, fourth, and fifth cervical vertebrae. *Interior oblique portion:* Anterior surface of bodies of first two or three thoracic vertebrae. *Vertical portion:* Anterior surface of bodies of first three thoracic and last three cervical vertebrae.	Tubercle on anterior arch of atlas. Anterior tubercles of transverse processes of fifth and sixth cervical vertebrae. Anterior surface of bodies of second, third, and fourth cervical vertebrae.
Longus capitis[a]	Anterior tubercles of transverse processes of third through sixth cervical vertebrae.	Inferior surface of basilar part of occipital bone.
Rectus capitis anterior[a]	Root of transverse process, and anterior surface of atlas.	Inferior surface of basilar part of occipital bone.
Rectus capitis lateralis[a]	Superior surface of transverse process of atlas.	Inferior surface of jugular process of occipital bone.
Scalenus anterior[a]	Anterior tubercles of transverse processes of third through sixth cervical vertebrae.	Scalene tubercle and cranial crest of first rib.
Scalenus medius[a]	Posterior tubercles of transverse processes of second through seventh cervical vertebrae.	Cranial surface of first rib between tubercle and subclavian groove.
Scalenus posterior[a]	By two or three tendons from posterior tubercles of transverse processes of last two or three cervical vertebrae.	Outer surface of second rib.
Platysma[b]	Fascia covering superior parts of Pectoralis major and Deltoid.	Inferior margin of mandible, and skin of lower part of face and corner of mouth.
Sternocleidomastoid[b]	*Medial or sternal head:* Cranial part of manubrium sterni. *Lateral or clavicular head:* Medial one third of clavicle.	Lateral surface of mastoid process, lateral one half of superior nuchal line of occipital bone.
Rectus capitis posterior major	Spinous process of axis.	Lateral part of inferior nuchal line of occipital bone.
Rectus capitis posterior minor	Tubercle on posterior arch of atlas.	Medial part of inferior nuchal line of occipital bone.
Obliquus capitis inferior	Apex of spinous process of axis.	Inferior and posterior part of transverse process of atlas.
Obiquus capitis superior	Superior surface of transverse process of atlas.	Between superior and inferior nuchal lines of occipital bone.
Trapezius, upper	See p. 282 for origins and insertions.	
Splenius capitis Splenius cervicis Iliocostalis cervicis Longissimus cervicis Longissimus capitis Spinalis cervicis Spinalis capitis Semispinalis cervicis Semispinalis capitis Multifidi, cervical Rotatores, cervical Interspinales, cervical Intertransversarii, cervical	See p. 138 for origins and insertions.	

[a]See illustration, p. 314.
[b]See illustration, p. 301.

316

Muscles	Acting bilaterally		Acting unilaterally		
	Extension	Flexion	Lateral flexion	Rotation	
				To same side	To opposite side
Longus colli		X	X	X	
Longus capitis		X		X	
Rectus capitis anterior		X		X	
Rectus capitis lateralis			X		
Scalenus anterior		X	X		X
Scalenus medius			X		X
Scalenus posterior			X		X
Platysma		X			
Sternocleidomastoid	X	X	X		X
Rectus capitis posterior major	X			X	
Rectus capitis posterior minor	X				
Obliquus capitis inferior				X	
Obliquus capitis superior	X		X		
Splenius cervicis	X		X	X	
Splenius capitis	X		X	X	
Trapezius, upper	X		X		X
Iliocostalis cervicis	X		X		
Longissimus cervicis	X				
Longissimus capitis	X		X	X	
Spinalis cervicis	X				
Spinalis capitis	X				
Semispinalis cervicis	X				X
Semispinalis capitis	X				
Multifidi, cervical	X				X
Rotatores, cervical	X				X
Interspinales, cervical	X				
Intertransversarii, cervical			X		

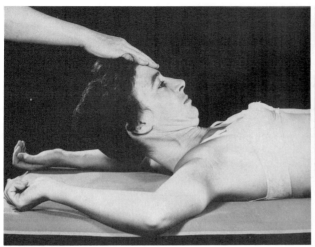 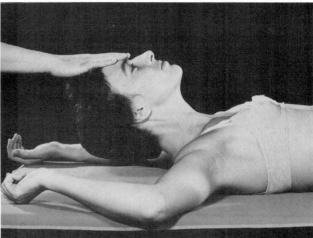

Patient: Supine with elbows bent and hands overhead, resting on table.

Fixation: Anterior abdominal muscles must be strong enough to give anterior fixation of thorax to pelvis before the head can be raised by the neck flexors. If abdominal muscles are weak, the examiner can give fixation by firm downward pressure on the thorax. Children approximately 5 years and under should have fixation of the thorax by the examiner.

Test: Flexion of the cervical spine by lifting the head from the table with the chin depressed and approximated toward the sternum.

Pressure: Against the forehead in a posterior direction.

Modified Test: In cases of marked weakness have patient make an effort to flatten the cervical spine on the table, approximating the chin toward the sternum.

Pressure: Against the chin in the direction of neck extension.

Note: The anterior vertebral flexors of the neck are the Longus capitis and colli and the Rectus capitis anterior. In this movement they are aided by the Sternocleidomastoid, anterior Scaleni, suprahyoids, and infrahyoids. The Platysma will attempt to aid when flexors are very weak.

Weakness: Hyperextension of the cervical spine resulting in a forward head position.

Contracture: A neck flexion contracture is rarely seen except unilaterally as in torticollis.

If anterior vertebral neck flexors are weak and the Sternocleidomastoid muscles strong, an individual can raise the head from the table (as illustrated), and can hold against pressure, but this is not an accurate test for neck flexors. Action is accomplished chiefly by the Sternocleidomastoids aided by the anterior Scaleni and the clavicular portions of the upper Trapezius.

Grading: Since most grades of 10 are based on adult standards, it is necessary to acknowledge when a grade less than 10 is normal for children of a given age. This is particularly true with respect to the strength of the anterior neck and anterior abdominal muscles. The size of the head and trunk in relation to the lower extremities, as well as the long span and normal protrusion of the abdominal wall, affect the relative strength of these muscles. Anterior neck muscles may grade about 3 in a 3-year-old child, about 5 in a 5-year-old, and gradually increase up to the 10 standard of performance by as early as 10 to 12 years of age. Many adults will exhibit no more than a grade of 6, but this need not be interpreted as neurogenic because usually it is found to be associated with faulty posture of the head and upper back.

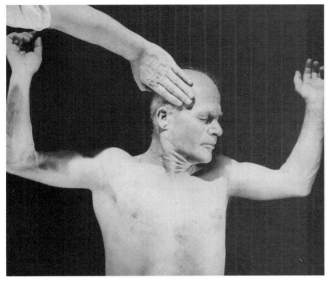 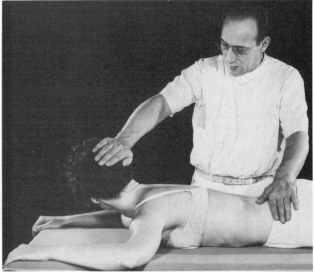

The muscles acting in this test are chiefly Sternocleidomastoid and Scaleni.

Patient: Supine with elbows bent and hands beside head, resting on table.

Fixation: If anterior abdominal muscles are weak, the examiner can give fixation by firm downward pressure on the thorax.

Test: Anterolateral neck flexion.

Pressure: Against the temporal region of the head in an obliquely posterior direction.

Note: With neck muscles just strong enough to hold, but not strong enough to flex completely, a patient can lift the head from the table by raising the shoulders. A patient will do so especially on the tests for right and left neck flexors because of the attempt to help by taking some weight on the elbow or hand in order to push the shoulder from the table. To avoid this, keep the patient's shoulder flat on the table.

Contracture and Weakness: A contracture of the right Sternocleidomastoid produces a right torticollis. The face is turned toward the left and the head is tilted toward the right. Thus, a right torticollis produces a cervical scoliosis convex toward the left. The left Sternocleidomastoid is elongated and weak. Contracture of the left Sternocleidomastoid, with weakness of the right, produces a left torticollis with a cervical scoliosis convex toward the right.

In an habitually faulty posture with forward head, the Sternocleidomastoid muscles remain in a shortened position, and tend to develop shortness.

The muscles included in this test are chiefly the Splenius capitis and cervicis, Semispinalis capitis and cervicis, and cervical Erector spinae. (See pp. 138 and 139.)

Patient: Prone with elbows bent and hands overhead, resting on table.

Fixation: None necessary.

Test: Posterolateral neck extension with face turned toward the side being tested. (See *Note.*)

Pressure: Against the posterolateral aspect of the head in an anterior direction.

Shortness: The right Splenius capitis and left upper Trapezius are usually short along with the Sternocleidomastoid in a left torticollis. The opposite muscles are short in a right torticollis.

Note: The upper Trapezius, which is also a posterolateral neck extensor, is tested with the face turned away from the side being tested. (See p. 287.)

MUSCLE	ORIGIN	INSERTION	ACTION	INNERVATION Motor	INNERVATION Sensory	ROLE IN DEGLUTITION
TONGUE						
Sup. longitudinal	Intrinsic	Intrinsic	Shortens tongue / Raises sides and tip of tongue	Hypoglossal XII	General sensation Ant. ⅔ — Trigeminal V; Post ⅓ — Glossopharyngeal IX; Base—Vagus X	**Bolus Preparation** During this phase the tongue and the buccinator muscles keep the food between the molar teeth where it is crushed and ground by the action of muscles of mastication. Alternate side to side movements and twisting of the tongue, performed chiefly by the intrinsic muscles and by the styloglossi acting unilaterally, aid in mixing the food with saliva and in sorting larger particles from the sufficiently ground portion which is ready to be rolled into a bolus and swallowed.
Transverse	Intrinsic	Intrinsic	Lengthens and narrows tongue			
Vertical	Intrinsic	Intrinsic	Flattens and broadens tongue			
Inf. longitudinal	Intrinsic	Intrinsic	Shortens tongue / Turns tip of tongue downward			
Genioglossus	Mental spine	Tongue & body of hyoid	Depresses tongue; protrudes & retracts tongue; elevates hyoid	Hypoglossal XII	Special sensation (taste) Ant. ⅔ — Facial VII; Post. ⅓ — Glossopharyngeal IX; Base—Vagus X	
Hyoglossus	Greater horn of hyoid	Tongue	Depresses and pulls tongue posteriorly			
Styloglossus	Styloid process	Tongue	Elevates and pulls tongue posteriorly			
Palatoglossus	Aponeurosis of soft palate	Tongue	Elevates and pulls tongue posteriorly; narrows fauces.	Pharyngeal plexus IX, X, XI		
SOFT PALATE						
Tensor veli palatini	Scaphoid fossa, spine of sphenoid, lateral auditory tube	Aponeurosis of soft palate	Tenses soft palate	Trigeminal V	Trigeminal V Glossopharyngeal IX	**Voluntary Stage** The tongue depressor muscles contract and form a groove in the posterior portion of the dorsum of the tongue which cradles the bolus. A movement initiated by the intrinsic muscles raises the anterior portion and then the posterior portion of the tongue to the hard palate. This sequential movement dislodges the bolus and squeezes it toward the fauces. In turn the base of the tongue is elevated and pulled posteriorly mainly by the action of the styloglossi muscles forcing the bolus through the fauces into the pharynx. Occurring simultaneously with this elevation of the base of the tongue is a moderate elevation of the hyoid bone and the larynx.
Levator veli palatini	Petrous portion, temporal bone; medial auditory tube	Soft palate	Elevates soft palate	Pharyngeal plexus IX, X, XI		
Uvulae	Posterior nasal spine; aponeurosis of palate	Uvula	Shortens soft palate			
FAUCES						
Palatoglossus	See above		Narrows fauces:	Pharyngeal plexus IX, X, XI	Glossopharyngeal IX	**Involuntary (Reflex) Stage** As the bolus passes through the fauces to the pharynx, branches of cranial nerves V, IX and X are stimulated producing impulses in the afferent limb of the swallow reflex. Upon reaching the brainstem, these impulses are transmitted across synapses to efferent fibers of cranial nerves IX, X and XI completing the reflex arc and effecting the following automatic events:
Palatopharyngeus	Aponeurosis of soft palate	Posterior thyroid cartilage; Posterolateral pharynx	Narrows fauces; Elevates larynx & pharynx	Pharyngeal plexus IX, X, XI		
SUPRAHYOID						
Digastric Ant. belly	Inferior border of mandible near symphysis	Intermediate tendon to body and cornu of hyoid	Elevates and pulls hyoid anteriorly / Assist in depressing the mandible	Trigeminal V		
Post. belly	Mastoid process		Elevates and pulls hyoid posteriorly	Facial VII		
Mylohyoid	Mylohyoid line of mandible	Body of hyoid & median raphe	Elevates hyoid & tongue; depresses mandible	Trigeminal V		
Geniohyoid	Median ridge of mandible	Body of hyoid	Elevates hyoid & tongue; depresses mandible	Ansa cervicalis C1, 2		
Stylohyoid	Styloid process of temporal bone	Body of hyoid	Elevates and pulls hyoid posteriorly	Facial VII		

INFRAHYOID

Muscle	Origin	Insertion	Action	Innervation
Thyrohyoid	Oblique line of thyroid cartilage	Greater horn of hyoid	Elevates the thyroid cartilage; depresses the hyoid	Ansa cervicalis C1, 2
Sternohyoid	Manubrium sterni; medial end of clavicle	Body of hyoid, inf. border	Depresses hyoid	Ansa cervicalis C1, 2, 3
Sternothyroid	Manubrium sterni; costal cartilage of 1st rib	Oblique line of thyroid cartilage	Depresses thyroid cartilage	Ansa cervicalis C1, 2, 3
Omohyoid — Sup. belly	Superior border of scapula near scapular notch	Intermediate tendon, by fascia to clavicle	Depresses the hyoid	Ansa cervicalis C1, 2, 3
Omohyoid — Inf. belly	Intermediate tendon by fascia to clavicle	Body of hyoid, inf. border	Depresses the hyoid	

LARYNX

Muscle	Origin	Insertion	Action	Innervation
Aryepiglottic	Apex of arytenoid cartilage	Lateral margin of epiglottis	Assists in closing inlet of larynx	Vagus X
Thyroepiglottic	Medial surface of thyroid cartilage	Lateral margin of epiglottis	Assists in closing inlet of larynx	Vagus X
Thyroarytenoid	Medial surface of thyroid cartilage	Muscular process of arytenoid cartilage	Assists in closing glottis; shortens vocal folds	Vagus X
Arytenoid-Oblique	Base of one arytenoid cartilage	Apex of opposite arytenoid cartilage	Assist in closing glottis by adducting arytenoid cartilages	Vagus X
Transverse	Posterior surface and lateral border of one arytenoid cartilage	Posterior surface and lateral border of opposite arytenoid cartilage		Vagus X
Lat. cricoarytenoid	Upper border of arch of cricoid cartilage	Muscular process of arytenoid cartilage	Adducts and medially rotates arytenoid cartilage assisting in closing glottis	Vagus X Mainly accessory XI, cranial root
Vocalis	Medial surface of thyroid cartilage	Vocal process of arytenoid cartilage	Regulates tension of vocal folds	
Post. cricoarytenoid	Posterior surface of lamina of cricoid cartilage	Muscular process of arytenoid cartilage	Abducts arytenoid cartilage widening glottis	
Cricothyroid-Straight	Anterior and lateral part of arch of cricoid cartilage	Anterior border, inferior horn of thyroid cartilage	Elevates cricoid arch and elongates vocal folds	
Cricothyroid-Oblique		Lower border of lamina of thyroid cartilage	Elevates cricoid arch and elongates vocal folds	

PHARYNX

Muscle	Origin	Insertion	Action	Innervation
Salpingopharyngeus	Auditory tube	Pharyngeal wall	Elevates pharynx	Pharyngeal plexus IX, X, XI
Palatopharyngeus	See above			Pharyngeal plexus IX, X, XI
Stylopharyngeus	Styloid process	Posterior border of thyroid cartilage; posterolateral wall of pharynx	Elevates pharynx and larynx	Glossopharyngeal IX
Superior constrictor	Medial pterygoid plate; pterygomandibular raphe; mandible	pharyngeal tubercle; pharyngeal raphe	Constrict, sequentially, nasopharynx, oropharynx, laryngopharynx	Pharyngeal plexus IX and X
Middle constrictor	Horns of hyoid	pharyngeal raphe		Pharyngeal plexus IX and X
Inferior constrictor	Thyroid and cricoid cartilages	pharyngeal raphe		Pharyngeal plexus IX and X
Cricopharyngeus	Arch of cricoid cartilage	Arch of cricoid cartilage	Acts as sphincter to prevent air entering esophagus; relaxes during swallowing	Pharyngeal plexus IX and X

The soft palate is elevated and brought into contact with the posterior pharyngeal wall by the contraction of the tensor and levator veli palatini muscles. This action closes off the nasopharynx ensuring passage of the bolus into the lumen of the laryngopharynx. This passage is facilitated when the lumen is expanded by the elevation of the pharyngeal wall and the cranial and anterior movement of the hyoid bone and the larynx. When the last of the bolus leaves the oral cavity, the oropharynx opening is closed by contraction of the palatopharyngeal muscles and the descent of the soft palate.

The cranial movement of the thyroid cartilage toward the hyoid bone and of these two structures, in turn, toward the base of the tongue results in tilting the epiglottis posteriorly. The weight of the bolus as it contacts the anterior surface of the epiglottis assists in increasing this posterior tilt. The change of position of the epiglottis aids in directing the bolus material around the sides of the larynx through the piriform sinuses and over the tip of the epiglottis into the hypopharynx. It also aids in preventing foodstuffs from entering the larynx. The major mechanism for protecting the larynx, however, is the concurrent sphincter-like closure of the laryngeal inlet to the vestibule and the closure of the vestibular and vocal folds of the glottis.

Occurring simultaneously with the above events is a sequential contraction of the superior, middle and inferior constrictors which strips the pharynx forcing the bolus toward the esophagus. Horizontally oriented fibers found between the inferior constrictor and the esophagus have been named the cricopharyngeus muscle. This muscle acts as a sphincter and functionally is related more to the esophagus then to the pharynx. It relaxes when the bolus reaches the caudal extent of the hypopharynx permitting the foodstuff to enter the esophagus.

321

RESPIRATORY MUSCLE CHART

Patient's Name _____ Clinic # _____

Left						Right			
				Examiner					
				Date					
				Inspiratory Muscles Primary					
				Diaphragm					
· · · ·	· · · ·	· · · ·	· · · ·	Levator costarum	· · · ·	· · · ·	· · · ·	· · · ·	
				External intercostals					
				Internal intercostals, anterior (1)					
				Accessory					
				Scaleni					
				Sternocleidomastoid					
				Trapezius					
				Serratus ant. & post. superior					
				Pectoralis major & minor					
				Latissimus dorsi					
				Erector spinae, thoracic					
· · · ·	· · · ·	· · · ·	· · · ·	Subclavius	· · · ·	· · · ·	· · · ·	· · · ·	
				Expiratory Muscles Primary					
				Abdominal muscles					
				Internal oblique					
				External oblique					
				Rectus abdominis					
				Transversus abdominis					
				Internal intercostals, posterior (2)					
· · · ·	· · · ·	· · · ·	· · · ·	Transversus thoracis	· · · ·	· · · ·	· · · ·	· · · ·	
				Accessory					
				Latissimus dorsi					
· · · ·	· · · ·	· · · ·	· · · ·	Serratus posterior inferior	· · · ·	· · · ·	· · · ·	· · · ·	
				Quadratus lumborum					
				Iliocostalis lumborum					

Notes: _____
_____
_____
_____
_____

(1) Also called parasternal or intercartilaginous
(2) Also called interosseus

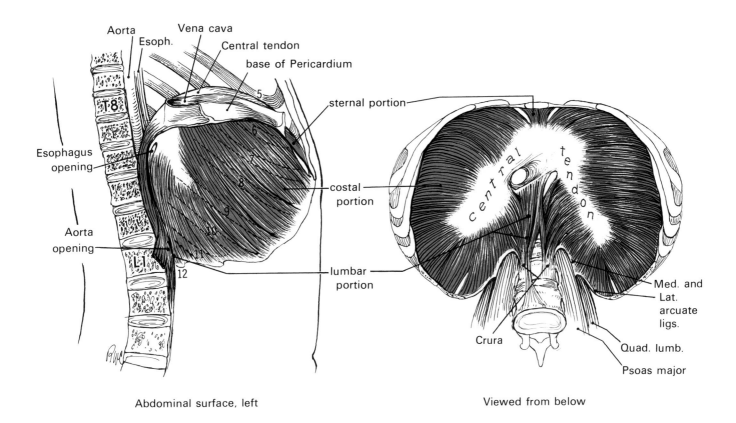

Aorta
Esoph.
Vena cava
Central tendon
base of Pericardium

T8

Esophagus opening

Aorta opening

L1

sternal portion

costal portion

lumbar portion

central tendon

Med. and Lat. arcuate ligs.

Crura

Quad. lumb.

Psoas major

Abdominal surface, left

Viewed from below

Origin of Sternal Part: Two fleshy slips from dorsum of xiphoid process.

Origin of Costal Part: Inner surfaces of lower six costal cartilages and lower six ribs on either side, interdigitating with Transversus abdominis.

Origin of Lumbar Part: By two muscular crura from the bodies of the upper lumbar vertebrae and by two fibrous arches on either side, known as medial and lateral arcuate ligaments, which span from the vertebrae to the transverse processes and from the latter to the 12th rib.

Insertion: Into central tendon. This tendon is a thin strong aponeurosis with no bony attachment. Since the anterior muscular fibers of the Diaphragm are shorter than the posterior muscular fibers, the central tendon is situated closer to the ventral part of the thorax than to the dorsal.

Action: The dome-shaped Diaphragm separates the thoracic and abdominal cavities and is the principal muscle of respiration. During inspiration, the muscle contracts and the dome descends increasing the volume and decreasing the pressure of the thoracic cavity, while decreasing the volume and increasing the pressure of the abdominal cavity. The descent of the dome or central tendon of the Diaphragm is limited by the abdominal viscera, and when descent occurs the central tendon becomes the more fixed portion of the muscle. With continued contraction, the vertical fibers attached to the ribs elevate and evert the costal margin. The dimensions of the thorax are constantly enlarged craniocaudally, anteroposteriorly, and transversely. During expiration, the Diaphragm relaxes and the dome ascends decreasing the volume and increasing the pressure of the thoracic cavity, while increasing the volume and decreasing the pressure of the abdominal cavity.

Note: In cases of pulmonary pathology such as emphysema, the dome of the Diaphragm is so depressed that the costal margin or base of the thorax cannot be expanded.

Nerve: Phrenic, C3, **4**, 5.

Respiratory Muscles

Respiration refers to the exchange of gases between the cells of an organism and the external environment. Numerous neural, chemical, and muscular components are involved, but this section relates specifically to the role of muscles.

Respiration consists of ventilation and circulation. Ventilation is the movement of gases into and out of the lungs, while circulation is the transport of these gases to the tissues. Although movement of gases in the lungs and tissues is by diffusion, their transport to and from the environment and throughout the body requires work by the respiratory and cardiac pumps.

The respiratory pump is comprised of the muscles of respiration and the thorax, which is made up of the ribs, scapulae, clavicle, sternum and thoracic spine. This musculoskeletal pump provides the necessary pressure gradients to move gases into and out of the lungs in order to ensure adequate diffusion of oxygen and carbon dioxide within the lung.

The work of breathing performed by respiratory muscles in overcoming lung, chest wall, and airway resistances normally occurs only during inspiration. Muscular effort is required to enlarge the thoracic cavity and lower intrathoracic pressure. Expiration results from the elastic recoil of the lungs upon relaxation of the inspiratory muscles. The muscles of expiration are active, however, when the demands of breathing are increased. Heavy work, exercise, blowing, coughing, and singing all involve significant expiratory muscle work. Also, in conditions like emphysema when the elastic recoil is impaired, techniques such as pursed-lip breathing are employed to enhance expiration and minimize effort.

The *Respiratory Muscle Chart* shows the division of muscles according to their *major* inspiratory or expiratory ventilatory roles. This division, however, does not mean that the listed muscles function only in that singular capacity. Abdominal muscles, the chief expiratory muscles, play a role in inspiration, while inspiratory intercostals and the Diaphragm perform an importance "braking" action during expiration.

The further division, on the chart, into primary and accessory muscles shows the numerous muscles that can be recruited to assist in the ventilatory process. Exactly which muscles participate and the extent of their participation depends not only on the demands of breathing but, also, on individual differences in breathing habits or needs.

The fact that breathing can be altered by changes in position, emotional state, activity level, disease, and even tight garments means that there are numerous varieties in patterns of breathing. For example, Duchenne remarked that normal breathing of women in the mid-19th century was "of the costosuperior type" because of compression from corsets on the lower part of the chest (37).

According to Shneerson: "It is better to regard the respiratory muscles as being capable of recruitment according to the pattern of ventilation, posture, wakefulness or stage of sleep, muscle strength, air flow resistance, and compliance of the lungs and chest wall" (38).

Some authorities dispute the accessory role of certain muscles, particularly the upper Trapezius and Serratus anterior. Other muscles are also often omitted in writings on accessory respiratory muscles. The Rhomboid, which is not included in the accompanying chart, has a role in stabilizing the scapula to assist the Serratus in forced inspiration.

All the muscles listed on the chart have the capacity to be recruited when needed to facilitate breathing. Many of them perform vital roles in stabilizing parts of the body so that there is adequate force to move air into and out of the lungs. As the work of breathing increases, larger volumes of gas must be moved more quickly and greater pressure generation is required. The ventilatory muscles work harder, and additional muscles are recruited to meet the demands of breathing.

The following quotation emphasizes the importance of *all* respiratory muscles: "The distance runner struggling for air . . . may use even the platysma for expanding his chest, and the patient in paroxysms of cough probably contracts every muscle of the trunk, thorax, and pectoral girdle during forced expiration" (39). Although the numerous muscles of the upper airways, especially the intrinsic and extrinsic muscles of the larynx, are not discussed here, it should be noted that they play an important role in permitting the free flow of air to and from the lungs. (See p. 321 for laryngeal muscles.)

In some individuals and under certain circumstances, accessory muscles may be used as primary. If the Diaphragm or intercostals are paralyzed, breathing is still possible through increased use of accessory muscles. The importance of accessory muscles was well documented in the case of a patient with a permanent tracheostomy, who had no movement in his Diaphragm or intercostal muscles. He had, surprisingly, a very large vital capacity, breathing with Scaleni supplied by cervical nerves, and Sternocleidomastoid and upper Trapezius supplied by the spinal accessory nerve (40).

Of the more than 20 primary and accessory muscles shown on the chart, almost all of them have a postural function. Only the Diaphragm and anterior intercostals may be purely respiratory. Twenty of these muscles have all or part of their origins or insertions on the ribs or costal cartilages. Any muscle attached to the rib cage is able to influence the mechanics of breathing to some degree. These muscles must be able to help support the skeletal structures of the ventilatory pump and be able to generate pressures that ensure continued adequate gas exchange at the alveoli.

These pressures can be substantial. Normally, in order to double air flow, a fourfold increase in pressure is required. If air flow is to remain constant in face of a twofold decrease in the radius of an airway, there must be a sixteenfold increase in pressure (39).

Respiratory complications can arise from a variety of obstructive and restrictive diseases and neuromuscular and skeletal disorders. Once a diagnosis is made, treatment is designed to preserve existing lung function and to eliminate or reduce the problem that is compromising respiratory function. The goal is to improve a patient's ability to ventilate the lungs.

Of primary importance is the need to lessen the work of breathing and reduce the energy expenditure (oxygen consumption) of respiratory muscles. Depending on the particular respiratory disorder, it may be the elastic, the resistive and/or the mechanical work of breathing that needs to be alleviated. Respiratory failure can result when the increased work of breathing leads to alveolar hypoventilation and hypoxia.

A variety of techniques, procedures, and mechanical devices are used to assist lung function. Although treatment must be specific to the type of ventilatory problem manifested, certain principles and practices are basic to respiratory therapy.

Reduce Patient's Fear. The first step in reducing the work of breathing and instituting effective treatment is to reduce a patient's fear and anxiety level in order to obtain the patient's confidence and compliance. Existing respiratory problems are severely exacerbated by breath-holding, breathlessness, and increased tension in accessory muscles that frequently accompany a fearful state. When the confidence and cooperation of a patient are obtained, other treatment measures will be far more effective.

Improve Relaxation. Relaxation brings about a decrease in the oxygen consumption of skeletal muscles and an increase in compliance of the chest wall. When indicated, diaphragmatic breathing exercises may aid relaxation and give a patient a better sense of control over respiration. These exercises emphasize abdominal rather than the rib cage expansion and are helpful when there is overuse of the accessory muscles of the neck and upper chest. Practicing a pattern of deep breathing and sighing can reduce the work of breathing and help relax a patient who has attacks of breathlessness or breath-holding.

Improve Posture. Optimal breathing capability derives from a posture of optimal muscle balance. A balanced musculature is most efficient in terms of energy expenditure.

Imbalance of the musculature resulting from tightness, weakness, or paralysis may adversely affect the volumes and pressures that can be attained and maintained. Very weak and protruding abdominal muscles are not able to generate maximum expiratory pressures to meet increased demands of breathing brought on by exertion or illness. Weakness of upper back Erector spinae and middle and lower Trapezius muscles interferes with the ability to straighten the upper back, thus limiting the ability to raise and expand the chest and maximize lung capacity. Postural problems associated with kyphosis, kyphoscoliosis, osteoporosis, and pectus excavum restrict breathing and result in decreased chest wall compliance.

Improve Strength and Endurance of Respiratory Muscles. "Strength is needed for sudden respiratory movements such as coughing and sneezing, and brief spells of extreme exertion, whereas endurance is necessary for more prolonged exercise or to overcome an increase in air flow resistance or a decrease in compliance" (38).

Muscles that are strong and well-conditioned are more efficient and require less oxygen to do a given amount of work than poorly conditioned muscles. Although there are mixed reports as to the efficacy of muscle strength training of respiratory muscles, such training may be beneficial if respiratory muscle weakness limits exercise or diminishes inspiratory capacity.

The stronger the abdominal muscles, the greater their ability to compress the abdomen and generate additional pressure during expiration. Exercises to strengthen these muscles can help improve coughing and other expulsive maneuvers that are required to clear airways and facilitate breathing.

If there is marked weakness of these abdominal muscles, exercises should be supplemented with a support that will reduce the downward pull of the abdomen and help keep the Diaphragm in a position that is most advantageous for both inspiration and expiration. Such assistance often helps minimize breathing problems associated with obesity.

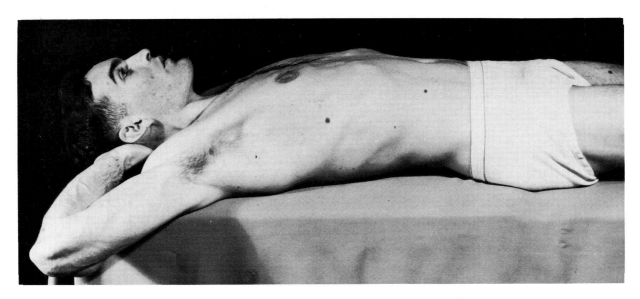

Normal inspiration: Intercostal and diaphragmatic.

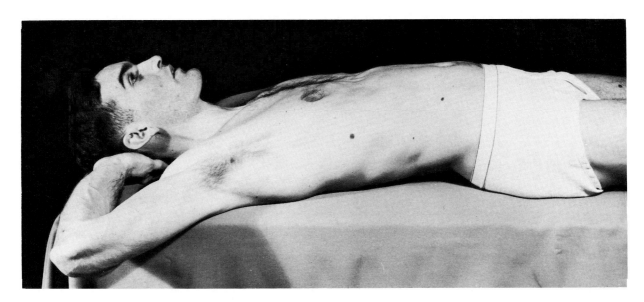

Inspiration: Diaphragmatic.

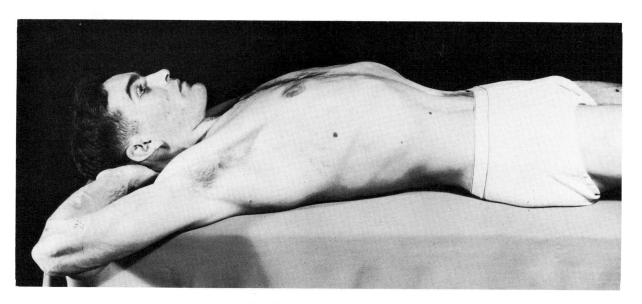

Inspiration: Intercostal

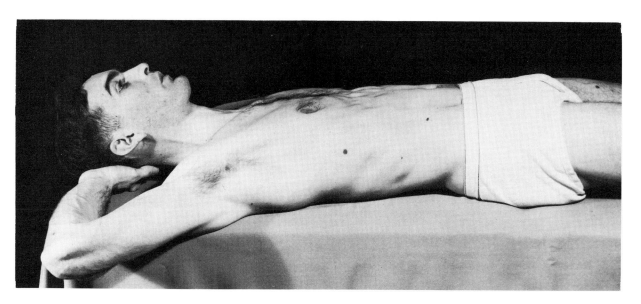

Forced expiration: Intercostal, abdominal, and accessory muscles.

Respiratory muscle fatigue may precipitate respiratory failure. Endurance training is intended to increase the capacity of muscles to resist fatigue. Training has been shown to benefit about 40% of patients suffering chronic air flow obstruction, and slight improvements in endurance have been observed in cystic fibrosis patients (38).

In disorders of the respiratory muscles, "Respiratory failure is usually closely related to the degree of respiratory muscle weakness but occasionally occurs with only mild impairment of muscle function" (38). Because of the high risk of respiratory failure associated with weak respiratory muscles, a program of exercises to strengthen these muscles may be of critical importance but must be very conservative, and closely monitored.

Improve Coordination. The oxygen cost of performing a task can be greater than normal in a person who moves in an uncoordinated fashion. When inefficient patterns of breathing and movement are identified, corrective treatment can be instituted and, gradually, the work of breathing will be reduced.

Improve Overall Fitness. Improve cardiovascular fitness through whole-body exercises such as walking and bicycle riding in order to strengthen ventilatory capability and efficiency. Exercises that involve the legs rather than the arms are preferred initially so that accessory muscles can be used to aid breathing.

Reduce Weight. Respiratory problems associated with obesity are often very severe. According to Cherniack, the oxygen cost of breathing in an obese person is about three times the normal cost (41). Unlike some skeletal and neuromuscular respiratory disorders, obesity is a condition that can sometimes be reversed and respiration greatly improved.

PRIMARY MUSCLES OF RESPIRATION

Diaphragm. The Diaphragm (see p. 323), by virtue of its attachment and actions, serves as a pressure partitioner and force transmitter. Normal length and strength of this muscle are essential for these functions. Limited or excessive excursion of the Diaphragm reduces its effectiveness in inspiration and expiration.

In certain respiratory conditions, such as emphysema, the Diaphragm is not able to return to a dome-shaped contour upon relaxation but is held, instead, in a shortened, flattened position. There is reduced pressure-generating capability and inspiratory capacity because the lungs remain in a partially inflated state at resting level. Also, the ability of the Diaphragm to act as

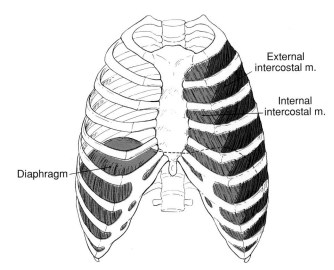

External intercostal m.

Internal intercostal m.

Diaphragm

a force transmitter and assist in emptying the lungs is reduced.

The abdominal viscera, supported by abdominal muscles, normally limit the downward descent of the Diaphragm during inspiration and assist its upward movement during expiration. Under abnormal circumstances, there can be a reverse action of the Diaphragm. A dramatic example of this was seen in an infant who had poliomyelitis and was placed in a respirator. The muscles of the abdomen, which are normally weak in an infant, were paralyzed. During the positive pressure phase, air was forced out of the lungs and the Diaphragm moved upward. During the negative pressure phase, air was drawn into the lungs with a momentary expansion of the rib cage, followed by excessive descent of the Diaphragm into the abdominal cavity. The abdomen ballooned as the viscera moved downward. By virtue of the attachment of the Diaphragm to the inner wall of the chest, the ribs were drawn down and inward, causing the rib cage to "cave in" as the Diaphragm descended into the abdominal cavity, completely defeating the function of this muscle.

Within hours, a support in the form of a tiny corset was made and applied to restrict the ballooning of the abdomen, and to help prevent the excessive descent of the Diaphragm and the devastating effect on the rib cage.

The Intercostal Muscles. The External intercostals arise from the lower borders of the ribs and attach to the upper borders of the ribs below. Similarly, the Internal intercostals have their origins on the inner surfaces of ribs and costal cartilages and insertions on the upper borders of adjacent ribs below. There are two layers of these rib cage muscles "everywhere except anteriorly in the interchondral region and posteriorly in the areas medial to the costal angle" (27).

These muscles play an important postural, as well as respiratory, role. They stabilize and maintain the shape and integrity of the rib cage.

Anatomically, they appear to be extensions of the External and Internal oblique muscles.

Debate persists as to the *exact* respiratory function of these muscles. It seems that at least the exposed anterior portion of the Internal intercostals (parasternal, intercartilaginous) acts as an inspiratory muscle along with the External intercostals, elevating the ribs and expanding the chest. The posterior portion (interosseous) of the Internal intercostals depresses the ribs and acts in an expiratory capacity.

Some have suggested that the function of these muscles varies with lung volume and depth of respiration as the position and slope of the ribs to which they are attached changes. These muscles are always active during speech. During controlled expiration, they perform an important "braking action" that minimizes the static recoil of the lungs and chest wall. Singers make much use of this expiratory action of the intercostals.

Breathing is possible when intercostals are paralyzed, but there is diminished sucking and blowing capacity. There is also limited rib cage movement and decreased ability to stabilize the rib cage.

The Abdominal Muscles. The abdominal muscles are the Internal obliques, External obliques, Rectus abdominis, and Transversus abdominis. (See pp. 147–151.) These muscles are the chief expiratory muscles but are also active towards the end of inspiration. The particular muscles that are most important at the end of inspiration and beginning of expiration are those with little or no flexor action. Specifically, the lower fibers of the Internal obliques and Transversus are most active, along with the lateral fibers of the External obliques.

These muscles must be able to contract sufficiently to raise intra-abdominal pressure to meet increased demands of breathing—especially sudden expulsive acts. Pressure so generated is transmitted to the thoracic cage by the Diaphragm to assist in emptying the lungs.

The Transversus arises from the cartilages of the lower six ribs and interdigitates with the Diaphragm. The Quadratus lumborum, by virtue of its insertion on the 12th rib, anchors the rib cage and so aids diaphragmatic action in inspiration as well as expiration.

The External oblique muscles cover a major portion of the lower thorax since some fibers interdigitate with the lower serrations of the Serratus anterior. Increased abdominal activity, particularly of the External oblique, reduces fluctuations of thoracic cage volume and helps to maintain constancy of pressure.

ACCESSORY MUSCLES OF RESPIRATION

Scalenes. The anterior, medial and posterior scalenes are accessory muscles of inspiration that function as a unit. By elevating and firmly fixing the first and second ribs, they aid deep inspiration. The scaleni have been observed to be active during quiet breathing and have been classified by some researchers as primary rather than accessory.

The scaleni may become active during *expiratory* efforts, also. According to Egan, "It is felt that the expiratory function of the scalene muscles is to fix the ribs against the contraction of the abdominal muscles and to prevent herniation of the apex of the lung during coughing" (42). (See also pp. 314 and 316–317.)

Sternocleidomastoid. This muscle is considered by many to be the most important accessory muscle of inspiration. For the Sternocleidomastoid to act in this capacity, the head and neck must be held in a stable position by the neck flexors and extensors. This muscles "pulls from its skull insertions and elevates the sternum, increasing the A-P diameter of the chest" (42). It contracts during moderate and deep inspiration. When lungs are hyperinflated, the Sternocleidomastoids are especially active. Electrical activity is sometimes evident during quiet inspiration (38). They are not active during expiration. (See pp. 310 and 316–317.)

Serratus Anterior. This muscle arises from the upper eight or nine ribs and inserts on the costal surface of the medial border of the scapula. Its primary action is to abduct and rotate the scapula and hold the medial border firmly against the rib cage.

Some studies have "disproved" a respiratory role for the Serratus anterior muscle. Gray's Anatomy (37th ed.) notes, however, that one such study (Catton and Gray 1957) "ignored the effects of fixing the scapula by grasping, e.g., a bedrail or railing, as asthmatics and athletes certainly do!" (43).

When the scapula is stabilized in adduction by the Rhomboids, thereby fixing the insertion, the Serratus can assist in forced inspiration. It helps to expand the rib cage by pulling the origin toward the insertion. Because it takes a stronger Serratus to move the rib cage than to move the scapula, a person with only fair strength may be able to move the scapula in abduction but would have difficulty expanding the rib cage with the scapula fixed in adduction. Consequently, weakness in this muscle diminishes its ability to be recruited to meet increased inspiratory needs. (See p. 288.)

Pectoralis Major. This is a large fan-shaped muscle that is active in deep or forced inspiration and not active in expiration. Egan considers this muscle to be the third most important accessory muscle and describes its mechanism of action as follows: "If the arms and shoulders are fixed, as by leaning on the elbows or firmly grasping a table, the pectoralis major can use its insertion as an origin and pull with great force on the anterior chest, lifting up ribs and sternum and increasing thoracic A-P diameter" (42).

Pectoralis Minor. The Pectoralis minor assists in forced inspiration by raising the ribs, thereby moving the origin toward the insertion. The insertion must be fixed by stabilizing the scapula in optimal position. The scapula must be stabilized in a position that prevents anterior tilt with depression of the coracoid process down and forward. This stabilization is accomplished by the lower and middle Trapezius. (See pp. 286 and 284.)

Upper Trapezius. The Trapezius muscle is discussed in detail on pp. 282 and 287. The ventilatory role of the upper Trapezius is to assist forced inspiration by helping to elevate the thoracic cage. The insertion of the upper fibers onto the lateral third of the clavicle ensures the participation of this portion of the muscle whenever clavicular breathing is needed for ventilation.

Latissimus Dorsi. Although its respiratory role is essentially in forceful expiration, studies have shown that the Latissimus dorsi also has a role in deep inspiration. The anterior fibers, which are active during trunk flexion, assist in expiration; the posterior fibers, active during trunk extension, assist in inspiration. (See p. 279.)

Erector Spinae (Thoracic). Thoracic Erector spinae muscles extend the thoracic spine and aid inspiration by raising the rib cage to permit full expansion of the chest. (See pp. 138–139.)

Iliocostalis Lumborum. This Erector spinae muscle inserts onto the inferior angles of the lower six or seven ribs and can assist as an accessory muscle of expiration. (See p. 138.)

Quadratus Lumborum. This accessory muscle fixes the posterior fibers of the Diaphragm by holding down the 12th rib so that it is not elevated along with the others during respiration. (See p. 143.)

The following muscles listed on the *Respiratory Muscle Chart* are those that cannot be tested manually and are inaccessible to palpation.

Serratus Posterior Superior. This inspiratory muscle is attached to ribs 2–5 and has its origin on the spines of the seventh cervical and two or three upper thoracic vertebrae. It lies beneath the fibers of the Rhomboids and Trapezius. It expands the chest by raising the ribs to which it is attached.

Serratus Posterior Inferior. This muscle inserts on the lower four ribs and has its origin on the spines of the lower two thoracic and upper two or three lumbar vertebrae. It acts to draw the ribs back and downward. Usually, it is considered an accessory muscle of expiration, although some list it as an inspiratory muscle (38, 44).

Levatores Costarum. These are 12 strong fan-shaped muscles that are parallel with the posterior borders of the external intercostals. Their action is to elevate and abduct the ribs and extend and laterally flex the vertebral column. They are considered inspiratory. They arise from the transverse processes of the seventh cervical and upper 11 thoracic vertebrae and insert onto the rib immediately below each vertebra.

Transversus Thoracis. This muscle, and other muscles of the innermost layer of the thorax, act in an expiratory capacity to decrease the volume of the thoracic cavity. The Transversus thoracis (Triangularis sterni) is an expiratory muscle on the ventral thoracic wall. It narrows the chest by depressing the second through sixth ribs. It arises from the xiphoid cartilage and sternum and inserts onto the lower borders of the costal cartilages of these ribs. Its caudal fibers are continuous with the Transversus abdominis.

Also in this layer are the Intercostales intimi and the Subcostales. The latter muscles on the lower dorsal thoracic wall bridge two or three intercostal spaces, and they act to draw the ribs together.

Subclavius. This is a shoulder girdle muscle with its origin on the first rib and cartilage and insertion on the undersurface of the clavicle. It draws the clavicle down and stabilizes it. The action of this muscle suggests it is important in the avoidance of clavicular breathing when this is not appropriate.

chapter 10

Painful Conditions of the Upper Back, Neck, and Arm

TREATMENT CONCEPTS

This introduction contains a brief overview of the various topics that will be covered in this chapter. The purpose of this section is to present some of the concepts and clinical approaches to evaluation and treatment that are pertinent to the discussion of painful musculoskeletal problems contained in this and the next chapter.

Mechanical Causes of Pain. Pain—whether it is in the muscle, joint, or nerve itself—is a response of the nerve. Regardless of where the stimulus may arise, the sensation of pain is conducted by nerve fibers. The mechanical factors that give rise to pain must, therefore, directly affect nerve fibers. There are two such factors to be considered in problems of faulty body mechanics.

Pressure on nerve root, trunk, nerve branches, or nerve endings may be caused by some adjacent firm structure such as bone, cartilage, fascia, scar tissue, or taut muscle. Pain resulting from an enlarged ligamentum flavum or protruded disc exemplifies nerve root pressure. The "scalenus anticus syndrome" in cases of arm pain, and the "piriformis syndrome" in cases of sciatica are examples of nerve irritation associated with tautness of the respective muscles.

Tension on structures containing nerve endings sensitive to deformation, as found in stretch or strain of muscles, tendons, or ligaments, can cause pain that is slight or excruciating, depending on the severity of the strain. Forces within the body that exert an injurious tension resulting in *strain* of soft tissue usually arise from a prolonged distortion of bony alignment or from a sudden muscle pull.

Distribution of pain along the course of the involved nerve and the areas of cutaneous sensory disturbance are aids in determining the site of the lesion. Pain may be localized below the level of direct involvement or may be widespread because of reflex or referred pain. In a root lesion, pain tends to extend from the origin of the nerve to its periphery, and cutaneous sensory involvement is on a dermatome basis.

A peripheral nerve involvement is often distinguished by pain below the level of the lesion. Most peripheral nerves contain both sensory and motor fibers. Symptoms of pain or tingling usually appear in the cutaneous areas supplied by the nerve before numbness or weakness is apparent. There are, however, numerous muscles that are supplied by nerves that are *purely motor* to the muscle, and symptoms of weakness appear without prior or concurrent symptoms of pain or tingling. (For further details, see p. 378.)

Spasm. *Muscle spasm* is an involuntary contraction of muscle, or of a segment within a muscle, that occurs as a result of painful nerve stimulation. Irritation from root, plexus, or peripheral nerve branch level will tend to cause spasm of a number of muscles, while spasm due to irritation of the nerve endings within a muscle may be limited to the muscle involved, or may be widespread due to reflex pain mechanisms.

Treatment of muscle spasm depends on the type of spasm. Relief of spasm resulting from *initial nerve irritation* of the root, trunk, or peripheral branch must depend on relief of the nerve irritation causing it. Aggressive treatment of the muscle or muscles in spasm will tend to aggravate the symptoms. For example, one should avoid the use of heat, massage, and stretching of Hamstring muscles in cases of acute sciatica. Rigid immobilization of the extremity is also contraindicated.

Protective spasm may occur secondary to injury of underlying structures such as ligament or bone. This protective "splinting," such as often occurs following a back injury, prevents movement and further irritation of the injured structure. Protective spasm should be treated by the application of a protective support in order to relieve the muscles of this extraordinary function. Muscle spasm tends to subside rapidly and pain diminishes when a support is applied. As the muscles relax, the support maintains this function of protection to permit healing of whatever underlying injury gave rise to the protective muscle response.

Besides the relief from restriction of motion, the support gives added relief by putting pressure on the muscles in spasm. The positive response to direct pressure on the muscle distinguishes this type of spasm from that due to initial nerve irritation. In the low back, where protective muscle spasm frequently occurs, a brace with a lumbar pad, or a corset with posterior stays bent to conform to the contour of the low back, may be used for both immobilization and pressure.

In most instances one may assume that the underlying disturbance is severe enough to require the use of a support for at least a few days in order to permit healing. However, it is not uncommon to find, when the acute onset of pain is caused by a sudden exaggeration of movement, that a rigid posture persists because of the fear of movement, rather than because of the continued need for protective reaction. Because there is this possibility, it is often useful to apply heat and gentle massage as a diagnostic aid in determining the extent of protective reaction.

Segmental muscle spasm is an involuntary contraction of the *uninjured* segment of a muscle as a result of an injury to the muscle. The contraction of this part puts tension on the injured part and a condition of strain is present. Pain associated with tension within the muscle may be outlined by the margins of the muscle, or may be widespread due to reflex or referred pain mechanisms. Treatment requires immobilization in a position that relieves tension on the affected muscle. A positive response may also be obtained by gentle, localized massage to the area in spasm.

Muscle spasm associated with tendon injury differs from the above when the tension is exerted on the tendon rather than on a part of the muscle. Tendons contain many nerve endings sensitive to stretch, and pain associated with tendon injury tends to be severe.

Adaptive Shortening. *Adaptive shortening* is tightness that occurs as a result of the muscle remaining in a shortened position. Unless the opposing muscle is able to pull the part back to neutral position, or some outside force is exerted to lengthen the short muscle, it will remain in a shortened condition.

Tightness or shortness represents a slight to moderate decrease in muscle length, and results in a corresponding restriction of range of motion. It is considered to be reversible, but stretching movements must be done gradually to avoid damage to tissue structures. A period of several weeks is usually necessary for restoration of mobility in muscles exhibiting moderate tightness.

Stretch Weakness. *Stretch weakness* is defined as weakness that results from muscles remaining in an elongated condition, however slight, beyond the neutral physiological rest position, but *not* beyond the normal range of muscle length. The concept relates to the duration of the faulty alignment rather than to the severity of it. (It does not refer to overstretch, which means beyond the normal range of muscle length.)

Many cases of stretch weakness have responded to treatment that supported the muscles in a favorable position, even though the muscles had been weak or partially paralyzed for a long time, even as long as several years after onset of the initial problem. (See below and p. 123). Return of strength in such instances indicates that damage to the muscles was not irreparable.

Muscles exhibiting stretch weakness should not be treated by stretching or movement through the full range of joint motion in the direction of elongating the weak muscles. The condition has resulted from continuous stretching and responds to immobilization in physiological rest position for a sufficient period of time to allow for recovery to occur.

Stretch weakness may be superimposed on normal muscles, or on muscles initially affected by a lesion of the peripheral nerve, anterior horn cell, or central nervous system. The following are examples of the various types of involvement.

A familiar example of stretch weakness superimposed on *normal muscle* is the foot-drop that may develop in a bed-ridden patient as a result of bed clothes holding the foot in plantar flexion. Weakness in the dorsiflexors results from the continuous stretch on these muscles even though there is no neurological involvement.

The following is an example of stretch weakness superimposed on a *peripheral nerve* injury. A woman was lifting a heavy rock while she was gardening. Her hands were in supination. The rock suddenly fell, turning her forearms into pronation. She felt a sharp pain in her right upper forearm. Weakness developed in the muscles supplied by the radial nerve below the level of the Supinator. She was examined by several doctors including a neurosurgeon who said that he had seen some cases, and knew of others reported in the literature, in which the radial nerve had been similarly involved at the level where it passes through the Supinator.

The patient was first seen by a physical therapist *18 months after onset.* The wrist extensors and Extensor digitorum showed marked weakness but not complete paralysis, grading poor and poor +. A splint was applied, and in 2 weeks the strength had improved to grades of poor + and fair +. Then the condition reached a stalemate. The patient had started doing more work with the hand, and left the splint off most of the time. Three months went by, but rather than give up, it was decided by the patient, the doctor, and the physical therapist that a period of more complete immobilization be tried. A plaster cock-up splint including extension of the metacarpophalangeal joints was applied. This protected wrist extensors and the Extensor digitorum but allowed use of the interphalangeal joints in flexion and extension. The splint was removable but the patient was cautioned to keep it on as much of the 24 hours as possible, and not to move the wrist and fingers into full flexion at any time when the splint was removed. After 2 weeks, wrist and finger muscles were much improved. The patient played the piano and typed for the first time in 2 years.

Stretch weakness superimposed on muscles affected by *anterior horn cell* involvement was seen numerous times in poliomyelitis patients. The following is one example. This patient was first seen *4 years after onset.* She was admitted for treatment of scoliosis and an arm problem. The patient also had a foot-drop but treatment had not been planned for that condition. Examination revealed a questionable trace of strength in the Tibialis anterior muscle. The doctor in charge was persuaded to put a removable plaster cast on the foot, holding it in slight dorsiflexion and inversion. During treatments (given daily or at least three times a week) the foot was not allowed to drop below right angle. In 3 months the muscle strength had returned to fair −, and in 6 months it had improved to a grade of good. The patient was discharged wearing a brace during the day and using the half-shell cast at night. Later the brace and cast were discarded and the only correction was an inner wedge on the heel of the shoe. Under normal activity, the muscle had retained a strength of good − as indicated by an examination 2 years later.

Stretch weakness superimposed on a lesion of the *central nervous system* has been observed in multiple sclerosis patients, especially with regard to the wrist extensors and ankle dorsiflexors. Stretching opposing muscles that have become shortened, and applying a support in the form of a cock-up splint for the wrist or an orthosis for the ankle have resulted in improvement in strength and functional ability.

Another type of central nervous system lesion with superimposed weakness is exemplified by the following case. A child who had a right hemiplegia at birth, was first seen *at the age of 12* for a wrist drop. The hand was put into a cock-up splint and left for several months in that position, day and night except for treatment periods. The muscles showed excellent return of strength. The following data taken from her record are especially interesting because this patient was seen occasionally over a long period of time.

Patient's Age (years)	Grades of Muscle Strength	
	Extensor carpi radialis	Extensor carpi ulnaris
12	P −	F
13	G +	G +
16	N	N
20	N	N
24	G	G

Stretch weakness of less dramatic nature is seen frequently in cases of occupational and postural strain. The muscles most often affected have been one-joint muscles: Gluteus medius and minimus, Iliopsoas, hip external rotators, abdominal muscles, and middle and lower Trapezius.

Stretch weakness, being the result of persistent tension on the muscle, must be treated by relief of tension. Realignment of the part, bringing it into a neutral position, and use of supportive measures to help restore and maintain such alignment until weak muscles recover strength are important factors in treatment. Any opposing tightness that tends to hold the part out of alignment must be corrected in order to relieve tension on weak muscles. Faulty occupational positions that impose continuous tension on certain muscles must also be adjusted or corrected. Care must be taken not to overwork a muscle that has been subjected to a prolonged tension stress. As the muscles improve in strength and are capable of maintaining the gain, the patient is expected to use the muscles by working to maintain proper muscle balance and good alignment.

Stability or Mobility. In the treatment of abnormal conditions of joints and muscles, one must determine the overall objectives of treatment based on whether *stability* or *mobility* is the desired outcome for optimal function. Joint structures are so designed that along with greater mobility there is less stability, and along with greater stability there is less mobility.

It is quite generally accepted that along with growth from childhood to adulthood, there is a "tightening up" of the ligamentous structures, with a corresponding decrease in flexibility of muscles. This change affords greater stability and strength for adults than for children.

The individual with "relaxed" ligaments, often referred to as the "loosely knit" type, does not have the stability in standing that a less flexible individual has. A knee that goes into hyperextension, for example, is not mechanically as stable for weight bearing as one that is held in normal extension.

Lack of stability of the spine in the flexible individual can lead to problems when work requires prolonged sitting or standing, or the need to lift or carry heavy objects. Muscles do not succeed in functioning for both *movement* and the *support* normally afforded by the ligaments. When symptoms occur, they will at first appear as fatigue, and later as pain. Often a young adult with excellent strength, but excessive spinal flexibility will require a back support to relieve painful symptoms.

Under some circumstances, function is improved and pain is alleviated by range of motion being restricted to the point of complete fixation. Such conditions as Marie-Strümpell arthritis of the spine, if fused in good alignment, and postoperative fusions of the spine, hip, foot, or wrist all exemplify this principle.

From a mechanical standpoint, there are two types of faults relating to *alignment* and *mobility*: 1) undue compression on articulating surfaces of bone, and 2) undue tension on bones, ligaments, or muscles. Eventually, two types of bony changes may occur. Excessive compression produces an eroding effect on the articulating surface, while traction may result in an increase in bony growth at the point of attachment.

Lack of mobility is closely associated with persistent faulty alignment as a factor in causing undue compression. When mobility is lost there is stiffness and a certain alignment remains constant. This may be due to restriction of motion by *tight muscles,* or due to the inability of *weak muscles* to move the part through the arc of motion. Muscle tightness is a constant factor tending to maintain the part in faulty alignment regardless of the position of the body. Muscle weakness is a less constant factor because changing the body position can bring about a change in alignment of the part. When there is normal movement in joints, wear and tear on joint surfaces tends to be distributed; however, if there is limitation of range, the wear will take place only on the joint surfaces that represent the arc of use. If the part that is restricted by muscle tightness is protected against any movement that may cause strain, other parts that must compensate for such restriction will suffer the strain instead.

Excessive joint mobility results in tension on the ligaments that normally limit the range of motion, and can result in undue compression on the margins of the articulating surfaces when the excessive range is longstanding.

Musculoskeletal Structures. The musculoskeletal system is composed of striated *muscles,* various types of *connective tissue,* and the *skeleton.* This system provides the essential components for stability in weight bearing, strength, flexibility, and voluntary movement.

The bones of the skeleton are joined together by *ligaments,* which are strong fibrous bands or sheets of connective tissue. They are flexible, but not extensible. Some ligaments limit motion to such an extent that the joint is immovable; some allow freedom of movement. Ligaments are classified as capsular, extracapsular, and intracapsular. They contain nerve endings that are important in reflex mechanisms and in the perception of movement and position. They may differ from the standpoint of mechanical function. For example, collateral ligament refers to an extracapsular type that remains taut throughout the range of joint motion; cruciate ligament (as in the knee joint) becomes slack during some movements and taut during other movements.

Skeletal muscle fibers are classified primarily into two types: Type I (red slow twitch) and Type II (white fast twitch). The types of fibers are intermingled in most muscles, but usually one type predominates, depending on the contractile properties of the muscle as a whole. Type I fibers seem to predominate in some postural muscles such as the Erector spinae and Soleus. Type II fibers often predominate in limb muscles where rapid powerful forces are needed. However, there is variability in these ratios in the population, especially as related to development and aging.

Muscles, which constitute about 40% of body weight, are attached to the skeleton by aponeuroses, fasciae, or tendons. *Aponeuroses* are sheets of dense connective tissue, glistening white in color. They furnish the broad origins for the Latissimus dorsi muscles. The External and Internal oblique muscles are attached to the linea alba by means of aponeuroses. The Palmaris longus inserts into and tenses the palmar aponeurosis.

Fascia is of two types, *superficial* which lies beneath the skin and permits free movement of the skin; and *deep* which envelopes, invests, and separates muscles. Some deep fascia furnishes attachments for muscles; for example, the Iliotibial tract is a strong band of deep fasciae that provides attachments for the Tensor fasciae latae into the tibia and for the Gluteus maximus into the femur and tibia. The thoracolumbar fascia furnishes attachment for the Transversus abdominis.

Tendons are white fibrous bands that attach muscles to bones. They have great tensile strength, but are practically inelastic and resistant to stretch. Tendons have few blood vessels, but are supplied with sensory nerve fibers that terminate in organs of Golgi near the musculotendinous junction. In injuries that involve a severe stretch, the muscle is most likely to be affected. Sometimes the tendinous attachment to the bone is affected. For example, the Peroneus brevis attachment at the base of the fifth metatarsal may be disrupted in an inversion injury of the foot. Tendons can rupture. When the Achilles tendon ruptures there is retraction of the Gastrocnemius and Soleus muscles with spasm and acute pain.

Treatment Modalities. The therapeutic effects of *heat* include relief of pain and muscle spasm, decreased joint stiffness, increased extensibility of collagen tissue, increased blood flow, and some assistance in resolution of inflammatory infiltrates (45). The relaxing properties of superficial heat make it an effective modality in the treatment of tight or contracted muscles, by relieving pain and spasm and facilitating stretch.

However, heat should *not* be applied to muscles that are weak as a result of stretch because further relaxation of the muscles is not indicated. For example, in upper back pain, when weakness of the middle and lower Trapezius is the chief concern, heat should be avoided. The use of heat may increase rather than decrease the pain.

Heat should not be used in most acute conditions, nor over areas where sensation and circulation are impaired. Whirlpool type of heat is not advocated when there is swelling because it necessitates a dependent position of the arm or leg during treatment. If heat causes an increase in pain or feels "uncomfortable," it usually means that the type of heat is wrong, or that it is excessive in duration or intensity. An adverse response to heat may accompany overdosage.

If used with care, *deep heat,* such as ultrasound, can be effective by increasing extensibility of tight connective tissue, increasing blood flow, or assisting in the resolution of a chronic inflammatory process.

The therapeutic effects of *cold* include alleviation of the cycle of pain and muscle spasm secondary to skeletal and joint pathology, reduction of spasticity, and reduction of edema and bleeding by promoting vasoconstriction.

Many types of *electrical stimulation* modalities are currently available for use in treatment programs for pain control, muscle reeducation, or management of edema. Some are effective, if used judiciously, as an adjunct in a well-planned treatment program. Others, however, are of questionable value and remain controversial.

Treatment Procedures. *Traction* is a force used therapeutically for the purpose of producing elongation or stretch of joint structures and/or muscles. Properly applied, the force pulls in the direction of separation or distraction of extremity joints or vertebral bodies. Traction may be applied manually, or a mechanical traction device, static weights, or positional distraction may be used. Therapeutic effects include relief of pain and spasm, reduction or prevention of adhesions, stretching of tight musculature, and improved circulation.

Massage is often underrated and underutilized as a therapeutic procedure. When applied correctly, it can be very effective in the management of musculoskeletal conditions. The purposes for which it is used are chiefly to improve circulation, promote relaxation of muscles, help loosen scar tissue, and stretch tight muscles and fasciae. A gentle relaxing massage is effective in relieving muscle spasm (as seen in protective spasm).

Prior application of gentle, superficial heat often improves the response. Because of the relaxing effect of massage, it should not be used when dealing with stretched muscles that are weak. (See below for treatment of paralyzed muscles.)

The technique utilized, the area of application, direction and duration of the massage should be appropriate to the soft tissue dysfunction, patient tolerance, and desired outcome of treatment. Stretching massage is invaluable in the corrective treatment of muscles and fasciae shortened by longstanding postural faults or immobilization. The patient response elicited is often that of "a hurt that feels good," and the effective stretch enables the tight muscles to "let go." Relief of symptoms is sometimes almost immediate, confirming the appropriateness of this approach. The correct technique employs firm-but-gentle kneading strokes specific to the tight tissues ("soft tissue mobilization"). Sometimes it is more effective to stroke from the direction of origin toward insertion. One must avoid excessive stretching, as it will result in exaggerated soreness.

Massage is also appropriate when the goal is to relieve excessive edema that restricts motion. Swelling usually occurs distally following surgery, trauma, and prolonged dependency and disuse. The part should be in an elevated position, and massage should be carefully applied using firm, smooth pressure in a distal to proximal direction (toward the heart).

Exercise. Muscles possess the capacity to contract and to be elongated. The quality of elasticity of muscles depends on a combination of these two characteristics. Exercises are used to strengthen weak muscles, and to lengthen short muscles for the purpose of restoring, as nearly as possible, the elasticity upon which normal muscle function depends. Exercises are also used to increase endurance, improve coordination, and restore function.

Stretching movements must be done gradually to avoid damage to tissue structures. Tightness that has occurred over a period of time must be given a reasonable time for correction. Several weeks is usually necessary for restoration of mobility in muscles exhibiting moderate tightness.

Treatment of muscle weakness due to stretch and disuse requires consideration of the underlying causes. In cases of faulty body mechanics there are numerous instances of muscle stretch weakness, while the element of disuse atrophy is much less common.

Muscles that are *paralyzed or weakened by disease or injury* require special care in handling and in treatment. Muscles that are undergoing dener-vation atrophy are more delicate than normal muscles and can be injured by treatment that would not be injurious to normal muscles. "Trauma to the delicate atrophic fibers in the first months of atrophy undoubtedly hastens the pro-cess of degeneration" (46).

Muscles that are incapable of movement need treatment to stimulate circulation and to help keep the muscles pliable. Mild heat and massage are indicated, but the massage must be *gentle*. Paralyzed or denervated muscles are extremely vulnerable to secondary involvement by careless handling or overtreatment. Sunderland states that one of the objectives of treatment is "To main-tain paralyzed muscles at rest and protect them from being overstretched or permanently short-ened by interstitial fibrosis" (47).

The rational approach to treatment consists of maintaining a functional range of motion in order to prevent joint stiffness, to move joints to full range of motion in the direction of stretching normal mus-cles, but to use great care when moving in the direc-tion of elongating the weak or paralyzed muscle. Weak muscles that have lost strength, when sub-jected to stretching procedures, have regained strength when the only change in treatment has been to restrict the range of stretching.

Supports. Supports are used for various reasons: 1) to immobilize a part, 2) to correct faulty align-ment, 3) to relieve strain on weak muscles, 4) to facilitate function, or 5) to restrict movement in a given direction. Correction of alignment faults associated with weakness often requires support-ive measures, but such measures may not be effec-tive if tightness exists in muscles opposing the weak ones. Application of a support in a faulty position will not relieve strain. The contracted muscle must be stretched. A support that is adjustable and can help maintain the correction obtained by treatment may facilitate and hasten recovery.

The question frequently arises whether per-sons with weak abdominal muscles should be advised to wear a support or would it be relied upon to such an extent that the muscles will get weaker? If muscle and posture testing procedures are employed, trial and error can be minimized in regard to determining when to use supportive measures. The degree of weakness and the extent of faulty alignment help determine whether a sup-port is necessary. Extreme weakness due to strain or fatigue may require temporary bed rest, or restriction of movement of the affected part by the application of a support. Moderate weakness may or may not require support—depending to a great extent on the occupation of the individual. Mild weakness of muscles will usually respond to local-ized exercise without support or reduction of func-tional activity. In terms of abdominal muscle strength, adults who grade fair or less are consid-ered to be in need of support.

It is often difficult to convince an individual that wearing a support will help bring about an increase in the strength of the weak muscles. Such a statement appears contrary to general knowl-edge that exercise and activity will increase mus-cle strength. One must explain to the patient that instead of the particular muscle weakness being caused by lack of exercise, it is caused by contin-uous strain. The support will relieve the postural strain and allow the muscles to function in more nearly normal position.

Whenever a support has been applied, the question arises, how long will the support be needed? The support will need to be permanent *only* if the part supported has been irreparably weakened; for example, by paralysis or injury. However, the majority of conditions of muscle weakness associated with postural faults can be corrected, and consequently supports need be only *temporary* until muscle strength has been restored. If no treatment other than the support is used, the individual may become dependent on the support and reluctant to remove it. But if it is understood that therapeutic exercises are to supplement the wearing of the support so that later it may be abandoned, then supports become only an aid to correction rather than a permanent part of treatment.

GUIDELINES FOR THE CLINICIAN

Be guided by the age-old adage "Thou shalt do no harm."

Obtain the patient's confidence and cooperation.

Listen carefully to the patient.

Observe posture, body language, and spontaneous movements that provide valuable diagnostic clues.

Apply your basic knowledge of anatomy, physi-ology, and body mechanics in musculoskeletal evaluations and treatments of patients.

Consider whether the patient's occupational or recreational activities alleviate or aggravate existing problems.

Educate your patients; help them understand the nature of their problems, encourage them to help themselves, and discourage unnecessary depen-dence on the therapy or the therapist.

Be patient with your patients. It often takes more than one session to overcome anxiety and "guarding" against pain.

Be guided by the patient's reaction to previous treatments.

Start treatments in a gentle manner.

Understand that a muscle weakened by injury or disease must be handled with more care than a normal muscle.

Grasp with firmness, yet gentleness, when applying traction. Avoid pinching, twisting, or pulling the skin over the part that is held.

Expect treatments to progress gradually according to each patient's tolerance and response.

Avoid the attitude that "More is better." It is preferable to undertreat than overtreat since reactions to treatment are often delayed. One may not know until the next day whether the previous treatment was "too much."

Recognize that continuation of treatment is contraindicated if any of the following symptoms appear: swelling, redness, abnormal temperature of the part, marked tenderness, loss of range of motion, or persistent pain.

Remember that it is essential to obtain relaxation before attempting to stretch tight muscles. Stretching that is too vigorous may retard rather than hasten recovery.

Avoid application of heat over areas of impaired sensation or impaired circulation.

Involve the patient in setting treatment goals and planning a home program.

Be accountable. Document your assessment, evaluation, treatment plan, and follow-up care.

PAINFUL CONDITIONS OF UPPER BACK

The reasons for, and source of, pain in the upper back remain a matter of conjecture. Unlike areas where muscles are supplied by nerves that are both sensory and motor, the Rhomboids and Serratus anterior are supplied by nerves that are motor only. Consequently, the usual sensory symptoms associated with stretched or tight muscles are not present (see p. 378.) The spinal accessory nerve to the Trapezius is motor only but there may be some sensory innervation via spinal nerve branches (see p. 388).

Pain may occur in and around joints, however, or in closely related areas as a result of changes in alignment of the scapula and shoulder girdle; or it may be most pronounced in the area of muscle attachments to bone.

The loss of normal movement in one area may result in excessive movement in another area. Contracted Rhomboids limit the excursion of the scapula in the direction of abduction, and excessive strain on the posterior shoulder joint may result when raising the arm forward in flexion. Whatever the cause of related pain, the treatment of choice is restoration of muscle balance to facilitate normal movement through stretching tight muscles and strengthening weak muscles, and use of supports when indicated.

Middle and Lower Trapezius Strain. Middle and lower Trapezius strain refers to the painful upper back condition that results from gradual and continuous tension on the middle and lower Trapezius muscles. The condition is rather prevalent, and is one that is usually chronic. It does not have an acute onset unless associated with injury, but chronic symptoms may reach a point of being very painful.

Symptoms of pain do not appear early. The weakness may be present for some time without many complaints. However, it appears that complaints of pain are associated with traction by the muscle on its bony attachments along the spine. Patients may complain of a sore spot, or palpation may elicit pain or acute tenderness in the areas of vertebral or scapular attachments of the middle and lower Trapezius.

The stretch weakness of the muscles that precedes the chronic muscle strain may result from a habitual position of forward shoulders or round upper back, or the combination of these two faults. It may occur also as a result of shoulders being pulled forward by overdeveloped, short anterior shoulder-girdle muscles. Repetitive movements associated with some sports, such as baseball, may contribute to overdevelopment of shoulder adductor muscles. Occupations, such as typing, piano playing, and many others that require continuous movement with arms in a forward position, contribute to the stretching of the Trapezius muscles. A draftsman, for example, who sits on a high stool, bent forward over his work, is subjected to such a strain. Although the chief problem is one of undue tension on the posterior muscles, there is also undue compression on the anterior surfaces of the bodies of the thoracic vertebrae.

Recumbency or change of sitting posture may remove the element of continuous tension on the Trapezius, but in individuals who have tightness in the shoulder adductors and the coracoclavicular

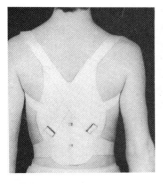 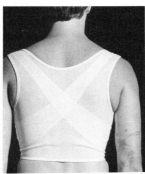

Shoulder support with stays in back to help support the upper back and hold shoulders back.

An elastic vest-type support that helps hold the shoulders back.

fascia, tension is continuously present. Change of position of the individual does not change the alignment of the part when such tightness exists. Pain is relieved very little if at all by recumbency.

Tests for length of the shoulder adductors and internal rotators should be done to determine whether tightness exists. (See pp. 63 and 64.) If tightness is present, gradual stretching of the tight muscles and fascia is indicated. There should be some effective relief of pain in a short time if gentle treatment is given daily.

When there is marked weakness of the middle and lower Trapezius, whether opposing tightness exists or not, a shoulder support is often indicated. It can effectively assist in the effort to hold the shoulders back in a position that relieves tension on the muscles.

Heat and massage to the upper back over the area of muscle stretch should be *avoided*. Such measures merely serve to relax the already stretched muscles. After a support has been applied, and along with treatment to correct opposing muscle tightness, exercises should be given to strengthen the lower and middle Trapezius muscles. The exercise of pulling elbows

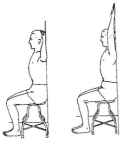

back against the wall with arms up beside the head, and pulling arms back against the wall in a diagonally overhead position are the two movements specific for strengthening these muscles. Rhomboid exercises are contraindicated in cases of middle and lower Trapezius strain. (See p. 339)

For patients (usually older people) who have a fixed kyphosis of the spine, little correction can be obtained. Some correction of the forward shoulders may be possible, but the basic faults cannot be altered. A Taylor-type brace (see p. 353) may be used to prevent progression of the deformity and to give some relief from painful symptoms.

For some women, the weight of heavy breasts that are not adequately supported contributes to the faulty position of the upper back, neck, and shoulders. (See page 344 for further details.)

Subjects with a round upper back often develop symptoms in the posterior neck. As the thoracic spine flexes into a kyphosis, the head is carried forward, eyes seek eye level to preserve the erect position of the head, and the cervical spine is extended (see pp. 66 and 91). Symptoms associated with this problem are described under *Tightness of Posterior Neck Muscles*, p. 341.

Contracted Rhomboids. Rhomboids may shorten as a result of forceful exercises in the direction of adduction, elevation, and downward rotation of the scapula. They may also become shortened as a result of weakness or paralysis of the Serratus anterior, which is a direct opponent of the Rhomboids. Massage and stretching of the Rhomboids is indicated. Placing the arm forward in flexion of the shoulder normally brings the scapula in the direction of abduction. When Rhomboids are contracted it is difficult to obtain an abducted position merely by positioning the arm. In order to stretch the Rhomboids it is necessary to apply some pressure against the vertebral border of the scapula in the direction of abduction.

Pain in Cases of Serratus Paralysis. During a time of hospital affiliation, the Kendalls examined and treated numerous cases of Serratus anterior paralysis. Depending upon the etiology, some patients had pain associated with the paralysis but not in the area of the muscle itself. Some patients did not complain of pain before, during, or for a while after the onset of paralysis. Early complaints were about the inability to use the arm normally. In some cases, when onset was gradual, there were no complaints until weakness became more and more pronounced. When the effects of Serratus weakness created secondary problems involving other structures, there were complaints of pain or discomfort in areas other than the Serratus muscle, e.g., neck or shoulder. Significant to such history is the fact that *the long thoracic nerve to the Serratus is purely motor*. (See p. 378.)

Middle and Upper Back Pain from Osteoporosis. Thoracic kyphosis is a primary deformity found in osteoporosis, usually accompanied by compensatory extension of the cervical spine.

Complaints of upper, middle, and low back pain are common, and can best be treated by gentle efforts to reduce the postural deformity and prevent further progression before it becomes a fixed structural fault. If a support can be tolerated, the patient should be encouraged to use one to help maintain the best possible alignment. As tolerated, exercises should be done to help maintain functional range of motion and develop strength.

NECK

The muscle problems associated with pain in the posterior neck are essentially of two types, one associated with muscle tightness and the other with muscle strain. Symptoms and treatment indications differ according to the underlying fault. Both types are quite prevalent; the one associated with muscle tightness usually has a gradual onset of symptoms, while the one associated with muscle strain usually has an acute onset.

Tightness of Posterior Neck Muscles. Neck pain and headaches associated with tightness in the posterior neck muscles are found most often in patients who have a forward head and round upper back. As shown on pages 66 and 91, the compensatory head position associated with a slumped, round upper back results in a position of extension of the cervical spine.

The faulty mechanics associated with this condition consist chiefly of undue compression posteriorly on the articulating facets and posterior surfaces of the bodies of the vertebrae, stretch weakness of anterior vertebral neck flexors, and tightness of neck extensors including the upper Trapezius, Splenius capitis, and Semispinalis capitis.

Headaches associated with this muscle tightness comes under two headings, *occipital headache*, and *tension headache*. The greater occipital nerve, which is both sensory and motor, supplies the Semispinalis and Splenius capitis muscles. It pierces the Semispinalis capitis and the Trapezius near their attachments to the occipital bone. This nerve also innervates the scalp posteriorly up to the top of the head. In the occipital headache, there usually is pain and tenderness on palpation in the area where the nerve pierces the muscles and pain in the scalp in the area supplied by the nerve. In the tension headache, besides the faulty postural position of the head and neck and the tightness of the posterior neck muscles, there usually is an element of stress that makes the condition fluctuate with the times of increased or decreased stress. In any event, the tight muscles usually respond to treatment that helps relax the muscles.

Symptoms in addition to pain may occur along with tension headaches, "Occasionally, muscle contraction headaches will be accompanied by nausea, vomiting, and blurred vision, but there is no preheadache syndrome as with migraine" (48).

From another source comes the statement that this forward-head position has been found "to cause an alteration in the rest position of the mandible, upper thoracic respiration with subsequent hyperactivity of the respiratory accessory muscles, and mouth breathing with a loss of the rest position of the tongue. . . and may lead to eventual osteoarthrosis and remodeling of the temporomandibular joint" (49).

On palpation, the posterior muscles are tight; movements of the neck are often limited in all directions except in extension. Pain may be less in intensity when the patient is recumbent, but it tends to be present regardless of the position the patient assumes.

The patient should use a pillow that permits a comfortable position of the neck, but *should not* sleep without a pillow because the head will drop back in extension of the neck. On the other hand, the use of too high a pillow should be discouraged because it can result in an increased forward head position. A commercially available or home-made cervical pillow, can provide the needed comfort and keep the neck in good position. It should be flattened in the center to provide support posteriorly and laterally. Active treatment consists of heat, massage, and stretching. At first the massage should be gentle and relaxing, progressing to deeper kneading. The stretching of the tight muscles must be very gradual, using both active and assisted movements. The patient should actively try to stretch the posterior neck muscles by efforts to flatten the cervical spine; i.e., pulling the chin down and in. (See p. 67.) This action compares with the effort to flatten the lumbar spine in cases of lordosis. This exercise may be done in supine, sitting, or standing positions, not in prone position. *Exercises that hyperextend the cervical spine are contraindicated.*

Because the faulty head position is usually compensatory to a thoracic kyphosis, which in turn may result from postural deviations of the low back or pelvis, it is frequently necessary to begin treatment by correction of the associated faults. Treatment for the neck may need to begin with exercises to strengthen the lower abdominal muscles, and with the use of a good abdominal support that permits the patient to assume a better upper back and chest position.

Unilateral tightness in posterolateral neck muscles is increasingly commonplace as a result of holding a telephone on the shoulder. The shoulder is elevated and the head is tilted toward the same side (see illustration, p. 346). The scapular muscle that is the most direct opponent of the upper Trapezius is the lower Trapezius which acts to depress the scapula posteriorly. The most direct opponent of the upper Trapezius acting to depress the shoulder and shoulder girdle directly downward in the coronal plane is the Latissimus dorsi. Tests for strength of this muscle often reveal weakness on the side of the elevated shoulder, and exercises to strengthen this muscle are indicated along with exercises to stretch the lateral neck flexors. (See p. 67 for Latissimus exercise, and for exercises to stretch lateral neck flexors.)

Upper Trapezius Strain. The upper Trapezius is that part of the Trapezius muscle extending from the occiput to the lateral third of the clavicle and the acromion process of the scapula. A strain of this muscle results in pain, usually acute, in the posterolateral region of the neck.

The stress that gives rise to this condition is often a combination of tension on, and contraction of, the muscle. Stretching sideways to reach for an object while holding the head tilted in the opposite direction can cause such an attack. (A typical example may be someone on the floor reaching to recover an object that rolled under a desk, or sitting in the front seat of a car reaching to recover an object from the back seat.) The abduction of the arm requires scapular fixation by action of the Trapezius, and the sideways tilt of the head puts tension on the muscle at the same time.

The muscle develops a "knot" or cramp, better described as segmental spasm in the muscle. (See p. 333.) The application of heat or massage to the entire area tends to increase the pain since the muscle is strained. The part to be treated is the part in spasm. Since it is difficult to localize heat effectively to the small area, massage alone is indicated. Start with gentle kneading massage, and increase as tolerated.

Either an improvised collar or a sling, or both, may be used if the condition remains very painful

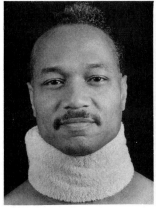 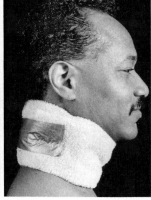

and does not respond favorably to the massage. A simple collar can be made from a small towel which is folded lengthwise to the correct width, wrapped securely around the neck, and held in place by a strip of strong tape. The collar can be made more firm by placing a strip of cardboard inside the towel. The collar may be needed for only two or three days to give relief.

ARM

Localized or radiating pain in the arm is often the result of faulty alignment that causes compression or tension on nerves, blood vessels, or supporting soft tissues. The faulty alignment may be primarily in the neck, upper back, or the shoulder girdle but more often all three areas are involved and treatment must be directed to overall correction.

Thoracic Outlet Syndrome. Thoracic outlet syndrome results from compression of the subclavian artery or brachial plexus within the channel bordered by the Scalenus anterior and posterior muscles and the first rib. The diagnosis is often puzzling and controversial because it encompasses numerous similar clinical entities including Scalenus anticus, hyperabduction, costoclavicular, costodorsal outlet, Pectoralis minor, and cervical rib syndromes.

Symptoms are varied and may be neurogenic or vascular in origin. Parasthesias and diffuse "aching" pain over the whole arm are common. The condition is aggravated by carrying, lifting, or engaging in activities such as playing a musical instrument.

When muscle atrophy is present, it usually affects all the intrinsic muscles of the hand. Tendon reflexes are not altered. Arterial compression is a less common cause than once thought, but symptoms such as coldness, aching in the muscles and loss of strength with continued use can reflect vascular compromise. "The proper diagnostic test should be the production of the neurologic symptoms by arm abduction, whether or not there is a change in the pulse or the appearance of a bruit" (50).

Unless symptoms are severe and clearly defined, conservative treatment should emphasize increasing the space of the thoracic outlet by improving the posture, correcting the muscle imbalance, and modifying the occupational, recreational, and sleeping habits that adversely affect the posture of the head, neck and upper back. Cooperation by the patient in carrying out treatment is essential to success. The patient should be taught self-stretching exercises to relieve tightness in the Scaleni, Sternocleidomastoid, Pectoral muscles, and neck extensors. (See

p. 67 and exercise sheet, p. 117.) Learning to do diaphragmatic breathing will lessen the involvement of accessory respiratory muscles, some of which are muscles that are in need of stretching. Sleeping in a prone position should be avoided. Activities that involve raising the arms overhead should be kept to a minimum. Research has shown that "with conservative therapy [and] . . . exercises designed to correct slumping shoulder posture, . . . at least two out of three patients improve to a satisfactory degree" (50).

Coracoid Pressure Syndrome. Coracoid Pressure Syndrome[*] is a condition of arm pain in which there is compression of the brachial plexus. It is associated with muscle imbalance and faulty postural alignment (15).

At the level of the attachment of the Pectoralis minor to the coracoid process of the scapula, the three cords of the plexus and the axillary artery and vein pass between these structures and the rib cage. (See figure, opposite.) In normal alignment of the shoulder girdle there should be no compression on the nerves or blood vessels. Forward depression of the coracoid process, which occurs in some types of faulty postural alignment, tends to narrow this space.

The coracoid process may be tilted down and forward because of tightness in certain muscles, or because weakness of other muscles allows it to ride into that position. The painful arm conditions are more often found where the tightness factor predominates.

The muscle that acts to depress the coracoid process anteriorly is chiefly the Pectoralis minor. The upward pull of the Rhomboids and Levator scapulae posteriorly aid in the upward shift of the scapula that goes along with the anterior tilt. Tightness of the Latissimus dorsi affects the position indirectly through its action to depress the head of the humerus. Tightness of the sternal part of the Pectoralis major acts in a similar manner. In some instances, tightness of the Biceps and Coracobrachialis, which originate on the coracoid process along with the Pectoralis minor, appears to be a factor. Muscle tightness may be ascertained by the shoulder adductor and internal rotator length tests. (See pp. 63 and 64.)

Weakness of the lower Trapezius contributes to the faulty shoulder position. Stretch weakness of this muscle allows the scapula to ride upward and tilt down anteriorly, and favors an adaptive shortening of the Pectoralis minor.

---

* This syndrome was reported by the authors in 1942. It was presented at a Joint Meeting of the Baltimore and Philadelphia Orthopedic Society, March 17, 1947, by E. David Weinberg, M.D., and referred to in an article by Dr. Irvin Stein entitled Painful conditions of the shoulder joint. Phys Ther Rev, 1948; 28(6).

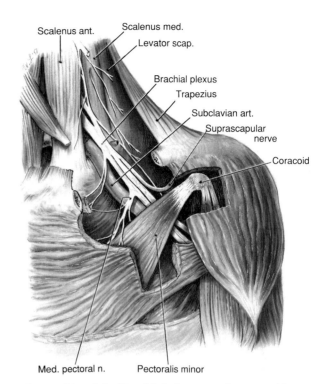

Relationship of the Brachial plexus to the coracoid process and Pectoralis minor muscle.

In the acute stage, moderate or even slight pressure over the coracoid process usually elicits pain down the arm. Soreness is acute in that spot, and in the area described by the Pectoralis minor muscle along the chest wall.

The pain down the arm may be generalized or may be predominately of lateral or medial cord distribution. There may be tingling, numbness, or weakness. The patient often complains of loss of grip in the hand. Evidence of circulatory congestion with puffiness of the hand and engorgement of the blood vessels may be present. In cases of marked disturbance, the hand may be somewhat cyanotic in appearance. The patient will complain of increased pain when wearing a heavy overcoat, trying to lift a heavy weight, or carrying a suitcase with that arm. Pressure can also be caused by a backpack or a shoulder bag.

Frequently the area extending from the occiput to the acromion process, which corresponds to the upper Trapezius muscle, is found to be sensitive and painful. This muscle is in a state of protective spasm in an effort to lift the weight of the shoulder girdle to relieve pressure on the plexus. It tends to remain in a state of contraction unless effective treatment is instituted.

Treatment in the acute stage consists first of applying a sling (p. 345B) that supports the weight of the arm and shoulder girdle, relieving

343

pressure on the plexus, and taking the workload off the upper Trapezius. Heat and massage may be applied to the upper Trapezius and to other muscles that exhibit tightness. Massage should be gentle and relaxing, progressing after a few treatments to gentle kneading and stretching. Slow passive stretching of the Pectoralis minor can be initiated (see p. 68). If tightness is also present in the Pectoralis major and/or Latissimus, the involved arm should be placed carefully overhead, *if tolerated,* to place the muscles on a slight stretch. Gentle traction is applied with one hand while massage is applied with the other. A shoulder support (see p. 340) is usually needed to help maintain the correction of alignment and relieve strain on the lower Trapezius muscle during the recovery period.

Among women who have very large breasts, the faulty alignment may be accentuated by pressure from brassiere straps. Treatment includes obtaining an uplift, long brassiere (one with a diaphragm band 2 or 3 inches wide) that has been reinforced with feather-bone stays. The reinforced brassiere supports the weight of the breasts from below. Straps should carry no weight if the support is effective. See photographs below.

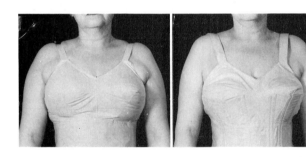

After strain has been relieved by support and by stretching of tight opposing muscles, specific exercises are indicated for the middle and lower Trapezius. (See figures, p. 68 and exercise sheet, p. 117.) If the overall posture is faulty, general postural correction is needed.

Certain exercises are *contraindicated.* Head and shoulder raising from a back-lying position, as in trunk curls, should be avoided because this movement rounds the upper back, depresses the coracoid anteriorly, increasing compression in the anterior shoulder region. Forceful shoulder extension exercises that involve Rhomboid, Pectoralis minor, and Latissimus action depress the head of the humerus and coracoid process, and exaggerate the existing faults. (See photo above right.)

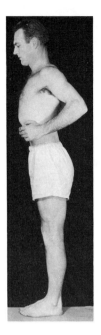

In faulty posture with round upper back and forward head, the scapulae are depressed anteriorly. Pushing the elbows back as in the accompanying photograph, should be *avoided* because it tends to increase the existing postural faults.

Teres Syndrome. The quadrilateral (or quadrangular) space in the axilla is bounded by the Teres major, Teres minor, long head of the Triceps, and the humerus. The axillary nerve emerges through this space to supply the Deltoid and the Teres minor. The area of sensory distribution of the cutaneous branch of the axillary nerve is shown on p. 380.

"Teres syndrome" was described in *Posture and Pain* (15). In a book published in 1980, there is a very interesting discussion of this syndrome in which it is called "Quadrilateral Space Syndrome" (51). Another text recognizes the involvement of the axillary nerve in this space in connection with sports injuries (50).

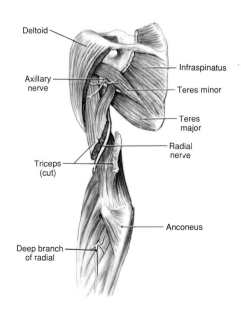

This syndrome is characterized by shoulder pain and by limitation of shoulder joint motion, particularly rotation and abduction. Pain extends into the area of cutaneous distribution of the sensory branch of the axillary nerve. Tenderness may be elicited by palpation of the quadrilateral space between the Teres major and minor. A slight or moderate pressure over the space may elicit sharp pain radiating into the area of the Deltoid muscle.

The Teres major, which is a medial rotator, is usually tight and holds the humerus in internal rotation. In standing, the arm tends to hang at the side in a position of internal rotation, i.e., the palm of the hand faces more toward the back than toward the side of the body (see p. 90). There is an element of tension on the posterior cord and axillary branch produced by the position of the arm. Pain that is more marked during active motion is indicative of friction on the axillary nerve by the Teres muscles in movement. Internal *or* external rotation, whether done actively *or* passively, is painful. With limitation of external rotation, abduction movements are also painful because the humerus does not rotate outward as it normally should during abduction. The pain is not unlike that encountered in cases of subdeltoid bursitis.

Treatment consists of heat and massage to the areas of muscle tightness, and active assisted exercises to stretch the medial rotators, and the adductors of the humerus. Stretching of the arm overhead in flexion or abduction and in external rotation is done very gradually.

With tightness in the Teres major, the scapula is pulled in abduction as the arm is raised in flexion or abduction and externally rotated. To insure that stretching is localized to the Teres, it is necessary to press against the axillary border of the scapula when raising the arm in order to restrict excessive abduction of the scapula. If the scapula moves excessively in the direction of abduction, the Teres, which is a scapulohumeral muscle, will not be stretched, and the Rhomboids, which attach the scapula to the vertebral column, will stretch too much (See p. 68.).

Pain from Shoulder Subluxation. Shoulder pain resulting from traction on the shoulder joint due to loss of tone and malalignment of the joint requires special treatment considerations. The cause may be paresis secondary to stroke, trauma to the brachial plexus, or a lesion of the axillary nerve. Effective management requires maintaining joint approximation during rest and during treatment to restore motion and improve motor control.

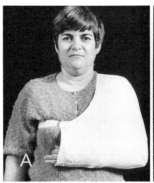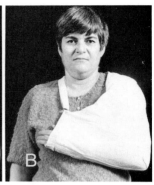

In figure A, the sling supports the arm with the humerus held firmly in the glenoid fossa. The weight of the arm is carried by the shoulder girdle and there is no pressure by the sling hanging on the neck.

In figure B, the weight of the arm is carried by the neck and opposite shoulder girdle. In cases of lateral neck strain, the shoulder needs to be supported on the side of strain. The sling accommodates for use in that manner.

A special sling called a shoulder-arm support (52) helps provide joint approximation and support to protect the subluxed shoulder when the patient is sitting or standing. (See figure A, above.) When used to hold the humerus in the glenoid, the shoulder girdle carries the weight of the arm and the sling does not hang on the neck. Careful measurement should be taken in order for the sling to provide the best approximation of the joint and prevent further stretch, instability, and pain in the weakened upper extremity. Measurements are taken with the elbow bent at right angle. A tape measure is held at the top of the shoulder, looped down around the forearm and back up to the shoulder. The number of inches determines the size.

The patient should be taught how to protect the shoulder when out of the sling. Proper alignment and approximation can be maintained when sitting in an armchair by having the affected arm supported on the arm rest. In this position, the patient can use the opposite hand to press downward on top of the shoulder making the humerus feel snug in the glenoid cavity. Teach the patient to relax the arm in this position on the arm rest and to *avoid* shrugging the shoulder. Shoulder joint approximation must be maintained during active assisted exercises to restore joint motion and function (53). In other words, do not let the joint be subluxed at any time.

Cervical Nerve Root Pressure. Just as sciatic pain caused by a protruded lumbar disc is basically a neurological problem, so also is arm pain due to cervical nerve root pressure. Faulty posture of the cervical spine may act as a contributory factor in cases when the onset is not associated with sudden trauma. Extension of the cervical spine as seen in a typical forward head position (see p. 66) produces undue compression on the facets and posterior surfaces of the bodies of the cervical vertebrae.

When the condition is acute, significant relief may be obtained by the use of moist heat (comfortably warm) to relieve protective muscle spasm, and gentle massage to help relax the muscles, along with low-level manual or mechanical traction to relieve compression. The use of a collar is often necessary in early intervention. It can provide appropriate support to help immobilize the cervical spine, prevent hyperextension, and help to transmit the weight of the head to the shoulder girdle. When symptoms are subacute or chronic, treatment should also include exercises to correct any underlying faults in alignment or muscle balance. Conservative treatment may be adequate or it may be an adjunct to surgical measures. (See figure, p. 342.)

Cervical Rib. A cervical rib is a rare congenital bony abnormality which may or may not give rise to symptoms of nerve irritation.

A painful arm condition appearing in young or middle-aged adults is occasionally found to be related to the presence of a cervical rib. The posture of the individual with a cervical rib often determines whether or not painful symptoms will occur. The appearance of symptoms only after the person has reached adulthood may be explained by the fact that the posture of the individual has gradually become more faulty in alignment, thus causing the relationship of the rib and adjacent nerve trunks to change unfavorably.

The faulty alignment most likely to cause irritation is the type characterized by a round upper back and forward head. Care of a patient with painful symptoms due to a cervical rib requires postural correction of upper back and neck. This treatment may relieve the symptoms completely and obviate the need for surgical procedures.

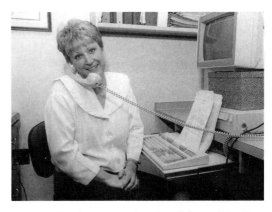

Resting a telephone on the shoulder with the neck in lateral flexion and the shoulder elevated can give rise to neck and/or arm pain. (See unilateral tightness of neck, p. 341.)

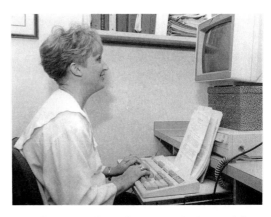

In this photograph, subject is sitting with upper back round and head raised to look at a monitor that is placed too high on the table. Holding the head in this position can precipitate painful posterior neck problems.

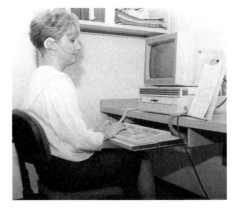

The height of the monitor, keyboard, and easel should be adjusted to the individual needs of the worker to keep stress and strain to a minimum. The use of a headphone or speaker phone helps prevent the faulty head position that leads to unilateral tightness in the neck.

chapter 11

Painful Conditions of the Low Back and Lower Extremities

THE LOW BACK ENIGMA

The etiology of many common painful conditions remains obscure. Low back pain, which is one of the most common, continues to puzzle the experts. The literature is replete with statements about the difficulty of making a definitive diagnosis.

The inability to pinpoint the problems has resulted in an array of solutions. With modern technology, an amazing amount of information is available but still inconclusive with respect to adequate diagnosis. DeRosa and Porterfield state that "... at present, identifying with any certainty the exact tissues involved in most low back pain is virtually impossible" (54).

The result is that, in the area of conservative (nonsurgical) treatment, signs and symptoms are largely the basis for determining treatment. However objective the signs may be, the *interpretation* of their significance varies. Various systems of treatment evolve from the interpretations—supported by evidence of success.

It is frequently quoted that a high percentage (as high as 80%) of low back pain cases recover within 2 weeks with or without treatment. In view of these statistics, it is no wonder that there is a high success rate regardless of the approach or system of treatment. But there is no doubt in the minds of those who have been relieved of severe pain, that treatment has helped. Treatment may come in various forms: bed rest and medication; successful mobilization (manipulation); immediate application of a support that provides immobilization; or gentle treatment that employs various pain-relieving modalities and procedures.

Regardless of the approach to treatment, there are constant references in the literature to the need for postural correction as a part of treatment. Sometimes immediate care involves correction of alignment, but lasting correction and prevention of future problems are even more important aspects of care. It is this area of treatment with which this text is primarily concerned.

Correction of postural faults involves examination of alignment and tests for length and strength of muscles. Preservation of good alignment depends upon establishing and maintaining good muscle balance. This was the basic thesis as stated by the original authors of this text in a pamphlet entitled *Study and Treatment of Muscle Imbalance in Cases of Low Back and Sciatic Pain* (1936), and in *Posture and Pain* (1952) (55, 15).

This chapter focuses on evaluation and treatment based on the findings of tests for alignment, range of motion, muscle length, and muscle strength. It does not put labels on most of the types of painful low back conditions other than to name the associated alignment and muscle imbalance problems. In order to present the complexities of postural alignment, all of Chapter 4 has been devoted to this subject, and detailed descriptions of the various tests referred to in this chapter are found in Chapters 3 and 6–8.

Evaluation of faulty posture must include examination of the related parts and not be limited to the areas where symptoms appear. A mechanical or functional strain causing an imbalance in one part of the body will soon result in compensatory changes in other parts of the body. The mechanics of the low back is inseparable from that of the overall posture but especially that of the pelvis and the lower extremities. Pain manifested in the leg may be due to an underlying problem in the back. Conversely, the symptoms appearing in the low back may be due to underlying faulty mechanics of the feet, legs, or pelvis. More often, however, symptoms and faults appear in the same area.

An imbalance may begin with abdominal muscle weakness or strain resulting from surgery or obesity. Among women, pregnancy may be the cause. Low back pain has often followed childbearing, and patients have received complete relief of pain by treatment to strengthen abdominal muscles and correct faulty posture.

In adults, very few activities require strenuous use of abdominal muscles while most activities tend to strengthen the back muscles. An important factor to be considered as a predisposing cause of shortening of back muscles and relaxation of abdominal muscles is that Erector spinae muscles are numerous and short and attached to a strong bony framework, while abdominal muscles are long with strong fascial attachments but without a supporting bony framework. In addition, abdominal muscles bear the strain of weight of abdominal viscera and, for women, muscle stretch and strain accompanying pregnancy.

The low back problems described in this chapter are those associated with anterior, posterior, and lateral pelvic tilt. The lower extremity pain problems are those associated with a tight or with a stretched Tensor fasciae latae and Iliotibial band, with sciatic pain associated with protrusion of a disc or with a stretched Piriformis, with pain and weakness in the region of the posterior Gluteus medius, and with knee and foot problems in which faulty alignment and muscle imbalance are important factors.

LOW BACK PAIN

Conditions addressed in this category include lumbosacral strain, sacroiliac strain, and, briefly, facet slipping and coccyalgia. Lumbosacral strain may be postural in origin. The other three are not considered primarily posture problems, but there often are associated alignment and muscle imbalance problems that affect these conditions.

Lumbosacral Strain

Lumbosacral strain is the most common type of low back problem. The word "strain," which denotes an injurious tension, does not cover the mechanical faults that are present, however. There are essentially two problems: *Undue compression* on bony structures, present especially in weight-bearing (standing or sitting); and *undue tension* on muscles and ligaments in weightbearing and during movements. (See also p. 333.)

A back may have *good alignment* in weightbearing, but if the *low back muscles are tight* they will be subjected to undue tension in a sudden or unguarded attempt to bend forward. Acute muscle strain may follow.

A back may have very *faulty alignment*, such as a *lordosis without tightness of low back muscles*. Movement may not cause a strain, but standing for any length of time may give rise to pain. Compressive stress resulting from faulty alignment, if marked or constant, may evoke painful symptoms. This type of posture is more common among women than among men. The fault is often associated with weakness of the abdominal muscles. The onset of symptoms usually is gradual rather than acute, and symptoms often remain more or less chronic. Pain is less if the person is active than if standing still and is relieved by recumbency or sitting.

When a combination of *faulty alignment and muscle tightness* is present, both position and movement may give rise to pain. Pain tends to be constant although it may vary in intensity with change of position. Stresses which would not be excessive under ordinary circumstances may give rise to pain. An apparently inconsequential act may cause an acute onset of pain.

Anterior Pelvic Tilt. Four groups of muscles support the pelvis in anterior-posterior alignment. The low back extensors pull upward on the pelvis posteriorly, the Hamstrings pull downward posteriorly, the abdominal muscles pull upward anteriorly, and the hip flexors pull downward anteriorly. When there is good muscle balance, the pelvis is maintained in good alignment. With imbalance, the pelvis tilts anteriorly or posteriorly. With *anterior pelvic tilt*, the low back arches forward into a position of *lordosis*. There is undue compression posteriorly on the vertebrae and the articulating facets, and there is undue tension on the anterior longitudinal ligament in the lumbar area.

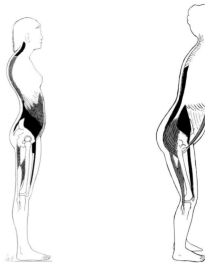

Kyphosis-lordosis posture. Hip flexion with trunk inclined forward

The muscle imbalances associated with an anterior tilt may include all or part of the following: *Weak anterior abdominal muscles; Tight hip flexor muscles (chiefly Iliopsoas); Tight low back muscles; Weak hip extensor muscles.*

The figures above show these muscle imbalances. Figure A has a marked lordosis; the lordosis in figure B would also be marked if the subject were to assume an erect posture. When all four muscle groups are involved, correction of the anterior pelvic tilt requires that the anterior abdominal muscles and the hip extensors be strengthened, and that the tight low back and hip flexor muscles be stretched. Any one of the above may be a primary factor but the tight low back and weak hip extensor muscles are least likely to be the primary cause.

Frank Ober stated "It is well known that a lordotic spine may be a painful spine, but this, of course, is not true in every case" (20). Farni and Trueman have emphasized the common association of increased lumbar lordosis and low back pain (56). It is true that some individuals with a lordosis complain of low back pain while others with a more severe lordosis may not complain of any pain. A lordosis may be habitual, but if the muscles of the back are flexible enough that position can be changed from time to time, symptoms may not develop. However, a back so tight that the lordotic position is fixed tends to be a painful back in any position of the body.

The best index in regard to painful low back is not the degree of lordosis or other mechanical defect visible on examination of alignment but the extent of muscle tightness that maintains a fixed anteroposterior alignment, and the extent of

350

muscle weakness that allows the faulty position to occur and to persist.

Weak Anterior Abdominal Muscles. Weakness of anterior abdominal muscles *allows* the pelvis to tilt forward. The muscles are incapable of exerting the upward pull on the pelvis that is needed to help maintain a good alignment. As the pelvis tilts forward, the low back is drawn into a position of lordosis.

The individual with a lordosis in which abdominal muscle weakness is the main problem usually complains of pain across the low back. In early stages it is described as fatigue and later as an ache which may or may not progress to being acutely painful.

Pain is usually worse at the end of day and is relieved by recumbency to such an extent that after a night's rest the individual may be free of symptoms. Sleeping on a firm mattress allows the back to flatten and this change from the lordotic position gives relief and comfort to the patient.

The back may be eased in sitting by resting against the back of the chair, avoiding the erect sitting position which tends to arch the low back. Relief of pain can come, also, from the use of a proper *support* that helps to correct the faulty alignment and relieve strain on the weak abdominal muscles. (The William's Flexion Brace and the Goldthwait Brace were designed to support the abdomen and correct the lordosis.) (See also p. 353.)

When marked weakness exists, the patient should be started on an exercise program and should continue the use of the support for a period of time while working to build up muscle strength. This advice is contrary to that often-repeated admonition that the muscles will get weaker if a support is used. Weakness from wearing a support will only occur if the patient does not exercise to build up the muscles. *Use of the support helps to maintain alignment and relieve stretch and strain of the weak muscles until they regain strength through exercise.*

Abdominal muscle weakness is present for varying lengths of time following pregnancy. Being cognizant of this fact, physicians often give patients a list of exercises intended to strengthen these muscles. Unfortunately, these lists have included sit-ups and double-leg-raising exercises that should not be given when abdominal muscles are very weak. (See pp. 158–159 and 166 for exercises to strengthen abdominal muscles.)

If there is tightness of the back extensors or hip flexors, it is necessary to treat these muscles to restore normal length before the abdominals can be expected to function optimally. (See pp. 53 and 55, and 117–118 for stretching exercises.)

Tight One-Joint Hip Flexors (Chiefly Iliopsoas). Tight one-joint hip flexors *cause* an anterior tilt of the pelvis in standing. The low back goes into a lordosis as the subject stands erect. Occasionally, a subject inclines forward from the hips, avoiding an erect position that would result in a marked lordosis. (See facing page.)

The severity of the lordosis depends directly on the extent of tightness in the hip flexors. Stress on the low back in the lordotic position is often relieved by giving in to the tight hip flexors. In standing, this is accomplished by bending the knees slightly. In sitting, the hips are flexed and hip flexors are slack. Some people can sit for long periods of time without pain or discomfort but have pain when standing for brief periods. One should examine for hip flexor shortness in such cases. Lying on the back or on the side with hips and knees flexed relaxes the pull of the tight hip flexors on the low back. Patients often seek these means to relieve pain in the back and legitimately so in the acute stage. However, the problem is that giving in to the tightness by flexing the hips in these various positions aggravates the underlying muscle problem permitting further adaptive shortening of the very muscles that are causing the problem.

When knees are bent to relieve discomfort in the back, an effort should be made not to bend them more than necessary. After the hip flexors are stretched through appropriate stretching exercises, it is not necessary to flex the hips and knees in order to be comfortable when lying on the back.

In the back-lying position with hips flexed enough to allow the back to flatten, the patient is more comfortable on a firm mattress than on a soft one. On a soft mattress, the pelvis sinks down and tilts anteriorly, causing a lordotic position of the low back.

Lying on the abdomen is not tolerated because the tight hip flexors hold the back in a lordotic position. However, the prone position can be made comfortable by placing a firm pillow directly under the abdomen to help flatten the low back and allow slight flexion of the hips.

A back support can provide some relief to a painful back that is held in a lordosis by tight hip flexors but it cannot help stretch the tight hip flexors. (See p. 53 for hip flexor stretching exercises, and p. 158–159 for exercises to strengthen lower abdominal muscles.)

Trying to accomplish stretching of tight hip flexors by occasional periods of treatment is difficult if occupation requires staying in a sitting position. The patient must realize that it may be necessary to do stretching of the tight muscles daily in order to counteract the effects of a continuous sitting position.

Tight Two-Joint Hip Flexors. The degree of tightness that is usually seen in the two-joint hip flexors (Rectus femoris and Tensor fasciae latae) *does not cause* a lordosis in standing. The reason is that the muscles are not elongated over the knee joint when the knee is straight. (Tightness would have to be severe to be tight over both joints.)

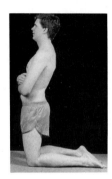

Tightness *does cause* a lordosis in the kneeling position, however. When someone complains that only the kneeling position causes pain in the low back, it is important to examine for two-joint hip flexor shortness. (See hip flexor length test, pp. 33–35).

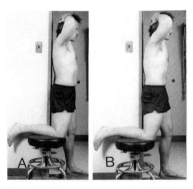

Sometimes this tightness is very marked, and stretching should be done in a manner that does not put stress on the patella during knee flexion. For that reason, it is recommended that the knee be placed in flexion, figure A, so the patella can ride over the knee joint before starting further stretching. Proceed to stretch hip flexors by pulling up and in with the lower abdominal muscles to posteriorly tilt the pelvis and extend the hip joint as in B.

Tight Low Back Muscles. Tight low back muscles *cause* an anterior tilt of the pelvis and hold the low back in a position of lordosis. While these muscles cross over joints of the vertebral column, they do not cross over another joint at which the muscles can give in to the tightness. Regardless of what position the body assumes, the low back

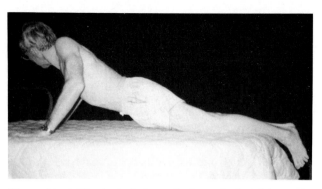

The subject illustrated above had marked tightness in hip flexors which limited hip joint extension. He also had limitation of back extension. In order to push up from the table, movement had to take place at the knee joint. As an exercise this movement would not be appropriate for this subject.

will remain in a degree of extension that corresponds to the degree of tightness of these muscles. In forward bending, the low back remains in an anterior curve and does not straighten. (See p. 47).

In cases in which tightness of the low back muscles is a primary factor, pain may be chronic but often has an acute onset. Pain is increased by, and tends to have its onset in, movement rather than standing or sitting positions. The problem tends to be more common among men than among women.

Pain may be relieved or made worse by recumbency. The relief of pain in recumbency is due to removing part of the strain caused by movement or muscle action in maintaining the upright position. Increase of pain in recumbency occurs if the body weight in the supine position imposes a strain on the back muscles. During bed rest in the acute stage, some relief is obtained by giving in to the back by putting a small roll under the back. It should *conform to the contour* and give support to the low back. Along with giving some support, the pressure against the low back offers some relief. When a back support in the form of a corset or brace is indicated, it is sometimes advisable to use the support when recumbent as well as when weight bearing.

In addition to the relief that comes from restriction of motion, pain is relieved by pressure from the support against the low back. Steel stays in back supports (illustrated on facing page) should be bent in to conform to the back, and a pad may be added if it gives additional comfort.

The relief of pain that may accompany immobilization, and the fear of repeating the movement that brought on the acute attack, may have so impressed the patient that there is reluctance to cooperate in treatment to restore movement. Recovery depends upon cooperation by the patient, and this will not be obtained unless the patient understands the procedure.

Giving in to the lordotic position and supporting the back in that position for the relief of pain should not be construed as the goal of treatment. Stretching the low back muscles to restore normal flexibility and building up abdominal muscle strength are long term goals. (See p. 55 for stretching low back, and pp. 158–159 for strengthening lower abdominal muscles.)

Below are several forms of abdominal and back supports.

Adhesive strapping may be used for those needing only temporary support, or used until a more rigid support can be obtained.

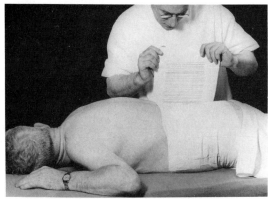

A piece of muslin is placed under the abdomen with the patient in prone position. The adhesive strips are anchored to the muslin on either side. A series of thin wooden applicators, placed on an additional patch of adhesive, is then placed over the tape on the low back.

The applicators are broken by gentle pressure so they conform to the apex of the curve in the low back, and then several more strips of adhesive are applied. The muslin acts as an abdominal support, and, by anchoring the adhesive to it, there is less chance of irritation from the tape.

People who have a lordosis often complain of having a "weak back." The term is used because of the feeling of aching and fatigue in the low back, and because of the inability to lift heavy objects without pain. This type of back is *mechanically weak* and inefficient because of the faulty alignment, but *low back muscles are not weak.* The connotation of the word "weak" is that the back muscles are weak and in need of strengthening exercises. On the contrary, the muscles are strong, overdeveloped, and short, *and back extension exercises are contraindicated.*

The lordosis posture with tight low back muscles tends to give rise to pain in movement or position. Change of position of the body does not give relief if tightness is marked. The back remains immobilized in faulty alignment by the muscle tightness whether the patient is standing, sitting, or lying.

Years ago it was not uncommon to find muscle tightness in the low back. Environmental and cultural factors affect postural habits. Low back muscle tightness, sufficient to hold the low back in a fixed anterior curve, is no longer a common finding. It is possible that sitting at work, sitting in cars, and the emphasis on exercises that flex the spine (especially the knee-bent sit-ups), have reversed the problems and created some new ones with respect to low back pain.

Weak Hip Extensor Muscles. Hip extensors consist of the one-joint Gluteus maximus and the two-joint Hamstring muscles. Weakness of these muscles is seldom found as the primary factor in anterior pelvic tilt, but when found in conjunction with hip flexor shortness or abdominal muscle weakness, the pelvic tilt and lordosis tend to be more exaggerated than if the hip extensor weakness were not present.

Slight to moderate weakness of the Gluteus maximus and Hamstring muscles will *allow* the pelvis to tilt forward in the standing position. Weakness of the Hamstrings alone would not

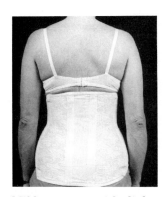
Mild support with light steels

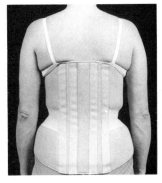
Moderate support with heavy steels

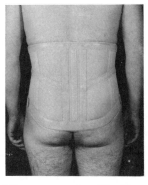
Firm support with Bennett Brace

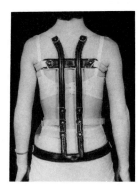
Taylor Brace for upper and lower back support

affect the pelvic position to the same extent. *Marked weakness* or paralysis of the hip extensors presents the opposite picture. With extreme weakness, the only stable position of the hips is obtained by displacing the pelvis forward and the upper trunk backward (as in sway-back posture) distributing the body weight over the center of gravity with the hip joint locked in extension and the pelvis in posterior tilt. (See p. 223 for comparable example of marked hip abductor weakness.)

Hamstring weakness more often results from overstretching than from lack of exercise. The first step in strengthening these muscles is to *avoid* the movements or positions that overstretch them. Exercises to strengthen Hamstrings can then be added in the form of resisted knee flexion with the hip flexed, or prone knee flexion with the hip extended. In prone position the knee should not be flexed to the extent that this two-joint muscle is placed in an ineffective shortened position. The optimal position for strengthening and testing is at an angle of approximately 50° to 70° of knee flexion in the prone position. (See p. 39 for normal Hamstring length, and pp. 208–209 for optimal test and exercise positions.)

In the standing position, Hamstring muscles may feel *taut* whether they are stretched or short. On postural examination, this tautness usually is interpreted as tight Hamstrings with the result that treatment to stretch the Hamstrings is ordered as a corrective measure. When this tautness is associated with stretched Hamstrings, stretching is contraindicated. Accurate testing for Hamstring length, as described in *Chapter 3* is necessary for accurate diagnosis and for prescription of therapeutic exercises. Faulty postural alignment is indicative of Hamstring length: a lordosis and hyperextended knees suggest the presence of stretched Hamstrings; in flat-back and sway-back postures, Hamstrings tend to be short.

Posterior Pelvic Tilt. Two types of posture exhibit posterior pelvic tilt, hip joint extension, and weakness of the Iliopsoas muscle: The *flat-back*, as the name implies, is a straight back in both the lumbar and thoracic areas except that there is some degree of flexion in the upper thoracic area that accompanies the forward head position. The *sway-back* posture is one in which there is a posterior displacement (swaying back) of the upper trunk and an anterior displacement (swaying forward) of the pelvis. There is a long kyphosis extending into the upper lumbar region and a flattening of the low lumbar region. The posterolateral fibers of the External oblique are elongated. (See accompanying illustrations and pp. 160 and 161.)

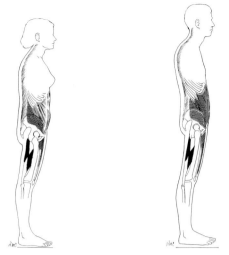

Flat-back Posture   Sway-back Posture

Sway-back Posture. In the past, the words "lordosis" and "sway-back" were used interchangeably in referring to the curvature in the low back and lower thoracic areas. The postural differences between the lordosis and the sway-back postures were recognized in *Posture and Pain*, but the name sway-back was not applied until the third edition of *Muscles, Testing and Function* published in 1983. Separating the use of these terms also differentiated these two postures. They are distinctly different with respect to the anteroposterior tilting of the pelvis, the position of the hip joint, and the accompanying muscle imbalances that exist. Weakness of the Iliopsoas is a constant finding in the sway-back posture in contrast to being strong in the lordotic posture. As determined by the lower abdominal muscle test, the external oblique is usually weak in both the lordotic and sway-back postures.

The postures resemble each other by the fact that there is a curve in the back. In the lordotic posture, there is an increase in the anterior curve in the low back; in the sway-back posture, there is an increased posterior curve in the thoracic and thoracolumbar regions. In the lordotic posture, strain is usually felt across the low back; in the sway-back posture, strain is more often in the area of the thoracolumbar junction.

Treatment requires that the spine be held in good alignment with the low back in a normal anterior curve and the upper back in correction of the long kyphosis. A properly fitted support should be considered if the posture has reached a stage of being painful, or if the upper back and lower abdominal muscles are too weak to maintain postural correction. Exercises to strengthen the Iliopsoas, and exercises for the lower abdominal muscles, are usually indicated for the subject

354

with sway-back posture. Supine, with low back held flat on table, alternate (but not double) leg raising may be used for hip flexor strengthening.

From the neutral position of the pelvis, the range of motion in the direction of the posterior tilt is less than in the direction of anterior tilt. The same four muscle groups support the pelvis anteriorly and posteriorly: anterior abdominal muscles; hip flexors (chiefly Iliopsoas); low back muscles; and hip extensors.

Flat-back Posture. When describing the flat-back posture, it is necessary to recognize two types, one that is flexible (the more common), and the rigid flat low back. Since normal flexion is defined as a flattening or straightening of the lumbar spine, both types of flat-back posture exhibit normal flexion. In the flexible back, extension is not limited; in the rigid back, extension is limited. (The latter is not included in the following discussion.)

The flexible flat-back posture appears to be more common among certain cultures than among others. Asians seem to exhibit this type of posture more frequently than most Americans or Europeans. This type of flat-back does not give rise to as many problems of low back pain as does the lordotic back, or the sway-back posture. The range of motion in extension is usually normal and may be excessive.

The low back muscles are strong; abdominal muscles, especially the lower, tend to be stronger than average; hip extensors are usually strong and Hamstrings often show shortness. Consistently, the one-joint hip flexors are weak. This weakness is not evident when doing the usual *group* hip-flexor test in sitting, but is evident when doing the supine test for Iliopsoas (see p. 214) or the test requiring completion of hip joint flexion in sitting (see p. 215). If Hamstrings are tight, stretching exercises are indicated. (See p. 54.)

Following is a statement made by the original senior author of this text in a 1936 publication.

> In my experience I have not come in contact with a patient having a normally *flexible* so-called flat-back, with a balance between the strength of the back and abdominal muscles, who has complained of chronic low back pain. . . . The weight-bearing line of the body is nearly normal in these patients and they do not exhibit the type of chronic low back pains associated with extreme faulty posture (55).

Careful consideration must be given to examination findings when planning a course of treatment. It is a mistake to assume that extension exercises are indicated—they may be unnecessary or may be contraindicated. The flat-back posture is one in which the hip joint is in extension and the Hamstrings are strong and, usually, short.

If this type of posture exists without low back pain, it is not necessary to change it. If the back is painful, and restoring the normal anterior curve is indicated, the measure of choice should be strengthening the weak hip flexors. The problems with back extension from prone position are that it involves strong hip joint extension and extensor muscle action to stabilize the pelvis to the thigh in order for the trunk to be raised, and the hip extension stretches the already weak Iliopsoas.

If low back extension is indicated, for whatever reason, it can be done in a sitting position, or by the stabilization action of the low back during alternate leg raising in a prone position—raising the leg only about 10° in extension.

Excessive Flexion (or Hyperflexion). Excessive flexion of the lumbar spine is not uncommon. It is seen as a kyphosis of the low back in sitting, but rarely does it appear as a kyphosis in standing. (See photograph, p. 37.) In most cases of excessive low back flexion, the back extensor muscles are not weak, but Hamstrings are often tight. (See pp. 47 and 49.)

Some individuals who have *excessive flexion in sitting* will *stand in a lordotic position*. Certain exercises promote excessive flexion of the low back at the same time that they strengthen and tend to shorten the hip flexors. Notably, the curled-trunk sit-up from a bent-knee position creates a demand for complete curling of the trunk including the lumbar spine, and exercises the Iliopsoas in hip joint flexion almost to completion of range of motion.

When the low back is painful and there is hypermobility in flexion, the treatment of choice is a support that prevents excessive range of motion. If Hamstrings are tight and exercises are done to stretch them, one should avoid forward bending, and wear the back support while doing passive or active straight leg raising. (See p. 54.)

Lateral Pelvic Tilt. Problems of postural low back pain associated with lateral pelvic tilt are common, but many go undetected. The mechanical problem is chiefly one of undue compression at the articulating facets of the spine on the high side of the pelvis. The sore spot that corresponds with the area of greatest compression is usually over the articulating facet of the fifth lumbar vertebra on the high side.

Muscle imbalances are usually present in the lateral or posterolateral trunk, and the lateral or anterolateral thigh muscles in cases of lateral pelvic tilt. The posterolateral trunk muscles and lumbodorsal fascia are tighter on the high side of the pelvis while the leg abductors and Tensor fasciae latae are tighter on the low side of the pelvis. On the high side, the leg assumes a position of postural adduction in relation to the pelvis, and the abductors, particularly the posterior part of the Gluteus medius, show weakness. (See figure, p. 222.) An imbalance may be noted, also, in the hip adductors. The pattern most frequently seen in right-handed individuals is that of tight left Tensor, weak right Gluteus medius, and stronger right hip adductors and right lateral trunk muscles.

Left-handed individuals tend to show the reverse of this pattern. However, their acquired patterns of muscle imbalances tend to be less fixed than in right-handed individuals. Equipment and tools are most often designed for right-handed use if there is an element of asymmetry involved, and left-handed people are required to use the instruments in a right-handed manner.

As a result of faulty lateral alignment and muscle imbalances, pain may appear in the low back or in the leg. Careful examination often will reveal problems in both areas regardless of the area of chief complaint.

Treatment is primarily concerned with realignment. Essentially, treatment consists of the application of a straight raise on the heel of the shoe on the low side of the pelvis. Seldom is it necessary or advisable to use a lift more than 1/8 or 3/16 inch thick. A firm rubber and leather heel pad that can be inserted into a shoe often suffices.

The difference in level of the posterior spines, as seen when the patient is standing with knees straight, should provide the basis for determining the need for, and the amount of, shoe lift. *Apparent leg length* measurements taken in the supine position for use as a basis for determining the side of application of the lift are unfortunately often misleading. (See analysis of fallacy in this regard, p. 103.)

If there is tightness in the Tensor fasciae latae on one side, the faulty alignment will not be automatically corrected by the application of a shoe lift. It may be necessary to treat this tightness even though no specific symptoms are present in the area. Such treatment should either precede or accompany the use of a shoe lift. It may consist merely of active stretching exercises or of assisted stretching. (See pp. 60 and 117.)

Gluteus Medius Weakness. Discomfort, aching, or, in some instances, pain may be present in the area of the posterior Gluteus medius muscle. It may start as an annoying discomfort in standing. It may progress to being an ache in standing

or in side-lying. In side-lying, it may hurt whether lying on the affected or the unaffected side. Habitually standing with weight on one leg more than the other gives rise to stretch weakness which, if it persists, can result in the complaint of discomfort or pain. Treatment may be as simple as breaking the habit of standing with weight shifted toward the affected side.

The weakness of the Gluteus medius, which is usually present on the high side of the pelvis, must be corrected in order to maintain good lateral alignment. The shoe raise on the opposite side which is used to level the pelvis at once removes the element of tension on the weaker medius *provided* the subject stands evenly on both feet and avoids standing in adduction on the side of the weak medius. As a general rule, specific exercises for the Gluteus medius are not necessary for individuals who are normally active. The exercise involved in the ordinary functional activity of walking usually suffices for strengthening this muscle.

A minimum of 6 weeks is usually advisable for wearing a lift. Whether it is needed longer depends, to a great extent, on how long the immediate postural problem has existed, whether any actual leg length difference exists, and whether occupational activities or postural habits can be changed to permit maintenance of good alignment.

Though it may be slight, some degree of rotation of the pelvis on the femurs usually accompanies a lateral pelvic tilt. The pelvis tends to rotate forward on the side of a high hip. In other words, there usually is counterclockwise rotation of the pelvis when the right hip is high and the right leg is in postural adduction on the pelvis. The rotation tends to disappear when the pelvis is leveled laterally.

Sacroiliac Strain

The kind of joint and the amount of movement permitted by the sacroiliac joint is central to any discussion regarding recognition and treatment of sacroiliac strains.

The Sacroiliac Joint. Basmajian describes two areas of articulation in the sacroiliac joint. As seen from the side, the wings of the sacrum present anterior areas and posterior areas. The anterior area is shaped like an ear and is referred to as the auricular surface. Its articulation with the ilium is called the *synovial sacroiliac joint*. The posterior area is rough and is referred to as the tuberosity. This articulation with the ilium is called the *fibrous sacroiliac joint* and "it gives attachment to strong interosseus and strong posterior sacroiliac ligaments that bind the bones together and permit only a minimum of movement" (57).

This distinction helps clarify the confusion that results when the joint is variously described as a syndesmosis (immovable), as a synchondrosis (slightly movable), or as a synovial (freely movable) joint.

It is recognized that movement occurs during childbirth and that some of the recurring sacroiliac problems for women are the result of a single or subsequent deliveries. Hippocrates believed that the joint was immobile except during pregnancy (58).

According to anatomists: Gray refers to this joint as a synchondrosis (13); Sabotta states that it is an almost immovable joint and that the tuberosities are united anteriorly by a joint and posteriorly by a syndesmosis (59).

Orthopedists, as a group, have had more experience than those in other branches of medicine in dealing with problems of the sacroiliac joint. The following excerpts, many direct quotes, express views of outstanding orthopedists dating from 1918 to 1986.

Davis: "A small amount of movement is possible in most cases . . ."(60).

Jones & Lovett: ". . . the consensus of opinion is that sacroiliac relaxation is a rare phenomenon" (61).

Ober, in *Lovett's Lateral Curvature of the Spine*: "The strong joint between the sacrum and the ilium through which the whole body weight is transmitted is a synchondrosis. That they permit some motion is well established, but this amount of motion is small" (62).

Steindler: "It is a true joint, with articular facets, synovial lining, and capsule; but it is so irregular in its surface, with its numerous interlocking elevations and indentations, that practically no motion is possible in this joint under normal conditions" (63).

Hoppenfeld: "For all intents and purposes, the sacroiliac and pubic symphysis are practically immovable joints, and, while they may become involved pathologically, they seldom restrict function or cause pain" (21).

Cyriax, prominent in the field of physical medicine and rehabilitation, states, "Movement does occur at the sacroiliac joint; at the extremes of trunk flexion and extension, rotation takes place between the sacrum and the ilium. . . . No muscles span the joint. There is no intra-articular meniscus. All in all, there is little that can go wrong." "The only condition encountered with any frequency is ankylosing spondylitis" (64). According to Hinwood, "The joint moves only a few millimeters and in a three-dimensional manner" (65).

The following quotes are from two physical therapists.

Saunders: "The fact that the sacroiliac joint moves is not a matter of speculation. . . . Since the sacroiliac joint is a synovial joint, it can be injured in the same manner as any other synovial joint" (66). The term synovial joint implies a freely movable joint. When applied to the sacroiliac joint, the term should be qualified to insure that it does not imply that the sacroiliac joint is freely movable.

Norkin: "The sacroiliac joint is part synovial and part fibrous" (67). The fact that there are two joint surfaces described, with different types of joint linings (one synovial, the other, a thin cartilaginous layer) does not mean that, functionally, one is dealing with two independently movable joints. The sacroiliac, regarded functionally as one joint, is only very slightly movable.

When the range of motion is stated in terms of millimeters, the amount is very small:

Cyriax states that ". . . rotation takes place between the sacrum and the ilium, but it is limited to 0.25 mm" (64).

Lovett refers to a study by Klein who found that ". . . 25 kg of force applied to the symphysis with the sacrum fixed produced a rotation of the ilia on the sacrum, which on the average, measured by the excursion of the symphysis, was 3.9 mm in man and 5.8 in woman. Measured at the sacroiliac joint this excursion was about one sixth of this amount; that is, in man the average amount of sacroiliac motion, measured at the posterior part of the joint, was about 0.6 mm." (61).

Cox states that, "It is now generally accepted that motion occurs in both the sacrum and the ilium; however, this motion is only in the range of 1 to 2 mm and is thus very hard to measure" (58).

For those who need to think in terms of inches, 1 millimeter is approximately 1/25 inch. Surely these measurements put this joint clearly in the classification of an almost immovable or, at best, a slightly movable joint. When one considers, also, that the sacroiliac joints and the symphysis pubis, like the saggital suture of the skull, hold the two halves of the body together, the concept of an almost immovable joint is a very important one.

Rationale for Treatment. Sacroiliac strains do exist. As stated by the authors of *Posture and Pain* "Because the normal range of motion of the joint is small, it takes very little more to be excessive. A tension sufficient to cause ligamentous strain may not appear on x-ray" (15).

Treatment varies from the conservative approach of nothing other than the application of support in the form of a belt, corset, or brace to the use of sophisticated mobilization techniques.

In all probability, most sacroiliac strains are the result of undue tension on the ligaments without any displacement. There is no way of knowing how many cases never seek professional help but clear up spontaneously. Very often the application of a belt or other support gives immediate relief. This response to immobilization is strong indication of a strain only.

There are wide variations of opinions with respect to the need for mobilization. In some cases it may be the treatment of choice and be appropriate; in other cases it may be unnecessary and unwarranted. If a belt does not offer relief, and mobilization does, it is plausible that a minor displacement was corrected by the manipulation. Many individuals will be helped by a support following the mobilization treatment. A person who is subject to recurrent attacks is in greater need of a support to protect the joint from becoming too mobile than the person who has had a simple strain.

The sacroiliac joint is supported by strong ligaments. There are no muscles that cross directly over the joint to support it. There would be no useful function for elastic, contractile tissue such as muscle to act on a joint that has almost no movement. However, weakness or tightness of muscles elsewhere can affect the sacroiliac joint. When motion is restricted in an adjacent area such as the back or the hip joints, stress on the sacroiliac joints is increased during any forward-bending movements.

Sacroiliac strain in subjects with flat-back posture and tight Hamstrings tends to be more common among men than among women. On the other hand, sacroiliac strain in subjects with a lordosis is found more often among women. Sacroiliac strain may be bilateral, but more often it is unilateral. There may be more pain in sitting than in standing or walking. The strain can be brought on by sitting in unsupported flexion of the lumbosacral region (e.g., sitting on the floor tailor fashion, squatting, or sitting on a chair or sofa that is too deep from front to back).

Usually there is tenderness over the affected sacroiliac area; there may be diffuse, not easily defined pain through the pelvis, buttock, and into the thigh; pain may be referred to the lower abdomen and groin area; and, at times, there may be associated sciatic symptoms. In some cases there is pain on hip flexion.

For immobilization with a belt, commercial belts are usually available and adequate for men. With women it is more difficult to keep a belt from riding up out of a position of support.

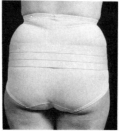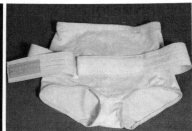

The photographs above show a panty girdle with a strap about 3 inches wide attached to the girdle by three strips of velcro. One piece is attached at the center posteriorly, and one on either side anterolaterally. The strap stays in place both in sitting and in standing. If there is a low back problem, for which the subject is wearing a corset, the strap can be attached to that garment.

Facet Slipping

The joints or facets that connect one vertebra with another may show abnormal deviations of alignment, referred to as facet slipping. Conceivably, a slipping may occur at the limit of range in flexion or in hyperextension. As a fault in hyperextension, it may result from either a sudden movement in that direction, or from a severe and persistent lumbar lordosis. The latter has been seen in x-ray (68). The vertebral interspaces are diminished and the lordosis is so marked that the compression force has caused joint structures to give way and permit the "over-riding" of one facet on another.

The suddenness of onset, acuteness of pain, and absence of previous neuromuscular symptoms suggest that some cases of acute low back pain may be due to facet slipping. The patient's description of "hearing a click like something slipping out of place" suggests that an alignment fault has occurred. Usually these incidents are of momentary duration, and as such are not confirmed by x-ray. The diagnosis is based necessarily on subjective rather than objective findings.

The movement of the body, and the direction of stress denote the direction of the alignment fault. Most often it occurs during flexion and the patient reports being unable to straighten up.

When the stress results from hyperextension movements, the so-called "catch in the back" may be muscle spasm or may involve excessive motion in the form of facet slipping.

The faults of alignment and mobility that result in excessive joint motion are the basic factors to be considered in correcting or preventing faults of this type.

Coccyalgia

Coccyalgia or coccygodynia refers to pain in the coccyx or neighboring area. Numerous factors, including trauma, are responsible for coccyalgia. Faulty position of the body may have no relation to onset of symptoms but may result secondarily and become an important factor.

One who has persistent coccyalgia tends to sit in a very erect position with hyperextension (lordosis) of the spine in an effort to avoid undue pressure on the painful coccyx. Years of sitting in such a position can result in tightness in the low back and weakness of the Gluteus maximus muscles.

Conservative treatment consists of providing some padding for the coccyx by use of a corset that is worn low to hold the buttocks close together. Preferably, it is a corset with back laces that cross over and tighten by lateral straps.

The corset should be tightened while the patient is in the standing position. The gluteal muscles thus form a padding for the coccyx in the sitting position. A soft pad may be incorporated in the corset. Pain may be alleviated by this simple procedure.

LIFTING

Low back pain is often caused or triggered by the act of lifting. For this reason, a brief discussion of this topic is included in this chapter.

Much has been written about how to lift, about conditions in the workplace that need to be corrected, and about problems as they affect the lifter. The weight of the object to be lifted, the frequency and the duration of lifting, the level from which an object must be lifted are all matters of concern with respect to how the lifter is affected.

Because of the many variables involved in lifting, there cannot be *one* correct way to lift. There are some points of agreement, however, that relate to the lifter and to the object to be lifted:

Stand as close to the object as possible.
Stand with feet apart and one foot slightly in front of the other.
Bend knees.
Begin the lift slowly without jerking.
Avoid twisting in the forward-bent position.

There is also agreement that lifting from floor height presents many hazards. It is preferable that objects not be at floor level, but if there is no choice, then an assistive device should be used if possible.

There are differences of opinion about whether to squat or stoop, and whether the low back should be straight or curved anteriorly (in the direction of a lordosis). Squatting involves moderate knee bending; stooping involves bending forward from the hips or waist or both, and slight knee bending.

The squat lift has been advocated as a means of placing the load more on the legs and reducing it on the back. However, the squat position for lifting places the Quadriceps at a mechanical disadvantage and subject to severe strain. Furthermore, many people have knee problems that prohibit lifting from a squat position. Some who may tolerate the position but lack the necessary strength may be able to build up Quadriceps strength for a job that requires this type of lifting; others may not be able to do so. Deep knee bending has been discouraged in exercise programs for a long time and the squat position should not approach deep knee bending for lifting.

In many instances, the squat lift is not an option and there is no alternative but to stoop. Lifting an infant up from a playpen, helping a patient get up from a chair to stand, and lifting objects from the level of the thighs to a higher position are examples of situations when stooping is required.

The mechanics of lifting is important, but the body mechanics of the lifter is even more important. How to lift must take into consideration the ability or vulnerability of the lifter. Of major concern are the mobility, stability, and strength of the lifter. In the general population, there are wide variations in the mobility of the low back ranging from excessive to limited. Excessive flexion and excessive extension both represent potential problems related to lifting. Limitation of motion to the extent of stiffness in the low back presents the problem of undue strain elsewhere if not in the low back itself.

In forward bending, some people exhibit *excessive flexion* (hyperflexion) in which the lumbar spine curves convexly in a posterior direction and assumes a position of lumbar kyphosis. This condition is not uncommon. Although the low back muscles remain strong, the posterior ligaments are stretched and the back is vulnerable to strain when lifting. When this condition exists, the treatment of choice is a support that prevents excessive flexion when lifting. The alternative is to attempt to hold the back in a neutral position by strong co-contraction of back and abdominal muscles.

Some exhibit *excessive extension* in which the lumbar spine curves convexly in an anterior direction and assumes a position of marked lordosis. Pope et al. referring to the work of Farni: ". . . as the lumbar lordosis increases, the plane of the L5 and S1 disc becomes more vertical and subject to greater shear and cyclic torsional forces, while nonlordotic segments are subject to compressive forces" (56, 69). Pope et al. referring to the work of Farfan: "Bending and torsional loads are of particular interest, since the bulk of experimental findings suggest that these, and not the compressive loads, are the most damaging to the discs" (69, 70).

The *normal anterior curve* in the low back is a slight curve, convex anteriorly. It is not a stable position—movement can take place in either an anterior or posterior direction. Furthermore, there is no stability afforded by ligamentous restraint in either direction. Trunk muscles must be called upon to stabilize the trunk.

When it is advocated that the back be held in a normal anterior curve (or in some degree of lordosis) during lifting, the question arises about precisely what muscles must come into play to hold that *exact* position. If the back muscles contract, *unopposed*, the anterior curve and anterior pelvic tilt increase, and the potential for overwork of the muscles and injury to the low back also increases and predisposes the subject to an added problem. Chaffin, referring to work by Poulson et al. and Tishauer et al.: ". . . lumbar muscles (like all skeletal muscles) suffer ischemic pain when statically contracted for prolonged periods of moderate to heavy loading" (71–73).

The opposing force that prevents an increase in the curve must be provided by anterior abdominal muscles, most specifically the lower abdominals. Tests and exercises specific to these muscles should be applied. Weakness of lower abdominal muscles is a common finding among otherwise strong individuals and this weakness presents a potential hazard in regard to lifting. Strengthening the abdominal muscles can affect more than merely the stability of the back. Pope et al. find, ". . . intradiscal pressure fell when abdominal pressure was increased. Thus in the standing posture intradiscal pressure is decreased coincident with increased abdominal muscular activity" (69).

The accompanying photographs are of a weightlifter who had developed a backache and had to stop weightlifting until he built up strength in his abdominal muscles. He had returned to lifting weights and demonstrated the manner in which he would pick up a heavy object from the floor. For those who have weakness of the abdominal muscles and continue weightlifting, it is advisable to use a support that provides abdominal and back stabilization.

Many individuals will exhibit a *flat low back* in the forward bent position. Flexion of the lumbar spine is movement in the direction of straightening the low back, and a flat low back represents normal flexion. When the low back flexes to, *but not beyond*, the point of flattening, there is stability afforded by this limitation of motion just as there is stability at the knee joint if it does not

hyperextend. In the back this limitation provides a "built-in chair-back" that gives stability when lifting with the back straight.

The potential for *strain* of low back muscles and ligaments exists with hyperflexion; the potential for *ischemic pain* exists with the lordotic back; and *disc problems* may result from either (74).

From the standpoint of prevention, one must assess how some exercises adversely affect the body in relation to potential hazards in lifting. The knee-bent sit-up is conducive to excessive low back flexion, and to overdevelopment and shortening of the hip flexors. Among adolescents when legs are long in relation to the trunk and there is a tendency for tightness in the Hamstrings, for-

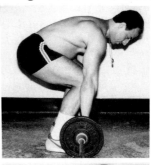

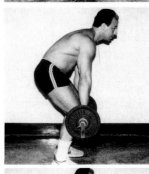

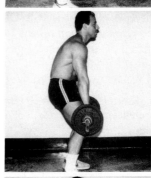

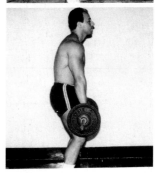

ward bending to reach to or beyond the toes often results in excessive back flexion. Press-ups in the prone position that emphasize back extension to the point of fully extending the elbows encourages excessive range of motion in extension.

With emphasis on maintaining or restoring good body mechanics and muscle balance, or compensating for deficits by such means as necessary bracing, there will be fewer problems of low back pain from lifting.

LEG PAIN

The conditions discussed under this heading include pain associated with a tight Tensor fasciae latae and Iliotibial band, stretched Tensor fasciae latae and Iliotibial band, and sciatica associated with a protruded intervertebral disc or with a stretched Piriformis.

Tight Tensor Fasciae Latae and Iliotibial Band

A condition, sometimes mistakenly diagnosed as sciatica, is that of pain associated with a tight Tensor fasciae latae and Iliotibial band. The dermatome area of cutaneous distribution corresponds closely with the area of pain.

Pain may be limited to the area covered by the fascia along the lateral surface of the thigh or may extend upward over the buttocks involving the gluteal fascia as well.

Palpation over the full length of the fascia lata, from its origin on the iliac crest to the insertion of the iliotibial band into the lateral condyle of the tibia, may elicit pain or tenderness. There is tenderness especially along the upper margin of the trochanter, and at the point of insertion near the head of the tibia.

Painful symptoms may be limited to the area of the thigh or may appear in the area supplied by the peroneal nerve. A review of the anatomy of the lateral aspect of the knee shows the relationship of the peroneal nerve to the muscles and fascia in this area.

The peroneal branch of the sciatic nerve passes obliquely forward over the neck of the fibula, crossing directly under the fibers of origin of the Peroneus longus muscle. It is well known that any prolonged pressure over this area, even though slight, must be avoided because of the danger of peroneal nerve paralysis. Even in the application of adhesive traction to the lower leg one must be extremely cautious to avoid either *pressure* over the nerve or *excessive* traction on the soft tissue at that point.

The mechanism by which the peroneal nerve is irritated in cases of tightness of the iliotibial band may be explained on the basis of either the

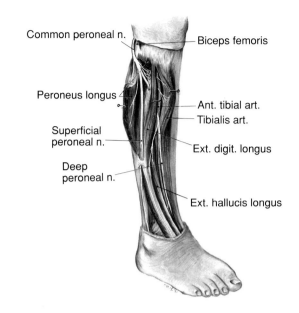

effect of pressure by the rigid bands of fascia or by the effects of traction on this part. When the fascia is drawn taut as in movements of walking, or on testing for tightness, the fascia is often observed to be extremely rigid.

The effect of traction is often seen in acute cases. With the patient side-lying with the affected leg uppermost, the mere dropping of the foot into inversion (downward toward the table) puts tension on the muscle and fascial band. Symptoms of nerve irritation in the area supplied by the peroneal nerve may be elicited by this simple movement of the foot. When the side-lying position is assumed for sleeping or for treatment, and pillows are placed between the legs to keep the leg in abduction, the foot should be supported, also, to prevent it from dropping into inversion. The failure to recognize the peripheral cause of this peroneal nerve irritation has often resulted in rather obscure explanations of this problem.

Tightness of the Tensor fasciae latae and Iliotibial band may be bilateral or unilateral, but it is more often unilateral when tightness is marked. Activities such as skating, skiing, or horseback riding may contribute to bilateral tightness.

Treatment Indications for Acute Symptoms. Heat may be applied to the lateral aspect of the thigh while the patient is in a position that gives in to the tightness. This is done by abducting the leg in back-lying or side-lying. To support the leg in abduction in side-lying, firm pillows are placed between the thighs and lower legs, making sure that the foot is also supported. A pillow at the back or abdomen helps balance the patient comfortably in this side-lying position. As soon as the patient can tolerate it, which may be during the first treatment or may be 2 or 3 days later, massage may be started. Massage should be *firm* but not deep. Often a superficial stroking is more irritating than firm gentle pressure. Massaging downward may be more effective than the usual upward stroke. Patients frequently describe their reaction to the massage as "a hurt that feels good." They are aware of a feeling of tightness and describe "wishing they could make the muscle let go" or that "it would feel good if somebody stretched it." Patients should avoid exposure to cold or drafts because even the slightest exposure often causes an increase in the pain.

The almost immediate relief of symptoms, in some instances, indicates that the condition is basically one of tight muscles and fascia. (These treatment reactions differ from those in sciatica. The same procedures applied to the painful area along the Hamstring muscles in cases of sciatic irritation would give rise to increased pain.)

For Subacute Stages. As acute pain subsides, succeeding treatments should be directed toward stretching the tight fascia. The position and movement for assisted stretching is illustrated on p. 117.

Self stretching in the standing position (as first described by Frank Ober (19)), may be done if the hip does not internally rotate or flex, but that is hard to control (see p. 60). Instead, more precise stretching should be used, as described and illustrated (p. 60).

The shoe correction indicated for correction of the lateral pelvic tilt associated with Tensor fasciae latae tightness also acts as an aid in the gradual stretching of the tight fascia. For this reason, such shoe alterations may not be tolerated until acute symptoms have subsided, and until some active treatment, in the form of heat and massage and stretching, has been instituted to relax and stretch the tight fascia.

Stretched Tensor Fasciae Latae and Iliotibial Band

Though the condition of pain associated with a contracted Tensor fasciae latae is the more common, there are instances of *strain* on the high side of the pelvis. When a leg is in a position of postural adduction, there is a continuous tension on the abductors of the thigh on that side. Symptoms of pain may become quite acute. If present, they are treated by relief of strain—that is, leveling the pelvis and correction of any opposing muscle tightness that may be causing the persistent tension. Since the chief opponent is the opposite Tensor, this problem may sometimes be resolved by treatment of the contracted muscles and fascia on the low side, even though symptoms of strain are present on the side that is higher.

There are instances in which the Tensor and the fascia lata are stretched by a fall sideways or by a sideways thrust in which the pelvis moves laterally on the fixed extremity, thrusting the hip joint into adduction.

On several occasions, adhesive taping has been successfully used in a way that *limits the adduction.* The accompanying illustrations explain the procedure. Adhesive tape, preferably 1 1/2 inches wide is cut in lengths that will extend from the area of the anterior-superior spine of the pelvis to just below the lateral knee joint.

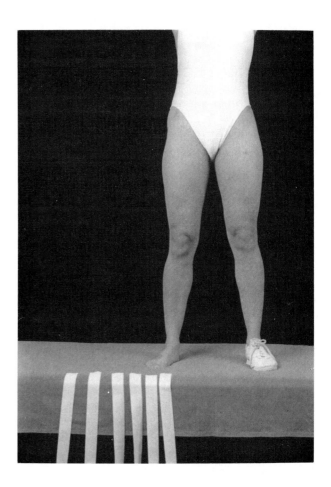

The subject removes the shoe on the affected side, or if both shoes are removed, a raise of about 1/2 inch is placed under the unaffected side. The subject stands with the feet apart to place the affected leg in some abduction. It is not expected that the tape will hold that same degree of abduction—there is always some give in the tape.

It is very important that patients be checked for skin sensitivity to adhesive tape, particularly if used during hot weather. Tincture of benzoin has been used on the skin each time the taping procedure has been used.

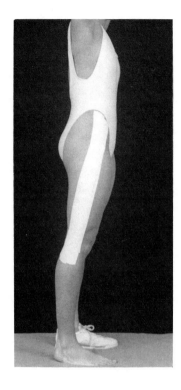

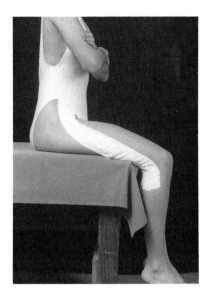

The tape is directed from anterolateral pelvis to posterolateral area of the knee in such a manner that hip and knee flexion will not be restricted in the sitting position.

Brief Case History. The subject caught her right heel on the edge of a step and averted a fall down a long flight of stairs by suddenly stepping down three steps with the left leg.

At first, pain was felt in the left hip. Two days later the left knee gave way. The left knee continued to be painful.

Four days after injury, patient was seen by an orthopedist who took an x-ray of the left knee. Five days later, patient was seen by another orthopedist who took x-rays of the hip and knee.

Two weeks after injury, patient was seen by a neurosurgeon who recommended disc surgery.

Four days later, patient was referred to a physical therapist. Following are the pertinent findings:

1. When lying supine, patient could not let knee extend without severe pain.
2. When patient was placed in a sitting position and tested for Quadriceps strength, the knee extended fully with no pain of any consequence.
3. When patient was again put in supine position and the thigh was supported to keep the hip in flexion, the patient extended the knee without pain.
4. Any attempt to extend the knee in the supine position while also extending the hip resulted in severe pain at the knee.
5. The test for strength of the Tensor fasciae latae was painful.
6. On palpation, the Tensor fasciae latae muscle appeared to be in spasm.

Impression. The site of injury appeared to be in the Tensor fasciae latae muscle with pain referred to the lateral knee via the fascia lata (i.e., the muscle in spasm placing tension on the iliotibial tract whenever the hip was extended).

Following the examination, the patient was given moist heat and massage (stroking downward) to the Tensor fasciae latae. The patient felt considerable relief of pain in the lying position, but there was pain in standing.

The anterolateral aspect of the left thigh was strapped from the crest of the ilium to just below the knee (in such a way as not to interfere with hip or knee flexion). The patient felt much relief of symptoms after strapping. (Nonallergic adhesive was used.)

Two days later, (and again 6 days after that), the strapping was checked to be sure there was no irritation, and to reinforce with more tape.

Three days later, no skin irritation was found and new strapping was applied.

Six days after that visit, the patient removed the strapping and was walking without a cane.

Approximately 5 weeks after the patient removed the strapping, a note received from her doctor stated, "The examination of (the patient's) leg assures me that she is well and there has been no residual. I feel that we can discharge her, and she can assume her general duties."

The procedure for the taping was the same as illustrated by the photographs above.

363

Sciatica

Sciatica refers to a neuritic type of pain along the course of the sciatic nerve. Pain extends down the posterior thigh and lower leg to the sole of the foot, and along the lateral aspect of the lower leg to the dorsum of the foot.

Sciatica may occur in connection with various infections or inflammatory disease processes, or may be due to some mechanical factor of compression or tension.

The symptoms may originate from a lesion of one or more of the nerve roots that later join through a plexus to form the sciatic nerve. A protruded intervertebral disc is an example of mechanical irritation that is present at the level where the nerve roots emerge from the spinal canal. Distribution of pain tends to extend from the root origin to the terminal nerve endings with the result that it is quite widespread. An L5 lesion, for example, may give rise, not only to symptoms down the course of the sciatic nerve, but also to pain in the region of the posterior and lateral thigh supplied by the inferior and superior gluteal nerves.

Symptoms of sciatica may arise from irritation anywhere along the course of the sacral plexus, the sciatic nerve trunk, or its peripheral nerve branches. Sciatica may arise as reflex pain from irritation of peripheral nerve endings. Unless so severe as to set up a reflex mechanism, a lesion along the course of the nerve or its branches may often be distinguished from a root lesion by the localization of pain to the distribution below the level of the lesion.

Other than at the root, there are two commonly recognized sites of lesions giving rise to sciatic pain: 1) the sacroiliac region where the spinal nerves emerge through the sacral foramen; and 2) at the level of the Piriformis muscle where the sciatic nerve trunk emerges through the sciatic notch and passes either through or under the Piriformis muscle.

This discussion about sciatica is concerned with faulty body mechanics in relation to disc protrusion, and with sciatic symptoms associated with the Piriformis syndrome. There will be no discussion of sciatica in relation to the sacroiliac strain other than to suggest that the faulty mechanics causing this strain may put tension on the sacral plexus because of the close association of the involved structures in this area.

Protruded Intervertebral Disc. The basic concepts about flexion and extension movements of the spine in relation to disc protrusion play an important role in determining treatment. The following quotes are pertinent to this topic.

Nordin and Frankel state, "The forward inclination of the spine makes the disc bulge on the concave side. Hence, when the spine is flexed the disc protrudes anteriorly and is retracted posteriorly" (75). Pope et al. record the findings of Brown et al. and Roaf (64). Brown et al. reported disc bulging anteriorly during flexion, posteriorly during extension, and toward the concavity of the spinal curve during lateral bend (76). Roaf stated that the bulging of the annulus is always on the concave side of the curve, and that during flexion and extension the nucleus does not change in shape or position (77).

This information is contrary to what many people believe or have been taught. However, in the analysis of low back problems and sciatica, this concept is important.

Strong back muscles are essential for posture and function. Although low back muscles are seldom weak, back extension exercises are frequently prescribed. Overemphasis on back extension can contribute to an increase in a lordotic position. Quoting again from Nordin and Frankel, "The erector spinae muscles are intensely activated by arching the back in the prone position. Loading the spine in extreme positions such as this one produces high stresses on spine structures, so this hyperextended position should be avoided" (75).

Good strength in abdominal muscles is also important to counterbalance the back muscles and stabilize the trunk in good postural alignment and during activities such as lifting. Unfortunately, abdominal muscles are often weak, especially the lower abdominals, and not enough attention is paid to doing appropriate exercises.

If a disc has ruptured and is pressing on a nerve root with intractable pain and no relief has been obtained from conservative measures, there may be no alternative to surgery. However, there are many cases of sciatica in which clinical findings suggest a disc lesion, but the fluctuation of symptoms suggest that the protrusion is not constant. Conservative treatment of many such cases has brought about effective relief of symptoms without surgery. In instances when, for some reason, the patient declines operation or the doctor does not elect to do surgery, conservative treatment becomes the necessary alternative.

The rationale for conservative treatment is based on the premise that any bending, torsional loads, or compressive force, whether due to muscle spasm, tightness of back muscles, or stress of superimposed weight on the lumbar spine, may be factors in causing the disc protrusion.

Two measures provide effective conservative treatment: First, immobilization of the back for relief of acute muscle spasm and for restriction of motion; and, second, use of an hourglass type of support for the low back which acts to transmit the weight of the thorax to the pelvis and relieve stress on the lumbar spine (in much the same manner as a cervical collar is used to relieve pressure on the cervical spine).

To treat by immobilization, and for relief of superimposed body weight, a fitted support is reinforced with strong lateral and posterior stays. Following relief of acute symptoms, therapeutic measures may be instituted to correct any underlying muscle imbalance or faults in alignment.

Acute sciatic symptoms associated with protrusion of a ruptured disc often occur as a result of a sudden twist and extension of the spine from a forward bent position such as twisting the trunk while lifting a weight. That such a type of stress should be related to this type of lesion is not surprising in view of the fact that "rotation of the lumbar spine takes place at the intervertebral disc" (13).

Sciatic symptoms that have been acute or subacute often cause the body to be drawn into such faulty alignment that secondary symptoms of compression and muscle strain are added to the original problem. These secondary symptoms may, on occasion, persist after the original underlying problems have subsided.

Piriformis Muscle and Its Relation to Sciatic Pain. Albert Freiberg, described the Piriformis muscle and its relation to sciatic pain, and furnished an interesting explanation for a possible cause of sciatic symptoms (78). Though there may be numerous cases in which sciatic pain is associated with a *contracted* Piriformis, as he described, it is the opinion of the authors that irritation of the sciatic nerve by the Piriformis muscle is often associated with a *stretched* Piriformis.

The Piriformis arises with a broad origin from the anterior aspect of the sacrum and inserts into the superior border of the greater trochanter. This muscle has three functions *in standing*. It acts as an external rotator of the femur, aids slightly in tilting the pelvis down laterally, and aids in tilting the pelvis posteriorly by pulling the sacrum downward toward the thigh.

In a faulty position with a leg in postural adduction and internal rotation in relation to an anteriorly tilted pelvis, there is marked stretching of the Piriformis muscle along with other muscles that function in a similar manner. The mechanics of this position are such that the Piriformis muscle and the sciatic nerve are thrust into close contact. The figure below shows the relationship of the sciatic nerve to the Piriformis muscle.

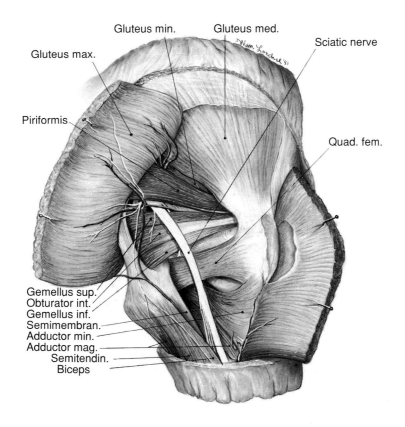

365

Evaluation. The following points should be considered in the diagnosis of sciatic pain associated with a stretched Piriformis.

1. Do the sciatic symptoms diminish or disappear in non-weight bearing?
2. Do internal rotation and adduction of the thigh in the flexed position, with patient supine, increase sciatic symptoms?
3. Do the symptoms diminish in standing if a straight raise is placed under the opposite foot?
4. Does the patient seek relief of symptoms by placing the leg in external rotation and abduction, both in the lying and standing positions?

The test movement to place the Piriformis on maximum stretch (point 2) is done in the following manner: The patient is supine on a table. The knee and hip of the affected leg are flexed to right angles. Flexion of the knee rules out any confusion with pain due to irritation of the Hamstring muscles. The examiner then internally rotates and adducts the thigh passively.

In regard to point 3 above, it has been a frequent clinical observation that, during the course of examination, a lift applied under the foot of the affected side would increase symptoms, while a lift placed under the foot of the unaffected side would give some immediate relief in the affected leg.

Shoe corrections, for cases suggesting irritation due to a stretched, rather than a contracted, Piriformis, consist of a straight raise (usually 1/8 to 1/4 inch) on the heel of the *unaffected* side to relieve tension on the abductors of the affected side; and an inner wedge on the heel on the *affected* side to correct the internal rotation of the leg. Heat, massage, and stretching of low back muscles if they are contracted, abdominal muscle exercise if abdominal weakness is present, and instructions for correcting the faulty position of the pelvis in standing are used as indicated.

KNEE PROBLEMS

The habitual position of the knee in standing indicates which areas are subjected to undue pressure and which are subjected to undue tension. Symptoms of muscle and ligamentous strain are associated with the areas of undue tension, while symptoms of bony compression are related to the areas of pressure. The postural faults may appear separately, or in various combinations. For example, postural bowlegs results from the combination of hyperextension of the knees, medial rotation of the hips, and pronation of the feet. Medial rotation and slight knock-knee are frequently seen in combination. Lateral rotation is often seen with severe knock-knee. (See p. 97.)

This text does not deal with treatment of congenital or acquired deformities of the feet and knees. An excellent reference for such treatment is found in the chapter by Joseph H. Kite in Basmajian's Therapeutic Exercise (best in the *3rd* edition) (79).

Medial Rotation of Hip and Pronation of Feet. The position of the knees in which the patellae face slightly inward results from medial rotation at the hip joints. As a *functional or apparent* (i.e., not structural) malalignment, it is usually accompanied by pronation of the feet. (See p. 94.) The initial problem may be at the hip or at the foot and may result from weakness of the hip external rotators, or from weakness of the muscles and ligaments that support the longitudinal arches of the feet. Whichever of these predisposes to the fault, the end result is usually that both conditions exist if the initial problem is not corrected. A tight Tensor fasciae latae may be a contributing cause, and sitting in reverse tailor (or "W") position may predispose toward faulty hip, knee, and foot positions. (See figure below.)

There may be a *structural* malalignment in which there is a lateral tibial torsion accompanying the hip medial rotation. In either event, there tends to be pronation of the foot, but with tibial torsion there is more out-toeing of the foot.

The malalignment affects the knee joint adversely, causing ligamentous strain anteromedially and joint compression laterally.

Treatment consists of shoe alterations and/or orthoses that support the longitudinal arch; exercises for foot inverters (see foot exercises, p. 374); strengthening exercises for hip lateral rotators; and stretching of the Tensor fasciae latae, if it is tight (see pp. 60 and 117).

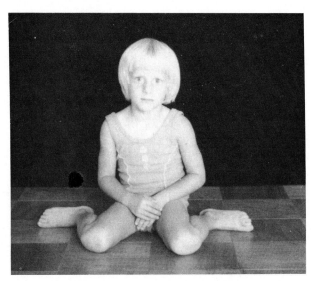

Reverse tailor or "W" position

Knee Hyperextension. Hyperextension of the knee joint results in undue compression anteriorly, and undue tension on muscles and ligaments posteriorly. Pain may occur in either area. (See pp. 95 and 96.) Pain in the popliteal space is not uncommon in adults who have stood with knees in hyperextension.

Hyperextension may cause further problems if uncorrected. The Popliteus is a short (one-joint) muscle that acts somewhat as a broad posterior knee joint ligament. Its action is to flex the knee and rotate the leg medially on the thigh. (See p. 211.) If it is stretched by knee hyperextension, it allows the lower leg to rotate laterally on the femur in flexion or in hyperextension.

Prevention or correction of hyperextension is based on instruction in good postural alignment, and cooperation by the subject in avoiding positions of knee hyperextension in standing. Specific exercises for knee flexors may be indicated. Bracing may be required in cases that do not respond otherwise, and in severe cases.

Knee Flexion. Knee flexion is a less common finding than the three above-mentioned problems except that it is fairly common among older people. Habitually standing with knees flexed (see figure p. 95) can cause problems at the knee and along the Quadriceps muscle. It is a position that requires constant muscular effort to keep the knees from flexing further. Pain is most often associated with muscle strain of the Quadriceps, or with the effect of traction by the Quadriceps (through its patellar tendon insertion) on the tibia.

Sometimes knee flexion is a position assumed to ease a painful low back that is otherwise pulled into a lordotic curve by tight hip flexors. There may also be actual shortness of the Popliteus and the one-joint Hamstring, namely the short head of the Biceps femoris. If hip flexors and knee flexors are tight, appropriate stretching exercises should be instituted.

Effect on Posture. Unilateral knee flexion creates concerns beyond the area of the knee. The effect on the posture may be seen in the figures on right. With the left knee flexed, the right foot is more pronated than the left, the right thigh is medially rotated, the pelvis tilts down on the left, the spine curves convexly toward the left, the right hip is high, and the right shoulder is low.

Bowlegs. In children, a position of bowlegs may be either *actual* or *apparent*, i.e., structural or postural. An actual bowing is of the shaft (femur or tibia or both) and is usually due to rickets. An apparent bowing occurs as a result of a combination of joint positions that permit faulty alignment without any structural defect in the long bones. It results from a combination of medial rotation of the hip, hyperextension of the knee joint, and pronation of the foot. (See pp. 95 and 97.)

Hyperextension alone does not result in a position of postural bowlegs; the medial rotation component is required. Medial rotation of the thigh plus pronation of the foot do not result in the bowing unless accompanied by hyperextension. Thus, on testing, the apparent postural bowing will disappear in non-weight bearing, or in standing if the knees are held in neutral extension.

Correction depends upon use of appropriate shoe corrections, exercises to correct pronation, exercises to strengthen hip lateral rotators, and cooperation by the subject in avoiding a position of knee hyperextension.

There are instances in which postural bowing and hyperextension are compensatory for knock-knees, as described on p. 98. Paradoxically, the correction of this type of postural bowing must be based on correction of the underlying knock-knee problem.

Correction of *structural* bowing depends chiefly on timely intervention and effective bracing. An outer wedge on the heel or sole usually is not indicated because there is a tendency for the foot to pronate as the legs bow outward.

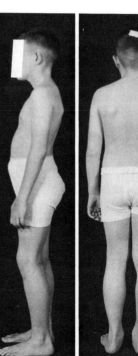
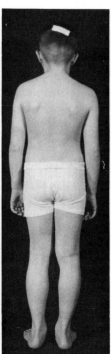
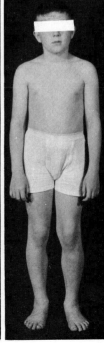

Knock-Knees. Tension on the medial ligaments, and compression on the lateral surfaces of the knee joint are present in knock-knee. Discomfort and pain associated with the tension on the ligaments is annoying, but is often tolerated for a long time before becoming incapacitating. The pain associated with compression, on the other hand, is slow to develop, but is often intolerable when it manifests itself. Evidence of arthritic changes may appear in x-ray.

Tightness of the Tensor fasciae latae and iliotibial band is frequently seen in conjunction with knock-knees, even in young children. Heat, massage, and stretching of the muscle and fascia lata is often needed along with shoe corrections in order to bring about a realignment.

In *treatment* of early *mild* knock-knee, an inner border wedge on a shoe tends to realign the extremity thus relieving strain medially and compression laterally. There is danger in using too high an inner wedge because the overcorrection of the foot may be overcompensated for by an increase in knock-knee. A 1/8 to 3/16 inch inner heel wedge is usually adequate. A *moderate* degree of knock-knee may benefit from a knee support in addition to shoe corrections. The support should have lateral steel uprights with a joint at the knee. *Severe* knock-knee requires bracing or may require surgery.

FOOT PROBLEMS

The foot has *two longitudinal arches* that extend lengthwise from the heel to the ball of the foot. The *inner* or *medial* longitudinal arch is made up of the calcaneus, astragalus, scaphoid, three cuneiform, and three medial metatarsal bones. The *outer* or *lateral* longitudinal arch is made up of the calcaneus, cuboid, and two lateral metatarsal bones. The outer arch is lower than the inner and tends to be obliterated in weight bearing. Any references to "the longitudinal arch" will mean the inner arch.

There are two *transverse metatarsal arches*, one across the midsection and one across the ball of the foot. The *posterior metatarsal* arch is at the proximal end (or base) of the metatarsal bones. It is a structural arch with wedge-shaped bones at the apex of the arch. The *anterior metatarsal* arch is at the distal ends (or heads) of the metatarsals.

Painful foot conditions may be roughly divided into three groups: those dealing with longitudinal arch strain, those dealing with metatarsal arch strain, and those dealing with faulty positions of the toes. The three types of painful conditions may exist in the same foot, but more often one type predominates over the others.

Examination of faulty and painful feet should include the following:

> Examine the overall postural alignment for any evidence of superimposed strain on the feet such as occurs in cases of postural faults in which the body weight is borne too far forward over the balls of the feet (see p. 77A).
> Check the alignment of the feet in standing with and without shoes.
> Observe the manner of walking with and without shoes.
> Test for muscle weakness or tightness of toe and foot muscles.
> Check regarding unfavorable occupational influences.
> Examine the shoes for overall fit, etc. (see p. 372) and check for places of wear on the sole and heel. Faulty weight distribution in standing or walking is often revealed by excessive wear on certain parts of the shoe.

Treatment may be considered as being of two types, corrective and palliative. Ideally, treatment should be corrective, but in view of the fact that many painful foot conditions occur in older people whose bony, ligamentous, and muscular structures cannot adjust to corrective measures, it is necessary to use measures designed to obtain relief with the minimum of correction.

Faulty and Painful Foot Conditions and Treatment Indications

There is a familiar saying, "If your feet hurt, you hurt all over." For those whose occupation requires constant standing, or those engaged in activities that place great stress on the feet, the statement is especially applicable.

In older people, feet may become painful because of the loss of normal padding on the soles of the feet. *Insoles* that cushion the foot markedly improve comfort and function. The insole must be thin enough to fit in the shoe without crowding the foot, but thick enough to offer a firm, resilient cushion.

To the extent that foot pain or discomfort is relieved, the insole may indirectly help to alleviate the discomfort elsewhere that resulted from a painful foot condition.

Pronation Without Flatness of the Longitudinal Arch. This type of fault is most often found among women who wear high heels. In weight bearing, there may be some symptoms of foot strain in the longitudinal arch, but more often the pronation causes strain medially at the knee. In the foot itself, the anterior arch is subjected to more strain than the longitudinal arch.

Occasionally, the longitudinal arch is higher than average. This situation may require the use of an arch support that is higher than usual so that the support may conform to the foot and provide a uniform base of support.

Treatment for pronation consists of the use of an inner heel wedge, or an orthosis that provides the same type of correction. As a general principle, patients should be discouraged from wearing a high heel if there are symptoms of foot or knee pain, but it may be inadvisable to recommend shoes with little or no heel because the foot tends to pronate more in the flat-heeled shoe. With a medium heel, the longitudinal arch is increased and a heel wedge or arch support will help correct pronation.

Regarding shoe correction, on a heel of medium height, a 1/16 inch inner wedge is usually used, while a 1/8 inch wedge is the usual adjustment on a low heel. A high heel cannot be altered by use of an inner wedge without interfering with stability.

Pronation with Flatness of the Longitudinal Arch.

This position of the foot is comparable to a position of dorsiflexion and eversion. In weight bearing the position of pronation with flatness of the longitudinal arch is usually accompanied by an out-toeing of the forefoot. Excessive tension is exerted on the muscles and ligaments on the inner side of the foot that support the longitudinal arch. Undue compression is exerted on the outer side of the foot in the region of the sinus tarsi where the astragalus and calcaneus articulate.

The Tibialis posterior and Abductor hallucis are usually weak. Toe extensor muscles and the Flexor brevis digitorum may also be weak. The peroneal muscles tend to be tight if pronation is marked.

Supportive treatment consists of using an inner heel wedge and a longitudinal arch support. When the heel has a wide base, a wedge of 1/8 inch thickness is most often used. When the fault is severe, the patient should be discouraged from wearing a shoe without a heel. This type of fault is more prevalent among men and children than among women.

Metatarsal Arch Strain.

This type of strain is usually the result of wearing high heels, or of walking on hard surfaces in soft-soled shoes. It may also result from an unusual amount of running, jumping, or hopping. An interesting and unusual example of the latter was observed in a child about 10 years of age who had won a hop-scotch tournament. The foot on which she did most of her hopping had developed metatarsal strain and a callus on the ball of the foot.

In cases of metatarsal arch strain, the Lumbricales, the Adductor hallucis (transverse and oblique), and the Flexor digiti minimi are most noticeably weak. If asked to flex the toes and cup the front part of the foot, the patient can flex the end joints of the toes only; there is little or no flexion of the metatarsophalangeal joints.

Stretching of the toe extensors is indicated if tightness exists. Supportive treatment consists of the use of a metatarsal pad or a metatarsal bar. If there are calluses under the heads of the second, third, and fourth metatarsals a pad is usually indicated; if there are calluses under the heads of all the metatarsals, a bar is indicated.

In-toeing Position of the Foot.

An in-toeing position of the feet, like the out-toeing, may be related to faults at various levels. The term *pigeon-toes* may be considered as synonymous with in-toeing.

If the legs are internally rotated at hip level, the patellae face inward, the feet point inward, and there is usually pronation of the feet. When there is in-toeing related to medial torsion of the tibia, the patellae face forward and the feet point inward. If the problem is within the foot itself, the hips and knees may be in good alignment, but there is anterior foot varus (adduction of the forefoot). (See photo, p. 370.)

As a general rule, children do not exhibit muscle tightness. However, it is not uncommon to find that the Tensor fasciae latae, which is an internal rotator, is tight in children who exhibit medial rotation from hip level. Stretching of the Tensor may be indicated but it should be done carefully.

Children who develop this medial rotation from hip level often sit in reverse tailor or "W" position. (See photograph, p. 366.) Encouraging the child to sit in a cross-legged position tends to offset the effects of the other position.

The shoe correction used in cases of in-toeing associated with internal rotation of the extremity is a small, essentially semicircular patch placed on the outer side of the sole at about the base of the fifth metatarsal (see fig C, p. 373). To mark the area for the patch, the shoe is held upside down and bent sharply at the sole in the manner it bends in walking. The patch extends about equally forward and backward from the apex of the bend. It is cut so that it is of a given thickness (either 1/8 or 3/16 inch, depending on the size of the shoe) along the outer border. It tapers off to zero toward the front, center and back of the sole.

In-toeing associated with internal rotation of the extremity tends to be more marked in walking than in standing, and the shoe correction helps to change the walking rather than the standing pattern. The effect of changing the walking pattern in turn helps to correct the standing position.

The patch, by its convex shape, pivots the foot outward as the sole of the shoe is brought in con-

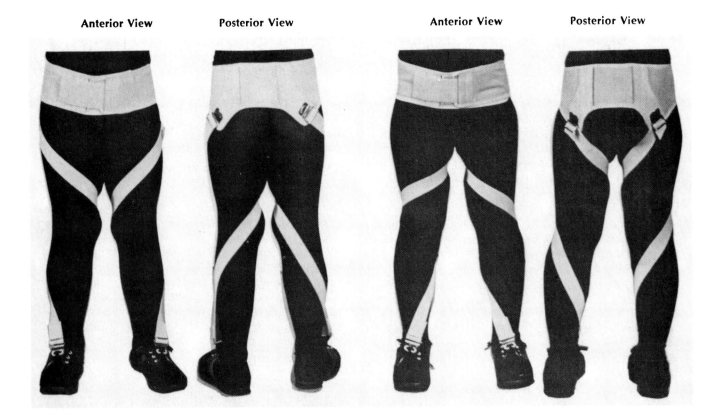

Anterior View   Posterior View   Anterior View   Posterior View

TWISTER

THE ELASTIC ROTATION LEG CONTROL is designed to exert a counter-rotation force on the legs and feet to correct excessive internal or external rotation. This appliance is recommended for children with mild to moderate rotation problems and is frequently combined with other forms of treatment such as shoe corrections and ankle braces. The simple fitting procedure of lacing the shoe hooks to the shoes, securing the pelvic belt with its Velcro fastener, extending the elastic straps as shown above, and adjusting the strap tension for the position desired produces an effective rotation control usually requiring only a short patient adjustment period. Courtesy C.D. Denison Orthopaedic Appliance Corp. (52).

tact with the floor in the usual transfer of weight forward. Before marking the shoe for alteration, a leather patch may be taped to the sole of the shoe and tested for position by observing the child's walk.

An in-toeing position due to malalignment of the forefoot in relation to the rest of the foot is similar to a mild clubfoot except that there is no supination of the heel or equinus. As a matter of fact, there may be pronation of the heel along with the adduction.

Inflare shoes may be comfortable but will not be corrective. The child should be fitted with shoes that have been made on a straight last. A stiff inner counter extending from the base of the first metatarsal to the end of the great toe should be added to the shoe. The outer counter should be stiff from the heel to the cuboid.

When shoe alterations fail to bring about a correction of the in-toeing, a "twister" is used.

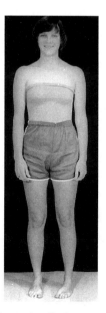

Anterior foot varus

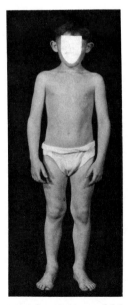

External rotation of hips and out-toeing of feet

370

Out-toeing Position of the Feet. Out-toeing may be the result of external rotation of the entire extremity from hip level, tibial torsion in which the shaft of the tibia has developed a rotation, or may be a fault of the foot itself in which the fore-foot abducts in relation to the posterior part of the foot.

In young children in whom the problem is from hip level, a *twister* may be used. Usually, results are obtained within a relatively short period of time, i.e., a matter of several months (see facing page).

The external rotation of the extremity (see figure on facing page) does not automatically cause difficulty in standing, but walking in an out-toed position tends to put strain on the longitudinal arch as weight is transferred from heel to toes.

If tibial torsion is present as an established fault in an adult, no effort should be made to have the individual walk with the feet straight ahead because such "correction" of the foot position would result in a faulty alignment of the knees.

Abduction of the forefoot is the result of a breakdown of the longitudinal arch. In children, measures that correct the arch position will help to correct the out-toeing. Wearing corrective shoes may be advisable because they typically have an inflare last. In adults, however, if the fault is established, corrective shoes do not change the alignment of the foot but rather cause undue pressure on the foot. Usually it is necessary to have the patient wear shoes that have been made over a straight last or even an outflare last. The patient can tolerate some arch support and inner wedge alterations if these are indicated, but the alignment of the shoe must necessarily conform to that of the foot to avoid pressure.

Toeing out in walking may result from tightness of the tendo Achillis, in which case stretching of the plantar flexor muscles is indicated. (See p. 52 for stretching exercises.)

Supinated Foot. A supinated foot is a very uncommon postural fault (see p. 94). It is essentially the reverse of a pronated foot—the arch is high and weight is borne on the outer side of the foot. Shoe corrections are essentially the opposite of those applied to a pronated foot. An outer wedge on the heel, a reverse modified Thomas heel, and an outer sole wedge are usually indicated.

If knock-knee is associated with supination of the foot, shoe corrections as described above may increase the deformity of the knee. Careful consideration should be given to associated faults.

Hallux Valgus. A hallux valgus is a position of faulty alignment of the big toe in which the end of the toe deviates toward the midline of the foot, (see figure, p. 98) sometimes to the point of overlapping the other toes. The Abductor hallucis

muscle is stretched and weakened, and the Adductor hallucis muscle is tight.

Such cases may require surgery if the fault cannot be corrected or pain alleviated by conservative means. However, in early stages it may be possible to affect considerable correction.

The patient should wear shoes that have a straight inner border, and should avoid the use of shoes with cut out toe space. A "toe-separator" which is a small piece of rubber that is inserted between the big toe and the second toe, aids considerably in holding the big toe in more normal alignment. As a pure palliative procedure for the relief of pain due to pressure, a bunion-guard is often useful.

Because excessive pronation often is the cause of the hallux valgus, prevention or correction require that the arch be supported. "Excessive" means that there is marked relaxation of the supporting arch structures that require firm support. Rigid orthoses are needed in such instances.

Hammer Toes. The position of hammer toes (as illustrated) is one in which the toes are extended at the metatarsophalangeal and distal interphalangeal joints, and flexed at the proximal interphalangeal joints. Usually there are calluses under the ball of the foot and corns on the toes as a result of pressure from the shoe.

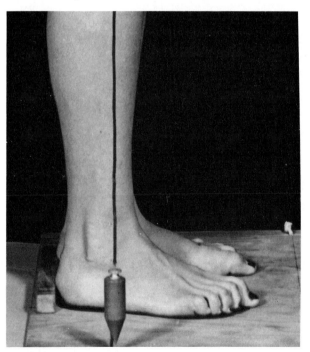

Massage and stretching may aid in correcting the faulty alignment of the toes in the early stage, and benefit may be obtained from a metatarsal bar. An inside metatarsal bar may be more effective, but an outside metatarsal bar may be more comfortable. (See figure, p. 373.)

SHOES

The protection and support given by shoes are important considerations with regard to the postural alignment in standing. Various factors predispose toward faulty alignment and foot strain, and create the need for adequate shoe support. The flat, unyielding floors and sidewalks of our environment, the use of heels that decrease the stability of the foot, and prolonged periods of standing, as required in some occupations, are some of the contributing causes of foot problems.

There are a number of factors relating to the size, shape, and construction of a shoe that need to be considered.

Length. *Overall length* should be adequate for comfort and normal function.

Length from the heel to the ball: Feet vary in arch and toe length, some having a longer arch and shorter toes while others have a shorter arch and longer toes. No special type of shoe is suited to all individuals, and one must find a shoe that fits in respect to arch length as well as over-all length.

Width. A shoe that is too narrow cramps the foot; one that is too wide fails to give proper support or may cause blisters by rubbing against the foot.

Width of the heel cup: The shoe should fit snugly around the heel of the foot. It is often a problem to find a shoe with a heel cup narrow enough in proportion to the rest of the shoe.

Width of the shank: The shank is the narrow part of the sole under the instep. The shank should not be too wide, but should permit the contour of the leather upper part of the shoe to be molded around the contour of the arch of the foot. If the shank is too wide, the arch of the foot does not have the support given by the shoe counter.

Toe width: This needs to allow for good toe position and to permit action of the toes in walking. The toe box (or toe counter) helps to give space to this part of the foot and keeps the pressure of the shoe off the toes.

Shape of the Shoe. A normal foot should be able to assume a normal position in a properly fitted shoe. Any distortion in shape that tends to pull the foot out of good alignment is not desirable. It is a fairly common fault that shoes flare in too much. This design is based on the assumption that strain on the long arch is relieved because it is raised by an inward twist of the forefoot. The foot of a growing child may conform to the abnormal shape if such shoes are worn for a period of years. Because an adult's foot is not as flexible as a child's and is not easily forced out of its usual

alignment, a shoe with an inflare is likely to cause excessive pressure on the toes.

Heel Counter. A *heel counter* is a reinforcement of stiff material inserted between the outer and inner layers of leather that form the back of a shoe. It serves two purposes; to provide lateral support for the foot, and to help preserve the shape of the shoe. As the height of the heel increases, the lateral stability of the foot decreases and the counter becomes especially important for balance.

When the leather surrounding the heel is not reinforced it will usually collapse after a short period of wear and shift laterally in whatever direction the wearer habitually thrusts the weight. When this has happened the feet can no longer be held in a good alignment by such shoes.

Shoes that have a cut-out back and depend upon a strap to hold the heel in place offer even less stability than do shoes with enclosed heels and no counter. The shoe itself does not show as much deterioration with wear because the strap merely shifts sideward with the heel, and there is no heel leather to break down. In flat-heeled shoes, the effect on the wearer may be minimal, but the lack of lateral support in a higher heel cannot persist indefinitely without some ill effects. The effects may be felt more at the knee than in the foot itself.

Strength of the Shank. A good *shank* is of prime importance both for the durability of the shoe itself and for the well-being of the person who wears it. When a shoe has a heel of any height the part of the shoe under the instep is off the floor. The shank must then be an arch-like support that bridges the space between the heel and the ball of the foot. If the shank is not made of a strong enough material it will sag under a normal

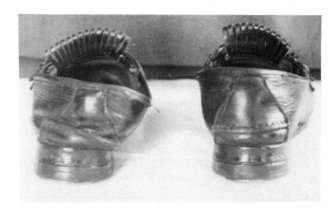

Shoes without stiff heel-counter: The absence of a stiff counter in the heel allows the foot to deviate inward or outward. The shoe breaks down and any existing fault tends to become more pronounced.

load when the shoe is worn. Such a sag permits a downward shift of the arch of the foot, and tends to drive the toe and heel of the shoe apart. The extreme of this type of deterioration in a flat heeled shoe is sometimes seen in the rounded, rocker-bottom shape that results, the shank being lower than the tip of the toe or back of the heel.

A strip of steel reinforcing the shank provides the strength required to preserve the shoe as well as to protect the wearer from foot strain. (Left figure, p. 374.) Both low- and high-heeled shoes require a strong shank. Fortunately most high-heeled shoes are made with good shanks. Low-heeled shoes often are not. A prospective buyer can judge the shank of a shoe to some extent by placing the shoe on a firm surface and pressing downward on the shank. If such moderate pressure makes it bend downward, it is safe to assume it will break down under the weight of the body.

In heel-less shoes such as sandals or some tennis shoes, the firmness of the shank is of little importance for a person with no foot problems. Because the whole foot is supported by the floor or ground, support from the shoe is not a major consideration, unless the foot is being subjected to unusual strain from activity (as in athletics) or strain from prolonged standing.

Sole and Heel of the Shoe. *Thickness* and *flexibility* are the two important factors in judging the *sole* of a shoe. For prolonged standing especially on hard floors of wood, tile, or concrete, a thick sole of leather or rubber is desirable. It has some resiliency and is able to cushion the foot against the effects of the hard surface.

For people who are required to do a great deal of walking, a firm sole is desirable. The repeated movement of transferring weight across the ball of the foot in walking is a source of continuous strain. A firm sole that restricts an excessive bend at the junction of the toes with the ball of the foot guards against unnecessary strain. The sole should not be so stiff, however, that there is a restriction of normal movement in walking.

When a child is learning to walk, the shoes should have no heel and a sole flat and firm enough to give stability. The sole should be fairly flexible, however, to allow the proper development of the arch through walking.

The height of the heel is important in relation to strain of the arches of the foot. Wearing a heel changes the distribution of body weight, shifting it forward. The proportion of weight borne on the ball of the foot increases directly with the height of the heel. Continuous wearing of high heels eventually results in anterior foot strain.

The effects of a fairly high heel can be offset, but only to a limited degree, by the use of metatarsal pads and by wearing shoes that help to counteract the tendency of the foot to slide forward toward the toe of the shoe. A shoe that laces at the instep or a pump with a high-cut *vamp* (preferably elasticized) helps to restrain the foot from sliding forward by providing an evenly-distributed and uniform pressure if the shoe fits well.

When the foot is allowed to slip forward in the shoe, the toes are wedged into too small a space and subjected to considerable deforming pressure.

From the standpoint of normal growth and development as well as normal function, it is advisable that a person use a well-constructed shoe with a low heel. However, there are individuals, especially women with a painful condition of the longitudinal arch, who benefit from wearing shoes with heels of medium height. The higher heel mechanically increases the height of the longitudinal arch, and a flexible foot that is subject to longitudinal arch strain may be relieved of symptoms by using a heel about 1 1/2 inches high.

SHOE CORRECTIONS AND ORTHOSES

Since correction of faulty foot conditions is largely dependent on supports and shoe alterations, brief descriptions of some of these are pertinent to this discussion.

A *heel wedge* is a small piece of leather made in the shape of half of the heel. It is usually applied between the leather or rubber heel lift and the heel proper. It is of a given thickness, usually

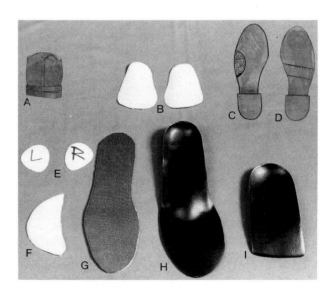

A, inner heel wedge
B, metatarsal supports
C, toe-out patch
D, metatarsal bar
E, metatarsal pads
F, longitudinal arch support (cookie)
G, insole
H and I, rigid orthotic devices.

1/16 to 1/8 inch at the side and tapers off to nothing at the midline of the heel. An *inner wedge* is so placed that the thickness appears on the inner side of the heel and it serves to tilt the shoe slightly outward. In an *outer wedge* the thicker part is at the outer side of the heel and tends to tilt the shoe inward.

A *sole wedge* made in the shape of one-half of the sole (cut lengthwise) may be an inner or an outer wedge.

A *Thomas heel* is a heel extended on the inner side for the purpose of medial longitudinal arch support. A *Reverse Thomas Heel* is extended on the outer side for correction of a supinated foot.

A *longitudinal arch support* is a support put inside the shoe under the medial longitudinal arch of the foot. It is often made of firm rubber and leather. In many instances, however, a more rigid support is needed. Such devices need to be custommade for each individual. Semi-rigid or rigid supports are fabricated from a neutral suspension cast, designed to hold the subtalar joint in neutral position while locking the midtarsal joint.

A *metatarsal pad* is a small firm rubber pad made in an essentially triangular shape. It is placed proximal to the heads of the metatarsals and acts to reduce the hyperextension of the metatarsophalangeal joints of the second, third, and fourth toes. To indicate the position of the support *in relation to the foot* and *in relation to the shoe* a metatarsal pad was inserted in a shoe and an x-ray of the foot was taken with the shoe on.

A *metatarsal bar* is a strip of leather extending across the sole of the shoe. It acts to lift the metatarsals proximal to the heads as does the pad, but is more rigid and affects the position of all the toes rather than just the second, third, and fourth. (See D in figure, p. 373.)

A *long counter* is an extended counter that is added on the inner or outer side of the shoe.

The foot muscles cannot be expected to compensate for or correct a condition in which there

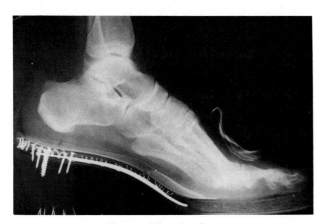
X-ray of foot in shoe

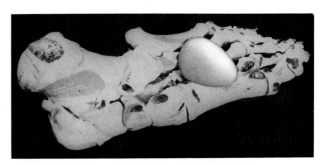
Metatarsal pad on bones of sole of foot

is faulty bony alignment and ligamentous relaxation. Strong muscles will help preserve good alignment, but supports are necessary for correction of faulty alignment. The support should relieve strain on the muscles. For tight muscles that maintain a persistent faulty alignment of the foot or toes, stretching is indicated. Effective shoe corrections do much to bring about the gradual stretching of the tight muscle.

Normal use of the foot usually provides sufficient exercise for strengthening the muscles. Except among individuals who have been bedridden or who do very little walking, it is safe to assume that the average person does not lack exercise of the feet.

CORRECTIVE FOOT EXERCISES FOR PRONATED FEET

Lying on back:
1. Curl toes down and hold while pulling foot up and in.
2. With legs straight and together, try to touch soles of feet together.

Sitting in chair:
3. With left knee crossed over right, move left foot in half circle, down, in, and up, then relax. (Do not turn foot outward.) Repeat with right foot.
4. With knees apart, place soles of feet together and hold while bringing knees together.
5. Place towel on floor. With feel parallel and about 6 inches apart, grip towel with toes and pull inward (in adduction) with both feet, bunching towel between feet.
6. With small ball (about 1 1/4 to 1 1/2 inches in diameter) cut in half, placed under anterior arch of foot, grip toes down over ball.

Standing:
7. With feet straight ahead or slightly outtoeing, roll weight to outer borders of feet by pulling up under arches.

Walking:
8. Walk along a straight line on the floor, pointing toes straight ahead, and transferring weight from heel along outer border of foot to toes.

chapter 12

Plexuses, and Spinal Nerve and Muscle Charts

NERVE COMPRESSION AND TENSION

Peripheral nerves are subject to trauma in many areas of the body and from a wide variety of causes. Some trauma may be *invasive* in nature and may be accidental such as lacerations, piercing wounds, injections of medications, or nerves cut or injured during surgery. Some invasive trauma may be caused by necessary procedures such as a nerve resection or rhizotomy.

Numerous neurological problems arise from *noninvasive* trauma that can cause compression or tension (traction) on a nerve. The trauma may be sudden or gradual, the latter occurring as a result of maintained positions or repetitive movements. Involvement may vary from being widespread throughout an extremity to being localized to a single nerve branch; it may be transitory or result in permanent deficits.

Trauma may result from an *external force causing compression* on a nerve. Examples include the following:

Radial, median, or ulnar nerve (or a combination of these) as in "Saturday night palsy" from an arm hanging over the back of bench or chair.
Radial or median nerve (or both) from crutch paralysis.
Radial, median, and ulnar nerves from a tourniquet. (See chart, *Case #1.*)
Median nerve from various sleeping positions, e.g., supine, arm overhead; side-lying on the arm in adduction (47).
Ulnar nerve from trauma to elbow.
Ulnar or median nerve from sudden or repeated trauma to hypothenar or thenar eminence.
Anterior interosseus nerve from (forearm) armband sling (80).
Brachial plexus from strap over shoulder.
Peroneal nerve by a cast, adhesive strapping, or garter producing pressure over the head of the fibula; or prolonged sitting with legs crossed and one knee resting on the other.

A transitory external compressive force is exemplified by a bump on the elbow, hitting the "funny bone" (so-named because it is the distal end of the humerus). The bruise hurts and causes tingling into the ring and little finger but the symptoms do not last long.

Trauma by an *external force causing tension* on nerves can occur to the brachial plexus, for example, as a result of an accident or a manipulation that puts excessive traction on the plexus. The long thoracic nerve is susceptible to stretch from carrying a heavy bag with strap over the shoulder.

Internal compression or tension affecting nerves usually occurs in areas of the body where the nerve is vulnerable because of close association with firm skeletal structures. Under ordinary conditions, a groove or a tunnel may be a protection, but if there is injury or inflammation with swelling and scar tissue, then the confined area becomes a source of entrapment. *Internal compression* is exemplified by pressure on:

Spinal nerve root from calcium deposits in the foramen.
Suprascapular nerve as it passes under the ligament and through the scapular notch (50, 81–83).
Brachial plexus from a cervical rib. (See posture in relation to cervical rib, p. 346.)
Brachial plexus from coracoid process and tight Pectoralis minor (see p. 343) (15, 47).
Axillary nerve in the quadrilateral space (see p. 344) (50, 51).
Median nerve as in carpal tunnel syndrome.
Nerve to (usually 4th) toe as in Morton's neuroma.

Internal tension on a nerve is exemplified by:

Suprascapular nerve as it passes through the scapular notch being subject to stretch with displacement of shoulder and scapula (84).
Peroneal nerve, secondary to spasm in the Tensor fasciae latae with resultant traction on the Iliotibial band to its insertion below the head of the fibula (see p. 361).
Peroneal nerve, secondary to traction on the leg by inversion of the foot (47, 83).

In some instances, there may be a combination of factors. Consider the case of a woman who awoke in the middle of the night with the sensation that she did not have a right arm. The whole arm had gone "dead." With her left arm she tried to find the arm, starting down at the right side of the body and finally found it extended overhead. She put the arm down, rubbed it briskly, and it was back to normal in a minute or two.

With the arm overhead, and the entire arm affected, there may have been both compression and tension on trunks of the brachial plexus and on the blood vessels from angulation under the coracoid process and the Pectoralis minor. In view of the quick response from stimulating the circulation by massaging the arm, the problem may have been primarily circulatory.

NERVE IMPINGEMENT

In this text, the word "impingement" is being used with reference to nerve irritation associated with muscles.

In the 1930's, there was great reluctance to speak about the possibility that, in addition to bone and other firm structures, muscles might play a role in causing irritation to nerves. In an article by Albert H. Freiberg, published in 1934, regarding the Piriformis muscle, he stated, "That pressure of a muscle belly upon the trunk of the sciatic nerve can be productive of pain and tenderness must be looked upon as unproved at present" (78). The author was cautious and almost apologetic about suggesting that the muscle could play that kind of a role.

During that same era, one of the original authors of *Muscles, Testing and Function*, Henry O. Kendall, rather courageously offered such explanations for several clinical entities. Most instances were related to muscles that were pierced by a peripheral nerve, and in which movement and alteration of muscle length were factors in causing a friction type of irritation to the nerve. Symptoms of pain or discomfort could be elicited by having the muscle actively contract, by stretching it, or by repetitive movements.

The authors are cognizant of the fact that explaining peripheral nerve pain on the basis of pressure or friction by muscles is still a controversial issue with respect to certain syndromes, notably the Piriformis (50, 85). However, the concept is well recognized with respect to nerve involvement with numerous muscles:

> Supinator with radial nerve (50, 86).
> Pronator with median nerve (50, 84, 86).
> Flexor carpi ulnaris with ulnar nerve (47).
> Lateral head of Triceps with radial nerve (50, 86).
> Trapezius with greater occipital nerve (47).
> Scalenus medius with C5 and C6 root of the plexus, and long thoracic nerve (47).
> Coracobrachialis with musculocutaneous (50, 84).

Under normal conditions and through normal range of motion, it may be presumed that a muscle will not cause irritation to a nerve that lies in close proximity to it or pierces it. However, a muscle that is drawn taut becomes firm and has the potential for exerting a compressive or friction force. A muscle that has developed adaptive shortness moves through less range and becomes taut before reaching normal length; a stretched muscle moves through more than normal range before becoming taut. A taut muscle, especially a weight-bearing muscle, can cause friction on a nerve during repetitive movements.

In mild cases, the symptoms may be discomfort and dull ache rather than sharp pain when the muscles contract or are elongated. Sharp pain may be elicited on vigorous movements, but it tends to be intermittent because the subject finds ways to avoid the painful movements.

Recognizing this phenomenon in early stages can increase the likelihood of finding means to counteract or prevent the more painful or disabling problems that develop later. Physical therapists who deal with stretching and strengthening exercises have the opportunity to observe early signs of impingement among their patients.

The axillary nerve emerges through the quadrilateral space that is bounded by the Teres major, Teres minor, the long head of the Triceps, and the humerus. When stretching a tight Teres major, a patient may complain of a shooting pain in the area of cutaneous sensory distribution of the axillary nerve. The assumption is that the axillary nerve is being compressed or stretched against the tight Teres major. The pain that results from direct irritation to the nerve is in contrast to the discomfort that is often associated with the usual stretching of tight muscles. (See cutaneous nerve distribution, pp. 380–381, and Teres syndrome, p. 344.)

The femoral nerve pierces the Psoas major muscle. During assisted stretching exercises, a patient with tight Iliopsoas muscles may complain of pain along the anteromedial aspect of the leg in the area of cutaneous sensory distribution of the saphenous nerve. (See cutaneous nerve distribution, p. 382.)

The greater occipital nerve pierces the Trapezius muscle and fascia. Movements of head and neck in the direction of contracting or stretching the Trapezius may elicit pain in the area of the back of the head and cervical region. (See occipital headache, p. 341.)

NERVES TO MUSCLES: MOTOR AND SENSORY

Following is a brief description of the relationship of the nerves and muscles. The material is chiefly from *Gray's Anatomy* (13).

Axillary. Leaves the axilla through the space bounded by the surgical neck of the humerus, Teres major, Teres minor, and long head of the Triceps, and supplies the Deltoid and Teres minor.

Femoral. Pierces the Psoas major at the distal part of the lateral border. It supplies the Iliacus, Pectineus, Sartorius, and Quadriceps. The largest and longest branch of the femoral nerve is the *saphenous* nerve which supplies the skin over the medial side of the leg.

Genitofemoral. Passes through the Psoas muscle. The *femoral* branch of the Genitofemoral supplies the skin over the proximal part of the anterior surface of the thigh.

Greater Occipital. Crosses obliquely between the Obliquus inferior and the Semispinalis capitis, piercing the latter and the Trapezius near the attachment to the Occipital bone. It supplies the back of the head, and scalp over top of head. It communicates with the *smaller occipital* sensory nerve, which supplies the skin over the side of the head behind the ear.

Iliohypogastric. Penetrates the posterior part of the Transversus abdominis near crest of ilium. The *lateral cutaneous* branch pierces the Internal and External oblique just above the iliac crest and supplies the skin over part of the gluteal region. The *anterior cutaneous* branch pierces the Internal oblique and passes through an opening in the aponeurosis of the External, and supplies the skin over the hypogastric region.

Median. Passes between two heads of the Pronator teres, and under the flexor retinaculum. It is distributed to the forearm and hand. See *Spinal Nerve and Muscle Chart*, p. 389 for list of muscles innervated.

Musculocutaneous. Pierces the Coracobrachialis and supplies this muscle as well as the Biceps and Brachialis.

Obturator. (From L2, 3, 4.) The *posterior* branch pierces the anterior part of the External oblique and divides into two branches. Through its muscular branch, it supplies the Obturator externus, Adductor magnus and, sometimes, the Adductor brevis; and through its *articular* branch, it is distributed to the synovial membrane of the knee joint.

Peroneal. Passes between the Biceps femoris and the lateral head of the Gastrocnemius to the head of the fibula, and deep to the Peroneus longus. (See illustration, p. 361.) It supplies the ankle dorsiflexors and everters. (See p. 393.)

Radial. The *Posterior interosseus* branch divides into a muscular and an articular branch. The muscular branch supplies the Extensor carpi radialis brevis and the Supinator before passing between the superficial and deep layers of the Supinator muscle. After passing through the Supinator, it supplies the remaining muscles which are innervated by the radial nerve. (See p. 389.)

Sciatic. (From L4, 5 and S1, 2, 3.) In most instances, the sciatic nerve lies beneath the Piriformis muscle and crosses the Obturator internus, Gemelli, and Quadratus femoris. (See illustration, p. 365.) Variations exist, however, in which the muscle is split and one (usually the peroneal) or both parts of the sciatic nerve pass through the muscle belly. (See *Spinal Nerve and Muscle Chart*, p. 393 for muscles supplied by the Sciatic nerve.)

Some muscles are supplied by nerves that are purely motor. In some instances, there may be a sensory branch that goes to a joint or joints but not to the muscle.

NERVES TO MUSCLES: MOTOR ONLY

For years, the senior author has been gathering information about which muscles are supplied by purely motor nerves. Some typewritten pages listing the peripheral nerves and whether they were sensory, motor, or both date back to the late thirties, but had no reference source noted; a 1932 Dorland's Medical Dictionary had a table of nerves that included the information; an article on Serratus anterior paralysis stated, "The long thoracic nerve or external respiratory nerve of Bell is almost unique in that it arises directly from the spinal nerve roots, carries no known sensory fibers, and goes to a single muscle of which it is the sole innervation of consequence" (87). Later, a table was found in Taber's dictionary (88). The 1988 edition of Dorland's dictionary did not have the tables that were included in an earlier edition, but the information was found in conjunction with the description of each nerve (89). Finally, scattered bits of information have come from some of the many books and articles on nerve injuries, compression, and entrapments (80–84, 90, 91).

Surprisingly, as the information has been compiled, a very interesting pattern has developed. The accompanying chart shows that the nerves from the roots, trunks, and cords of the brachial plexus to muscles are motor nerves. In addition, the anterior and posterior interosseus nerves, which are branches of the median and radial nerves, respectively, are purely motor to the muscles they supply (84, 88, 90, 91). Several of the nerves have sensory branches to joints. Of the suprascapular nerve, Hadley et al state, ". . . and gives off motor branches to that muscle and sensory branches to the shoulder and acromioclavicular joints" (81).

The following statements indicate the clinical significance of muscles being supplied by purely motor nerves. With reference to the suprascapular nerve, Dawson et al state, "Since there is no cutaneous territory for this nerve, there are no characteristic sensory symptoms or findings in any lesion of this nerve" (50).

Conway et al. state: ". . . entrapment of the posterior interosseous nerve is purely motor and has no associated sensory loss or dysesthetic pain" (83).

The lack of sensory fibers provides the explanation for lack of sensory symptoms in the muscles that are supplied by nerves that are only motor. (See discussion and examples, pp. 339–340.)

Nerves to Muscles: Motor and Sensory or Motor

SOURCE		SPINAL SEGMENT	NERVE	MOTOR/SENSORY TO MUSCLE	MUSCLE
Cervical Plexus	Cervical Nerves	C2, 3, 4	Spinal accessory	Motor	Sternocleidomastoid, Trapezius
Brachial Plexus	Plexus Roots	C4, 5	Dorsal scapular	Motor	Levator, Rhomboids
		C5, 6, 7	Long thoracic	Motor	Serratus anterior
	Superior Trunk	C5, 6	Subclavian	Motor[a]	Subclavius
		C5, 6	Suprascapular	Motor[b]	Supraspinatus, Infraspinatus
	Posterior Cord	C5, 6	Subscapular, upper and lower	Motor	Subscapularis, Teres major
	Posterior Cord	C6, 7, 8	Thoracodorsal	Motor	Latissimus dorsi
	Lateral Cord	C5, 6, 7	Lateral pectoral	Motor[b]	Pectoralis minor
	Medial Cord	C7, 8, T1	Medial pectoral	Motor	Pectoralis major, Pectoralis minor
Terminal Branches		C5, 6	Axillary	Motor and sensory	Deltoid, Teres minor
		C5, 6, 7	Musculocutaneous	Motor and sensory	Coracobrachialis, Biceps, Brachialis
		C5, 6, 7, 8, T1	Radial	Motor and sensory	17 muscles
		C6, 7, 8, T1	Median	Motor and sensory	12 muscles
		C8, T1	Ulnar	Motor and sensory	18 muscles
Branch of Radial Nerve		C5, 6, 7, T1	Interosseus, posterior	Motor[c]	9 muscles
Branch of Median Nerve		C7, 8, T1	Interosseus, anterior	Motor[c]	Pronator quadratus, Flexor pollicis longus, Profundus, 1 and 2
Lumbar Plexus	Ventral Primary Ramus	T12, L1	Iliohypogastric	Motor and sensory	Internal oblique, Transversus abdominis
		L1, 2, 3, 4	Lumbar plexus	Motor and sensory	Quadratus lumborum, Psoas major, Psoas minor
	Posterior Division	L2, 3, 4	Femoral	Motor and sensory	Iliacus, Pectineus, Sartorius, Quadriceps
	Anterior Division	L2, 3, 4	Obturator	Motor and sensory	Hip adductors
Lumbosacral Plexus	Posterior Division	L4, 5, S1	Gluteal, superior	Motor[d]	Gluteus medius, Gluteus minimus, Tensor fasciae latae
	Posterior Division	L5, S1, 2	Gluteal, inferior	Motor	Gluteus maximus
	Posterior Division	L4, 5, S1, 2	Peroneal	Motor and sensory	Short head of Biceps, Tibialis anterior, Toe extensors, Peroneals
	Anterior Division	L4, 5, S1, 2, 3	Tibial	Motor and sensory	Semimembranosus, Semitendinosus, Long head of Biceps; 19 ankle and foot muscles
Sacral Plexus	Ventral Primary Ramus	L4, 5, S1, 2, 3	Sacral plexus	Motor and sensory	Piriformis, Gemelli superior and inferior, Obturator internus, Quadratus femoris

[a]Sensory to sternoclavicular joint.
[b]Sensory to acromioclavicular joint and shoulder joint.
[c]Sensory to wrist and intercarpal joints.
[d]Sensory to hip joint.

Cutaneous Nerves of the Upper Limb: Anterior View

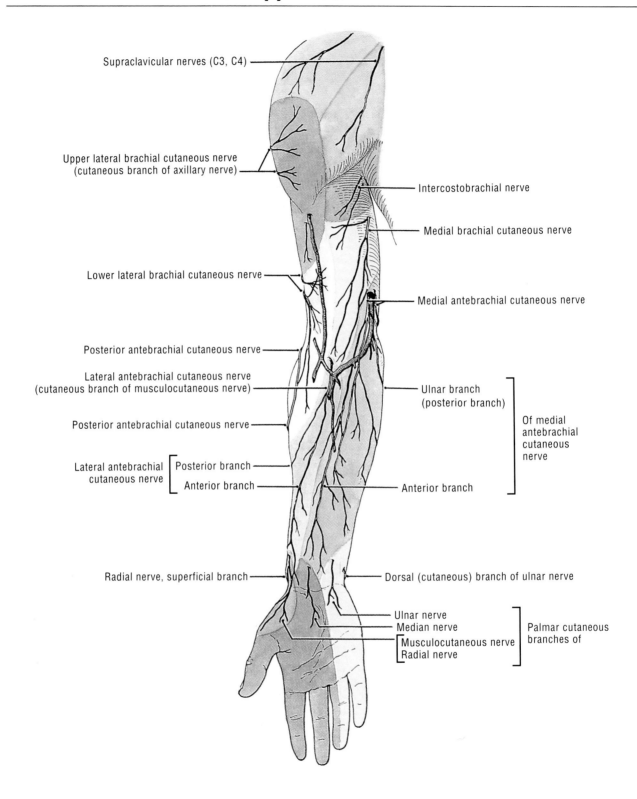

Supraclavicular nerves (C3, C4)

Upper lateral brachial cutaneous nerve (cutaneous branch of axillary nerve)

Lower lateral brachial cutaneous nerve

Posterior antebrachial cutaneous nerve

Lateral antebrachial cutaneous nerve (cutaneous branch of musculocutaneous nerve)

Posterior antebrachial cutaneous nerve

Lateral antebrachial cutaneous nerve
Posterior branch
Anterior branch

Radial nerve, superficial branch

Intercostobrachial nerve

Medial brachial cutaneous nerve

Medial antebrachial cutaneous nerve

Ulnar branch (posterior branch)

Of medial antebrachial cutaneous nerve

Anterior branch

Dorsal (cutaneous) branch of ulnar nerve

Ulnar nerve
Median nerve
Musculocutaneous nerve
Radial nerve

Palmar cutaneous branches of

Of the five terminal branches of the brachial plexus—musculocutaneous, median, ulnar, radial, and axillary nerves—the first four contribute cutaneous branches to the hand.

The posterior cord of the plexus is represented by five cutaneous nerves. One of these, the upper lateral brachial cutaneous nerve, is a branch of the axillary nerve.

From Grant's Atlas of Anatomy (92) with permission.

Cutaneous Nerves of the Upper Limb: Posterior View

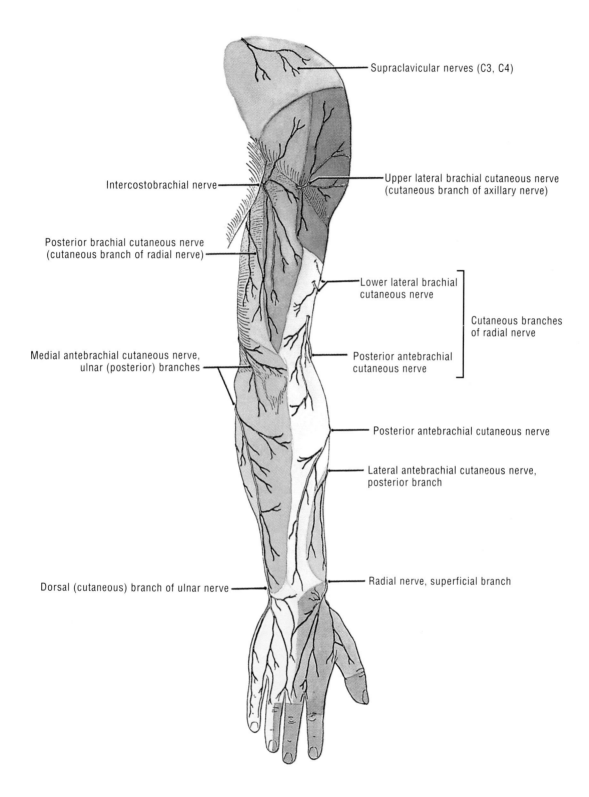

Supraclavicular nerves (C3, C4)

Upper lateral brachial cutaneous nerve
(cutaneous branch of axillary nerve)

Intercostobrachial nerve

Posterior brachial cutaneous nerve
(cutaneous branch of radial nerve)

Lower lateral brachial
cutaneous nerve

Cutaneous branches
of radial nerve

Medial antebrachial cutaneous nerve,
ulnar (posterior) branches

Posterior antebrachial
cutaneous nerve

Posterior antebrachial cutaneous nerve

Lateral antebrachial cutaneous nerve,
posterior branch

Dorsal (cutaneous) branch of ulnar nerve

Radial nerve, superficial branch

The other branches of the posterior cord are: the posterior brachial cutaneous nerve, the lower lateral brachial cutaneous nerve, the posterior antebrachial cutaneous nerve, and the superficial branch of the radial nerve.

From Grant's Atlas of Anatomy (92) with permission.

Cutaneous Nerves of the Lower Limb

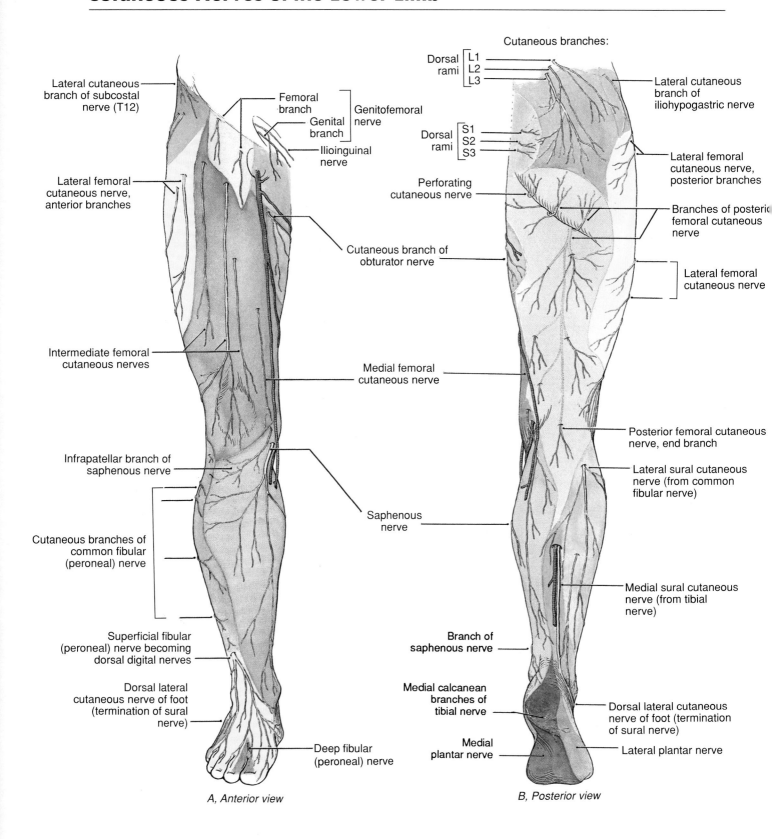

Lateral cutaneous branch of subcostal nerve (T12)

Lateral femoral cutaneous nerve, anterior branches

Intermediate femoral cutaneous nerves

Infrapatellar branch of saphenous nerve

Cutaneous branches of common fibular (peroneal) nerve

Superficial fibular (peroneal) nerve becoming dorsal digital nerves

Dorsal lateral cutaneous nerve of foot (termination of sural nerve)

Femoral branch

Genital branch

Genitofemoral nerve

Ilioinguinal nerve

Cutaneous branch of obturator nerve

Medial femoral cutaneous nerve

Saphenous nerve

Deep fibular (peroneal) nerve

A, Anterior view

Cutaneous branches:

Dorsal rami [L1, L2, L3]

Dorsal rami [S1, S2, S3]

Perforating cutaneous nerve

Lateral cutaneous branch of iliohypogastric nerve

Lateral femoral cutaneous nerve, posterior branches

Branches of posterior femoral cutaneous nerve

Lateral femoral cutaneous nerve

Posterior femoral cutaneous nerve, end branch

Lateral sural cutaneous nerve (from common fibular nerve)

Medial sural cutaneous nerve (from tibial nerve)

Branch of saphenous nerve

Medial calcanean branches of tibial nerve

Medial plantar nerve

Dorsal lateral cutaneous nerve of foot (termination of sural nerve)

Lateral plantar nerve

B, Posterior view

Note in B, *Sural* is Latin for the calf. The medial sural cutaneous nerve is here joined just proximal

to the ankle by a communicating branch (not labeled) of the lateral sural cutaneous nerve to form the sural nerve. The level of the junction is variable, here being very low.

From Grant's Atlas of Anatomy (92) with permission.

The word "plexus" comes from the Latin word that means a braid. A nerve plexus results from the dividing, reuniting, and intertwining of nerves into a complex network. When describing the origins, components, and terminal branches of a plexus, the words "nerves," "roots," and "cord" are used with dual meanings. There are spinal nerves and peripheral nerves, roots of the spinal nerves and roots of the plexus, the spinal cord and cords of the plexus. To avoid confusion, appropriate modifying words are used in the descriptions below.

The *spinal cord* lies within the vertebral column extending from the first cervical vertebra to the level of the second lumbar vertebra. Each of the 31 pairs of *spinal nerves* arises from the spinal cord by two *spinal nerve roots*. The *ventral root* composed of motor fibers, and the *dorsal root* composed of sensory fibers, unite at the intervertebral foramen to form the spinal nerve. (See p. 384 at top.) A *spinal segment* is the part of the spinal cord that gives rise to each pair of spinal nerves. Each spinal nerve contains motor and sensory fibers from a single spinal segment.

Shortly after the spinal nerve exits through the foramen, it divides into a *dorsal primary ramus* and a *ventral primary ramus*. The dorsal rami are directed posteriorly, and the sensory and motor fibers innervate the skin and extensor muscles of the neck and trunk. The ventral rami, except those in the thoracic region, contain the nerve fibers that become part of the plexuses. (Four plexuses are described and illustrated on the following pages.) Emerging from the plexuses at various levels or as terminal branches are the *peripheral nerves*. As a result of the interchange of fibers within the plexus, peripheral nerves contain fibers from at least two, and, in some instances, as many as five, spinal segments.

The *cervical plexus* is formed by the ventral primary rami of spinal nerves C1 through C4 with a small contribution from C5. Peripheral nerves arising from it innervate most of the anterior and lateral muscles of the neck, and supply sensory fibers to part of the head and much of the neck.

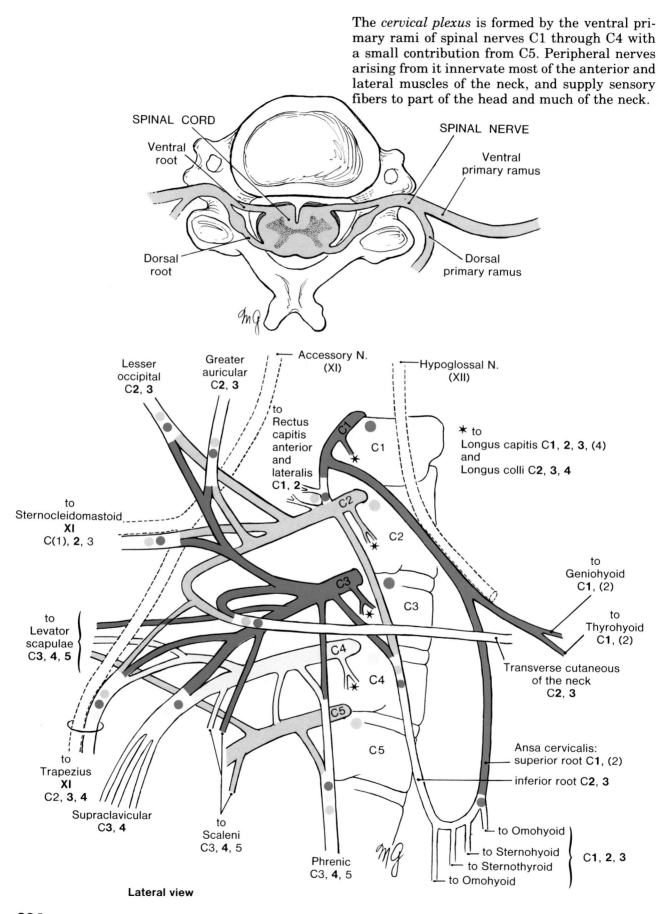

Lateral view

The *brachial plexus* arises just lateral to the Scalenus anterior muscle. The ventral rami of C5, 6, 7, and 8, and the greater part of T1, plus a communicating loop from C4 to C5 and one from T2 (sensory) to T1 form, successively, the roots, trunks, divisions, cords, and branches of the plexus.

Ventral rami containing C5 and C6 fibers unite to form the *superior* (upper) *trunk*, C7 fibers form the *middle trunk*, and C8 and T1 fibers unite to form the *inferior* (lower) *trunk*. Next the trunks separate into *anterior* and *posterior divisions*. The anterior divisions from the superior and middle trunks, composed of C5, 6, and 7 fibers, unite to form the *lateral cord*; the anterior division from the inferior trunk, composed of C8 and T1 fibers, forms the *medial cord*; the posterior divisions from all three trunks, composed of fibers from C5 through C8 (but not T1), unite to form the *posterior cord*.

The cords then divide and reunite into *branches* that become *peripheral nerves*. The posterior cord branches into the axillary and radial nerves. The medial cord, after receiving a branch from the lateral cord, terminates as the ulnar nerve. One branch of the lateral cord becomes the musculocutaneous nerve; the other branch unites with one from the medial cord to form the median nerve. Other peripheral nerves exit directly from various components of the plexus and some directly from the ventral rami. (See left column and top of *Spinal Nerve and Muscle Chart*, p. 389.)

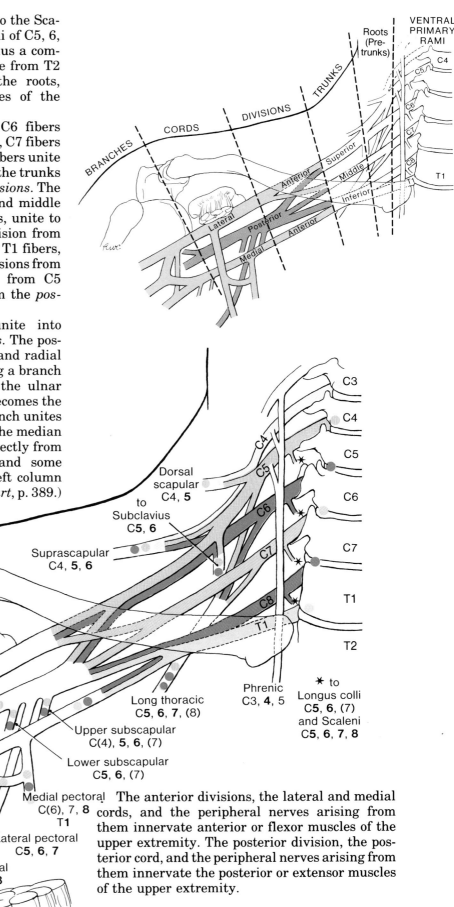

The anterior divisions, the lateral and medial cords, and the peripheral nerves arising from them innervate anterior or flexor muscles of the upper extremity. The posterior division, the posterior cord, and the peripheral nerves arising from them innervate the posterior or extensor muscles of the upper extremity.

385

The *lumbar plexus* is formed by the ventral primary rami of L1, 2, 3, and a part of L4 with, frequently, a small contribution from T12. Within the substance of the Psoas major muscle, the rami branch into anterior and posterior divisions. Peripheral nerves from the anterior divisions innervate adductor muscles on the medial side of the thigh; those from the posterior divisions innervate hip flexors and knee extensors on the anterior aspect of the thigh.

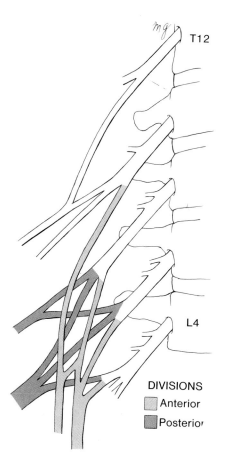

T12

L4

DIVISIONS
- Anterior
- Posterior

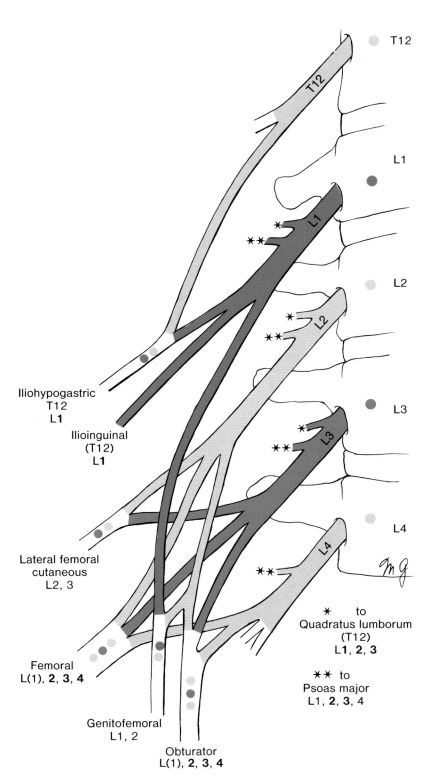

T12

L1

L2

L3

L4

Iliohypogastric
T12
L1

Ilioinguinal
(T12)
L1

Lateral femoral
cutaneous
L2, 3

Femoral
L(1), **2, 3, 4**

Genitofemoral
L1, 2

Obturator
L(1), **2, 3, 4**

✱ to
Quadratus lumborum
(T12)
L1, 2, 3

✱✱ to
Psoas major
L1, **2, 3, 4**

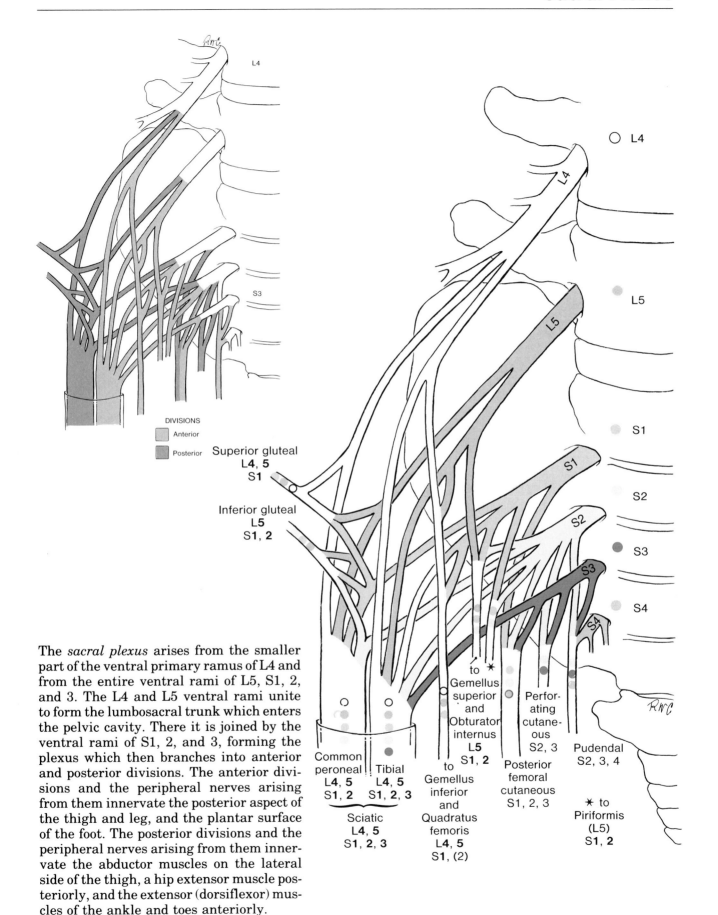

DIVISIONS

Anterior

Posterior

Superior gluteal
L4, 5
S1

Inferior gluteal
L5
S1, 2

to
Gemellus
superior
and
Obturator
internus
L5
S1, 2

Common
peroneal
L4, 5
S1, 2

Tibial
L4, 5
S1, 2, 3

to
Gemellus
inferior
and
Quadratus
femoris
L4, 5
S1, (2)

Sciatic
L4, 5
S1, 2, 3

Perfor-
ating
cutane-
ous
S2, 3

Posterior
femoral
cutaneous
S1, 2, 3

Pudendal
S2, 3, 4

✳ to
Piriformis
(**L5**)
S1, 2

L4

L5

S1

S2

S3

S4

The *sacral plexus* arises from the smaller part of the ventral primary ramus of L4 and from the entire ventral rami of L5, S1, 2, and 3. The L4 and L5 ventral rami unite to form the lumbosacral trunk which enters the pelvic cavity. There it is joined by the ventral rami of S1, 2, and 3, forming the plexus which then branches into anterior and posterior divisions. The anterior divisions and the peripheral nerves arising from them innervate the posterior aspect of the thigh and leg, and the plantar surface of the foot. The posterior divisions and the peripheral nerves arising from them innervate the abductor muscles on the lateral side of the thigh, a hip extensor muscle posteriorly, and the extensor (dorsiflexor) muscles of the ankle and toes anteriorly.

Spinal Nerve and Muscle Charts

The recording of test results is an important part of muscle examinations. Records are important from the standpoint of diagnosis, treatment, and prognosis. An examination performed without recording the details can be of value at the moment, but one has an obligation to the patient, to the institution if one is involved, and to oneself to record the findings.

Charts used for recording should permit complete tabulation of test results, and the arrangement of the information should facilitate interpretation.

SPINAL NERVE AND MUSCLE CHARTS

There are two charts in this category, one for the neck, Diaphragm, and upper extremity (p. 389), the other for the trunk and lower extremity (p. 393). Each chart has an accompanying anatomical drawing of the spinal nerves and motor points (pp. 391 and 392). These charts have been designed especially for use as an aid in differential diagnosis of lesions of the spinal nerves. The motor involvement as determined by manual muscle tests can aid in determining whether there is a lesion of the nerve at root, plexus, or peripheral level. The chart may be useful, also, in determining the level of a spinal cord lesion.

In the upper and lower extremity charts the names of the muscles appear in the left column and are grouped, as indicated by heavy black lines, according to their innervations listed to the left of the muscle names. The space between the column of muscle names and the nerves is used for recording the grade of muscle strength.

The Sternocleidomastoid and the Trapezius muscles are listed on the *Spinal Nerve and Muscle Chart*, p. 389, and the *Cranial Nerve and Muscle Chart*, p. 310. While these muscles receive their motor innervation mainly from the spinal portion of the 11th cranial nerve (accessory), additional spinal nerve branches are distributed to them: C2, C3 to the Sternocleidomastoid and C2, C3, C4 to the Trapezius. It has not been determined, in man, whether these cervical spinal nerve branches consist of motor and sensory or only sensory fibers. Clinical findings in cases of pure accessory nerve lesions have led neurologists to assume that these spinal nerve fibers are chiefly concerned in the innervation of the caudal part of the Trapezius, its cranial and middle parts as well as the Sternocleidomastoid being supplied predominantly by the accessory nerve (93). Some authors report that these cervical nerves supply chiefly the upper part of the Trapezius. In still other individuals it would appear that these nerve fibers do not contribute any motor fibers to the Trapezius, the motor innervation of the entire muscle being dependent on the spinal portion of the accessory nerve. Apparently, considerable individual variations exist in the innervation of the Trapezius (94).

Peripheral Nerve Section. Peripheral nerves and their segmental origins are listed across the top of the center of the chart and follow the order of proximal-distal branching insofar as possible. For the peripheral nerves that arise from cords of the brachial plexus, the appropriate cord is indicated. The key at the top of the charts explains the abbreviations used.

Below this section, in the body of the chart, the dots indicate the peripheral nerve supply to each muscle. (See p. 410 for sources of material for this section.)

Spinal Segment Section. In this section, a number denotes the spinal segment origin of nerve fibers innervating each of the muscles listed in the left column. (See pp. 406–409 for sources of material for this section.)

Sensory Section. On the right side of the charts are diagrams showing the dermatomes and the distribution of cutaneous nerves for the upper extremity on the one chart, and for the trunk and lower extremity on the other. The dermatome illustrations are redrawn from Keegan and Garrett on the extremity charts (95), and from Gray on the cranial chart (13). The cutaneous nerve illustrations are redrawn from Gray (for cranial chart, see p. 310).

It is possible to use the illustrations for charting areas of sensory involvement by shading or using colored pencil to outline the areas of the involvement for any given patient. Only drawings of the right extremity are used on the extremity charts but labeling can indicate, when necessary, that the recorded information pertains to the left side.

SPINAL NERVE AND MUSCLE CHART
NECK, DIAPHRAGM AND UPPER EXTREMITY

Name _____   Date _____

KEY

D.	= Dorsal Prim. Ramus
V.	= Vent. Prim. Ramus
P.R.	= Plexus Root
S.T.	= Superior Trunk
P.	= Posterior Cord
L.	= Lateral Cord
M.	= Medial Cord

Peripheral nerve column legend (order left→right): D. Cervical (1–8); V. Cervical (1–8); V. Cervical (1–4); Phrenic (3,4,5); Long Thor. P.R. (5,6,7,(8)); Dor. Scap P.R. (4,5); N. to Subcl. S.T. (5,6); Suprascap S.T. (4,5,6); U. Subscap P. ((4),5,6,(7)); Thoracodor P. ((5),6,7,8); L. Subscap P. (5,6,(7)); Lat. Pect. L. (5,6,7); Med. Pect. M. ((6),7,8); Axillary P. (5,6); Musculocu. P. ((4),5,6,7); Radial P. (5,6,7,8); Median L.M. (5,6,7,8); Ulnar M. (7,8)

Group	Muscle	Nerve	C1	C2	C3	C4	C5	C6	C7	C8	T1
Cervical nerves	HEAD & NECK EXTENSORS	D. Cervical	1	2	3	4	5	6	7	8	1
	INFRAHYOID MUSCLES	V. Cervical	1	2	3						
	RECTUS CAP ANT. & LAT.	V. Cervical	1	2							
	LONGUS CAPITIS	V. Cervical	1	2	3	(4)					
	LONGUS COLLI	V. Cervical		2	3	4	5	6	(7)		
	LEVATOR SCAPULAE	V. Cervical / Dor. Scap			3	4	5				
	SCALENI (A. M. P.)	V. Cervical			3	4	5	6	7	8	
	STERNOCLEIDOMASTOID	V. Cervical	(1)	2	3						
	TRAPEZIUS (U. M. L.)	V. Cervical		2	3	4					
	DIAPHRAGM	Phrenic			3	4	5				
Brachial Plexus — Root	SERRATUS ANTERIOR	Long Thor.					5	6	7	8	
	RHOMBOIDS MAJ & MIN	Dor. Scap				4	5				
Trunk	SUBCLAVIUS	N. to Subcl.					5	6			
	SUPRASPINATUS	Suprascap				4	5	6			
	INFRASPINATUS	Suprascap				(4)	5	6			
P Cord	SUBSCAPULARIS	U. Subscap / L. Subscap					5	6	7		
	LATISSIMUS DORSI	Thoracodor						6	7	8	
	TERES MAJOR	L. Subscap					5	6	7		
M&L	PECTORALIS MAJ (UPPER)	Lat. Pect.					5	6	7		
	PECTORALIS MAJ (LOWER)	Lat. Pect. / Med. Pect.						6	7	8	1
	PECTORALIS MINOR	Med. Pect.						(6)	7	8	1
Axil.	TERES MINOR	Axillary					5	6			
	DELTOID	Axillary					5	6			
Musculo-cutan	CORACOBRACHIALIS	Musculocu.						6	7		
	BICEPS	Musculocu.					5	6			
	BRACHIALIS	Musculocu.					5	6			
Radial	TRICEPS	Radial						6	7	8	1
	ANCONEUS	Radial							7	8	
Lat. M	BRACHIALIS (SMALL PART)	Radial					5	6			
	BRACHIORADIALIS	Radial					5	6			
	EXT CARPI RAD L	Radial					5	6	7	8	
	EXT CARPI RAD B	Radial						6	7	(8)	
	SUPINATOR	Radial					5	6	(7)		
Post Inter	EXT DIGITORUM	Radial						6	7	8	
	EXT DIGITI MINIMI	Radial						6	7	8	
	EXT CARPI ULNARIS	Radial						6	7	8	
	ABD POLLICIS LONGUS	Radial						6	7	8	
	EXT POLLICIS BREVIS	Radial						6	7	8	
	EXT POLLICIS LONGUS	Radial						6	7	8	
	EXT INDICIS	Radial						6	7	8	
Median	PRONATOR TERES	Median						6	7		
	FLEX CARPI RADIALIS	Median						6	7	8	
	PALMARIS LONGUS	Median						(6)	7	8	1
	FLEX DIGIT SUPERFICIALIS	Median							7	8	1
	FLEX DIGIT PROF I & II	Median							7	8	1
A Inter	FLEX POLLICIS LONGUS	Median						(6)	7	8	1
	PRONATOR QUADRATUS	Median							7	8	1
	ABD POLLICIS BREVIS	Median						6	7	8	1
	OPPONENS POLLICIS	Median						6	7	8	1
	FLEX POLL BREV (SUP. H)	Median						6	7	8	1
	LUMBRICALES I & II	Median						(6)	7	8	1
Ulnar	FLEX CARPI ULNARIS	Ulnar							7	8	1
	FLEX DIGIT. PROF. III & IV	Ulnar							7	8	1
	PALMARIS BREVIS	Ulnar							(7)	8	1
	ABD DIGITI MINIMI	Ulnar							(7)	8	1
	OPPONENS DIGITI MINIMI	Ulnar							(7)	8	1
	FLEX DIGITI MINIMI	Ulnar							(7)	8	1
	PALMAR INTEROSSEI	Ulnar								8	1
	DORSAL INTEROSSEI	Ulnar								8	1
	LUMBRICALES III & IV	Ulnar							(7)	8	1
	ADDUCTOR POLLICIS	Ulnar								8	1
	FLEX POLL BREV. (DEEP H.)	Ulnar								8	1

SENSORY

Dermatomes redrawn from Keegan and Garrett Anat Rec 102. 409. 437. 1948
Cutaneous Distribution of peripheral nerves redrawn from *Gray's Anatomy of the Human Body*. 28th ed

SPINAL NERVE AND MOTOR POINT CHARTS

Drawings which show the course of the nerves from spinal cord to motor points appear on pp. 391 and 392. These illustrations facilitate interpretation of the muscle test findings as recorded on the *Spinal Nerve and Muscle Chart*, and aid in determining the site or level of a lesion. Every effort has been made to preserve anatomical accuracy in showing the course of the nerves in relation to the muscles. Cross-section illustrations were used to check the position of the nerves at various levels (96). For the most part, the motor point location, which is the site where a nerve enters the muscle it innervates, was based on the work of Brash (97).

Anterior divisions of the plexuses and their branches are shown in yellow; posterior divisions and their branches, in green. The motor points are designated as black dots.

USE OF CHARTS IN DIFFERENTIAL DIAGNOSIS

Muscle strength grades are recorded in the column to the left of the muscle names. The grades may be in numeral or letter symbols. (See p. 188.)

For the cases that follow, except *Case #6*, only a brief interpretation of the manual muscle test is presented. No significance need be attached to the fact that letter grades were used in some instances and numerals in others. Either system may be used and grades can be translated as indicated on the *Key to Grading Symbols*, p. 188.

After the grades have been recorded, the nerve involvement is plotted, when applicable, by circling the dot under peripheral supply and the number(s) under spinal segment distribution that corresponds with each involved muscle.

The involvement of peripheral nerves and/or parts of the plexus is ascertained from the encircled dots by following the vertical lines upward to the top of the chart, or the horizontal lines to the left margin. (See p. 389.) When there is evidence of involvement at spinal segment level, the level of lesion may be indicated by a heavy black line drawn vertically to separate the involved from the uninvolved spinal segments. (See p. 398.)

As a rule, muscles graded good (8) and above may be considered as not being involved from a neurological standpoint. This degree of weakness may be the result of such factors as inactivity, stretch weakness, or lack of fixation by other muscles. It should be borne in mind, however, that a grade of good might indicate a deficit of a spinal segment that minimally innervates the muscle.

Weakness with grades of fair or less may occur as a result of inactivity, disuse atrophy, immobilization, or from neurological problems. Faulty posture of the upper back and shoulders, may cause weakness of the middle and lower Trapezius. It is not uncommon to find bilateral weakness of these muscles with grades as low as fair −. It is unlikely that there is a neurological problem with involvement of the spinal accessory nerve in cases of isolated weakness of these muscles unless there is involvement of the upper Trapezius also.

The use of the *Spinal Nerve and Muscle Charts* is illustrated by the case studies on pages 394–403.

For the cases that follow, except *Case #6*, only a brief interpretation of the manual muscle test is presented.

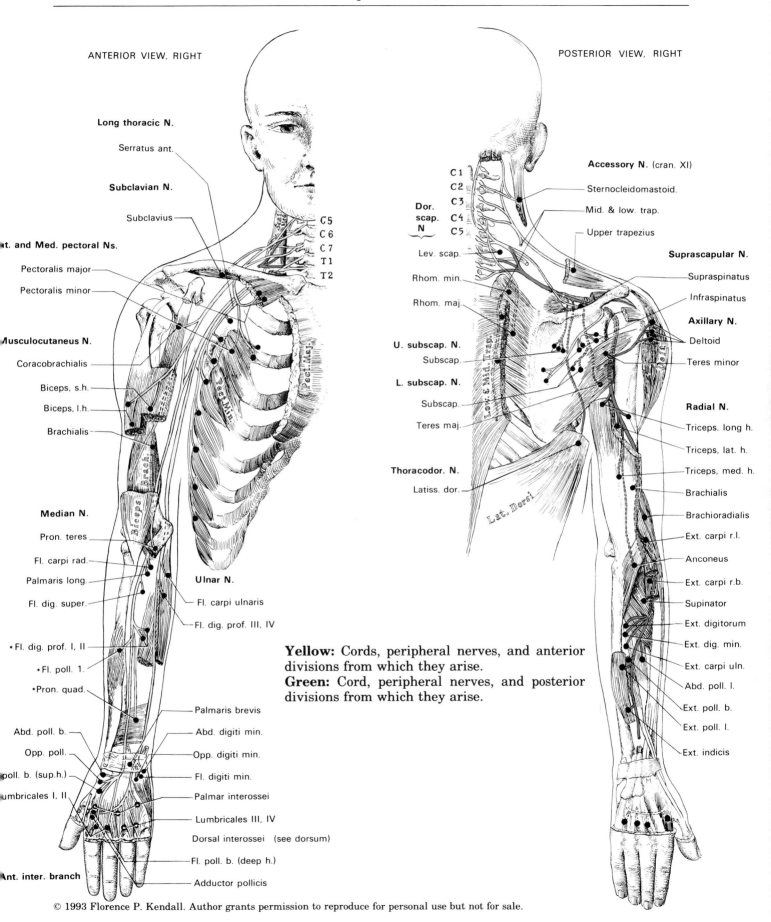

ANTERIOR VIEW, RIGHT

POSTERIOR VIEW, RIGHT

Long thoracic N.

Serratus ant.

Subclavian N.

Subclavius

...t. and Med. pectoral Ns.

Pectoralis major

Pectoralis minor

Musculocutaneus N.

Coracobrachialis

Biceps, s.h.

Biceps, l.h.

Brachialis

Median N.

Pron. teres

Fl. carpi rad.

Palmaris long.

Fl. dig. super.

*Fl. dig. prof. I, II

*Fl. poll. 1.

*Pron. quad.

Abd. poll. b.

Opp. poll.

...poll. b. (sup.h.)

...umbricales I, II

Ant. inter. branch

C5
C6
C7
T1
T2

Ulnar N.

Fl. carpi ulnaris

Fl. dig. prof. III, IV

Palmaris brevis

Abd. digiti min.

Opp. digiti min.

Fl. digiti min.

Palmar interossei

Lumbricales III, IV

Dorsal interossei (see dorsum)

Fl. poll. b. (deep h.)

Adductor pollicis

C1
C2
C3
C4
C5

Dor.
scap.
N

Lev. scap.

Rhom. min.

Rhom. maj.

U. subscap. N.

Subscap.

L. subscap. N.

Subscap.

Teres maj.

Thoracodor. N.

Latiss. dor.

Accessory N. (cran. XI)

Sternocleidomastoid.

Mid. & low. trap.

Upper trapezius

Suprascapular N.

Supraspinatus

Infraspinatus

Axillary N.

Deltoid

Teres minor

Radial N.

Triceps. long h.

Triceps, lat. h.

Triceps, med. h.

Brachialis

Brachioradialis

Ext. carpi r.l.

Anconeus

Ext. carpi r.b.

Supinator

Ext. digitorum

Ext. dig. min.

Ext. carpi uln.

Abd. poll. l.

Ext. poll. b.

Ext. poll. l.

Ext. indicis

Yellow: Cords, peripheral nerves, and anterior divisions from which they arise.
Green: Cord, peripheral nerves, and posterior divisions from which they arise.

Spinal Nerve and Motor Point Chart

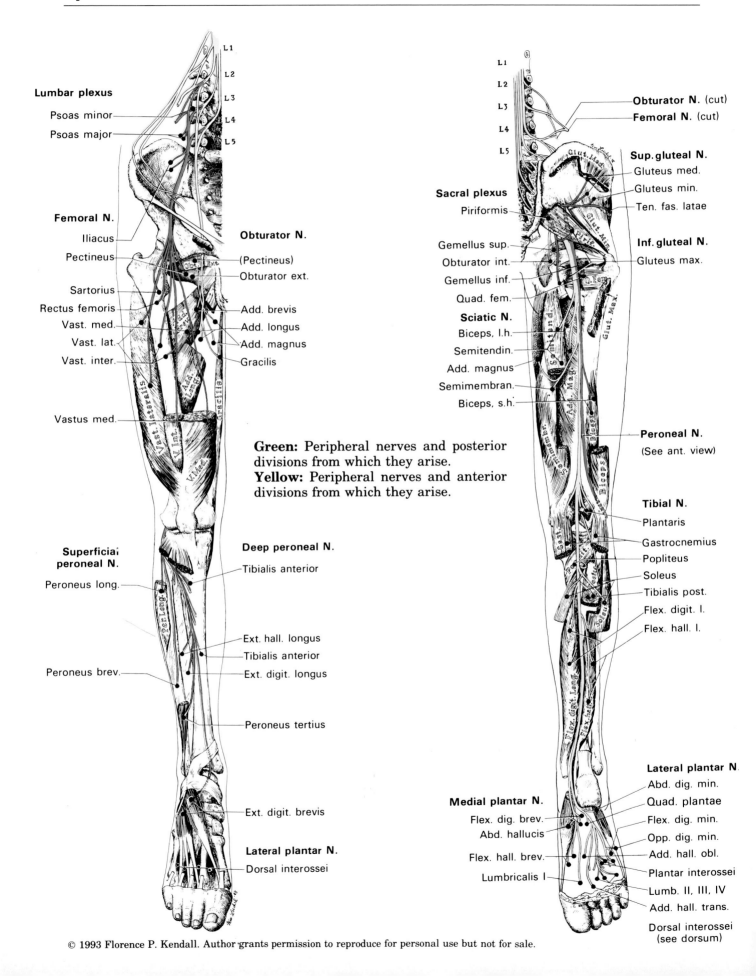

Lumbar plexus
Psoas minor
Psoas major

Femoral N.
Iliacus
Pectineus
Sartorius
Rectus femoris
Vast. med.
Vast. lat.
Vast. inter.
Vastus med.

Obturator N.
(Pectineus)
Obturator ext.
Add. brevis
Add. longus
Add. magnus
Gracilis

L1
L2
L3
L4
L5

Green: Peripheral nerves and posterior divisions from which they arise.
Yellow: Peripheral nerves and anterior divisions from which they arise.

Superficial peroneal N.
Peroneus long.
Peroneus brev.

Deep peroneal N.
Tibialis anterior
Ext. hall. longus
Tibialis anterior
Ext. digit. longus
Peroneus tertius
Ext. digit. brevis

Lateral plantar N.
Dorsal interossei

L1
L2
L3
L4
L5

Obturator N. (cut)
Femoral N. (cut)

Sup. gluteal N.
Gluteus med.
Gluteus min.
Ten. fas. latae

Sacral plexus
Piriformis
Gemellus sup.
Obturator int.
Gemellus inf.
Quad. fem.

Inf. gluteal N.
Gluteus max.

Sciatic N.
Biceps, l.h.
Semitendin.
Add. magnus
Semimembran.
Biceps, s.h.

Peroneal N.
(See ant. view)

Tibial N.
Plantaris
Gastrocnemius
Popliteus
Soleus
Tibialis post.
Flex. digit. l.
Flex. hall. l.

Medial plantar N.
Flex. dig. brev.
Abd. hallucis
Flex. hall. brev.
Lumbricalis I

Lateral plantar N.
Abd. dig. min.
Quad. plantae
Flex. dig. min.
Opp. dig. min.
Add. hall. obl.
Plantar interossei
Lumb. II, III, IV
Add. hall. trans.
Dorsal interossei (see dorsum)

SPINAL NERVE AND MUSCLE CHART
TRUNK AND LOWER EXTREMITY

Name _____   Date _____

SENSORY

PERIPHERAL NERVES — KEY

D	Dorsal Primary Ramus
V	Ventral Primary Ramus
A	Anterior Division
P	Posterior Division

Peripheral Nerve columns (left to right):
D — T1-12, L1-5, S1-3
V — T1,2,3,4
V — T5,6
V — T7,8
V — T9,10,11,12
V — Iliohypogastric T12 L1
V — Ilioinguinal T(12) L1
V — Lumb. Plex. T(12) L1,2,3,4
A — Femoral L(1)2,3,4
A — Obturator L1,2,3,4
P — Sup. Glut. L4,5,S1
P — Inf. Glut. L5,S1,2
V — Sac. Plex. L4,5,S1,2,3
P — Sciatic L4,5,S1,2
P — Sciatic L4,5,S1,2
A — C. Peroneal L4,5,S1,2
A — Tibial L4,5,S1,2,3

Group	Muscle	Peripheral Nerve	Spinal Segment (L1 L2 L3 L4 L5 S1 S2 S3)
Thoracic Nerves	ERECTOR SPINAE	D	1 2 3 4 5 1 2 3
	SERRATUS POST SUP	V (T1,2,3,4)	
	TRANS THORACIS	V (T1,2,3,4; T5,6; T7,8)	
	INT INTERCOSTALS	V (T1,2,3,4; T5,6; T7,8; T9,10,11,12)	
	EXT INTERCOSTALS	V	
	SUBCOSTALES	V	
	LEVATOR COSTARUM	V	
	OBLIQUUS EXT ABD	V (T5,6; T7,8; T9,10,11,12)	
	RECTUS ABDOMINIS	V	
	OBLIQUUS INT ABD	V; Iliohypogastric	1
	TRANSVERSUS ABD	V; Iliohypogastric; Ilioinguinal	1
	SERRATUS POST INF	V (T9,10,11,12)	
Lumb. Plexus	QUAD LUMBORUM	Lumb. Plex.	1 2 3
	PSOAS MINOR	Lumb. Plex.	1 2
	PSOAS MAJOR	Lumb. Plex.	1 2 3 4
Femoral	ILIACUS	Femoral	(1) 2 3 4
	PECTINEUS	Femoral; Obturator	2 3 4
	SARTORIUS	Femoral	2 3 (4)
	QUADRICEPS	Femoral	2 3 4
Obturator Ant.	ADDUCTOR BREVIS	Obturator	2 3 4
	ADDUCTOR LONGUS	Obturator	2 3 4
	GRACILIS	Obturator	2 3 4
Obturator Post.	OBTURATOR EXT	Obturator	3 4
	ADDUCTOR MAGNUS	Obturator; Sciatic	2 3 4 5 1
Gluteal Sup.	GLUTEUS MEDIUS	Sup. Glut.	4 5 1
	GLUTEUS MINIMUS	Sup. Glut.	4 5 1
	TENSOR FAS LAT	Sup. Glut.	4 5 1
Gluteal In.	GLUTEUS MAXIMUS	Inf. Glut.	5 1 2
Sacral Plexus	PIRIFORMIS	Sac. Plex.	(5) 1 2
	GEMELLUS SUP	Sac. Plex.	5 1 2
	OBTURATOR INT	Sac. Plex.	5 1 2
	GEMELLUS INF	Sac. Plex.	4 5 1 (2)
	QUADRATUS FEM	Sac. Plex.	4 5 1 (2)
Sciatic P.	BICEPS (SHORT H)	Sciatic	5 1 2
Sciatic Tibial	BICEPS (LONG H)	Sciatic	5 1 2 3
	SEMITENDINOSUS	Sciatic	4 5 1 2
	SEMIMEMBRANOSUS	Sciatic	4 5 1 2
Common Peroneal Deep	TIBIALIS ANTERIOR	C. Peroneal	4 5 1
	EXT HALL LONG	C. Peroneal	4 5 1
	EXT DIGIT LONG	C. Peroneal	4 5 1
	PERONEUS TERTIUS	C. Peroneal	4 5 1
	EXT DIGIT BREVIS	C. Peroneal	4 5 1
Common Peroneal Sup.	PERONEUS LONGUS	C. Peroneal	4 5 1
	PERONEUS BREVIS	C. Peroneal	4 5 1
Tibial	PLANTARIS	Tibial	4 5 1 (2)
	GASTROCNEMIUS	Tibial	1 2
	POPLITEUS	Tibial	4 5 1
	SOLEUS	Tibial	5 1 2
	TIBIALIS POSTERIOR	Tibial	(4) 5 1
	FLEX DIGIT LONG	Tibial	5 1 (2)
	FLEX HALL LONG	Tibial	5 1 2
Tibial Med Pl	FLEX DIGIT BREVIS	Tibial	4 5 1
	ABDUCTOR HALL	Tibial	4 5 1
	FLEX HALL BREVIS	Tibial	4 5 1
	LUMBRICALIS I	Tibial	4 5 1
Tibial Lat Plant	ABD DIGITI MIN	Tibial	1 2
	QUAD PLANTAE	Tibial	1 2
	FLEX DIGITI MIN	Tibial	1 2
	OPP. DIGITI MIN	Tibial	1 2
	ADDUCTORS HALL	Tibial	1 2
	PLANT INTEROSSEI	Tibial	1 2
	DORSAL INTEROSSEI	Tibial	1 2
	LUMB II,III,IV	Tibial	(4) (5) 1 2

Dermatomes redrawn from
Keegan and Garrett Anat Rec 102. 409. 437. 1948
Cutaneous Distribution of peripheral nerves
redrawn from *Gray's Anatomy of the Human Body.* 28th ed

Name **CASE #1**　　　　Date

LEFT MUSCLE

KEY →
- **D.** = Dorsal Prim. Ramus
- **V.** = Vent. Prim. Ramus
- **P.R.** = Plexus Root
- **S.T.** = Superior Trunk
- **P.** = Posterior Cord
- **L.** = Lateral Cord
- **M.** = Medial Cord

PERIPHERAL NERVES

	MUSCLE STRENGTH GRADE	Cervical T.	Cervical 1-8	Cervical 1-8	Cervical 1-4	Phrenic 3,4,5	Long Thor. 5,6,7,(8)	Dor. Scap 4,5	N. to Subcl. 5,6	Suprascap 4,5,6	U. Subscap. (4),5,6,(7)	Thoracodor (5),6,7,8	L. Subscap. 5,6,(7)	Lat. Pect. 5,6,7	Med. Pect. (6),7,8	Axillary (4),5,6,7	Musculocu. 5,6	Radial 5,6,7,8	Median 5,6,7,8,1	Ulnar 7,8,1	SPINAL SEGMENT C1-T1
HEAD & NECK EXTENSORS		●																			1 2 3 4 5 6 7 8 1
INFRAHYOID MUSCLES			●																		1 2 3
RECTUS CAP ANT. & LAT.			●																		1 2
LONGUS CAPITIS			●																		1 2 3 (4)
LONGUS COLLI				●																	2 3 4 5 6 (7)
LEVATOR SCAPULAE			●				●														3 4 5
SCALENI (A. M. P.)				●																	3 4 5 6 7 8
STERNOCLEIDOMASTOID			●																		(1) 2 3
TRAPEZIUS (U. M. L.)			●																		2 3 4
DIAPHRAGM					●																3 4 5
SERRATUS ANTERIOR						●															5 6 7 8
RHOMBOIDS MAJ & MIN							●														4 5
SUBCLAVIUS								●													
SUPRASPINATUS									●												
INFRASPINATUS									●												
SUBSCAPULARIS										●		●									
LATISSIMUS DORSI											●										
TERES MAJOR												●									
PECTORALIS MAJ (UPPER)													●								
PECTORALIS MAJ (LOWER)													●	●							
PECTORALIS MINOR														●							
TERES MINOR															●						
DELTOID															●						
CORACOBRACHIALIS																●					
BICEPS																●					5 6
BRACHIALIS																●					5 6
TRICEPS																	●				6 7 8 1
ANCONEUS																	●				7 8
BRACHIALIS (SMALL PART)																	●				5 6
BRACHIORADIALIS																	●				5 6
EXT CARPI RAD L																	●				5 6 7 8
EXT CARPI RAD B																	●				6 7 (8)
SUPINATOR																	●				5 6 (7)
EXT DIGITORUM																	◉				6 7 8
EXT DIGITI MINIMI																	◉				6 7 8
EXT CARPI ULNARIS																	◉				6 7 8
ABD POLLICIS LONGUS																	◉				6 7 8
EXT POLLICIS BREVIS																	◉				6 7 8
EXT POLLICIS LONGUS																	◉				6 7 8
EXT INDICIS																	◉				6 7 8
PRONATOR TERES																		●			6 7
FLEX CARPI RADIALIS																		●			6 7 8
PALMARIS LONGUS																		●			(6) 7 8 1
FLEX DIGIT SUPERFICIALIS																		◉			7 8 1
FLEX DIGIT PROF I & II																		◉			7 8 1
FLEX POLLICIS LONGUS																		◉			(6) 7 8 1
PRONATOR QUADRATUS																		◉			7 8 1
ABD POLLICIS BREVIS																		◉			6 7 8 1
OPPONENS POLLICIS																		◉			6 7 8 1
FLEX POLL BREV (SUP. H)																		◉			6 7 8 1
LUMBRICALES I & II																		◉			(6) 7 8 1
FLEX CARPI ULNARIS																			●		7 8 1
FLEX DIGIT. PROF. III & IV																			◉		7 8 1
PALMARIS BREVIS																			◉		(7) 8 1
ABD DIGITI MINIMI																			◉		(7) 8 1
OPPONENS DIGITI MINIMI																			◉		(7) 8 1
FLEX DIGITI MINIMI																			◉		(7) 8 1
PALMAR INTEROSSEI																			◉		8 1
DORSAL INTEROSSEI																			◉		8 1
LUMBRICALES III & IV																			◉		(7) 8 1
ADDUCTOR POLLICIS																			◉		8 1
FLEX POLL BREV. (DEEP H.)																			◉		8 1

SENSORY

Case 1: The radial, median, and ulnar nerves are all involved at approximately the same level of the forearm just below the elbow. (Refer to *Motor Point Chart*, opposite.) This type of involvement may be the result of pressure from a tourniquet, bandaging, or a cast. While the etiology is not clear-cut in this particular instance, the history does indicate that bandaging may have been a factor.

Dermatomes redrawn from Keegan and Garrett Anat Rec 102. 409. 437. 1948
Cutaneous Distribution of peripheral nerves redrawn from *Gray's Anatomy of the Human Body.* 28th ed

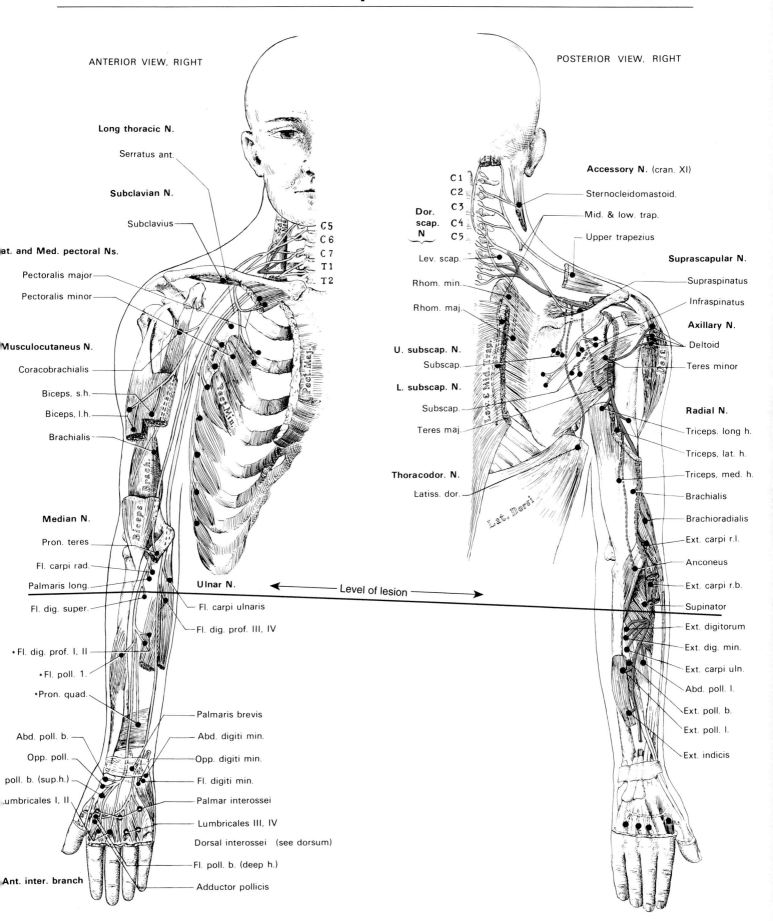

ANTERIOR VIEW, RIGHT

POSTERIOR VIEW, RIGHT

Long thoracic N.

Serratus ant.

Subclavian N.

Subclavius

Lat. and Med. pectoral Ns.

Pectoralis major

Pectoralis minor

Musculocutaneus N.

Coracobrachialis

Biceps, s.h.

Biceps, l.h.

Brachialis

Median N.

Pron. teres

Fl. carpi rad.

Palmaris long.

Fl. dig. super.

* Fl. dig. prof. I, II

*Fl. poll. 1.

*Pron. quad.

Abd. poll. b.

Opp. poll.

poll. b. (sup.h.)

umbricales I, II

Ant. inter. branch

C5
C6
C7
T1
T2

Ulnar N.

Fl. carpi ulnaris

Fl. dig. prof. III, IV

Palmaris brevis

Abd. digiti min.

Opp. digiti min.

Fl. digiti min.

Palmar interossei

Lumbricales III, IV

Dorsal interossei (see dorsum)

Fl. poll. b. (deep h.)

Adductor pollicis

C1
C2
C3
C4
C5

Dor. scap. N

Lev. scap.

Rhom. min.

Rhom. maj.

U. subscap. N.

Subscap.

L. subscap. N.

Subscap.

Teres maj.

Thoracodor. N.

Latiss. dor.

Level of lesion

Accessory N. (cran. XI)

Sternocleidomastoid.

Mid. & low. trap.

Upper trapezius

Suprascapular N.

Supraspinatus

Infraspinatus

Axillary N.

Deltoid

Teres minor

Radial N.

Triceps. long h.

Triceps, lat. h.

Triceps, med. h.

Brachialis

Brachioradialis

Ext. carpi r.l.

Anconeus

Ext. carpi r.b.

Supinator

Ext. digitorum

Ext. dig. min.

Ext. carpi uln.

Abd. poll. l.

Ext. poll. b.

Ext. poll. l.

Ext. indicis

Name **CASE #2**   Date

PERIPHERAL NERVES — KEY

D.	= Dorsal Prim. Ramus
V.	= Vent. Prim. Ramus
P.R.	= Plexus Root
S.T.	= Superior Trunk
P.	= Posterior Cord
L.	= Lateral Cord
M.	= Medial Cord

RIGHT MUSCLE

MUSCLE STRENGTH GRADE

Muscle	Spinal Segment
HEAD & NECK EXTENSORS	1 2 3 4 5 6 7 8 1
INFRAHYOID MUSCLES	1 2 3
RECTUS CAP ANT. & LAT.	1 2
LONGUS CAPITIS	1 2 3 (4)
LONGUS COLLI	2 3 4 5 6 (7)
LEVATOR SCAPULAE	3 4 5
SCALENI (A. M. P.)	3 4 5 6 7 8
STERNOCLEIDOMASTOID	(1) 2 3
TRAPEZIUS (U. M. L.)	2 3 4
DIAPHRAGM	3 4 5
SERRATUS ANTERIOR	5 6 7 8
RHOMBOIDS MAJ & MIN	4 5
SUBCLAVIUS	5 6
SUPRASPINATUS	4 5 6
INFRASPINATUS	(4) 5 6
SUBSCAPULARIS	
LATISSIMUS DORSI	
TERES MAJOR	
PECTORALIS MAJ (UPPER)	
PECTORALIS MAJ (LOWER)	
PECTORALIS MINOR	
TERES MINOR	
DELTOID	
CORACOBRACHIALIS	6 7
BICEPS	5 6
BRACHIALIS	5 6
TRICEPS	6 7 8 1
ANCONEUS	7 8
BRACHIALIS (SMALL PART)	5 6
BRACHIORADIALIS	5 6
EXT CARPI RAD L	5 6 7 8
EXT CARPI RAD B	6 7 (8)
SUPINATOR	5 6 (7)
EXT DIGITORUM	6 7 8
EXT DIGITI MINIMI	6 7 8
EXT CARPI ULNARIS	6 7 8
ABD POLLICIS LONGUS	6 7 8
EXT POLLICIS BREVIS	6 7 8
EXT POLLICIS LONGUS	6 7 8
EXT INDICIS	6 7 8
PRONATOR TERES	6 7
FLEX CARPI RADIALIS	6 7 8
PALMARIS LONGUS	(6) 7 8 1
FLEX DIGIT SUPERFICIALIS	7 8 1
FLEX DIGIT PROF I & II	7 8 1
FLEX POLLICIS LONGUS	(6) 7 8 1
PRONATOR QUADRATUS	7 8 1
ABD POLLICIS BREVIS	6 7 8 1
OPPONENS POLLICIS	6 7 8 1
FLEX POLL BREV (SUP. H)	6 7 8 1
LUMBRICALES I & II	(6) 7 8 1
FLEX CARPI ULNARIS	7 8 1
FLEX DIGIT. PROF. III & IV	7 8 1
PALMARIS BREVIS	(7) 8 1
ABD DIGITI MINIMI	(7) 8 1
OPPONENS DIGITI MINIMI	(7) 8 1
FLEX DIGITI MINIMI	(7) 8 1
PALMAR INTEROSSEI	8 1
DORSAL INTEROSSEI	8 1
LUMBRICALES III & IV	(7) 8 1
ADDUCTOR POLLICIS	8 1
FLEX POLL BREV. (DEEP H.)	8 1

Case 2: Radial nerve lesion below level of branches to Triceps following a fracture of the humerus. Initially, the Triceps was weak, but recovery was complete.

SENSORY

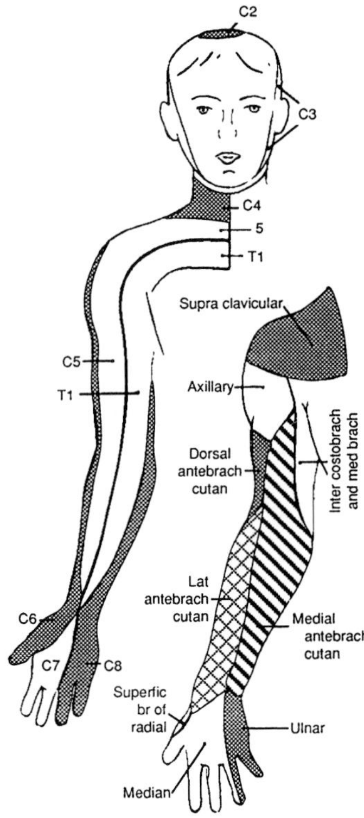

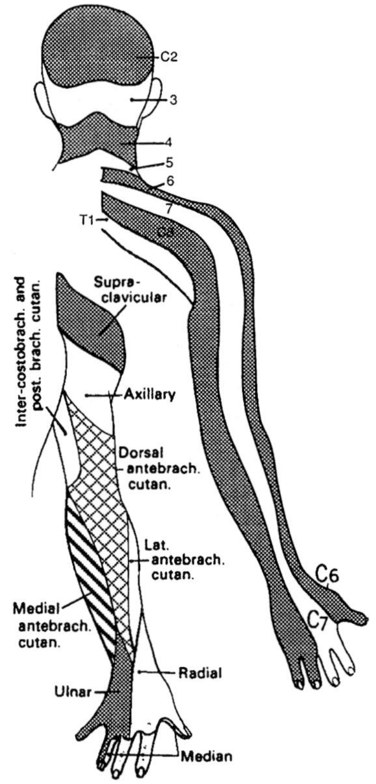

Dermatomes redrawn from Keegan and Garrett Anat Rec 102. 409. 437. 1948
Cutaneous Distribution of peripheral nerves redrawn from *Gray's Anatomy of the Human Body.* 28th ed

* Strength of i-p joint extension decreased due to loss of Ext. dig. strength.

Name *Case #3*

SPINAL NERVE AND MUSCLE CHART

TRUNK AND LOWER EXTREMITY

Date

LEFT

	MUSCLE STRENGTH GRADE	MUSCLE	D. T1-12, L1-5, S1-3	V. T1, 2, 3, 4	V. T5, 6	V. T7, 8	V. T9, 10, 11, 12	V. Iliohypogastric T12 L1	V. Ilioinguinal T(12) L1	V. Lumb. Plex. T(12) L1, 2, 3, 4	P. Femoral L(1) 2, 3, 4	A. Obturator L(1) 2, 3, 4	P. Sup. Glut. L4, 5, S1	P. Inf. Glut. L5, S1, 2	V. Sac. Plex. L4, 5, S1, 2, 3	P. Sciatic L4, 5, S1, 2	A. Sciatic L4, 5, S1, 2, 3	P. C. Peroneal L4, 5, S1, 2	A. Tibial L4, 5, S1, 2, 3					
		ERECTOR SPINAE	•																					
Thoracic Nerves		SERRATUS POST SUP		•																				
Thoracic Nerves		TRANS THORACIS		•	•	•																		
Thoracic Nerves		INT INTERCOSTALS		•	•	•	•																	
Thoracic Nerves		EXT INTERCOSTALS		•	•	•	•																	
Thoracic Nerves		SUBCOSTALES		•	•	•	•																	
Thoracic Nerves		LEVATOR COSTARUM		•	•	•	•																	
Thoracic Nerves		OBLIQUUS EXT ABD			(•)	•	•																	
Thoracic Nerves		RECTUS ABDOMINIS			•	•	•																	
Thoracic Nerves		OBLIQUUS INT ABD				•	•	•	(•)															
Thoracic Nerves		TRANSVERSUS ABD				•	•	•	(•)															
Thoracic Nerves		SERRATUS POST INF					•																	
Lumb. Plexus		QUAD LUMBORUM								•														
Lumb. Plexus		PSOAS MINOR								•														
Lumb. Plexus		PSOAS MAJOR								•														
Femoral		ILIACUS									•													
Femoral		PECTINEUS									•	(•)												
Femoral		SARTORIUS									•													
Femoral		QUADRICEPS									•													
Obturator Ant.		ADDUCTOR BREVIS										•												
Obturator Ant.		ADDUCTOR LONGUS										•												
Obturator Ant.		GRACILIS										•												
Obturator Post		OBTURATOR EXT										•												
Obturator Post		ADDUCTOR MAGNUS										•					•							
Gluteal Sup		GLUTEUS MEDIUS											•											
Gluteal Sup		GLUTEUS MINIMUS											•											
Gluteal Sup		TENSOR FAS LAT											•											
Gluteal In.		GLUTEUS MAXIMUS												•										
Sacral Plexus		PIRIFORMIS													•									
Sacral Plexus		GEMELLUS SUP													•						5	1	2	
Sacral Plexus		OBTURATOR INT													•						5	1	2	
Sacral Plexus		GEMELLUS INF													•					4	5	1	(2)	
Sacral Plexus		QUADRATUS FEM													•					4	5	1	(2)	
Sciatic P		BICEPS (SHORT H)														•					5	1	2	
Sciatic Tibial		BICEPS (LONG H)															•				5	1	2	3
Sciatic Tibial		SEMITENDINOSUS															•			4	5	1	2	
Sciatic Tibial		SEMIMEMBRANOSUS															•			4	5	1	2	
Common Peroneal Deep	3	TIBIALIS ANTERIOR																⊙		4	5	1		
Common Peroneal Deep	0	EXT HALL LONG																⊙		4	5	1		
Common Peroneal Deep	0	EXT DIGIT LONG																⊙		4	5	1		
Common Peroneal Deep	0	PERONEUS TERTIUS																⊙		4	5	1		
Common Peroneal Deep	0	EXT DIGIT BREVIS																⊙		4	5	1		
Common Peroneal Sup	2	PERONEUS LONGUS																⊙		4	5	1		
Common Peroneal Sup	2	PERONEUS BREVIS																⊙		4	5	1		
Tibial	—	PLANTARIS																	•	4	5	1	(2)	
Tibial	10	GASTROCNEMIUS																	•			1	2	
Tibial	—	POPLITEUS																	•	4	5	1		
Tibial	10	SOLEUS																	•		5	1	2	
Tibial	7	TIBIALIS POSTERIOR																	⊙	(4)	5	1		
Tibial	0	FLEX DIGIT LONG																	⊙		5	1	(2)	
Tibial	0	FLEX HALL LONG																	⊙		5	1	2	
Tibial Med Pl	10	FLEX DIGIT BREVIS																	•	4	5	1		
Tibial Med Pl	—	ABDUCTOR HALL																	•	4	5	1		
Tibial Med Pl	10	FLEX HALL BREVIS																	•	4	5	1		
Tibial Med Pl	8	LUMBRICALIS I																	•	4	5	1		
Tibial Lat Plant	—	ABD DIGITI MIN																	•			1	2	
Tibial Lat Plant	—	QUAD PLANTAE																	•			1	2	
Tibial Lat Plant	—	FLEX DIGITI MIN																	•			1	2	
Tibial Lat Plant	—	OPP. DIGITI MIN																	•			1	2	
Tibial Lat Plant	—	ADDUCTOR HALL																	•			1	2	
Tibial Lat Plant	—	PLANT INTEROSSEI																	•			1	2	
Tibial Lat Plant	—	DORSAL INTEROSSEI																	•			1	2	
Tibial Lat Plant	8	LUMB II,III,IV																	•	(4)	(5)	1	2	

KEY

- D Dorsal Primary Ramus
- V Ventral Primary Ramus
- A Anterior Division
- P Posterior Division

SENSORY

Case 3: The patient, on whom muscle and sensory tests were done 6 weeks after onset, had fallen through a glass door and sustained a laceration injury of the left leg. Muscle test findings indicated the following:

Involvement of the nerve branches to the Flexor digitorum longus and Flexor hallucis longus without involvement of the tibial nerve and its terminal branches.

Involvement of the superficial peroneal nerve; and of the deep peroneal nerve, probably below the level of a proximal branch to the tibialis anterior.

The weakness of the Posterior tibial muscle may have been due to trauma of the muscle rather than nerve involvement since it made complete recovery within 3 1/2 months after onset. By that time, the Flexor digitorum longus and Flexor hallucis longus had made good recovery, and made complete recovery by the end of 6 months. Progress was slow and muscle weakness, grading fair+, remained in all muscles supplied by the deep and superficial peroneal nerves.

(LEFT LEG)

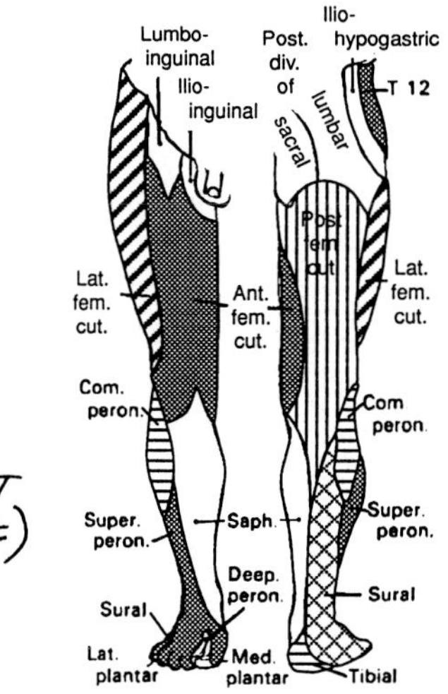

Lumbo-inguinal
Ilio-inguinal
Post. div. of
lumbar
sacral
Ilio-hypogastric
T 12
Lat. fem. cut.
Ant. fem. cut.
Post fem cut
Lat. fem. cut.
Com. peron.
Com peron.
Super. peron.
Saph.
Super. peron.
Deep. peron.
Sural
Sural
Lat. plantar
Med. plantar
Tibial

Dermatomes redrawn from Keegan and Garrett Anat Rec 102. 409. 437. 1948
Cutaneous Distribution of peripheral nerves redrawn from *Gray's Anatomy of the Human Body*. 28th ed

Name **CASE #4** Date

SENSORY

LEFT MUSCLE — MUSCLE STRENGTH GRADE

PERIPHERAL NERVES — KEY →

KEY	
D.	= Dorsal Prim. Ramus
V.	= Vent. Prim. Ramus
P.R.	= Plexus Root
S.T.	= Superior Trunk
P.	= Posterior Cord
L.	= Lateral Cord
M.	= Medial Cord

Peripheral nerve columns: Cervical (D. / T. / 1-8), Cervical (V. / 1-8), Cervical (V. / 1-4), Phrenic (V. / 3,4,5), Long Thor. (P.R. / 5,6,7,(8)), Dor. Scap. (P.R. / 4,5), N. to Subcl. (S.T. / 5,6), Suprascap. (S.T. / 4,5,6), U. Subscap. (P. / (4),5,6,(7)), Thoracodor. (P. / (5),6,7,8), L. Subscap. (P. / 5,6,(7)), Lat. Pect. (L. / 5,6,7), Med. Pect. (M. / (6),7,8), Axillary (P. / 5,6), Musculocu. (L. / (4),5,6,7), Radial (P. / 5,6,7,8), Median (L.M. / 5,6,7,8), Ulnar (M. / 7,8)

SPINAL SEGMENT columns: C1 C2 C3 C4 C5 C6 C7 C8 T1

	MUSCLE	Cervical			Phrenic	Long Thor.	Dor. Scap.	N. to Subcl.	Suprascap.	U. Subscap.	Thoracodor.	L. Subscap.	Lat. Pect.	Med. Pect.	Axillary	Musculocu.	Radial	Median	Ulnar	Spinal segment
	HEAD & NECK EXTENSORS	●																		1 2 3 4 5 6 7 8 1
Cervical nerves	INFRAHYOID MUSCLES		●																	1 2 3
	RECTUS CAP ANT. & LAT.		●																	1 2
	LONGUS CAPITIS		●																	1 2 3 (4)
	LONGUS COLLI	●																		2 3 4 5 6 (7)
	LEVATOR SCAPULAE		●				●													3 4 5
	SCALENI (A. M. P.)	●																		3 4 5 6 7 8
	STERNOCLEIDOMASTOID		●																	(1) 2 3
N?	TRAPEZIUS (U. M. L.)		●																	2 3 4
*	DIAPHRAGM				●															3 4 5
Brachial Plexus — Root	SERRATUS ANTERIOR					●														5 6 7 8
G	RHOMBOIDS MAJ & MIN						●													4 5
P	SUBCLAVIUS							●												5 6
?— Trunk	SUPRASPINATUS								●											4 5 6
T	INFRASPINATUS								●											(4) 5 6
— P Cord	SUBSCAPULARIS									●		●								5 6 7
G	LATISSIMUS DORSI										●									6 7 8
G	TERES MAJOR											●								5 6 7
G- M&L	PECTORALIS MAJ (UPPER)												●							5 6 7
G	PECTORALIS MAJ (LOWER)												●	●						6 7 8 1
G	PECTORALIS MINOR													●						(6) 7 8 1
Axil. — T	TERES MINOR														●					5 6
T	DELTOID														●					5 6
Musculo-cutan —	CORACOBRACHIALIS															●				6 7
P+	BICEPS															●				5 6
	BRACHIALIS															●				5 6
Radial — Lat.M	TRICEPS																●			6 7 8 1
G+	ANCONEUS																●			7 8
P	BRACHIALIS (SMALL PART)																●			5 6
F-	BRACHIORADIALIS																●			5 6
G	EXT CARPI RAD L																●			5 6 7 8
G	EXT CARPI RAD B																●			6 7 (8)
F+	SUPINATOR																●			5 6 (7)
N Post Inter	EXT DIGITORUM																●			6 7 8
N	EXT DIGITI MINIMI																●			
N	EXT CARPI ULNARIS																●			
N	ABD POLLICIS LONGUS																●			
N	EXT POLLICIS BREVIS																●			
N	EXT POLLICIS LONGUS																●			
N	EXT INDICIS																●			
Median — A Inter	PRONATOR TERES																	●		
N	FLEX CARPI RADIALIS																	●		
N	PALMARIS LONGUS																	●		
N	FLEX DIGIT SUPERFICIALIS																	●		
N	FLEX DIGIT PROF I & II																	●		
N	FLEX POLLICIS LONGUS																	●		
N	PRONATOR QUADRATUS																	●		7 8 1
N	ABD POLLICIS BREVIS																	●		6 7 8 1
N	OPPONENS POLLICIS																	●		6 7 8 1
N	FLEX POLL BREV (SUP. H)																	●		6 7 8 1
N	LUMBRICALES I & II																	●		(6) 7 8 1
Ulnar	FLEX CARPI ULNARIS																		●	7 8 1
N	FLEX DIGIT. PROF. III & IV																		●	7 8 1
—	PALMARIS BREVIS																		●	(7) 8 1
N	ABD DIGITI MINIMI																		●	(7) 8 1
N	OPPONENS DIGITI MINIMI																		●	(7) 8 1
N	FLEX DIGITI MINIMI																		●	(7) 8 1
N	PALMAR INTEROSSEI																		●	8 1
N	DORSAL INTEROSSEI																		●	8 1
N	LUMBRICALES III & IV																		●	(7) 8 1
N	ADDUCTOR POLLICIS																		●	8 1
N	FLEX POLL BREV. (DEEP H.)																		●	8 1

Case 4: Muscle test findings indicate a probable C5 lesion. The test findings in this case compare very closely with those in a known C5 lesion. *Note: Patient's breathing seemed slightly labored. Patient stated breathing was difficult for about a week after onset.

Dermatomes redrawn from Keegan and Garrett Anat Rec 102. 409. 437. 1948 Cutaneous Distribution of peripheral nerves redrawn from *Gray's Anatomy of the Human Body.* 28th ed

Case 5: Muscle test findings indicate a possible L5 lesion. Numerous muscles that receive innervation from L4 were normal in strength, leading to the assumption that L4 was not involved. The patient was able to stand on one foot at a time and rise on toes without any difficulty, hence the normal grade for the Gastrocnemius. With the innervation to this muscle from S1 and S2, the grade of normal rules out the probability of a disc below L5.

Subsequent examination by a neurologist confirmed a probable disc lesion, and patient had a complete recovery.

KEY

→		
D	Dorsal Primary Ramus	
V	Ventral Primary Ramus	
A	Anterior Division	
P	Posterior Division	

RIGHT — MUSCLE (MUSCLE STRENGTH GRADE)

Grade	Muscle
•	ERECTOR SPINAE
	SERRATUS POST SUP
	TRANS THORACIS
	INT INTERCOSTALS
	EXT INTERCOSTALS
	SUBCOSTALES
	LEVATOR COSTARUM
	OBLIQUUS EXT ABD
	RECTUS ABDOMINIS
	OBLIQUUS INT ABD
	TRANSVERSUS ABD
	SERRATUS POST INF
—	QUAD LUMBORUM
—	PSOAS MINOR
10	PSOAS MAJOR
10	ILIACUS
—	PECTINEUS
10	SARTORIUS
10	QUADRICEPS
	ADDUCTOR BREVIS
	ADDUCTOR LONGUS
10	GRACILIS
	OBTURATOR EXT
	ADDUCTOR MAGNUS
4	GLUTEUS MEDIUS
4	GLUTEUS MINIMUS
5	TENSOR FAS LAT
6	GLUTEUS MAXIMUS
	PIRIFORMIS
	GEMELLUS SUP
7	OBTURATOR INT
	GEMELLUS INF
	QUADRATUS FEM
7	BICEPS (SHORT H)
7	BICEPS (LONG H)
	SEMITENDINOSUS
	SEMIMEMBRANOSUS
4	TIBIALIS ANTERIOR
8	EXT HALL LONG
8	EXT DIGIT LONG
8	PERONEUS TERTIUS
8	EXT DIGIT BREVIS
7	PERONEUS LONGUS
7	PERONEUS BREVIS
—	PLANTARIS
10	GASTROCNEMIUS
10	POPLITEUS
10	SOLEUS
7	TIBIALIS POSTERIOR
6	FLEX DIGIT LONG
7	FLEX HALL LONG
7	FLEX DIGIT BREVIS
—	ABDUCTOR HALL
7	FLEX HALL BREVIS
8	LUMBRICALIS I
—	ABD DIGITI MIN
—	QUAD PLANTAE
—	FLEX DIGITI MIN
—	OPP. DIGITI MIN
—	ADDUCTOR HALL
—	PLANT INTEROSSEI
—	DORSAL INTEROSSEI
6	LUMB II, III, IV

Dermatomes redrawn from
Keegan and Garrett Anat Rec 102. 409. 437. 1948
Cutaneous Distribution of peripheral nerves
redrawn from *Gray's Anatomy of the Human Body.* 28th ed

SPINAL NERVE AND MUSCLE CHART
NECK, DIAPHRAGM AND UPPER EXTREMITY

Name: **CASE #6** Date:

RIGHT MUSCLE

MUSCLE STRENGTH GRADE

KEY
- D. = Dorsal Prim. Ramus
- V. = Vent. Prim. Ramus
- P.R. = Plexus Root
- S.T. = Superior Trunk
- P. = Posterior Cord
- L. = Lateral Cord
- M. = Medial Cord

PERIPHERAL NERVES

	Grade	Muscle	Cervical	Cervical	Cervical	Phrenic	Long Thor.	Dor. Scap.	N. to Subcl.	Suprascap	U. Subscap.	Thoracodor	L. Subscap.	Lat. Pect.	Med. Pect.	Axillary	Musculocu.	Radial	Median	Ulnar	Spinal Segment C1–T1
	—	HEAD & NECK EXTENSORS	●																		1 2 3 4 5 6 7 8 1
Cervical nerves	—	INFRAHYOID MUSCLES		●																	1 2 3
	—	RECTUS CAP ANT. & LAT.		●																	1 2
	—	LONGUS CAPITIS		●																	1 2 3 (4)
	—	LONGUS COLLI	●																		2 3 4 5 6 (7)
	N	LEVATOR SCAPULAE		●			●														3 4 5
	—	SCALENI (A. M. P.)	●																		3 4 5 6 7 8
	N	STERNOCLEIDOMASTOID		●																	(1) 2 3
	N	TRAPEZIUS (U. M. L.)		●																	2 3 4
	—	DIAPHRAGM				●															3 4 5
Brachial Plexus — Root	N	SERRATUS ANTERIOR					●														5 6 7 8
	N	RHOMBOIDS MAJ & MIN						●													4 5
Trunk	—	SUBCLAVIUS							●												5 6
	F	SUPRASPINATUS								●											4 5 6
	F+	INFRASPINATUS								●											(4) 5 6
P Cord	O?	SUBSCAPULARIS									●		●								5 6 7
	P?	LATISSIMUS DORSI										●									6 7 8
	O?	TERES MAJOR											●								5 6 7
M&L	O	PECTORALIS MAJ (UPPER)												●							5 6 7
	G	PECTORALIS MAJ (LOWER)												●	●						6 7 8 1
	G+	PECTORALIS MINOR													●						(6) 7 8 1
Axil.	P	TERES MINOR														●					5 6
	T	DELTOID														●					5 6
Musculo-cutan	P	CORACOBRACHIALIS															●				6 7
	O	BICEPS															●				5 6
	O	BRACHIALIS															●				5 6
Radial — Lat.M	P	TRICEPS																●			6 7 8 1
	—	ANCONEUS																●			7 8
	O	BRACHIALIS (SMALL PART)																●			5 6
	O	BRACHIORADIALIS																●			5 6
	O	EXT CARPI RAD L																●			5 6 7 8
	O	EXT CARPI RAD B																●			6 7 (8)
	O	SUPINATOR																●			5 6 (7)
Post Inter	O	EXT DIGITORUM																●			6 7 8
	O	EXT DIGITI MINIMI																●			6 7 8
	O	EXT CARPI ULNARIS																●			6 7 8
	O	ABD POLLICIS LONGUS																●			6 7 8
	O	EXT POLLICIS BREVIS																●			6 7 8
	O	EXT POLLICIS LONGUS																●			6 7 8
	O	EXT INDICIS																●			6 7 8
Median — A Inter	G	PRONATOR TERES																	●		6 7
	G	FLEX CARPI RADIALIS																	●		6 7 8
	G	PALMARIS LONGUS																	●		(6) 7 8 1
	N	FLEX DIGIT SUPERFICIALIS																	●		7 8 1
	N	FLEX DIGIT PROF I & II																	●		7 8 1
	N	FLEX POLLICIS LONGUS																	●		(6) 7 8 1
	G	PRONATOR QUADRATUS																	●		7 8 1
	G	ABD POLLICIS BREVIS																	●		6 7 8
	N	OPPONENS POLLICIS																	●		6 7 8
	G	FLEX POLL BREV (SUP. H)																	●		6 7 8
	N	LUMBRICALES I & II																	●		(6) 7 8 1
Ulnar	N	FLEX CARPI ULNARIS																		●	7 8 1
	N	FLEX DIGIT. PROF. III & IV																		●	7 8 1
	—	PALMARIS BREVIS																		●	(7) 8 1
	N	ABD DIGITI MINIMI																		●	(7) 8 1
	N	OPPONENS DIGITI MINIMI																		●	(7) 8 1
	N	FLEX DIGITI MINIMI																		●	(7) 8 1
	N	PALMAR INTEROSSEI																		●	8 1
	N	DORSAL INTEROSSEI																		●	8 1
	N	LUMBRICALES III & IV																		●	(7) 8 1
	N	ADDUCTOR POLLICIS																		●	8 1
	N	FLEX POLL BREV. (DEEP H.)																		●	8 1

SENSORY

Dermatomes redrawn from Keegan and Garrett Anat Rec 102. 409. 437. 1948
Cutaneous Distribution of peripheral nerves redrawn from *Gray's Anatomy of the Human Body*. 28th ed

400

CASE 6

A 30-year-old male fell from a moving automobile and was unconscious for about 20 minutes. He was treated in the emergency room of a local hospital for minor abrasions and then released. During the next 3 weeks he was seen and treated by several physicians because of paralysis and edema of his right arm and pains in his chest and neck (98).

Twenty-two days later, he was admitted to the University of Maryland Hospital. A neuromuscular evaluation, including a manual muscle test and an electromyographic study, was made at that time and showed extensive involvement of the right upper extremity.

The decision was made to defer surgical exploration and to treat the patient conservatively by the application of an airplane splint and follow-up therapy in the outpatient clinic. Unfortunately, the patient did not report to the outpatient clinic until 5 months later. Subsequently, a detailed manual muscle test (see facing page) as well as electrodiagnostic and further electromyographic studies were made.

Sensory and Reflex Tests. Sensation to pinprick was absent over the area of sensory distribution of the axillary, musculocutaneous, and radial nerves. There were no deep tendon reflexes of the Biceps or Triceps muscles.

Manual Muscle Test. The chart opposite indicates, at a glance, that the muscles supplied by the ulnar nerve were graded normal, those by the median were either normal or good, and those by the radial, musculocutaneous, and axillary were either poor or zero. At the brachial plexus level the involvement was more complicated, as noted by the grades ranging all the way from normal to zero. However, concurrent charting of the involved peripheral nerves and spinal segments furnished additional information and provided the basis for determination of the sites of the lesions as follows:

1. *A lesion of the posterior cord of the brachial plexus.* The muscles supplied by the upper and lower subscapular, thoracodorsal, axillary, and radial nerves, which arise from the posterior cord, show complete paralysis or major weakness.

   Involvement of the Subscapularis muscle places the site of lesion proximal to the point where the upper subscapular nerve arises ("c" in figure below).

2. *No involvement of the medial cord of the plexus.* The muscles supplied by the ulnar nerve, which is the terminal branch of the medial cord, graded normal. The sternal part of the Pectoralis major and the Pectoralis minor (C5–T1), and some muscles receiving median nerve supply (C6–T1) graded good. It is logical to assume that the slight weakness is attributable to the C5 and C6 deficit, and not to any involvement of the medial cord.

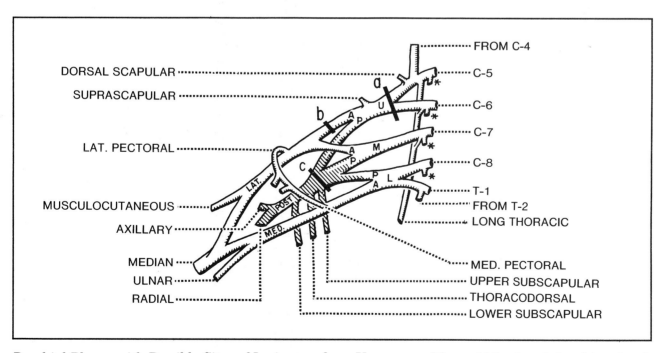

Brachial Plexus with Possible Sites of Lesions, **a, b, c**. U = upper; M = middle; L = lateral trunks; A = anterior divisions; P = posterior divisions; * = to longus coli and scaleni; lat = lateral cord; med = medial cord; post = posterior cord. Reprinted with permission of Phys Ther (98).

3. *A lesion of either the upper trunk (formed by C5 and C6 roots of the plexus) or the anterior division of the upper trunk before it joins with the anterior division of the middle trunk (C7) to form the lateral cord.* Confirmation of this statement requires an explanation of how it is ascertained that the lesion is in this area, and that it is no more proximal than "a" nor more distal than "b."

The complete paralysis of the Biceps and Brachialis (from C5 and C6) raises the question of the level of involvement of these muscles—musculocutaneous nerve (C5, C6, C7), lateral cord (C5, C6, C7), trunk, or spinal nerve root?

The fact that the Coracobrachialis showed some strength rules out complete involvement at the musculocutaneous level. A complete lesion at the level of the lateral cord (C5, C6, C7) is refuted by several findings that indicate that the C7 component is not involved.

The Flexor digitorum superficialis, the Flexor digitorum profundus I and II, and the Lumbricales I and II, which have C7, C8, and T1 supply through the median nerve, graded normal. Other muscles supplied by the median nerve, which have C6, C7, C8, and T1 supply, graded good and undoubtedly would have exhibited more weakness had C7 been involved.

The sternal part of the Pectoralis major and Pectoralis minor, which are supplied chiefly by the medial pectoral (C8 and T1) and to some extent by the lateral pectoral (C5, C6, and C7), graded good and good+. Had C7 been involved the weakness would undoubtedly have been greater.

The presence of some strength in the Coracobrachialis is thus explained on the basis of the C7 components being intact and further confirms that such is the case. The stretch weakness, superimposed on this muscle by the shoulder joint subluxation and the weakness of the Deltoid and Biceps, could account for the Coracobrachialis grading no more than poor.

Thus, with C7 not involved, the most distal point of lesion may be considered as "b."

The possibility of C5 and C6 being involved more proximal than "a" at the level of the roots of the plexus is ruled out because the Rhomboids and Serratus anterior muscles graded normal. Whether the lesion is proximal or distal to the point where the suprascapular nerve arises depends on whether the involvement of the Supraspinatus and Infraspinatus muscles is on a neurogenic or stretch weakness basis.

The Supraspinatus and Infraspinatus (C4, C5, C6) graded fair, and if this partial weakness resulted from a neurological deficit the lesion must be proximal to the point where the suprascapular nerve arises. Most logically, the presence of fair strength would then be interpreted as a result of regeneration in the 7 months since onset.

On the other hand, there is the possibility that the weakness in these muscles is of a secondary stretch weakness type, and that it was not neurogenic. The patient had not worn the airplane splint that was applied 23 days after injury, and there was subluxation of the joint and stretching of the capsule. The weakness was not as pronounced as in the other muscles supplied by C5 and C6, a fullness of contraction could be felt on palpation, and these muscles had been subjected to undue stretch. If the weakness resulted from stretch, the initial site of lesion would have been distal to the point where the suprascapular nerve arises.

Name: *CASE #7* Date:

LEFT

Case 7: A manual muscle test was done prior to surgery and findings indicated the following:

Slight involvement of the muscles supplied by the radial nerve below the level of the innervation to the Triceps.

Moderate involvement of the lateral cord below the level of the lateral pectoral nerve.

Probably complete involvement of the medial cord above the level of the medial pectoral nerve, interrupting C8 and T1 supply (inferior trunk).

The fact that the Pectoralis minor, Flexor carpi ulnaris, and the Flexor digitorum profundus III and IV show some strength can mislead one to assume that C8 and T1 are intact. These muscles, along with some of the intrinsic muscles of the hand, receive C7 innervation also, and there may be slight evidence of power in these muscles from C7 without the medial cord being intact.

At the time of surgery, it was found that the medial cord had been interrupted by a bullet above the level of the medial pectoral nerve as had been indicated by the muscle testing.

PERIPHERAL NERVES — KEY → D. = Dorsal Prim. Ramus

Grade (LEFT)	Region	Muscle	Nerve	Spinal segments
•		HEAD & NECK EXTENSORS	Cervical (D.) 1-8	
	Cervical nerves	INFRAHYOID MUSCLES	Cervical (V.) 1-8	
		RECTUS CAP ANT. & LAT.	Cervical (V.) 1-4	
		LONGUS CAPITIS	Cervical	
		LONGUS COLLI		
		LEVATOR SCAPULAE		
		SCALENI (A. M. P.)		
		STERNOCLEIDOMASTOID		
		TRAPEZIUS (U. M. L.)		
		DIAPHRAGM	Phrenic 3,4,5	
N	Brachial Plexus — Root	SERRATUS ANTERIOR	Long Thor. 5,6,7(8)	
N		RHOMBOIDS MAJ & MIN	Dor. Scap 4,5	
N	Trunk	SUBCLAVIUS	N. to Subcl. 5,6	
N		SUPRASPINATUS	Suprascap 4,5,6	
N		INFRASPINATUS	Suprascap 4,5,6	
N	P Cord	SUBSCAPULARIS	U. Subscap (4),5,6,(7)	
N		LATISSIMUS DORSI	Thoracodor (5),6,7,8	
N		TERES MAJOR	L. Subscap 5,6,(7)	
N	M&L / L	PECTORALIS MAJ (UPPER)	Lat. Pect. 5,6,7	
G-		PECTORALIS MAJ (LOWER)	Med. Pect. (6),7,8	
P		PECTORALIS MINOR	Med. Pect.	(6) 7 8 1
N	Axil.	TERES MINOR	Axillary 5,6	5 6
N		DELTOID	Axillary	5 6
G-	Musculo-cutan	CORACOBRACHIALIS	Musculocu. (4),5,6,7	6 7
F+		BICEPS	Musculocu.	5 6
		BRACHIALIS		5 6
N	Radial — Lat.M	TRICEPS	Radial	6 7 8 1
		ANCONEUS		7 8
—		BRACHIALIS (SMALL PART)		5 6
G-		BRACHIORADIALIS		5 6
N		EXT CARPI RAD L		5 6 7 8
N	Post Inter	EXT CARPI RAD B		6 7 (8)
N		SUPINATOR		5 6 (7)
G-		EXT DIGITORUM		6 7 8
N		EXT DIGITI MINIMI		6 7 8
F+		EXT CARPI ULNARIS		6 7 8
G-		ABD POLLICIS LONGUS		6 7 8
G-		EXT POLLICIS BREVIS		6 7 8
G-		EXT POLLICIS LONGUS		6 7 8
—		EXT INDICIS		6 7 8
P	Median — A Inter	PRONATOR TERES	Median 5,6,7,8,1	6 7
F+		FLEX CARPI RADIALIS		6 7 8
—		PALMARIS LONGUS		(6) 7 8 1
G-		FLEX DIGIT SUPERFICIALIS		7 8 1
F+		FLEX DIGIT PROF I & II		7 8 1
F+		FLEX POLLICIS LONGUS		(6) 7 8 1
P		PRONATOR QUADRATUS		7 8 1
F+		ABD POLLICIS BREVIS		6 7 8 1
F-		OPPONENS POLLICIS		6 7 8 1
P		FLEX POLL BREV (SUP. H)		6 7 8 1
O		LUMBRICALES I & II		(6) 7 8 1
F+	Ulnar	FLEX CARPI ULNARIS	Ulnar 7,8,1	7 8 1
P		FLEX DIGIT. PROF. III & IV		7 8 1
—		PALMARIS BREVIS		(7) 8 1
O		ABD DIGITI MINIMI		(7) 8 1
O		OPPONENS DIGITI MINIMI		(7) 8 1
O		FLEX DIGITI MINIMI		(7) 8 1
O		PALMAR INTEROSSEI		8 1
O		DORSAL INTEROSSEI		8 1
O		LUMBRICALES III & IV		(7) 8 1
O		ADDUCTOR POLLICIS		8 1
O		FLEX POLL BREV. (DEEP H.)		8 1

Cord annotations: Post. cord (Radial group); Med. + Lat. cord (Median group); Med. cord (Ulnar group).

SENSORY

Dermatomes redrawn from Keegan and Garrett Anat Rec 102. 409. 437. 1948

Cutaneous Distribution of peripheral nerves redrawn from *Gray's Anatomy of the Human Body*. 28th ed

403

SPINAL SEGMENT DISTRIBUTION TO NERVES AND MUSCLES

For anatomists and clinicians, the determination of the spinal segment distribution to peripheral nerves and muscles has proven to be a difficult task. The pathway of the spinal nerves is obscured by the intertwining of the nerve fibers as they pass through the nerve plexuses. Since it is almost impossible to trace the course of an individual nerve fiber through the maze of its plexus, information regarding spinal segment distribution has been derived mainly from clinical observation. The use of this empirical method has resulted in a variety of findings regarding the segmental origins of these nerves and the muscles they innervate. An awareness of possible variations is important in the diagnosis and the location of a nerve lesion. To focus attention on the range of variations that exists, the Kendalls tabulated information from six well-known sources.

The chart on p. 410 shows the spinal segment distribution to nerves; the charts on pp. 406–409 show the distribution to muscles.

The compilations derived from the charts became part of the *Spinal Nerve and Muscle Charts.*

The symbols used in tabulating the reference material were: a large X to denote a major distribution, a small x to denote a minor distribution, and a parenthetical (x) to denote a possible or infrequent distribution.

For the chart *Spinal Segment Distribution to Nerves* (p. 410), T2 was included in the brachial plexus by all of the sources but separate columns for T2 were not added to the upper extremity chart because T2 contains only cutaneous sensory fibers. The information in the compilation columns on the two charts (p. 410) has been converted from X's to numbers in the right column. This information regarding spinal segment distribution to nerves appears at the top of the upper and lower extremity *Spinal Nerve and Muscle Chart* under the heading *Peripheral Nerves.*

In the Kendall compilation of spinal segment supply to muscles as it appears in the last column on the right of the tabulation (see pp. 407 and 409), the x's represent an arithmetical summary. As a general rule, if five or six authorities agree that a spinal segment was distributed to a given muscle, the nerve supply was indicated by a large X; if three or four agree, by a small x; if only two agree, by a small x in parentheses; if mentioned by only one source, it was disregarded. (See Triceps tabulation as an example.)

Triceps

	C6	C7	C8	T1
Gray (13)		X	X	
deJong (99)	X	X	X	(x)
Cunningham (100)	X	X	X	
Spalteholz (101)	x	X	X	(x)
Foerster & Bumke (102)	(x)	X	X	x
Haymaker & Woodhall (103)		X	X	x
Totals	4	6	6	4
Kendall Compilation	x	X	X	x
of Triceps innervation	C6	C7	C8	T1

When one of the six sources did not specify the spinal segment, agreement by four or five sources was indicated by a large X. This occurred for the Popliteus and some intrinsic muscles of the foot.

While the tabulation of data focuses attention on the range of variations that exists among these sources, the arithmetical summary indicates the extent of their agreement. Only in the case of three thumb muscles (Opponens, Abductor brevis, and superficial head of the Flexor brevis) were the six authorities divided in their opinion, resulting in an apparent overstatement of the number of roots of origin. The method used in compiling the information resulted in all segments being listed with small x's, i.e., C6, 7, 8, and T1, without major emphasis on any one segment.

In most instances, the arithmetical summary preserved the major emphasis on the spinal segments that provide innervation to the muscles. When the summary did not do so, exceptions were made. For example, all sources included C3, 4, 5 innervation to the Diaphragm, but all placed emphasis on C4, so only C4 was given a large X. All sources included the following spinal segment innervations: C5 for the Supinator, C8 for the Extensor carpi radialis longus and brevis, L4 for the Adductor longus, and L4 as a component of the sacral plexus. However, all represented these innervations by a small x indicating a minor distribution, so the compilation preserved the lesser emphasis. All sources included T(12) innervation to the lumbar plexus but all indicated it was a minimal supply so T(12) remained in parentheses in the compilation.

Innervation was omitted in the compilation in two instances because there was a discrepancy between the spinal segment innervation to the *muscle* and that to the *peripheral nerve* supplying the muscle. C8 innervation, mentioned by two of the sources as supplying the Subscapularis, was omitted because there was no indication that the upper or lower subscapular nerve received C8 innervation. Likewise, C(4), included by two sources for the Teres minor, was omitted since there was no indication that the axillary nerve received C4 innervation. In two other instances, innervation was added in the compilation. C6 and C7 were added to the medial pectoral nerve. Above the communicating loop, the medial pectoral nerve is composed of C8 and T1 fibers. Below the loop, C7 and possible C6 fibers (branching from the lateral pectoral nerve) join the medial pectoral nerve. While the medial cord of the plexus is derived from C8 and T1, the ulnar nerve, as the terminal branch of this cord, is listed as having a C7 component in addition to C8 and T1. Numerous anatomists (99–101) record this information and some (104–106) indicate that the C7 component is variable.

The compilation was modified in regard to spinal segment distribution to the upper and lower portions of the Pectoralis major. In the muscle sections of the books used as references for the compilation, only one text (100) divided the Pectoralis major muscle into upper and lower portions and listed the spinal segment innervation to each portion. However, Gray (13), in the description of the lateral and medial pectoral nerves, indicated that the lateral pectoral supplies the more cranial part of the muscle while the medial pectoral, joined by two or three branches from the lateral, supplies the more caudal part. In addition, several other references (100, 103, 107) differentiate the peripheral supply to the upper and lower parts. In certain lesions of the cervical region of the spinal cord, it has been noted, clinically, that the upper part of the Pectoralis major has had normal strength while the lower part has been paralyzed. This observation suggests that there is a difference in spinal segment innervation to the parts of the muscle. On the basis of the above information, the compilation distinguishes between the upper and lower parts of the Pectoralis major in regard to spinal segment distribution.

The results of the compilation, pp. 407 and 409, have been used in the spinal segment column on the nerve-muscle charts. The X's have been converted to numbers that indicate the specific spinal segment. In the nerve-muscle charts, the major emphasis, as designated in the compilation by large X's, has been obtained by using *numbers* that are slightly larger than those used for minor emphasis; and the possible or infrequent innervation, by numbers in parentheses.

Spinal Segment Distribution To Muscles:

MUSCLE	GRAY[13]									deJONG[99]									CUNNINGHAM[100]								
	C1	C2	C3	C4	C5	C6	C7	C8	T1	C1	C2	C3	C4	C5	C6	C7	C8	T1	C1	C2	C3	C4	C5	C6	C7	C8	T1
HEAD & NECK EXTENSORS	X	X	X	X	X	X	X	X	x	X	X	X	X	X	X	X	X		X	X	X	X	X	X	X	X	X
INFRAHYOID MUSCLES	X	X	X																X	X	X						
RECTUS CAP. ANT. & LAT.	X	X								X	X								X	X							
LONGUS CAPITIS	X	X	X							X	X	X	X						X	X	X	X					
LONGUS COLLI		X	X	X	X	X	X					X	X	X	X					X	X	X	X	X	X		
LEVATOR SCAPULAE			X	X	(x)							X	X	X							X	X	X				
SCALENI (A.M.P.)			X	X	X	X	X	X					X	X	X	X	X				X	X	X	X	X	x	
STERNOCLEIDOMASTOID		X	X							(x)	X	X								X							
TRAPEZIUS (U.M.L.)			X	X							(x)	X	X								X	X					
DIAPHRAGM			x	X	x							x	X	x							(x)	X	X				
SERRATUS ANTERIOR					X	X	X							X	X	X	X							X	X	X	
RHOMBOIDS, MAJ. & MINOR					X								X	X							x	X	X				
SUBCLAVIUS					X	X							(x)	X	X								X	X			
SUPRASPINATUS					X								(x)	X	X								X	X			
INFRASPINATUS					X	X								X	X								X	X			
SUBSCAPULARIS					X	X								X	X								X	X			
LATISSIMUS DORSI						X	X	X							X	X	X							X	X	X	
TERES MAJOR					X	X								X	X	(x)							X	X			
PECTORALIS MAJ. (UPPER)		}			X	X	X	X	X		}			X	X	X	X	X					X	X	X	X	X
PECTORALIS MAJ. (LOWER)		}			X	X	X	X	X		}			X	X	X	X	X						X	X	X	X
PECTORALIS MINOR							X	X								X	X	X							X	X	X
TERES MINOR					X								(x)	X	X								X	X			
DELTOID					X	X								X	X								X	X			
CORACOBRACHIALIS						X	X							X	X									X	X		
BICEPS					X	X								X	X								X	X			
BRACHIALIS					X	X								X	X								X	X			
TRICEPS							X	X							X	X	X	(x)							X	X	X
ANCONEUS							X	X								X	X								X	X	
BRACHIALIS (SMALL PART)					X	X								X	X								X	X			
BRACHIORADIALIS					X	X								X	X								X	X			
EXT. CARPI RAD. L. & B.						X	X							(x)	X	X	(x)						X	X	X	X	
SUPINATOR						X								X	X								X	X			
EXT. DIGITORUM						X	X	X							X	X	X							X	X	X	
EXT. DIGITI MINIMI						X	X	X							X	X	X							X	X	X	
EXT. CARPI ULNARIS						X	X	X							X	X	X							X	X	X	
ABD. POLLICIS LONGUS						X	X								X	X	X							X	X	X	
EXT. POLLICIS BREVIS						X	X								X	X	X							X	X	X	
EXT. POLLICIS LONGUS						X	X	X							X	X	X							X	X	X	
EXT. INDICIS						X	X	X							X	X	X							X	X	X	
PRONATOR TERES						X	X								X	X								X	X		
FLEX. CARPI RADIALIS						X	X								X	X	(x)							X	X	X	
PALMARIS LONGUS						X	X								(x)	X	X								X	X	X
FLEX. DIGIT. SUPERFICIALIS							X	X	X							X	X	X							X	X	X
FLEX. DIGIT. PROF. I & II								X	X							X	X	X							X	X	X
FLEX. POLLICIS LONGUS								X	X						X	X	X	X							X	X	X
PRONATOR QUADRATUS								X	X							X	X	X							X	X	X
ABD. POLLICIS BREVIS						X	X								X	X										X	X
OPPONENS POLLICIS						X	X								X	X										X	X
FLEX. POLL. BREV. (SUP. H.)						X	X								X	X										X	X
LUMBRICALES I & II						X	X								X	X	X	X								X	X
FLEX. CARPI ULNARIS								X	X							(x)	X	X								X	X
FLEX. DIGIT. PROF. III & IV								X	X							X	X	X								X	X
PALMARIS BREVIS								X								(x)	X	X								X	X
ABD. DIGITI MINIMI								X	X							(x)	X	X								X	X
OPPONENS DIGITI MINIMI								X	X							(x)	X	X								X	X
FLEX. DIGITI MINIMI								X	X							(x)	X	X								X	X
PALMAR INTEROSSEI								X	X								X	X								X	X
DORSAL INTEROSSEI								X	X								X	X								X	X
LUMBRICALES III & IV								X									X	X								X	X
ADDUCTOR POLLICIS								X	X								X	X								X	X
FLEX. POLL. BREV. (DEEP H.)								X	X								X	X								X	X

SPALTEHOLZ[101] SPINAL SEGMENT										FORESTER & BUMKE[102] SPINAL SEGMENT										HAYMAKER & WOODHALL[103] (modified after Bing) SPINAL SEGMENT										COMPILATION by Kendalls SPINAL SEGMENT									
C1	C2	C3	C4	C5	C6	C7	C8	T1		C1	C2	C3	C4	C5	C6	C7	C8	T1		C1	C2	C3	C4	C5	C6	C7	C8	T1		C1	C2	C3	C4	C5	C6	C7	C8	T1	
x	x	x	x	x	x	x	x	x	x	X	X	X	X	X	X	X	X	X	X		X	X	X	X	X	X	X	X		X	X	X	X	X	X	X	X	X	X
x	x	x								(x)	X	X	(x)							X	X	X								X	X	X							
x	x									X	x									X										X	X								
x	x	x								X	X	X								X	X	X	X	X						X	X	X	(x)						
	x	x	x	x	x							X	X	X	x					X	X	X	X	X						X	X	X	X	X	X	(x)			
	(x)	x	x	x								x	X	x						X	X	X								X	X	X							
		(x)	x	x	x	x						X	X	X	X	x				X	X	X	X	X	X					x	X	X	X	X	X				
	x									(x)	X	X								X										(x)	X	x							
	x	x	x							X	X	X	x							X	X	X								x	X	X							
		x	X	x						(x)	x	X	x							x	X	x								x	X	x							
			x	X	X	(x)					x	X	X	(x)						X	X	X								X	X	X	x						
			x							x	x									x										x	X								
			x	x						x	X	X								x	X									X	X								
		(x)	x	(x)						x	X									X	x									x	X	x							
		(x)	X	x						x	X	x								X	x									(x)	X	X							
			x	x	(x)					x	X	X	x							X	X	X	X							X	X	x							
			(x)	X	x					x	X	x								x	X	X								x	X	x							
			x	X						x	X									X	X									x	X	x							
		(x)	X	X	X	x		}		x	X	X	X	x		}			X	X	X	X	X						X	X	X							
				x	x					x	X	x								X	X	X								(x)	X	X	x						
		x	X	(x)						(x)	X	x								X	x									X	X								
		X	x							(x)	X	X								X	x									X	X								
		x	X							X	x	(x)								x	X									X	X								
		x	x	(x)						X	X									X	X									X	X								
		x	x	(x)						x	X									X	X									X	X								
			x	X	X	(x)				(x)	X	X	x							X	X	x								x	X	X	x						
			(x)	X	x	(x)				(not listed)										X	X									X	X								
			x	x	(x)					x	X									X	X									X	X								
			x	x						x	X									x	X									X	X								
		(x)	x	x	x					x	X	(x)								x	X	x								x	X	X	x						
		(x)	x	x	x					x	X									x	X									x	X	(x)							
		(x)	x	X	X					x	X	(x)								X	x									x	X	X							
			x	x						(not listed)										X	x									x	X	X							
		(x)	x	X						x	X									X	x									x	X	X							
		(x)	x	x						x	X									X	X									x	X	X							
		(x)	x	x						x	X									X	x									x	X	X							
		(x)	x	x						x	X									X	x									x	X	X							
		(x)	x	x						X	x									X	x									x	X	X							
			X	x						x	X									x	X									X	X								
			x	x	(x)					(x)	X	(x)								x	X	x								X	X	x							
			x	x	x						X	x								x	X	x								(x)	X	X	x						
		(x)	(x)	X	x						x	X	X							x	X	X								X	X	X							
			x	x	X	x					x	X	X							x	X	X								x	X	X							
			x	x	x						X	X								x	X	X								(x)	x	X	X						
			x	x	X	x					x	X	x							x	X	X								x	X	X							
			x	X	(x)						x	X									X	x									x	x	X	x						
			x	x	(x)	(x)					x	X									X	x								x	x	X	X							
			x	X	x						x	X									X	X								x	x	X	X							
			x	x	x						x	X								x	X	X								(x)	x	X	X						
				x	x						X	x								x	X	x								x	X	x							
			x	x	X	x					X	X							x	X	X								x	X	X								
				(x)	x	(x)					x	X									x	X								(x)	X	X								
				(x)	x	(x)					x	X									x	X								(x)	X	X								
				(x)	x	(x)					x	X									x	X								(x)	X	X								
				(x)	x	(x)					x	X									x	X								(x)	X	X								
				(x)	x	x					x	X									x	X									X	X								
				(x)	x	x					x	X									x	X									X	X								
					x	x	x				x	X							x	X	X									(x)	X	X							
						x	X	x			x	X								x	X	X									X	X								

GRAY[13] — Spinal Segment

MUSCLE	T1,2,3,4	T5,6	T7,8	T9,10,11	T12	L1	L2	L3	L4	L5	S1	S2	S3
ERECTOR SPINAE	X	X	X	X	X	X	X	X	X	X	X	X	X
SERRATUS POST. SUP.	X												
TRANS. THORACIS	X	X	X										
INT. INTERCOSTALS	X	X	X	X									
EXT. INTERCOSTALS	X	X	X	X									
SUBCOSTALES		X	X	X									
LEVATOR COSTARUM	X	X	X	X									
OBLIQUUS EXT. ABD.			X	X	X								
RECTUS ABDOMINIS			X	X	X								
OBLIQUUS INT. ABD.				X	X	X							
TRANSVERSUS ABD.				X	X	X							
SERRATUS POST. INF.													
QUAD. LUMBORUM					X	X							
PSOAS MINOR						X							
PSOAS MAJOR							X	X					
ILIACUS							X	X					
PECTINEUS							X	X	X				
SARTORIUS							X	X					
QUADRICEPS							X	X	X				
ADDUCTOR BREVIS							X	X	X				
ADDUCTOR LONGUS							X	X	X				
GRACILIS								X	X				
OBTURATOR EXT.								X	X				
ADDUCTOR MAGNUS							X	X	X				
GLUTEUS MEDIUS									X	X	X		
GLUTEUS MINIMUS									X	X	X		
TENSOR FAS. LAT.									X	X	X		
GLUTEUS MAXIMUS										X	X	X	
PIRIFORMIS										X	X	X	
GEMELLUS SUPERIOR									X	X	X		
OBTURATOR INTERNUS									X	X	X		
GEMELLUS INFERIOR								X	X	X			
QUADRATUS FEMORIS								X	X	X			
BICEPS (LONG HEAD)										X	X	X	X
SEMITENDINOSUS									X	X	X	X	
SEMIMEMBRANOSUS									X	X	X	X	
BICEPS (SHORT HEAD)									X	X	X		
TIBIALIS ANTERIOR								X	X	X			
EXT. HALL. LONG.								X	X	X			
EXT. DIGIT. LONG.								X	X	X			
PERONEUS TERTIUS								X	X	X			
EXT. DIGIT. BREVIS								X	X	X			
PERONEUS LONGUS								X	X	X			
PERONEUS BREVIS								X	X	X			
PLANTARIS								X	X	X			
GASTROCNEMIUS											X	X	
POPLITEUS								X	X	X			
SOLEUS											X	X	
TIBIALIS POSTERIOR									X	X			
FLEX. DIGIT. LONG.									X	X	X		
FLEX. HALL. LONG.									X	X	X		
FLEX. DIGIT. BREVIS									X	X	X		
ABDUCTOR HALLUCIS									X	X	X		
FLEX. HALLUCIS BREVIS									X	X	X		
LUMBRICALIS I									X	X	X		
ABD. DIGITI MINIMI											X	X	
QUAD. PLANTAE											X	X	
FLEX. DIGITI MINIMI											X	X	
OPP. DIGITI MINIMI											X	X	
ADDUCTOR HALLUCIS											X	X	
PLANT. INTEROSSEI											X	X	
DORSAL INTEROSSEI											X	X	
LUMBRICALES II, III, IV											X	X	

deJONG[99] — Spinal Segment

MUSCLE	T1,2,3,4	T5,6	T7,8	T9,10,11	T12	L1	L2	L3	L4	L5	S1	S2	S3
ERECTOR SPINAE	X	X	X	X	X	X	X	X	X	X	X	X	X
SERRATUS POST. SUP.	X												
TRANS. THORACIS	X	X	X										
INT. INTERCOSTALS	X	X	X	X									
EXT. INTERCOSTALS	X	X	X	X									
SUBCOSTALES	(not listed)												
LEVATOR COSTARUM				X	X								
OBLIQUUS EXT. ABD.		X	X	X	X								
RECTUS ABDOMINIS			X	X	X								
OBLIQUUS INT. ABD.				X	X	X							
TRANSVERSUS ABD.			X	X	X	X							
SERRATUS POST. INF.				X	X								
QUAD. LUMBORUM	(not listed)												
PSOAS MINOR						X	X						
PSOAS MAJOR						(X)	X	X	X				
ILIACUS							X	X	X				
PECTINEUS							X	X					
SARTORIUS							X	X					
QUADRICEPS							X	X	X				
ADDUCTOR BREVIS							X	X	X				
ADDUCTOR LONGUS							X	X	X				
GRACILIS							X	X	X				
OBTURATOR EXT.								X	X				
ADDUCTOR MAGNUS							X	X	X	X			
GLUTEUS MEDIUS									X	X	X		
GLUTEUS MINIMUS									X	X	X		
TENSOR FAS. LAT.									X	X	X		
GLUTEUS MAXIMUS										X	X	X	
PIRIFORMIS										X	X	X	
GEMELLUS SUPERIOR										X	X	X	
OBTURATOR INTERNUS										X	X	X	
GEMELLUS INFERIOR									X	X	X		
QUADRATUS FEMORIS									X	X	X		
BICEPS (LONG HEAD)										X	X	X	X
SEMITENDINOSUS									X	X	X	X	
SEMIMEMBRANOSUS									X	X	X	X	
BICEPS (SHORT HEAD)										X	X	X	
TIBIALIS ANTERIOR									X	X	X		
EXT. HALL. LONG.									X	X	X		
EXT. DIGIT. LONG.									X	X	X		
PERONEUS TERTIUS									X	X	X		
EXT. DIGIT. BREVIS									X	X	X		
PERONEUS LONGUS									X	X	X		
PERONEUS BREVIS									X	X	X		
PLANTARIS									X	X	X		
GASTROCNEMIUS											X	X	
POPLITEUS									X	X	X		
SOLEUS											X	X	
TIBIALIS POSTERIOR									X	X	X		
FLEX. DIGIT. LONG.										X	X	X	
FLEX. HALL. LONG.										X	X	X	
FLEX. DIGIT. BREVIS									X	X	X		
ABDUCTOR HALLUCIS									X	X	X		
FLEX. HALLUCIS BREVIS									X	X	X		
LUMBRICALIS I									X	X	X		
ABD. DIGITI MINIMI											X	X	
QUAD. PLANTAE											X	X	
FLEX. DIGITI MINIMI											X	X	
OPP. DIGITI MINIMI	(not listed)												
ADDUCTOR HALLUCIS										X	X	X	
PLANT. INTEROSSEI											X	X	
DORSAL INTEROSSEI											X	X	
LUMBRICALES II, III, IV										X	X	X	

CUNNINGHAM[100] — Spinal Segment

MUSCLE	T1,2,3,4	T5,6	T7,8	T9,10,11	T12	L1	L2	L3	L4	L5	S1	S2	S3
ERECTOR SPINAE	X	X	X	X	X	X	X	X	X	X	X	X	X
SERRATUS POST. SUP.	X												
TRANS. THORACIS	X	X	X										
INT. INTERCOSTALS	X	X	X	X									
EXT. INTERCOSTALS	X	X	X	X									
SUBCOSTALES		X	X	X									
LEVATOR COSTARUM													
OBLIQUUS EXT. ABD.			X	X	X								
RECTUS ABDOMINIS			X	X	X								
OBLIQUUS INT. ABD.				X	X	X							
TRANSVERSUS ABD.				X	X	X							
SERRATUS POST. INF.													
QUAD. LUMBORUM						X	X	X					
PSOAS MINOR						X	(x)						
PSOAS MAJOR						X	X	X	(x)				
ILIACUS							X	X					
PECTINEUS							X	X					
SARTORIUS							X	X					
QUADRICEPS							X	X	X				
ADDUCTOR BREVIS							X	X	x				
ADDUCTOR LONGUS							X	X	x				
GRACILIS							X	X	x				
OBTURATOR EXT.								X	X				
ADDUCTOR MAGNUS								X	X	X	x		
GLUTEUS MEDIUS									X	X	X		
GLUTEUS MINIMUS									X	X	X		
TENSOR FAS. LAT.									X	X	X		
GLUTEUS MAXIMUS										X	X	X	
PIRIFORMIS											X	X	
GEMELLUS SUPERIOR										X	X	X	
OBTURATOR INTERNUS										X	X	X	
GEMELLUS INFERIOR										X	X	X	
QUADRATUS FEMORIS									X	X	X		
BICEPS (LONG HEAD)										X	X	X	X
SEMITENDINOSUS									X	X	X	X	
SEMIMEMBRANOSUS									X	X	X	X	
BICEPS (SHORT HEAD)									X	X	X	X	
TIBIALIS ANTERIOR									X	X	X		
EXT. HALL. LONG.									X	X	X		
EXT. DIGIT. LONG.									X	X	X		
PERONEUS TERTIUS									X	X	X		
EXT. DIGIT. BREVIS									X	X	X		
PERONEUS LONGUS									X	X	X		
PERONEUS BREVIS									X	X	X		
PLANTARIS									X	X	X		
GASTROCNEMIUS											X	X	
POPLITEUS									X	X	X		
SOLEUS										X	X	X	
TIBIALIS POSTERIOR										X	X		
FLEX. DIGIT. LONG.										X	X	X	
FLEX. HALL. LONG.										X	X	X	
FLEX. DIGIT. BREVIS									x	X	X		
ABDUCTOR HALLUCIS									x	X	X		
FLEX. HALLUCIS BREVIS									x	X	X		
LUMBRICALIS I									x	X	X		
ABD. DIGITI MINIMI											X	X	
QUAD. PLANTAE											X	X	
FLEX. DIGITI MINIMI											X	X	
OPP. DIGITI MINIMI											X	X	
ADDUCTOR HALLUCIS											X	X	
PLANT. INTEROSSEI											X	X	
DORSAL INTEROSSEI											X	X	
LUMBRICALES II, III, IV											X	X	

SPALTEHOLZ[101]			FORESTER & BUMKE[102]			SCHADE[108] & HAYMAKER & WOODHALL[103]			COMPILATION by Kendalls		
SPINAL SEGMENT			SPINAL SEGMENT			SPINAL SEGMENT			SPINAL SEGMENT		
THORACIC	LUMBAR	SACRAL	THORACIC	LUMBAR	SACRAL	THORACIC	LUMBAR	SACRAL	THORACIC	LUMBAR	SACRAL
T1,2,3,4 / T5,6 / T7,8 / T9,10,11 / T12	L1 / L2 / L3 / L4 / L5	S1 / S2 / S3	T1,2,3,4 / T5,6 / T7,8 / T9,10,11 / T12	L1 / L2 / L3 / L4 / L5	S1 / S2 / S3	T1,2,3,4 / T5,6 / T7,8 / T9,10,11 / T12	L1 / L2 / L3 / L4 / L5	S1 / S2 / S3	T1,2,3,4 / T5,6 / T7,8 / T9,10,11 / T12	L1 / L2 / L3 / L4 / L5	S1 / S2 / S3

Spinal Segment Distribution to Nerves: Neck, Diaphragm, and Upper Extremity

NERVE	CUNNINGHAM[100]	GRAY[13]	MORRIS[107]	SPALTEHOLZ[101]	deJONG[99]	HAYMAKER & WOODHALL[103]	COMPILATION BY KENDALLS	SPINAL SEGMENTS USED FOR SPINAL NERVE & MUSCLE CHART
Cervical Plex.					(Not listed)			Cervical Plex. C 1,2,3,4
Brachial Plex.					(Not listed)			Brach. Plex. C(4),5,6,7,8,T1
Phrenic								Phrenic C3,4,5
Long Thoracic								Long. Thor. C5,6,7,(8)
Dorsal Scapular								Dor. Scap. C4,5
N. to Subclavius								N. to Subclavius C5, 6
Suprascapular								Suprascap. C4, 5, 6
Upp. Subscap.								U. Subscap. C(4),5,6,(7)
Thoracodorsal								Thoracodor. C(5), 6, 7, 8
Low. Subscap.								L. Subscap. C5,6,(7)
Lat. Pectoral				(Not listed)	(Not listed)			Lat. Pect. C5,6,7
Med. Pectoral								Med. Pect.* C(6),7,8, T1
Axillary								Axillary C5,6
Musculocutan.								Musculocutan. C(4),5,6,7
Radial								Radial C5, 6, 7, 8 T1
Median								Median C5, 6, 7, 8 T1
Ulnar								Ulnar C7,8 T1

*See innervation to pectoral muscles, pp. 406–407.

Spinal Segment Distribution to Nerves: Trunk and Lower Extremity

NERVE	CUNNINGHAM[100]	GRAY[13]	MORRIS[107]	SPALTEHOLZ[101]	deJONG[99]	HAYMAKER & WOODHALL[103]	COMPILATION BY KENDALLS	SPINAL SEGMENTS USED FOR SPINAL NERVE & MUSCLE CHART
Iliohypogastric								Iliohypogastric T12, L1
Ilioinguinal								Ilioinguinal T(12), L1
Lumb. Plex.					(Not listed)			Lumb. Plex. T(12), L1, 2, 3, 4
Femoral								Femoral L(1), 2, 3, 4
Obturator								Obturator L(1), 2, 3, 4
Sup. Gluteal								Sup. Glut. L4, 5, S1
Inf. Gluteal								Inf. Glut. L5, S1, 2
Sac. Plex.					(Not listed)			Sac. Plex. L4, 5, S1, 2, 3
Sciatic								Sciatic L4, 5, S1, 2, 3
Common Peroneal								C. Peroneal L4,5,S1,2
Tibial								Tibial L4, 5, S1, 2, 3

Glossary

Abduction. See **Joint motions**.

Active insufficiency. The inability of a two-joint (or multi-joint) muscle to generate an effective force when placed in a fully shortened position. The same meaning is implied by the expression "the muscle has been put on a slack."

Adaptive shortening. Tightness that occurs as a result of a muscle remaining in a shortened position.

Adduction. See **Joint motions**.

Agonist. A contracting muscle whose action is opposed by another muscle (antagonist).

Alignment. The arrangement of body segments as seen in various postural positions. See *ideal alignment* and *faulty alignments* on pp. 75–98.

Anatomical position. Erect posture with face forward, arms at sides, forearms supinated so that palms of the hands face forward, and fingers and thumbs in extension. The anatomical position is the reference for terms relating to joint motions, planes, axes, surfaces, and directions, and is the zero position for measuring joint motion.

Antagonist. A muscle that works in opposition to another muscle (agonist); opponent.

Anterior. See **Direction** and **Surfaces**.

Anterior pelvic tilt. See **Pelvic tilt**.

Anterior-posterior plane. See **Planes**.

Assessment. See **Tests and Measurements**.

Asymptomatic. Having no subjective complaints; presenting no symptoms of disease or dysfunction.

Axes. Lines, real or imaginary, about which movement takes place. There are three basic types of axes at right angles to each other:

> **Coronal axis.** A horizontal line extending from side to side, about which the movements of *flexion and extension* take place.

> **Longitudinal axis.** A vertical line extending in a craniocaudal direction about which movements of *rotation* take place.

> **Sagittal axis.** A horizontal line extending from front to back, about which movements of *abduction and adduction* take place.

Axial line. A line of reference in the hand or foot. *In the hand*, the axial line extends in line with the third metacarpal and the third digit. *In the foot*, the axial line extends in line with the second metatarsal and the second digit.

Body mechanics. The science concerned with static and dynamic forces acting on the body; the efficient or inefficient use of these forces in relation to body positions and movements.

Bowlegs. Outward bowing of the legs.

> **Structural bowing** involves *actual bowing* of the bones of the lower extremities; genu varum.

> **Postural bowing** is an *apparent bowing* that results from a combination of pronation of the feet, hyperextension of the knees, and medial rotation of the hips.

Break test. A muscle strength test used to elicit the maximal effort exerted by a subject who is performing an isometric contraction as the examiner applies a gradual build-up of pressure to the point that the effort by the subject is overcome, i.e., the "breaking point." The break test is applicable for grading muscle strength of fair+ (6) through good+ (9) but not for grades of fair or below, nor for the grade of normal.

Center of gravity. That point on a body, freely acted upon by the earth's gravity, about which the body is in equilibrium; the point at which the three midplanes of the body intersect. In an ideally aligned posture, it is considered to be slightly anterior to the first or second sacral segment.

Circumduction. See **Joint motions**.

Clockwise rotation. See **Joint motions—Rotation**.

Compression. The force (or stress) that tends to shorten a body or squeeze it together. See **Tension, 2** for opposite meaning.

Concentric contraction. See **Contraction**.

Contractility. The property of a muscle that enables it to generate an effective force (produce tension). See **Tension, 1**.

Contraction. An increase in muscle tension, with or without change in overall length.

> **Concentric.** A shortening contraction; an isotonic contraction.

> **Eccentric.** A lengthening contraction.

> **Isometric.** Increase in tension without change in muscle length.

> **Isotonic.** Increase in tension with change in muscle length (in the direction of shortening); concentric contraction.

Contracture. A marked decrease in muscle length; range of motion in the direction of elongating the muscle is markedly limited.

> **Irreversible contracture.** A contracture that cannot be released by treatment because elastic tissue has been replaced by inelastic tissue.

Contraindication. A sign or symptom that indicates that a particular treatment or procedure is not appropriate.

Contralateral. On the opposite side.

Coronal axis. See **Axes**.

Coronal plane. See **Planes**.

Counterclockwise rotation. See **Joint motions—Rotation**.

Criteria. Standards upon which a decision can be based; established rules or principles for any given test.

Curves of the spine. Cervical, thoracic, lumbar (flexible curves), and sacral curve (fixed curve).

Normal curves. Slightly anterior in the cervical region, slightly posterior in the thoracic region, slightly anterior in the lumbar region, and posterior in the sacral region.

Abnormal curves. See **Kyphosis, Lordosis, Sway-back posture,** and **Scoliosis.**

Diagnosis. The identification and classification of a disease, injury, or dysfunction based on examination findings.

Musculoskeletal diagnosis is the identification and classification of musculoskeletal dysfunction.

Diagnostic. Useful in determining a diagnosis; pertaining to the art and science of distinguishing one injury, disease, or dysfunction from another.

Direction.

Anterior. Toward the front or ventral surface.

Posterior. Toward the back or dorsal surface.

Caudal. Downward, away from the head; (toward the tail).

Cranial. Upward, toward the head.

Distal. Farther from the center or median line, or from the trunk.

Proximal. Nearer to the center or median line, or to the trunk.

Lateral. Away from the midline.

Medial. Toward the midline.

Distal. See **Direction**.

Dorsiflexion. See **Joint motions**.

Dysfunction. Inability to function properly; functional impairment; or disability.

Eccentric contraction. See **Contraction**.

Evaluation. See **Tests and Measurements**.

Eversion. A combination of pronation and forefoot abduction; talipes valgus. (Eversion is more free in dorsiflexion than in plantar flexion.)

Examination. See **Tests and Measurements**.

Extensibility. The property of muscle that permits it to lengthen or be elongated.

Extension. See **Joint motions**.

External rotation. See **Joint motions—Lateral rotation**.

Fixation. Includes stabilization, support, and counterpressure; implies holding firm.

Flexibility. The ability to readily adapt to changes in position or alignment; may be expressed as normal, limited, or excessive.

Flexion. See **Joint motions**.

Frontal plane. See **Planes**.

Genu valgum. Knock-knees.

Genu varum. Bowlegs.

Goniometer. An instrument for measuring angles and determining range of joint motion.

Gravity line. A vertical line through the center of gravity: a line analogous to the intersection of the midsaggital and midcoronal planes.

Horizontal abduction. See **Joint motions**.

Horizontal adduction. See **Joint motions**.

Hyperextension. See **Joint motions**.

Ideal alignment. The alignment used as a standard when evaluating posture. (See pp. 71, 75, and 88.)

Impingement. An encroachment on the space occupied by soft tissue, such as nerve or muscle. In this text, impingement refers to nerve irritation (i.e., from pressure or friction) associated with muscles.

Indication. A sign or symptom that points out that a particular treatment or procedure is appropriate.

Internal rotation. See **Joint motions—Medial rotation**.

Intervening muscles. Muscles that hold an adjacent part (usually an arm or a leg) firmly fixed to the bone of insertion, thereby providing a longer lever for the purpose of testing and grading muscle strength. Examples: posterior Deltoid in Trapezius test, shoulder flexors in Serratus anterior test.

Inversion. A combination of supination and forefoot adduction; talipes varus. (Inversion is more free in plantar flexion than in dorsiflexion.)

Ipsilateral. On the same side.

Isometric contraction. See **Contraction**.

Isotonic contraction. See **Contraction**.

Joint Motions.

> **Abduction** and **Adduction**. Movement about a sagittal axis in a coronal plane; i.e., in a sideways direction. *Abduction* is movement away from, and *adduction* is movement toward, the midsaggital plane of the body, except for fingers, toes, and thumb. For fingers and toes, *abduction* is movement away from, and *adduction* is movement toward the axial line of the hand or foot. For the thumb, *abduction* is movement away from, and *adduction* is movement toward, the palm of the hand.

> **Circumduction.** A circular (conical) movement that results from a combination of flexion, extension, abduction, adduction, and rotation.

> **Dorsiflexion.** Ankle joint extension; opposite of plantar flexion. (Often mistakenly called flexion.) (See p. 22.)

> **Extension.** See **Flexion** and **Extension**.

> **Flexion** and **Extension**. In general, *flexion* means bending and *extension* means straightening. This meaning is applicable to the hinge joints in the body, i.e., the elbow joint, the finger joints, and

the knee joint. The meaning also is applicable to the thoracic spine. However, this simple definition does not suffice for other extremity joints, neck, and low back. Technically, *flexion* and *extension* are movements about a coronal axis in a sagittal plane (i.e., in anterior and posterior directions). *Flexion* is movement in the anterior direction, and *extension* is movement in the posterior direction for all extremity joints except the knee, ankle, foot, and toes. For these exceptions, *flexion* is movement in a posterior direction and *extension* in an anterior direction. See explanation, p. 13. In the neck and low back, flexion is movement of the spine in a posterior direction, i.e., moving from a position of anterior convexity to a straight position.

Horizontal abduction and **adduction.** Movements of the arm about a longitudinal axis in the transverse plane; *abduction* is movement away from the midline and *adduction* is movement toward the midline.

Hyperextension. 1. *Movement* beyond the normal range of joint motion in extension. **2.** A *position* of extension that is greater than normal postural alignment but not beyond the normal range of joint motion. It is seen as a lordotic position of the cervical spine in a typical forward-head posture, as a lordosis of the lumbar spine along with anterior pelvic tilt, and as hip joint extension in a sway-back posture.

Plantar flexion. Ankle joint flexion; opposite of dorsiflexion. (Often mistakenly called extension.) (See p. 22.)

Rotation. Movement about a longitudinal axis in a transverse plane.

> **Lateral or external rotation.** Turning the anterior surface of the extremity away from the midline of the body.

> **Medial or internal rotation.** Turning the anterior surface of the extremity toward the midline of the body.

> **Clockwise rotation.** Used in describing rotation of the thorax or pelvis. With the transverse plane as a reference and 12 o'clock at midpoint anteriorly, rotation forward on the left is clockwise rotation. (Also described as facing toward the right.)

> **Counterclockwise rotation.** Used in describing rotation of the thorax or pelvis. With the transverse plane as a reference and 12 o'clock at midpoint anteriorly, rotation forward on the right is counterclockwise rotation. (Also described as facing toward the left.)

Knock-knees. Knees touch with feet apart; genu valgum.

Kyphosis. An abnormal posterior curve, usually found in the thoracic region of the spine. As such, it is an *exaggeration of the normal posterior curve.* If used without any modifying word, it refers to a thoracic kyphosis. In the low back, there is, occasionally, a lumbar kyphosis which is a *reversal of the normal anterior curve.*

Lateral. See **Direction** and **Surfaces.**

Lateral flexion. Side bending; movement in which the body bends toward the side of concavity while the spine curves convexly toward the opposite side. (Curves of the spine are named according to the convexity; a curve to the right is lateral flexion toward the left.)

Lateral pelvic tilt. See **Pelvic tilt**.

Lateral rotation. See **Joint motions**.

Lordosis. An abnormal anterior curve, usually found in the lumbar region, and as such is an *exaggeration of the normal anterior curve* (avoid use of the term "normal lordosis"); often called "hollow back." It is accompanied by anterior pelvic tilt and hip joint flexion. If used without any modifying word, it refers to a lumbar lordosis. In the thoracic region, occasionally, there is a slight lordosis which is a *reversal of the normal posterior curve*. In a typical forward head position, the neck is in a position of extension that is greater than the normal anterior curve and as such resembles a lordosis.

Measurable test. A test that is quantifiable, based on a standard. One of the criteria for muscle length and strength tests.

Medial. See **Direction** and **Surfaces**.

Medial rotation. See **Joint motions**.

Median or midsagittal plane. See **Planes**.

Mobility. Ability to move freely.

Muscle balance. A state of equilibrium that exists when there is a balance of strength of opposing muscles acting on a joint, providing ideal alignment for movement and optimal stabilization.

Muscle imbalance. Inequality in strength of opposing muscles; a state of muscle imbalance exists when a muscle is weak and its antagonist is strong; leads to faults in alignment and inefficient movement.

Neutral position of the pelvis. One in which anterior-superior spines are in the same transverse plane, and the anterior-superior spines and the symphysis pubis are in the same vertical plane.

Normal. Conforming to a standard. See normal alignment, pp. 71, 75, and 88; normal flexibility according to age, pp. 48 and 112; normal range of motion, p. 25; and normal strength, pp. 186 and 190.

Normal flexion of lumbar spine. Straightening or flattening of the lumbar spine.

Ober test. A test for tightness of the Tensor fasciae latae and the Iliotibial band. (See p. 57.)

Objective. Pertaining to findings evident to the examiner. See **Sign**.

Optimal test position. Completed range of motion for one-joint muscles; a position within the mid-range of the overall length for *two-joint* muscles.

Overstretch. Stretch beyond the normal range of muscle length.

Overstretch weakness. Weakness in a two-joint (or multi-joint) muscle resulting from repetitive movements or habitual positions that *elongate the muscle beyond normal range of muscle length*.

Passive insufficiency. Shortness of a two-joint (or multi-joint) muscle; the length of the muscle is not sufficient to permit *normal elongation* over both joints simultaneously, e.g., short Hamstrings (34).

Passive range of motion. Movement through available, pain-free range of motion, performed by another individual without participation by the subject.

Pelvic tilt. An anterior (forward), a posterior (backward), or a lateral (sideways) tilt of the pelvis from neutral position. (See also **Neutral position of the pelvis.**)

> **Anterior tilt.** Pelvic tilt in which the vertical plane through the anterior-superior spines is anterior to the vertical plane through the symphysis pubis.

> **Posterior tilt.** Pelvic tilt in which the vertical plane through the anterior-superior spines is posterior to the vertical plane through the symphysis pubis.

> **Lateral tilt.** Pelvic tilt in which the crest of the ilium is higher on one side than on the other.

Planes. Two-dimensional, flat surfaces, real or imaginary, at right angles to each other.

> **Coronal (frontal or lateral) plane.** A vertical plane, extending from side to side, dividing the body into an anterior and a posterior portion.

> **Sagittal (anterior-posterior) plane.** A vertical plane, extending from front to back. The midsaggital (or median) plane divides the body into right and left halves.

> **Transverse plane.** A horizontal plane, dividing the body into upper (cranial) and lower (caudal) portions.

Plantar flexion. See **Joint motions.**

Plumb line. A line (piece of cord) to which is attached a plumb bob (a small lead weight). When suspended, it represents a vertical line. When used for analyzing standing posture, it must be suspended in line with fixed points, namely, midway between heels in posterior view, and just anterior to the lateral malleolus in a lateral view.

Posterior. See **Direction.**

Posterior pelvic tilt. See **Pelvic tilt.**

Practical test. A test that is relatively easy to perform and requires a minimum of equipment. One of the criteria for muscle length and strength tests.

Pressure. In muscle testing, the force applied by the examiner to elicit the strength of a muscle holding in *test position.* (Pertains to muscles grading fair + (6) or better.)

Pronation. A rotation movement. *Pronation of the forearm* occurs when the distal end of the radius moves from the anatomic lateral position (supination) to a medial position, causing the hand to face posteriorly. *Pronation of the foot* occurs when the foot rotates so that the sole of the foot faces in a somewhat lateral direction. In standing, weight is on the inner side of the foot.

Prone. Lying face downward; face-lying.

Protective muscle spasm. A reflex muscle spasm by which nature "splints" or immobilizes a part to avoid movement that would cause further irritation of the injured structure.

Proximal. See **Direction**.

"Put on a slack." Placing the muscle in a shortened position in which it is incapable of developing enough tension to exert an effective force. (Applies to two-joint muscles but not to one-joint muscles.) See **Active insufficiency**.

Range of motion. The range, usually expressed in degrees, through which a joint can move or be moved.

Referred pain. Pain that is felt at some distance from its source.

Reliable test. A test that produces the same results on successive trials. One of the criteria for muscle length and strength tests.

Resistance. A force tending to hinder motion; in muscle testing, refers to resistance by the examiner or by gravity during *test movements*.

Rotation. See **Joint motions**.

Round shoulders. Forward shoulders.

Round upper back. A kyphosis.

Sagittal axis. See **Axes**.

Sagittal plane. See **Planes**.

Scoliosis. Lateral curvature of the spine. The spine may curve toward one side only or may have compensatory curves. A lateral curve convex toward the right is a right curve and vice versa.

Shortness. Tightness; denotes a slight to moderate decrease in muscle length; movement in the direction of elongating the muscle is limited.

Sign. Indication of an abnormality, related to disease or dysfunction, that is evident to the examiner, i.e., objective evidence. Compare with **Symptom**.

Sit-up. The movement of coming from a supine to a sitting position by flexing at the hip joints. ("Trunk curl," which is spine flexion, should not be called a partial sit-up.)

Spasm. An involuntary muscle contraction.

Sprain. Injury to a joint with possible rupture of ligaments or tendons, but without dislocation.

Stability. Capacity to provide support; firmness in position.

Stabilization. Fixation; implies holding steady or holding down.

Strain. The effect of an injurious tension.

Stress. Any force that tends to distort a body. It may be in the direction of either pulling apart or pressing together.

Stretch. To elongate; increase in length. The implied meaning is that it is not beyond the normal length of the muscle. See also **Overstretch**.

Stretch weakness. Weakness that results from muscles remaining in an elongated condition, however slight, beyond the neutral physiological rest position, but *not* beyond the normal range of muscle length.

The concept relates to the duration of the faulty alignment rather than to the severity of it. See discussion p. 334; re multi-joint muscles, see **Overstretch weakness**.

Subjective. Perceived by the individual; not evident to the examiner. See **Symptom**.

Substitution. The action of muscles in attempting to function in place of other muscles that fail to perform because of weakness or pain.

Supination. A rotation movement. *Supination of the forearm* occurs when the distal end of the radius moves from a position of medial rotation (pronation) to the anatomic lateral position, causing the palm of the hand to face anteriorly. *Supination of the foot* occurs when the foot rotates so that the sole of the foot faces in a somewhat medial direction. In standing, weight is borne on the outer side of the foot.

Supine. Lying face upward; back-lying.

Surfaces.

> **Dorsal.** The posterior surface of the body, except that the front (or top) of the foot is the dorsal surface.

> **Lateral.** The outer side.

> **Medial.** The inner side.

> **Palmar (volar).** The palm of the hand.

> **Plantar.** The sole of the foot.

> **Ventral.** The anterior surface of the body.

Sway-back posture. A faulty postural alignment in which there is a posterior displacement (swaying back) of the upper trunk and an anterior displacement (swaying forward) of the pelvis. There is a long kyphosis extending into the upper lumbar region, and a flattening of the low lumbar region. The pelvis is in posterior tilt and the hip joints are extended. The head and neck are in a forward head position.

Symptom. An abnormality in function or sensation, perceived by the patient, and indicative of disease or dysfunction; i.e., subjective evidence. Compare with **Sign**.

Syndrome. A group of signs and symptoms that appear together as characteristic of a disease, lesion, or dysfunction.

Taut. Firm when fully elongated; not slack. Muscles become taut at the end of the available range of motion permitted by the muscle length, i.e., when stretched to their limit. See p. 184.

Tension. 1. As *applied to muscles*: the effective force generated by a muscle. **2.** As *applied to body mechanics*: the force (or stress) that tends to lengthen a body. Compression and tension are opposite in meaning. **3.** As *applied to headaches*: tightness of the posterior neck muscles.

Test movement. A movement of the part in a specified direction and through a specified arc of motion.

Test position. The position in which the part is placed by the examiner, and held (if possible) by the patient.

Tests and Measurements:

Test. A procedure for obtaining measurements to be interpreted according to a standard; e.g., a muscle length, muscle strength, range of motion, or alignment test.

Examination. A procedure that includes more than one type of test; e.g., a postural examination that includes a variety of tests.

Assessment. An appraisal of objective data from tests and examinations.

Evaluation. Interpretation of objective and subjective data for the purpose of determining a musculoskeletal diagnosis and the appropriate course of treatment.

Thomas Test. Definition from Jones and Lovett: "The Thomas flexion test is founded upon our inability to extend a diseased hip without producing a lordosis. If there is flexion deformity, the patient is unable to extend the thigh on the diseased side, and it remains at an angle" (61).

Tight. 1. Short, limiting the range of motion; i.e., the muscle *is* tight. **2.** Firm on palpation when drawn taut, i.e., the muscle *feels* tight; (may be true of a short or a stretched muscle).

Tightness. Shortness; denotes a slight to moderate decrease in muscle length; movement in the direction of lengthening the muscle is limited.

Tilt. Rotation about a transverse axis. See **Pelvic tilt**.

Transverse plane. See **Planes**.

Trendelenburg sign. Indication of hip abductor weakness as evidenced by the hip going into *adduction* when standing with full weight on the affected leg with the other foot off the floor. Initially, the Trendelenburg Test was used in diagnosing a dislocated hip. The Trendelenburg Gait is one in which the affected hip goes into *adduction* during each weight-bearing phase of the gait. This is in contrast to the *abducted* position of the hip joint in the gait associated with paralysis of hip abductors. See p. 222.

Useful test. A test that provides information of value for determining the proper course of treatment. One of the criteria for muscle length and strength tests.

Valgus. Knee (genu v.): knock-knees. Foot (talipes v.): pronation with forefoot abduction. Big toe (hallux v.): adduction of big toe (toward midline of foot), associated with a bunion.

Valid test. One that measures, quantitatively and qualitively, what it purports to measure. One of the criteria for muscle length and strength tests.

Varus. Knee (genu v.): bowlegs. Foot (talipes v.): supination with forefoot adduction.

Ventral. Front or anterior, as anterior surface of the body.

Bibliography

REFERENCES CITED IN TEXT

1. Paris SV. The Paris approach. Postgraduate advances in the evaluation and treatment of low back dysfunction. Berryville, Virginia: *Forum Medicum*, 1989. **p. ix**
2. Wright WG. Muscle function. New York: Paul B Hoeber, 1928. **p. xi**
3. Goldthwait JE et al. Essentials of body mechanics in health and disease. 4th ed. Philadelphia: JB Lippincott, 1945. **p. xi**
4. Posture and its relationship to orthopaedic disabilities. A report of the Posture Committee of the American Academy of Orthopaedic Surgeons, 1947:1. **p. 3**
5. Toffler A. Powershift. New York: Bantam Books, 1991. **p. 7**
6. Introducing the most significant aid to manual muscle testing ever devised: Myo-Metric II. [Advertising brochure.] **p. 7**
7. MicroFET: Technology applied to muscles. EMPI. [Advertising handout.] **p. 7**
8. Rheault W, Beal J, Kubick K, Novak T, Shepley J. Intertester reliability of the hand-held dynamometer for wrist flexion and extension. *Arch Phys Med Rehabil* 1989;70:909. **p. 7**
9. Brinkmann JR. Comparison of a hand-held to a fixed dynamometer in tracking strength change. [Abstract R226] In: Abstracts of papers accepted for presentation at the 67th Annual Conference of the American Physical Therapy Association, June 14–18, 1992. *Phys Ther* 1992;72(6)Suppl. **p. 7**
10. Rothstein JM. Muscle biology—clinical considerations. *Phys Ther* 1982;62(12)1825. **p. 7**
11. Inman VT, Saunders JB, de CM, Abbott LC. Observations on the function of the shoulder joint. *J Bone Joint Surg* 1944;26:1. **p. 17**
12. Stedman's medical dictionary. 25th ed. Baltimore: Williams & Wilkins, 1990. **p. 23**
13. Goss CM, ed. Gray's anatomy of the human body. 28th ed. Philadelphia: Lea & Febiger, 1966:277, 311, 319, 380–381, 968. **p. 29, 357, 365, 377, 388, 404**
14. Protractor and calipers: Prototype made for HO Kendall, 1953. Sample copies made by Chattanooga Group, 1992, **p. 32**
15. Kendall HO et al. Posture and pain. Baltimore: Williams & Wilkins, 1952:72–73, 156–159. **p. 33, 343, 344, 349, 357, 376**
16. Shober P. Lendenwirbelsaule und Kreuzschmerzen. Munch med Wschr 1937;84:336. **p. 51**
17. Macrae IF, Wright V. Measurement of back movement. *Ann Rheum Dis* 1969;28:584. **p. 51**
18. Miller SA, Mayer T, Cos R, Gatchel R. Reliability problems associated with the modified Schober technique for true lumbar flexion measurement. *Spine* 1992;17(3)345–348. **p. 51**
19. Ober FR. Back strain and sciatica. *JAMA* 1935; 104(18):1580–1581. **p. 56, 362**
20. Ober FR. Relation of the fascia lata to conditions of the lower part of the back. *JAMA* 1937;109(8):554–555. **p. 56, 58, 350**
21. Hoppenfeld S. Physical examination of the spine and extremities. East Norwalk, Connecticut: Appleton-Century-Crofts, 1976:167, 144. **p. 56**
22. Rothstein JM et al. The rehabilitation specialist's handbook. Philadelphia: FA Davis, 1991:64–65. **p. 56**
23. Guides to the evaluation of permanent impairment. Chicago: American Medical Association, 1984. **p. 56**
24. Daniels L, Worthingham C. Muscle testing—techniques of manual examination, 5th ed. Philadelphia: WB Saunders, 1986:54. **p. 56**
25. Palmer ML, Epler ME. Clinical assessment procedures in physical therapy. Philadelphia: JB Lippincott, 1990:247–248. **p. 26**
26. Norkin CC, White DJ. Measurement of joint motion: a guide to goniometry. Philadelphia: FA Davis, 1985:139. **p. 26**
27. Basmajian JV, De Luca DJ. Muscles alive. 5th ed. Baltimore: Williams & Wilkins, 1985:255, 414. **p. 71, 328**
28. Kendall HO, Kendall FP. Normal flexibility according to age groups. *J Bone Joint Surg* [Am] 1948;30-A:690. **p. 112**
29. Licht S. History. In: Basmajian JV. Therapeutic exercises 3rd ed. Baltimore: Williams & Wilkins, 1978:29. 4th ed. 1984:30. **p. 121**
30. Cailliet R. Exercises for scoliosis. In: Basmajian JV. Therapeutic exercise. 3rd ed. Baltimore: Williams & Wilkins, 1978:434. 4th ed. 1984:469. **p. 121**
31. American Academy of Orthopaedic Surgeons Staff. Instructional Course Lectures. Vol 34. St. Louis, Missouri: CV Mosby, 1985:103–104. **p. 121**
32. Boileau JC, Basmajian JV. Grant's methods of anatomy. 7th ed. Baltimore: Williams & Wilkins, 1965. **p. 164**
33. Nachemson A, Elfstron G. Intravital dynamic pressure measurements in lumbar discs. Stockholm: Almqvista Wiksell, 1970. **p. 166**
34. O'Connell AL, Gardner EB. Understanding the scientific basis of human motion. Baltimore: Williams & Wilkins, 1972:38. **p. 179**
35. Legg AT. Physical therapy in infantile paralysis. In: Mock. Principles and practice of physical therapy. Vol II. Hagerstown, Maryland: WF Prior, 1932:45. **p. 188**
36. Sobotta-Figge. Atlas of human anatomy. Vol 1. Munich: Urban & Schwarzenberg, 1974. **p. 314, 315**
37. Duchenne GB. Physiology of motion. Philadelphia: JB Lippincott, 1949:480. **p. 324**
38. Shneerson J. Disorders of ventilation. London: Blackwell Scientific Publications, 1988:22, 31, 155, 287, 289. **p. 324, 328, 330**
39. Youmans WD, Siebens AA. Respiration. In: Brobeck, ed. Best and Taylor's physiological basis of medical practice. 9th ed. Baltimore: Williams & Wilkins, 1973:6–30, 6–35. **p. 324, 325**
40. Guz A, Noble M, Eisele J, Trenchard D. The role of vagal inflation reflexes. In: Porter R, ed. Breathing: Hering-Breuer Centenary Symposium. A CIBA Foundation Symposium. London: JA Churchill, 1970:155, 235, 246, 287, 289. **p. 324**
41. Cherniack RM et al. Respiration in health and disease. 2nd ed. Philadelphia: WB Saunders, 1972:410. **p. 328**
42. Egan DF. Fundamentals of respiratory therapy. 3rd ed. St. Louis, Missouri: CV Mosby, 1977. **p. 329, 330**
43. Williams PL, Warwick R, Dyson M, Bannister L, eds. Gray's anatomy. 37th ed. New York: Churchill Livingstone, 1989:552–553, 563, 573, 564, 612. **p. 329**
44. Moore KL. Clinically oriented anatomy. 2nd ed. Baltimore: Williams & Wilkins, 1985. **p. 330**
45. Lehman JF, ed. Therapeutic heat and cold. Baltimore: Williams & Wilkins, 1982:404, 563–564. **p. 337**
46. Adams RD et al. Diseases of muscle. New York: Paul B Hoeber, 1953:15, 121, 415, 429, 441. **p. 338**
47. Sunderland S. Nerves and nerve injuries. 2nd ed. New York: Churchill Livingstone, 1978:692–694, 753, 906, 925, 970, 1011–1013, 1031. **p. 338, 376, 377**
48. Margolis S, Moses S, eds. Johns Hopkins medical handbook. New York: Rebus, 1992:128, 129. **p. 341**
49. Ayub E, Glasheen-Wray M, Kraus S. Head posture: a case study of the effects on the rest position of the mandible. *J. Orthop Sports Phys Ther* 1984;6:179–183. **p. 341**
50. Dawson DM, Hallett M, Millender LH. Entrapment neuropathies. 2nd ed. Boston: Little, Brown, 1990:218, 237, 245, 246, 270, 279, 311, 344–346, 348. **p. 343, 344, 376, 377, 378**

NOTE: Page numbers in bold type indicate page references in this text.

51. Cahill BR. Quadrilateral space syndrome. In: Omer GE, Spinner M. Management of peripheral nerve problems. Philadelphia: WB Saunders, 1980:602–606. **p. 344**

52. CD Denison Orthopaedic Appliance Corporation, 220 W 28th St, Baltimore, Maryland. **p. 345, 370**

53. Burstein D. Joint compression for treatment of shoulder pain. *Clin Man* 1985:5(2):9. **p. 345**

54. DeRosa CP, Porterfield JA. A physical therapy model for the treatment of low back pain. *Phys Ther* 1992; 72(4):263. **p. 349**

55. Kendall HO, Kendall FP. Study and treatment of muscle imbalance in cases of low back and sciatic pain. Baltimore: privately printed, 1936. **p. 349**

56. Fahrni WH, Trueman GE. Comparative radiological study of spines of a primitive population with North Americans and North Europeans. *J Bone Joint Surg* [Br] 1965;47-B:552. **p. 350**

57. Basmajian JV. Primary anatomy, 5th ed. Baltimore: Williams & Wilkins, 1964:29, 61. **p. 357**

58. Cox JM. Low back pain—mechanism, diagnosis, and treatment. 5th ed. Baltimore: Williams & Wilkins, 1990:215, 224, 225. (Hippocrates reference.) **p. 357**

59. Sabotta J. Atlas of human anatomy. New York: GE Stechert, 1933:142. **p. 357**

60. Davis G. Applied anatomy. Philadelphia: JB Lippincott, 1918:433. **p. 357**

61. Jones R, Lovett RW. Orthopedic surgery. 2nd ed. New York: William Wood and Co, 1929:693. **p. 357**

62. Ober FR, ed. Lovett's lateral curvature of the spine. 5th ed. Philadelphia: P Blakiston's Son & Co, 1931:13. **p. 357**

63. Steindler A. Diseases and deformities of the spine and thorax. St. Louis, Missouri: CV Mosby, 1929:547. **p. 357**

64. Cyriax J, Cyriax P. Illustrated manual of orthopaedic medicine. Boston: Butterworths, 1983:76. **p. 357**

65. Hinwood JA. Sacroiliac joint biomechanics. *Dig Chiro Econ* 1983;25(5):41–44. **p. 357**

66. Saunders HD. Evaluation, treatment and prevention of musculoskeletal disorders. 2nd ed. Edina, Minnesota: Educational Opportunities, 1985:86, 131. **p. 357**

67. Norkin CC, Levangie PK. Joint structure & function—a comprehensive analysis. Philadelphia: FA Davis, 1983:148. **p. 357**

68. Williams PC. Lesions of the lumbosacral spine. Part II. Chronic traumatic (postural) destruction of the lumbosacral intervertebral disc. *J Bone Joint Surg* 1937;19:690–703. **p. 358**

69. Pope M, Wilder D, Booth J. The biomechanics of low back pain. In: White AA, Gordon SL, eds. Symposium on idiopathic low back pain. St. Louis, Missouri: CV Mosby, 1982. **p. 359, 360**

70. Farfan HF. Mechanical disorders of the low back. Philadelphia: Lea & Febiger, 1973. **p. 360**

71. Chaffin DB. Occupational biomechanics of low back injury. In: White AA, Gordon SL, eds. Symposium on idiopathic low back pain. St. Louis, Missouri: CV Mosby, 1982. **p. 360**

72. Poulsen E, Jorgensen K. Back muscle strength, lifting and stoop working postures. *App Ergonomics* 1971:133–137. **p. 360**

73. Tichauer ER, Miller M, Nathan IM. Lordosimetry: a new technique for the measurement of postural response to materials handling. *Am Ind Hyg Assoc J* 1973:34:1–12. **p. 360**

74. Adams MA, Hutton WC. Prolapsed intervertebral disc: a hyperflexion injury. In: Industrial rehabilitation. American Therapeutics, 1989:1031–1038. Presented at the 8th Annual Meeting of the International Society for the Study of the Lumbar Spine. Paris, May 18, 1981. **p. 360**

75. Nordin M, Frankel V. Basic biomechanics of the musculoskeletal system. 2nd ed. Philadelphia: Lea & Febiger 1989:193, 201. **p. 364**

76. Brown T, Hanson R, Yorra A. Some mechanical tests on the lumbosacral spine with particular reference to the intervertebral disc. *J Bone Joint Surg* [Am] 1957;39-A:1135. **p. 364**

77. Roaf R. A study of the mechanics of spinal injuries. *J Bone Joint Surg* [Br] 1960;42-B:810. **p. 364**

78. Freiberg AH, Vinke TH. Sciatica and sacro-iliac joint. *J Bone Joint Surg* 1934;16:126–136. **p. 365**

79. Kite JH. Exercise in foot disabilities. In: Basmajian JV, ed. Therapeutic exercise, 3rd ed. Baltimore: Williams & Wilkins, 1978:485–513 [Au note: best in 3rd ed.] **p. 366**

80. O'Neill DB, Zarins B, Gelberman RH, Keating TM, Louis D. Compression of the anterior interosseous nerve after use of a sling for dislocation of the acromioclavicular joint. *J Bone Joint Surg* [Am] 1990;72-A(7)1100. **p. 376, 378**

81. Hadley MN, Sonntag VKH, Pittman HW. Suprascapular nerve entrapment. *J Neurosurg* 1986;64:843–848. **p. 376, 378**

82. Post M, Mayer J. Suprascapular nerve entrapment. *Clin Orthop Relat Res* 1987;223:126–135. **p. 376, 378**

83. Conway SR, Jones HR. Entrapment and compression neuropathies. In: Tollison CD, ed. Handbook of chronic pain management. Baltimore: Williams & Wilkins, 1989:433, 437, 438. **p. 376, 378**

84. Sunderland S. Nerve injuries and their repair: a critical appraisal. London: Churchill Livingstone, 1991:161. **p. 376, 377, 378**

85. Jankiewicz JJ, Hennrikus WL, Houkom JA. The appearance of the piriformis muscle syndrome in computed tomography and magnetic resonance imaging. *Clin Orthop Relat Res* 1991;262:207. **p. 377**

86. Spinner M. Management of nerve compression lesions of the upper extremity. In: Omer GE, Spinner M. Management of peripheral nerve problems. Philadelphia: WB Saunders, 1980. **p. 377**

87. Johnson JTH, Kendall HO. Isolated paralysis of the serratus anterior muscle. *J Bone Joint Surg* [Am] 1955;37-A:567; Ortho Appl J 1964;18:201. **p. 378**

88. Taber CW. Taber's Cyclopedic Medical Dictionary. Philadelphia: FA Davis, 1969:L-25, Appendix 45–50. **p. 378**

89. Dorland's illustrated medical dictionary, 27th ed. Philadelphia: WB Saunders, 1988:1118–1125. **p. 378**

90. Nakano KK. Neurology of musculoskeletal and rheumatic disorders. Boston: Houghton Mifflin, 1978:191, 200. **p. 378**

91. Geiringer SR, Leonard JA. Posterior interosseus palsy after dental treatment: case report. *Arch Phys Med Rehabil* 1985;66. **p. 378**

92. Agur AMR. Grant's atlas of anatomy. 9th ed. Baltimore: Williams & Wilkins 1991:263, 362, 363. **p. 380, 381, 382**

93. Brodal A. Neurological anatomy: in relation to clinical medicine. 3rd ed. New York: Oxford University Press, 1981. **p. 388**

94. Peele TL. The neuroanatomic basis for clinical neurology. 3rd ed. New York: McGraw-Hill, 1977. **p. 388**

95. Keegan JJ, Garrett FD. The segmental distribution of the cutaneous nerves in the limbs of man. *Anat Rec* 1948:102. **p. 388**

96. Eycleshymer AC, Shoemaker DM. A cross-section anatomy. New York: D Appleton and Co, 1923. **p. 390**

97. Brash JC. Neuro-vascular hila muscles. London: E & S Livingstone, 1955. **p. 390**

98. Coyne JM, Kendall FP, Latimer RM, Payton OD. Evaluation of brachial plexus injury. *J Am Phys Ther Assoc* 1968;48:733. **p. 401**

99. deJong RN. The neurologic examination. 3rd ed. New York: Harper & Row, 1967. **p. 404, 405**

100. Romanes GJ, ed. Cunningham's textbook of anatomy. 10th ed. London: Oxford University Press, 1964. **p. 404**

101. Spalteholz W. Hand atlas of human anatomy Vol II, III. 6th ed. in English. London: JB Lippincott. **p. 404**

102. Foerster O, Bumke O. Handbuch der Neurologie. Vol. V. Berlin: J Springer, 1936. **p. 404**

103. Haymaker W, Woodhall B. Peripheral nerve injuries. 2nd ed. Philadelphia: WB Saunders, 1953. **p. 404**

104. Brash JC, ed. Cunningham's Manual of Practical Anatomy. Vol 1. 11th ed. New York: Oxford University Press, 1948. **p. 405**

422

105. Hollinshead WH. Functional anatomy of the limbs and back. 3rd ed. Philadelphia: WB Saunders, 1969. **p. 405**
106. Tavores AS. L'Innervation des muscles pectoraux. *Acta Anat* 1954;21:132–141. **p. 405**
107. Anson BJ, ed. Morris human anatomy. 12th ed. New York: McGraw-Hill, 1966. **p. 405**
108. Schade JP. The peripheral nervous system. New York: American Elsevier, 1966. **p. 409**

SUGGESTED READINGS

Adams MA, Hutton WC. Prolapsed intervertebral disc—a hyperflexion injury. Spine 1982;7:3.

Andersson GBJ, Ortengren R, Nachemson AL, et al. Lumbar disc pressure and myoelectric back muscle activity during sitting. Scand J Rehabil Med 1974;6:104.

Andersson GBJ, Ortengren R, Nachemson AL, et al. The sitting posture: an electromyographic and discometric study. Orthop Clin North Am 1975;6:105.

Andersson GBJ, Ortengren R, Herberts P. Quantitative electromyographic studies of back muscle activity related to posture and loading. Orthop Clin North Am 1977;8:85.

Ardran GM, Kemp FH. The mechanism of the larynx. II, The epiglottes and closure of the larynx. Br J Radiol 1967;40:372.

Arnold GE. Physiology and pathology of the cricothyroid muscle. Laryngoscope 1961;71:687.

Atkinson M, Dramer P, Wyman SM., et al. The dynamics of swallowing. I, Normal pharyngeal mechanisms. J Clin Invest 1957;36:581.

Barun N, Arora N, Rochester D. Force-length relationship of the normal human diaphragm. J Appl Physiol 1982; 53(2):4405–412.

Basmajian JV. Electromyography of two-joint muscles. Anat Rec 1957;129:371.

Basmajian JV. Electromyography of iliopsoas. Anat Rec 1958;132:127.

Basmajian JV. Grant's method of anatomy. 9th ed. Baltimore: Williams & Wilkins, 1975.

Basmajian JV, Travill A. Electromyography of the pronator muscles in the forearm. Anat Rec 1961;139:45–49.

Basmajian JV, Wolf SL. Therapeutic exercise. 5th ed. Baltimore: Williams & Wilkins, 1990.

Batti'e MC, Bigos SJ, Sheehy A, Wortley MD. Spinal flexibility and individual factors that influence it. Phys Ther 1987;67:5.

Beattie P, Rothstein JM, Lamb RL. Reliability of the attraction method for measuring lumbar spine backward bending. Phys Ther 1987;67:364–368.

Bender JA, Kaplan HM. The multiple angle testing method for the evaluation of muscle strength. J Bone Joint Surg [Am] 1963;45-A:135.

Black SA. Clinical applications in muscle testing. Rehab Man 1990;3(1):30,32,61.

Blackburn SE, Portney LG. Electromyographic activity of back musculature during Williams' flexion exercises. Phys Ther 1981;61:878.

Blakely WR, Garety EJ, Smith DE. Section of the cricopharyngeus muscle for dysphagia. Arch Surg 1968;96:745.

Blankenship KL. Industrial rehabilitation—seminar syllabus. Stress and lift-pull indexes (Ch. 9). Proper lifting techniques (Ch. 10). American Therapeutics, Inc., 1989.

Blanton PL, Biggs NL, Perkins RC. Electromyographic analysis of the buccinator muscle. J Dent Res 1970;49:389.

Bohannon RW. Cinematographic analysis of the passive straight-leg-raising test for hamstring muscle length. Phys Ther 1982;62(9):1269–1274.

Bohannon RW, Gajdosik RL. Spinal nerve root compression—some clinical implications. Phys Ther 1987;67:3.

Bohannon RW, Gajdosik RL, LeVeau BF. Contribution of pelvic and lower limb motion to increases in the angle of passive straight leg raising. Phys Ther 1985;65(4):474–476.

Bosma JF. Deglutition: pharyngeal stage. Physiol Rev 1957;37:275.

Bouman HD, ed. An exploratory and analytical survey of therapeutic exercise: Northwestern University Special Therapeutic Exercise Project. Am J Phys Med 1967;46:1.

Bourn J, Jenkins S. Postoperative respiratory physiotherapy: indications for treatment. Physiother 1992;78(2):80–85.

Physiotherapy (The Journal of the Chartered Society of Physiotherapy) (British).

Brand PW, Beach RB, Thompson DE. Relative tension and potential excursion of muscles in the forearm and hand. J Hand Surg [Am] 1981;6:209.

Breig A, Troup JDG. Biomechanical considerations in the straight-leg-raising test. Spine 1979;4(3):242–250.

Brunnstrom, S. Clinical kinesiology. 3rd ed. Philadelphia: FA Davis, 1972.

Bullock-Saxton J. Normal and abnormal postures in the sagittal plane and their relationship to low back pain. Physiother Pract 1988;4(2):94–104.

Bunnell's Surgery of the hand, 4th ed. Boyes JH, ed. Philadelphia: JB Lippincott, 1964.

Campbell EJM. The respiratory muscles and the mechanics of breathing. Chicago: Year Book, 1958.

Campbell EJM, Agostini E, Davis JN. The respiratory muscles: mechanisms and neural control. 2nd ed. Philadelphia: WB Saunders, 1970.

Capuano-Pucci D, Rheault W, Aukai J, Bracke M, Day R, Pastrick M. Intratester and intertester reliability of the cervical range of motion device. Arch Phys Med Rehabil 1991;72:338–340.

Carmen DJ, Blanton PL, Biggs NL. Electromyographic study of the anterolateral abdominal musculature utilizing indwelling electrodes. Am J Phys Med 1972;51:113.

Cash JE, ed. Chest, heart and vascular disorders for physiotherapists. Philadelphia: JB Lippincott, 1975.

Cassella MC, Hall JE. Current treatment approaches in the nonoperative and operative management of adolescent idiopathic scoliosis. Phys Ther 1991;71:12.

Chusid JG. Correlative neuroanatomy and functional neurology. 15th ed. Los Altos, California: Lange Medical Publications, 1973.

Clapper MP, Wolf SL. Comparison of the reliability of the orthoranger and the standard goniometer for assessing active lower extremity range of motion. Phys Ther 1988;68(2):214–218.

Clayson SJ, Newman IM, Debevec DF, et al. Evaluation of mobility of hip and lumbar vertebrae of normal young women. Arch Phys Med Rehabil 1962;43:1.

Close JR. Motor function in the lower extremity. Springfield, Illinois: Charles C Thomas, 1964.

Close JR, Kidd CC. The functions of the muscles of the thumb, the index and long fingers. J Bone Joint Surg [Am] 1969;51-A:1601.

Close RI. Dynamic properties of mammalian skeletal muscles. Physiol Rev 1972;52:129.

Cohen-Sobel E, Levitz SJ. Torsional development of the lower extremity. J Am Podiatr Med Assoc 1991;81(7):344–357.

Cole TM. Goniometry: the measurement of joint motion. In: Krusen, Kottke, Elwood. Handbook of physical medicine and rehabilitation. 2nd ed. Philadelphia: WB Saunders, 1971.

Cooperman JM. Case studies: isolated strain of the tensor fasciae latae. J Orthop Sports Phys Ther 1983;5(4):201–203.

Cunningham DP, Basmajian JB. Electromyography of genioglossus and geniohyoid muscles during deglutition. Anat Rec 1969;165:401.

Currier DP. Maximal isometric tension of the elbow extensors at varied positions. Phys Ther 1972;52:1265.

Currier DP. Positioning for knee strengthening exercises. Phys Ther 1977;57:148.

Cyriax J. Textbook of orthopaedic medicine. Vol 1. 7th ed. Diagnosis of soft tissue lesions. London: Bailliere-Tindall, 1978.

Cyriax J, Cyriax P. Illustrated manual of orthopaedic medicine. London: Butterworth, 1983.

423

deJong RN. The neurological examination. 4th ed. New York: Harper & Row, 1979.

DeLuca CJ, Forrest WJ. Force analysis of individual muscles acting simultaneously on the shoulder joint during isometric abduction. J Biomech 1973;6:385.

DeRosa C, Porterfield JA. The sacroiliac joint. Postgraduate advances in the evaluation and treatment of low back dysfunction. Forum Medicum 1989.

Des Jardins TR. Cardiopulmonary anatomy and physiology. Albany, New York: Delmar, 1988.

DeSousa OM, Furlani J. Electromyographic study of the m. rectus abdominis. Acta Anat 1974;88:281.

DeSousa OM, Demoraes JL, (Demoraes Vieira FL.) Electromyographic study of the brachioradialis muscle. Anat Rec 1961;139:125.

DeSousa OM, Berzin F, Berardi AC. Electromyographic study of the pectoralis major and latissimus dorsi during medial rotation of the arm. Electromyography 1969;9:407.

Dickson RA, Lawton JL, Archer IA, Butt WP. The pathogenesis of idiopathic scoliosis. J Bone Joint Surg [Br] 1984;66-B(1):8–15.

Donelson R, Silva G, Murphy K. Centralization phenomenon—its usefulness in evaluating and treating referred pain. Spine 1990;15(3):211–213.

DonTigny RL. Anterior dysfunction of the sacroiliac joint as a major factor in the etiology of idiopathic low back pain syndrome. Phys Ther 1990;70(4):250–265.

Dostal WF, Soderberg GL, Andrews JG. Actions of hip muscles. Phys Ther 1986;66(3):351–361.

Downer AH. Physical therapy procedures. 3rd ed. Springfield, Illinois: Charles C Thomas, 1978.

Duval-Beaupere G. Rib hump and supine angle as prognostic factors for mild scoliosis. Spine 1992;17:1.

Eaton RG, Littler JW. A study of the basal joint of the thumb. J Bone Joint Surg [Am] 1969;51-A:661.

Ekholm J, Arborelius U, Fahlcrantz A, et al. Activation of abdominal muscles during some physiotherapeutic exercises. Scand J Rehabil Med 1979;11:75.

Elftman H. Biomechanics of muscle. J Bone Joint Surg [Am] 1966;48-A:363.

Eyler DL, Markee JE. The anatomy and function of the intrinsic musculature of the fingers. J Bone Joint Surg [Am] 1954;36-A:1.

Farfan HF. Mechanical disorders of the low back. Philadelphia: Lea & Febiger, 1973.

Farfan HF. Muscular mechanism of the lumbar spine and the position of power and efficiency. Orthop Clin North Am 1975;6:135.

Fast A. Low back disorders: conservative management. Arch Phys Med Rehabil 1988;69:880–891.

Fenn WO, Rahn H. Handbook of physiology. Section 3: Respiration. Vol 1. Washington, DC: American Physiological Society, 1964:377–384.

Fischer FJ, Houtz SJ. Evaluation of the function of the gluteus maximus muscle. Am J Phys Med 1968;47:182.

Fishman AP, ed. Pulmonary diseases and disorders. 2nd ed. New York: McGraw-Hill, 1988.

Flint MM. Abdominal muscle involvement during performance of various forms of sit-up exercise. Am J Phys Med 1965;44:224.

Flint MM. An electromyographic comparison of the function of the iliacus and the rectus abdominis muscles. J Am Phys Ther Assoc 1965;45:248.

Francis RS. Scoliosis screening of 3,000 college-aged women: The Utah Study—Phase 2. Phys Ther 1988;68(10):1513–1516.

Franco AH. Pes cavus and pes planus. Phys Ther 1987;67(5):688–693.

Frank JS, Earl M. Coordination of posture and movement. Phys Ther 1990;70(12):855–863.

Frese E, Brown M, Norton BJ. Clinical reliability of manual muscle testing—middle trapezius and gluteus medius muscles. Phys Ther 1987;67(7):1072–1076.

Fujiwara M, Basmajian JV. Electromyographic study of two-joint muscles. Am J Phys Med 1975;54:234.

Gajdosik R, Lusin G.L Hamstring muscle tightness. Phys Ther 1983;63(7):1085–1090.

Girardin Y. EMG action potentials of rectus abdominis muscle during two types of abdominal exercises. In: Cerquigleni S, Venerando A, Wartenweiler J. Biomechanics III. Baltimore: University Park Press, 1973.

Gleeson PB, Pauls JA. Obstetrical physical therapy—review of the literature. Phys Ther 1988;68(11):1699–1702.

Glennon TP. Isolated injury of the infraspinatus branch of the suprascapular nerve. Arch Phys Med Rehabil 1992;73:201–202.

Godfrey KE, Kindig LE, Windell EJ. Electromyographic study of duration of muscle activity in sit-up variations. Arch Phys Med Rehabil 1977;58:132.

Goldberg CJ, Dowling FE. Idiopathic scoliosis and asymmetry of form and function. Spine 1991;16(1):84–87.

Gose JC, Schweizer P. Iliotibial band tightness. J Orthop Sports Phys Ther 1989;9(4):399–406.

Gowitzke BA, Milner MM. Understanding the scientific basis of human motion. 2nd ed. Baltimore: Williams & Wilkins, 1980.

Gracovetsky S, Farfan HF, Lamy C. The mechanism of the lumbar spine. Spine 1981;6:249.

Gray ER. The role of leg muscles in variations of the arches in normal and flat feet. J Am Phys Ther Assoc 1969;49:1084.

Grieve GP. The sacro-iliac joint. Physiother 1976;62:384.

Guffey JS. A critical look at muscle testing. Clin 1991;11(2):15–19.

Halpern A, Bleck E. Sit-up exercise: an electromyographic study. Clin Orthop Relat Res 1979;145:172.

Hart DL, Stobbe TJ, Jaraiedi M. Effect of lumbar posture on lifting. Spine 1987;12(2):1023–1030.

Hasue M, Fujiwara M, Kikuchi S. A new method of quantitative measurement of abdominal and back muscle strength. Spine 1980;51:143.

Haymaker W. Bing's local diagnosis in neurological diseases. 15th ed. St. Louis: CV Mosby, 1969.

Hicks JH. The three weight-bearing mechanisms of the foot. In: Evans FG. Biomechanical studies of the musculoskeletal system. Springfield, Illinois: Charles C Thomas, 1961.

Hirano M, Koike Y, von Leden H. The sterno-hyoid muscle during phonation. Acta Otolaryngol 1967;64:500.

Houtz SJ, Lebow MJ, Beyer FR. Effect of posture on strength of the knee flexor and extensor muscles. J Appl Physiol 1957;11:475.

Hsieh C, Walker JM, Gillis K. Straight-leg-raising test. Phys Ther 1983;63(9):1429–1433.

Ingher RS. Iliopsoas myofascial dysfunction: a treatable cause of "failed" low back syndrome. Arch Phys Med Rehabil 1989;70:382–385.

Itoi E. Roentgenographic analysis of posture in spinal osteoporotics. Spine 1991;16(7):750–756.

Johnson JTH, Kendall HO. Localized shoulder girdle paralysis of unknown etiology. Clin Orthop 1961;20:151–155.

Joint motion, method of measuring and recording. Chicago: American Academy of Orthopaedic Surgeons, 1965.

Jonsson B, Olofsson BM, Steffner LCH. Function of the teres major, latissimus dorsi and pectoralis major muscles. Acta Morph Neerl Scand 1972;9:275.

Kaplan EB. Functional and surgical anatomy of the hand. 2nd ed. Philadelphia: JB Lippincott, 1965.

Keagy RD, Brumlik J, Bergan JJ. Direct electromyography of the psoas major muscle in man. J Bone Joint Surg [Am] 1966;48-A:1377.

Keller RB. Nonoperative treatment of adolescent idiopathic scoliosis. In: Barr JS, ed. The spine—instructional course lectures. Vol 30. 1989;129.

Kendall HO. Some interesting observations about the after care of infantile paralysis patients. J Excep Children 1937;3:107.

Kendall HO. Watch those T.V. exercises. TV Guide 1963;II-31:5.

Kendall HO, Kendall FP. Study and treatment of muscle imbalance in cases of low back and sciatic pain. Pamphlet. Baltimore: privately printed, 1936.

Kendall HO, Kendall FP. Care during the recovery period of paralytic poliomyelitis. U.S. Public Health Bulletin No 242. Washington, DC: U.S. Government Printing Office, 1939.

Kendall HO, Kendall FP. Gluteus medius and its relation to body mechanics. Physiother Rev 1941;21:131.

Kendall HO, Kendall FP. The role of abdominal exercise in a program of physical fitness. J Health Phys Ed 1943;480.

Kendall HO, Kendall FP. Unpublished report on the Posture Survey at U.S. Military Academy, West Point, 1945.

Kendall HO, Kendall FP. Physical therapy for lower extremity amputees. War Department Technical Manual TM-8-293:14/42 and 58/65, Washington, DC: U.S. Government Printing Office, 1946:12–48.

Kendall HO, Kendall FP. Orthopedic and physical therapy objectives in poliomyelitis treatment. Physiother Rev 1947;27:159.

Kendall HO, Kendall FP. Functional muscle testing. In: Bierman W, Licht S. Physical medicine in general practice, New York: Paul B Hoeber, 1952:339–384.

Kendall HO, Kendall FP. Posture, flexibility, and abdominal muscle tests (leaflet). Baltimore: Waverly Press, 1964.

Kendall HO, Kendall FP. Developing and maintaining good posture. J Am Phys Ther Assoc 1968;48:319.

Kendall HO, Kendall FP, Boynton DA. Posture and pain. Baltimore: Williams & Wilkins, 1952. Reprinted Melbourne, Florida: Robert E Krieger, 1971.

Kendall FP. Range of motion. The correlation of physiology with therapeutic exercise. New York: American Physical Therapy Association, 1956.

Kendall FP. A criticism of current tests and exercises for physical fitness. J Am Phys Ther Assoc 1965;45:187–197.

Kisner C, Colby LA. Therapeutic exercise—foundations and techniques. 2nd ed. Philadelphia: FA Davis, 1990.

Kleinberg S. Scoliosis—pathology, etiology, and treatment. Baltimore: Williams & Wilkins, 1951.

Klousen K, Rasmussen B. On the location of the line of gravity in relation to L5 in standing. Acta Physiol Scand 1968;72:45.

Koes BW, Bouter LM, vanMameren H, Essers AHM, Verstegen GMJR, Hofhuizen DM, Houben JP, Knipschild PG. The effectiveness of manual therapy, physiotherapy, and treatment by the general practitioner for nonspecific back and neck complaints. Spine 1992;17(1):28–35.

Kotby MN. Electromyography of the laryngeal muscles. Electroencephalog Clin Neurophysiol 1969;26:341.

Kraus H. Effects of lordosis on the stress in the lumbar spine. Clin Orthop 1976;117:56.

LaBan M, Raptou AD, Johnson EW. Electromyographic study of function of iliopsoas muscle. Arch Phys Med 1965;46:676–679.

Lieb FJ, Perry J. Quadriceps function. J Bone Joint Surg [Am] 1971;53-A:749.

Lilienfeld AM, Jacobs M, Willis M. A study of the reproducibility of muscle testing and certain other aspects of muscle scoring. Phys Ther Rev 1954;34(6):279–290.

Lindahl O. Determination of the sagittal mobility of the lumbar spine. Acta Orthop Scand 1966;37:241.

Lindahl O, Movin A. The mechanics of extension of the knee joint. Acta Orthop Scand 1967;38:226.

Lindstrom A, Zachrisson M. Physical therapy for low back pain and sciatica. Scand J Rehabil Med 1970;2:37.

Lipetz S, Gutin B. Electromyographic study of four abdominal exercises. Med Sci Sports 1970;2:35.

Loebl WY. Measurement of spinal posture and range of spinal movement. Ann Phys Med 1967;9:103.

Long C. Intrinsic-extrinsic muscle control of the fingers. J Bone Joint Surg [Am] 1968;50-A:973.

Loptata M, Evanich MJ, Lourenco RV. The electromyogram of the diaphragm in the investigation of human regulation of ventilation. Chest 1976;70(Suppl):162S.

Loring SH, Mead J. Action of the diaphragm on the rib cage inferred from a force-balance analysis. J Appl Physiol 1982;53;3:756–760.

Low JL. The reliability of joint measurement. Physiother 1976;62:227.

Mann R, Inman VT. Phasic activity of intrinsic muscles of the foot. J Bone Joint Surg [Am] 1964;46-A:469.

McCreary EK. The control of breathing in singing. [Research paper for Physiology Department] John A. Burns School of Medicine, Honolulu, Hawaii, 1982.

Mayhew TP, Norton BJ, Sahrmann SA. Electromyographic study of the relationship between hamstring and abdominal muscles during a unilateral straight leg raise. Phys Ther 1983;63(11):1769–1775.

Michelle AA. Iliopsoas. Springfield, Illinois: Charles C Thomas, 1962.

Mines, AH. Respiratory physiology. New York: Raven Press, 1981.

Moller M, Ekstrand J, Oberg B, Gillquist J. Duration of stretching effect on range of motion in lower extremities. Arch Phys Med Rehabil 1985;66:171–173.

Moore KL. Clinically oriented anatomy. Baltimore: Williams & Wilkins, 1980.

Moore ML. Clinical assessment of joint motion. In: Licht S. Therapeutic exercise. 2nd ed. Baltimore: Waverly Press, 1965.

Mulligan E. Conservative management of shoulder impingement syndrome. Athl Train 1988;23(4):348–353.

Nachemson A. Electromyographic studies on the vertebral portion of the psoas muscle. Acta Orthop Scand 1966;37:177.

Nachemson A. Physiotherapy for low back pain patients. Scand J Rehabil Med 1969;1:85.

Nachemson A. Towards a better understanding of low back pain: a review of the mechanics of the lumbar disc. Rheumatol Rehabil 1975;14:129.

Nachemson A. A critical look at the treatment for low back pain. Scand J Rehabil Med 1979;11:143.

Nachemson A, Lindh M. Measurement of abdominal and back muscle strength with and without low back pain. Scand J Rehabil Med 1969;1:60.

Nagler W, Pugliese G. Facet syndrome (letter to the editor). Arch Phys Med Rehabil 1989;70.

Ouaknine G, Nathan H. Anastomotic connections between the eleventh nerve and the posterior root of the first cervical nerve in humans. J Neurosurg 1973;38:189.

Paré EB, Schwartz JM, Stern JT. Electromyographic and anatomical study of the human tensor fasciae latae muscle. In: Proceedings of the 4th Congress of the International Society of Electrophysiological Kinesiology. Boston: Published by the organizing committee, 1979.

Partridge MJ, Walters CE. Participation of the abdominal muscles in various movements of the trunk in man. Phys Ther Rev 1959;39:791–800.

Patton NJ, Mortensen OA. A study of some mechanical factors affecting reciprocal activity in one-joint muscles. Anat Rec 1970;166:360.

Pearsall DJ, Reid JG, Hedden DM. Comparison of three noninvasive methods for measuring scoliosis. Phys Ther 1992;72:9.

Pearson AA, Sauter RW, Herrin GR. The accessory nerve and its relation to the upper spinal nerves. J Anat 1964;114-A:371.

Pennal CF, Conn GS, McDonald G, et al. Motion studies of the lumbar spine. J Bone Joint Surg [Br] 1972;54-B:442.

Physical Therapy, Journal of the American Physical Therapy Association. Special issues:
Pain. 1980;60:1. (Lister MJ, ed.)
Respiratory care. 1980;60:12. (Lister MJ, ed.)
Muscle biology. 1982;62:12. (Lister MJ, ed.)
Biomechanics. 1984;64:12. (Lister MJ, ed.)

Shoulder complex. 1986;66:12. (Lister MJ, ed.)

Clinical measurement. 1987;67:12. (Lister MJ, ed.)

Foot and ankle. 1988;68:12. (Rose SJ, ed.)

Clinical decision making. 1989;69:7. (Rose SJ, ed. em.)

Hand management in physical therapy. 1989;69:12. (Rothstein JM, ed.)

Physiotherapy. Journal of the Chartered Society of Physiotherapy. Special issues:

The hand. 1977;63:9. (Whitehouse J, ed.)

Update in respiratory care. 1992;78:2. (Whitehouse J, ed.)

Pruijs JEH, Keessen W, van der Meer R, van Wieringen JC, Hageman MAPE. School screening for scoliosis: methodologic considerations—Part 1: external measurements. Spine 1992;17(4):431–435.

Ralston HJ, Todd FN, Inman VT. Comparison of electrical activity and duration of tension in the human rectus femoris muscle. Electromyogr Clin Neurophysiol 1976;16:271.

Ramsey GH, Watson JS, Gramiak R, et al. Cinefluorographic analysis of the mechanism of swallowing. Radiology 1955;64:498.

Riddle DL, Finucane SD, Rothstein JM, Walker ML. Intrasession and intersession reliability of hand-held dynamometer measurements taken on brain-damaged patient. Phys Ther 1989;69(3):182–194.

Roberts RH, ed. Scoliosis. CIBA Found Symp 1972;24:1.

Rodgers MM, Cavanagh PR. Glossary of biomechanical terms, concepts, and units. Phys Ther 1984;64(12):1886–1902.

Root ML, Orien WP, Weed JH. Normal and abnormal function of the foot. Los Angeles: Clinical Biomechanics Corp, 1977:95–107.

Salminen JJ, Maki P, Oksanen A, Pentti J. Spinal mobility and trunk muscle strength in 15-year-old schoolchildren with and without low-back pain. Spine 1992;17(4):405–411.

Salter N, Darcus HD. The effect of the degree of elbow flexion on the maximum torques developed in pronation and supination of the right hand. J Anat 1952;86-B:197.

Saunders JB deCM, Davis C, Miller ER. The mechanism of deglutition. Ann Otol Rhinol Laryngol 1951;60:897.

Schuit D, Adrian M, Pidcoe P. Effect of heel lifts on ground reaction force patterns in subjects with structural leg-length discrepancies. Phys Ther 1989;69(8):663–670.

Schultz JS, Leonard JA Jr. Long thoracic neuropathy from athletic activity. Arch Phys Med Rehabil 1992;73:87–90.

Scoliosis: an anthology. (Articles reprinted from Physical Therapy) Alexandria, Virginia: American Physical Therapy Association, 1984.

Shaffer T, Wolfson M, Bhutani VK. Respiratory muscle function, assessment, and training. Phys Ther 1981;61:12.

Sharf M, Shvartzman P, Farkash E, Horvitz J. Thoracic lateral cutaneous nerve entrapment syndrome without previous lower abdominal surgery. J Fam Pract 1990;30:2.

Sharp JT, Draz W, Danon J, et al. Respiratory muscle function and the use of respiratory muscle electromyography in the evaluation of respiratory regulation. Chest 1976;70(Suppl):150S.

Sharrard WJW. The segmental innervation of the lower limb muscles in man. Ann R Coll Surg Engl 1964;35:106.

Shelton RL, Bosma JF, Sheets BV. Tongue, hyoid and larynx displacement in swallow and phonation. J Appl Physiol 1960;15:283.

Slonim NB, Hamilton LH. Respiratory physiology. St. Louis: CV Mosby, 1981.

Smidt GL, Rogers MW. Factors contributing to the regulation and clinical assessment of muscular strength. Phys Ther 1982;62(9):1283–1289.

Smith JW. Muscular control of the arches of the foot in standing: an electromyographical assessment. J Anat 1954;88-B:152.

Smith RL, Brunolli J. Shoulder kinesthesia after anterior glenohumeral joint dislocation. Phys Ther 1989;69(2):106–112.

Soderberg GL, Dostal WF. Electromyographic study of three parts of the gluteus medius muscle during functional activities. Phys Ther 1978;58(6):691–696.

Southwick WO, Keggi K. The normal cervical spine. J Bone Joint Surg [Am] 1964;46-A(8):1767–1777.

Speakman HGB, Weisberg J. The vastus medialis controversy. Physiother 1977;63:8.

Spitzer WO et al. Scientific approach to the assessment and management of activity-related spinal disorders: a monograph for clinicians—report of the Quebec Task Force on Spinal Disorders. Spine [European Edition] 1987;12:7s.

Stoff MD, Greene AF. Common peroneal nerve palsy following inversion ankle injury. Phys Ther 1982;62(10):1463–1464.

Stokes IAF, Abery JM. Influence of the hamstring muscles on lumbar spine curvature in sitting. Spine 1980;5(6):525–528.

Stone B, Beekman C, Hall V, Guess V, Brooks HL. The effect of an exercise program on change in curve in adolescents with minimal idiopathic scoliosis. Phys Ther 1979;59(6):759–763.

Straus WL, Howell AB. The spinal accessory nerve and its musculature. Rev Biol 1936;11:387.

Sullivan MS. Back support mechanisms during manual lifting. Phys Ther 1989;69(1):38–45.

Suzuki N. An electromyographic study of the role of muscles in arch support of the normal and flat foot. Nagoya Med J 1972;17:57.

Thomas HO. Diseases of the hip, knee and ankle joints. (Reproduction of 2nd ed, 1876.) Boston: Little, Brown, 1962.

Travell JG, Simons DG. Myofascial pain and dysfunction. Baltimore: Williams & Wilkins, 1983.

Trief PM. Chronic back pain: a tripartite model of outcome. Arch Phys Med Rehabil 1983;64:53–56.

Truex RC, Carpenter MG, eds. Strong and Elwyn's human neuroanatomy. 6th ed. Baltimore: Williams & Wilkins, 1969.

Urban LM. The straight-leg-raising test: a review. J Orthop Sports Phys Ther 1981;2(3):117–133.

Vander AJ, Sherman JH, Luciano DS. Human physiology: the mechanism of body function. 3rd ed. New York: McGraw-Hill, 1980.

Wadsworth CT, Krishnan R, Sear M, Harrold J, Nielsen DH. Intrarater reliability of manual muscle testing and hand-held dynametric muscle testing. Phys Ther 1987;67(9):1342–1347.

Walters CE, Partridge MJ. Electromyographic study of the differential action of the abdominal muscles during exercise. Am J Phys Med 1957;36:259.

Warfel JH. The head, neck and trunk. 5th ed. Philadelphia: Lea & Febiger, 1985.

Watkins MA, Riddle DL, Lamb RL, Personius WJ. Reliability of goniometric measurements and visual estimates of knee range of motion obtained in a clinical setting. Phys Ther 1991;71(2):90–97.

Weiss HR. The effect of an exercise program on vital capacity and rib mobility in patients with idiopathic scoliosis. Spine 1991;16:1.

Wells KF. Kinesiology, 4th ed. Philadelphia: WB Saunders, 1966.

White A, Panjabi M. Clinical biomechanics of the spine. Philadelphia: JB Lippincott, 1978.

Williams M, Lissner HR. Biomechanics of human motion. Philadelphia: WB Saunders, 1962.

Williams M, Stutzman L. Strength variation through the range of joint motion. Phys Ther Rev 1959;39:145.

Williams PC. The lumbosacral spine. New York: McGraw-Hill, 1965.

Wolf S. Normative data on low back mobility and activity levels. Am J Phys Med 1979;58:217.

Youdas JW, Carey JR, Garrett TR. Reliability of measurements of cervical spine range of motion—comparison of three methods. Phys Ther 1991;71(2):98–106.

Zimny N, Kirk C. A comparison of methods of manual muscle testing. Clin Man 1987;7(2):6–11.

426

Index

Page numbers in *italics* denote figures; those followed by "t" denote tables and charts.

Abdominal muscle tests, 133
  arm movements used in, 175
  effect of holding feet down during, 164, *164–165*
  for lower abdominals, 133, 154–155, *155*
  strength testing, 102
    of lateral flexors, 144
    of oblique flexors, 146, *146*
    in scoliosis, 122
    sit-ups for, 7–8
  for upper abdominals, 133, 162–163, *163*
Abdominal muscles, 70, *83. See also* specific muscles
  actions during leg lowering, 156, *156*
    during curled-trunk sit-up, 169–174, *170–174*
    during double leg raising, 137
  exercises for, 158, 159, 166
  in flat-back posture, 87
  imbalance of, 175
  in "military-type" posture, 86
  role in respiration, 324, 325, 327, 329
  weakness of, 133, 157, *157*, 165
    exercises for, 158, 159, 166, *166*, 351
    lifting and, 360
    lordosis and, 80
    low back pain due to, 349–351
    supports for, 351
    testing and grading of, 176
Abducens nerve (CN VI), *300*, 310t, 312t–313t
Abduction
  of carpometacarpal joint of thumb, 19
  in coronal plane, 11
  definition of, 14, *14*, 414
  of forefoot, 22, 371
  of hip joint, 21, *21*, 222–223, *223*
  horizontal
    definition of, 415
    of shoulder joint, 17
    in transverse plane, 11
  of metacarpophalangeal joint of thumb, 19
  of metacarpophalangeal joints of fingers, 18
  of scapula, 16, *16*
  of shoulder joint, 17
  of toes, 22
  of wrist (radial deviation), 18
Abductor digiti minimi (hand), 19, *391*
  actions of, 245, 296t–297t
  innervation of, 245, 296t, 389t
  origin and insertion of, 245, *245*
  spinal segment distribution to, 406t–407t
  testing strength of, 245, *245*
  weakness of, 245
Abductor digiti minimi (foot), *392*
  actions of, 232t–233t
  innervation of, 232t, 393t
  spinal segment distribution to, 408t–409t
Abductor hallucis, *191*, 191, *392*
  actions of, 191, 232t–233t
  contracture of, 191
  innervation of, 191, 232t, 393t
  origin and insertion of, 191
  spinal segment distribution to, 408t–409t
  stretched, 371
  testing strength of, 191
  weakness of, 191, 369
Abductor pollicis brevis, 19, *391*
  actions of, 238, 296t–297t

innervation of, 238, 296t, 389t
  origin and insertion of, 238, *238*
  testing strength of, 238, *238*
  weakness of, 238
Abductor pollicis longus, *391*
  actions of, 244, 296t–297t
  contracture of, 244
  innervation of, 244, 296t, 389t
  origins and insertion of, 244, *244*
  spinal segment distribution to, 406t–407t
  testing strength of, 244, *244*
  weakness of, 244
Accessory nerve (CN XI), *300*, 310t, 312t–313t, *384*, 388, *391*
Acetabulum, 20
Activity patterns, highly specialized or repetitive, 3
Adaptive shortening, 334
  consequences of, 334
  definition of, 334, 411
Adduction
  of carpometacarpal joint of thumb, 19
  in coronal plane, 11
  definition of, 14, *14*, 414
  of forefoot, 22
  of hip joint, 21, *21*, 222, 223, 228–230
  horizontal
    definition of, 415
    of shoulder joint, 17
    in transverse plane, 11
  of metacarpophalangeal joint of thumb, 19
  of metacarpophalangeal joints of fingers, 18–19
  of scapula, 16, *16*
  of shoulder joint, 17
  of toes, 22
  of wrist (ulnar deviation), 18
Adductor brevis, 33, *392*
  actions of, 228, 229, 232t–233t
  innervation of, 228, 232t, 378, 393t
  origin and insertion of, 228, *228*
  spinal segment distribution to, 408t–409t
Adductor hallucis, *191*, 191, *392*
  actions of, 191, 232t–233t
  contracture of, 191
  innervation of, 191, 232t, 393t
  origins and insertion of, 191
  spinal segment distribution to, 408t–409t
  tightness of, 371
  weakness of, 369
Adductor longus, 33, *392*
  actions of, 228, 229, 232t–233t
  innervation of, 228, 232t, 393t
  origin and insertion of, 228, *228*
  spinal segment distribution to, 408t–409t
Adductor magnus, *365*, *392*
  actions of, 228, 232t–233t
  innervation of, 228, 232t, 378, 393t
  origin and insertion of, 228, *228*
  spinal segment distribution to, 408t–409t
Adductor minimus, *365*
Adductor pollicis, *391*
  actions of, 237, 296t–297t
  contracture of, 237
  innervation of, 237, 296t, 389t
  origins and insertions of, 237, *237*
  spinal segment distribution to, 406t–407t

Constrictor pharyngis medius—*continued*
   actions of, 321t
   innervation of, 321t
   origin and insertion of, 321t
   role in deglutition, 321t
Constrictor pharyngis superior, *300*
   actions of, 321t
   innervation of, 321t
   origin and insertion of, 321t
   role in deglutition, 321t
Contractility, definition of, 412
Contraction
   concentric, 412
   definition of, 412
   eccentric, 412
   isometric, 412
   isotonic, 412
Contracture, 4. *See also* specific muscles
   definition of, 183, 412
   irreversible, 412
   on trunk extension test, 141
Contraindication, definition of, 412
Contralateral, definition of, 412
Coracobrachialis, *391*
   actions of, 267, 294t, 296t–297t
   innervation of, 267, 296t, 378, 379t, 389t
   involvement with musculocutaneous nerve, 377
   origin and insertion of, 267
   shortness of, 267
   spinal segment distribution to, 406t–407t
   testing strength of, 267, *267*
   weakness of, 267
Coracoid pressure syndrome, *343*, 343–344
   cause of, 343
   definition of, 343
   exercises contraindicated in, 344
   treatment of, 343–344
Corrugator supercilii, *300*
   innervation of, 310t, 312t–313t
   origin and insertion of, 302t
   testing of, 304, *304*
Counterpressure, 181
Cranial, definition of, 413
Cranial nerves (CN), *300*, 311
   cutaneous distribution of, *310*
   muscles and regions supplied by, 310t, 312t–313t
Cricoarytenoid
   lateral
      actions of, 321t
      innervation of, 321t
      origin and insertion of, 321t
      role in deglutition, 321t
   posterior
      actions of, 321t
      innervation of, 321t
      origin and insertion of, 321t
      role in deglutition, 321t
Cricopharyngeus
   actions of, 321t
   innervation of, 321t
   origin and insertion of, 321t
   role in deglutition, 321t
Cricothyroid
   actions of, 321t
   innervation of, 321t
   origins and insertions of, 321t
   role in deglutition, 321t
Criteria, definition of, 412
Crutch paralysis, 376

Deformities, 184

of foot and ankle, 197
Deglutition muscles, 320t–321t
Deltoid, 182, *391*
   actions of, 273, 294t, 296t–297t
   innervation of, 273, 296t, 344, *344*, 377, 379t, 389t
   origins and insertion of, 273
   spinal segment distribution to, 406t–407t
   testing strength of, 186
      anterior deltoid, 274–275, *274–275*
      middle deltoid, 273, *273*
      posterior deltoid, 274–275, *274–275*
   weakness of, 273
Depressor anguli oris, *301*
   innervation of, 310t, 312t–313t
   origin and insertion of, 302t
   testing of, 307, *307*
Depressor labii inferioris, *301*
   innervation of, 310t, 312t–313t
   origin and insertion of, 302t
   testing of, 306, *306*
Depressor septi, *301*
   innervation of, 310t, 312t–313t
   testing of, 304, *304*
Dermatomes, 333
   of neck and upper extremity, *389, 394, 396, 398, 400, 403*
   of trunk and lower extremity, *393, 397, 399*
Desks, 113–114
Diagnosis
   definition of, 413
   musculoskeletal, 413
Diagnostic, definition of, 413
Diaphragm, 322t, 323, *323*, 326, 328, *328*
   actions of, 323
   innervation of, 323, 389t
   origins and insertion of, 323
   spinal segment distribution to, 406t–407t
   spinal segment distribution to nerves of, 410t
   sternal, costal, and lumbar parts of, *323*
Digastric
   anterior belly of, *300, 315*
      actions of, 320t
      innervation of, 310t, 312t–313t, 320t
      origin and insertion of, 320t
      role in deglutition, 320t
   posterior belly of, *300, 315*
      actions of, 320t
      innervation of, 310t, 312t–313t, 320t
      origin and insertion of, 320t
      role in deglutition, 320t
Directions, 413
Distal, definition of, 413
Dorsal, definition of, 419
Dorsal digital nerves, *382*
Dorsal scapular nerve, 379t, *385, 401*
   muscles innervated by, 389t
   spinal segment distribution to, 410t
Dorsiflexion, 22, *22*, 52, 73
   definition of, 414
Dorsiflexors, 70
   innervation of, 378, 387
Double leg raising, 137, *137*, 164
   pelvic tilt during, 134
Drop-foot, 199, 201
Dynamometers, 6–7, *190*
Dysfunction, definition of, 413

Edema, massage for, 337
Elbow joint, 11, 18
   flexion of, 180
   "funny bone" at, 376
   movements of, 18
   nerve compression due to injury of, 376

in trunk extension test, 140–141
weakness of, 353–354
Hip flexors, 70, *83*
contracture of, 215
during curled-trunk sit-up, 172–174, *172–174*
in double leg raising, 137
in flat-back posture, 87
innervation of, 386
in kyphosis-lordosis posture, 84
in "military-type" posture, 86
muscles acting as, 33
normal range of motion for, 32
shortened, 34, *34*, 36, *36*, 215
effect on posterior pelvic tilt exercises, 159
effect on tests for hamstring length, 42–43, *42–43*
lordosis and, 80
trunk curl in presence of, 166, *166*
sit-up exercises for, 167–168
stretching of, 53, *53*, 118, 351–352
testing strength of, 7, 102, 188, 215, *215*
in scoliosis, 122
tests for length of, 30, 32–37, *33–37*
correct test, 37, *37*
error in testing, 37, *37*
excessive length, 35, *35*
normal length, 34, *34*
normal length of one-joint, shortness in two-joint
muscles, 35, *35*
in scoliosis, 122
shortness in one- and two-joint muscles, 34, *34*
shortness in one-joint, no shortness in two-joint muscles,
36, *36*
shortness in sartorius, 36, *36*, 36t
shortness in tensor fasciae latae, 36, 36t
tightness of
in one-joint muscles, 351–352
in two-joint muscles, 352, *352*
in trunk extension test, 140–141
weakness of, 215
in flat-back posture, 355
in sway-back posture, 85
Hip joint, 134
abduction of, 21, *21*, 222–223, *223*
adduction of, 21, *21*, 32, 222, 223, 228–230
extension of, 33
in faulty alignment, 89–90, *89–90*
in flat-back posture, 76, 87, *87*
flexion of, *20*, 20–21, 29, 134, 162, *163*, 180
in ideal alignment, 72–73, *75–76*, 83, *83*, 88, *88*
in kyphosis-lordosis posture, *76*, 80, 84, *84*
medial rotation of, with pronation of feet, 366, *366*
movements of, 20–21, *20–21*
during curled-trunk sit-up, 170–171, *170–171*
muscles involved in, 232t
normal joint ranges for, 30
opposing muscles of, 70
in sway-back posture, *76*, 85, *85*
while sitting, 99
Hip rotators, 70, 186
lateral
actions of, 218
contracture of, 219
innervation of, 218
origins and insertions of, 218, *218*
shortness of, 219
testing strength of, 219, *219*
weakness of, 219
medial
contracture of, 217
shortness of, 217
testing strength of, 217, *217*
weakness of, 217
Humerus, 17, 18
Hyoglossus, *300*

actions of, 320t
innervation of, 310t, 312t–313t, 320t
origin and insertion of, 320t
role in deglutition, 320t
Hyperextension, 13
definition of, 415
of knee, 21, *21*, 95, *95*, 204, 206, 207, *207*, 213, 367
of metacarpophalangeal joint, 181–182, 250, 255
of spine, 13, 24, 134, 355
Hypoglossal nerve (CN XII), *300*, 310t, 312t–313t, 320t, *384*
Hypoventilation, 325
Hypoxia, 325

Ideal alignment, 3, 72, *75, 76*, 83, *83. See also* Postural
alignment; Posture, standard
ankle in, 73
definition of, 414
feet in, 73–74
head and neck in, 74, *74*
hip and knee joints in, 72–73
knee joint in, 97, *97*
pelvis and low back in, 72
plumb line test for deviations of, 72
posterior views, 71–72, *88, 88*
shoulder joint and shoulder girdle in, 74
side views, 72, *75, 83*
in sitting position, 99, *99*
thoracic spine in, 74
Iliacus, *83*, 167, *392. See also* Iliopsoas
actions of, 232t–233t
innervation of, 214, 232t, 377, 379t, 393t
origins and insertion of, 214, *214*
spinal segment distribution to, 408t–409t
Iliocostalis cervicis, *139*
actions of, 317t
origins and insertions of, 138t
Iliocostalis lumborum, *139*
origins and insertions of, 138t
role in respiration, 322t, 330
Iliocostalis thoracis, 138t, *139*
Iliohypogastric nerve, 379t, *386*
distribution of, 378
lateral cutaneous branch of, *382*
muscles innervated by, 393t
spinal segment distribution to, 410t
Ilioinguinal nerve, *382, 386*
muscles innervated by, 393t
spinal segment distribution to, 410t
Iliopsoas, 70
actions of, 214, 232t–233t
contracture of, 214
lordosis associated with shortness of, 80
nerve impingement due to stretching of, 377
testing length of, 33
testing strength of, 214–215, *214–215*
tightness in, 351
weakness of, 214
posterior pelvic tilt due to, 354
Iliotibial band, *227*, 336
in faulty alignment, 89
length of, in scoliosis, 122
stretched, 362–363
stretching of, 60
tightness of, 361–362
knock-knees and, 368
Ober test for, 56–59
Immobilization, 4
Impingement
definition of, 414
of muscles on nerves, 376–377
In-toeing, 369–370

origin and insertion of, 253, *253*
spinal segment distribution to, 406t–407t
testing strength of, 253, *253*
weakness of, 253, *253*
Palsy
  Bell's, 311, 312t
  "Saturday night," 376
Patella, 21
Patellar tendon, 182
Patient positioning, 181
Pectineus, 33, *392*
  actions of, 228, 229, 232t–233t
  innervation of, 228, 232t, 377, 379t, 393t
  origin and insertion of, 228, *228*
  spinal segment distribution to, 408t–409t
Pectoral nerve
  lateral, 379t, *385*, *391*, *401*
    muscles innervated by, 389t
    spinal segment distribution to, 410t
  medial, 379t, *385*, *391*, *401*
    muscles innervated by, 389t
    spinal segment distribution to, 410t
Pectoralis major, *391*
  actions of, 276, 294t, 296t–297t
  differentiating parts of, 180
  innervation of, 276, 296t, 379t, 389t
  origins and insertions of, 276, *276*
  role in respiration, 322t, 330
  shortness of, 277
  spinal segment distribution to, 406t–407t
  testing strength of, 277, *277*
  tests for length of, 62, *62*, 142
  weakness of, 277
Pectoralis minor, *385*, *391*
  actions of, 278, 294t
  contracture of, 278
  innervation of, 278, 294t, 379t, 389t
  origins and insertion of, 278, *278*
  overdevelopment of, 65
  role in respiration, 322t, 330
  spinal segment distribution to, 406t–407t
  stretching of, 68, *68*, 344
  test for shortness of, 278, *278*
  testing strength of, 278, *278*
  tests for length of, 63, *63*, 142
  tightness of
    arm pain related to, 63, *343*, 343–344
    brachial plexus compression due to, 376
  weakness of, 278
Pelvic tilt, 15, 89–90, *89–90*
  anterior, 20, *20*, 72, *76*
    definition of, 417
    due to tight low back muscles, 352–353
    due to tight one-joint hip flexors, 351
    due to tight two-joint hip flexors, 352
    due to weak anterior abdominal muscles, 351
    due to weak hip extensors, 353–354
    low back pain and, 350–354
    muscle imbalance associated with, 350
    posterior pelvic tilt exercises for, *158–159*, 158–160
  definition of, 417
  during double leg raising, 134
  during sit-ups, 134
  in flat-back posture, *76*, *87*, 87
  in kyphosis-lordosis posture, *76*, *80*, 84, *84*
  in sway-back posture, *76*, *85*, *85*
  lateral, 20, *20*, *76*, 100, 102
    definition of, 417
    due to tensor fasciae latae tightness, 356, 362
    gluteus medius weakness and, 356
    handedness and, 356
    low back pain and, 355–356
    muscle imbalances in, 355–356
    rotation of pelvis on femurs with, 356

scoliosis and, 126, 128
    shoe corrections, 356, 362
    treatment of, 356
  in "military-type" posture, 86, *86*
  muscles involved in, 70, 83, *83*
  posterior, 20, *20*, 31, 72, *76*
    definition of, 417
    low back pain and, 354–355
  while sitting, 99
Pelvis
  in ideal alignment, 72, *75–76*, 83, *83*, 88, *88*
  movements during curled-trunk sit-up, 170–171, *170–171*
  neutral position of, 20, *20*, 31, 71, 72
    definition of, 416
  opposing muscles of, 70
  relationship to line of reference, 72
  rotation accompanying lateral pelvic tilt, 356
Peripheral nerves, 333, 383
  from brachial plexus, 385, 388, 389t
  from cervical plexus, 384
  compression or tension on, 376
  invasive trauma injuries of, 376
  from lumbar plexus, 386
  from sacral plexus, 387
  on spinal nerve and muscle charts, 388, 389t, 393t
  spinal segment distribution to, 404–405, 411t
Peroneal nerve, 361, 379t, *392*
  common, *361*, *382*, *387*, 393t
    muscles innervated by, 393t
    spinal segment distribution to, 410t
  compression or tension on, 376
  deep, *361*, *382*, *392*, 393t
  distribution of, 378
  spinal nerve and muscle chart indicating lesion of, 397t
  superficial, *361*, *382*, *392*, 393t
Peroneus brevis, 88, *88*, 203, *203*, *392*
  actions of, 203, 232t–233t
  contracture of, 203
  in faulty alignment, 89–90
  innervation of, 203, 232t, 379t, 393t
  origins and insertion of, 203
  in plantar flexion, 205
  spinal segment distribution to, 408t–409t
  testing strength of, 203
  weakness of, 203
Peroneus longus, 88, *88*, 203, *203*, 361, *361*, *392*
  actions of, 203, 232t–233t
  contracture of, 203
  in faulty alignment, 89–90
  innervation of, 203, 232t, 379t, 393t
  origins and insertions of, 203
  in plantar flexion, 205
  spinal segment distribution to, 408t–409t
  testing strength of, 203
  weakness of, 203
Peroneus tertius, 198, *198*, *392*
  actions of, 198, 232t–233t
  contracture of, 199
  innervation of, 198, 232t, 379t, 393t
  origins and insertion of, 198
  spinal segment distribution to, 408t–409t
  testing strength of, 199, *199*
  weakness of, 199
Phalanges
  of foot, 22
  of hand, 18–19
Pharyngeal plexus, *300*, 320t, 321t
Phrenic nerve, *384*, *385*
  muscles innervated by, 389t
  spinal segment distribution to, 410t
Physical examination, 5
Physical fitness tests, 7–8
  push-ups, 8
  sit-and-reach, 8